Pain Review

Pain Review

Steven D. Waldman, MD, JD

Clinical Professor, Department of Anesthesiology
University of Missouri–Kansas City School of Medicine
Kansas City, Missouri
Medical Director, Headache and Pain Center
Leawood, Kansas

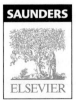

SAUNDERS

ELSEVIER

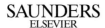

1600 John F. Kennedy Blvd.
Ste 1800
Philadelphia, PA 19103-2899

PAIN REVIEW

ISBN: 978-1-4160-5893-9

Notice

Knowledge and best practice in this field are constantly changing. As new research and experience broaden our knowledge, changes in practice, treatment, and drug therapy may become necessary or appropriate. Readers are advised to check the most current information provided (i) on procedures featured or (ii) by the manufacturer of each product to be administered, to verify the recommended dose or formula, the method and duration of administration, and contraindications. It is the responsibility of the practitioner, relying on his or her experience and knowledge of the patient, to make diagnoses, to determine dosages and the best treatment for each individual patient, and to take all appropriate safety precautions. To the fullest extent of the law, neither the Publisher nor the Author assumes any liability for any injury and/or damage to persons or property arising out of or related to any use of the material contained in this book.

The Publisher

Library of Congress Cataloging-in-Publication Data

Waldman, Steven D.
  Pain review / Steven D. Waldman. – 1st ed.
     p. ; cm.
  Includes bibliographical references.
  ISBN 978-1-4160-5893-9
1. Pain. I. Title.
  [DNLM: 1. Pain–therapy. 2. Musculoskeletal Diseases. 3. Nerve Block. 4. Nervous System Diseases.
5. Peripheral Nervous System. WL 704 W164p 2009]
  RB127.W3485 2009
  616′.0472–dc22

2008030147

Executive Publisher: Natasha Andjelkovic
Editorial Assistant: Isabel Trudeau
Publishing Services Manager: Tina Rebane
Senior Project Manager: Linda Lewis Grigg

Printed in USA

Last digit is the print number: 9 8 7 6 5 4 3 2 1

*Every long journey begins
with a first step*

—Confucius

To my children—David Mayo, Corey, Jennifer, and Reid—all of
whom are sick of hearing me invoke the above quote... but
have nevertheless steadfastly followed its
timeless wisdom in their daily lives!

Preface

Hypnopaedia: *the art or process of learning while asleep by means of lessons recorded on disk or tapes*

As a child, I was always fascinated by the advertisements on the back of the comic books that my brother Howard and I avidly read. Among the many ads for a myriad of amazing items and services was one featuring a picture of a white-bearded Russian scientist standing next to a sleeping woman, touting that for just $19.95 you could purchase lessons that could teach you to *Learn While You Sleep*. Given that the Russians had just launched Sputnik and had supposedly detonated a hydrogen bomb, I was completely convinced that this was something I could not live without. I must admit that part of my desire to buy *Learn While You Sleep* was that I hated school and was always looking for an easier way to complete my lessons.

While I was never able to con my parents into spending the $19.95 for the *Learn While You Sleep* lessons, they did buy me a pair of the x-ray vision glasses for the then-princely sum of $1.99. Needless to say, they didn't work nearly as well as I had hoped, and I began to wonder if the other things advertised on the back pages of my comics were as bogus. I didn't have to wonder too long as the full-size replica of a Sherman tank that my brother had ordered off the back of a Superman comic turned out to be little more than a big orange cardboard box. So much for *Learn While You Sleep*!

At this point, the reader might ask, "What does an old comic book ad for *Learn While You Sleep* have to do with a review text for pain management?" Well, as my brother Howard, with whom I have practiced pain management for the last 26 years, will tell you, I am still and always looking for an easier way to do things. When I started studying for my American Board of Anesthesiology recertification examination in pain management, there were no texts written to specifically help one review pain management in an organized and time-efficient manner, and I approached my publishers with the concept of creating such a review text. The result of our efforts is *Pain Review*.

In writing *Pain Review*, it was my goal to create a text that not only contained all of the material needed to review the specialty of pain management but also to organize that material into small, concise, easy-to-read chapters. I believe that by breaking up the overwhelming amount of knowledge related to pain management into smaller and more manageable packets of information, the task of reviewing the entire specialty becomes much less daunting. I have also made liberal use of illustrations, as in many chapters a picture is the best way to convey a concept or technique.

Whether you are getting ready to take your certification or recertification examination in pain management or simply want to learn more about the specialty, I hope that *Pain Review* will serve your needs and help with your studies.

Steven D. Waldman, MD, JD

Contents

Section 2

Neuroanatomy   163

Section 3

Painful Conditions   209

Section 4

Diagnostic Testing   **361**

Section 5

Nerve Blocks, Therapeutic Injections, and Advanced Interventional Pain Management Techniques   **385**

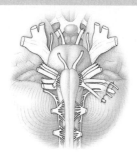

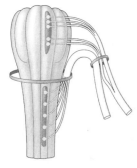

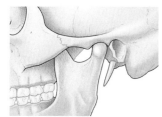

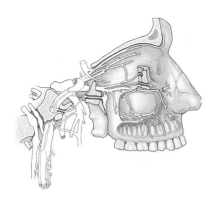

Anatomy

CHAPTER 1

Overview of the Cranial Nerves

Abnormal cranial nerve examination should alert the clinician to the possibility of not only central nervous system disease but also significant systemic illness. For this reason, a careful examination of the cranial nerves should be carried out in all patients suffering from unexplained pain. Abnormalities of the cranial nerves may affect one or more of the cranial nerves, and identification of these abnormalities may aid in the localization of a central nervous system lesion or may suggest a more diffuse process such as meningitis, pseudotumor cerebri, or the presence of systemic disease such as diabetes, sarcoidosis, botulism, myasthenia gravis, Guillain-Barré, vasculitis, and others. Common causes of specific cranial nerve abnormalities are listed in respective chapters that discuss each of the 12 cranial nerves. The 12 cranial nerves are listed here in Table 1-1.

To best understand cranial nerve abnormalities, it is useful to think about them in the context of their anatomy. Although the anatomy of the specific cranial nerves will be discussed in the individual chapters covering each cranial nerve, the following schema may be applied to all of the 12 cranial nerves. The efferent fibers of the cranial nerves arise deep within the brain in localized anatomic areas called the nuclei of origin. These nerves exit the brain and brainstem at points known as the superficial origins (Fig. 1-1). The afferent fibers of the cranial nerves arise outside the brain and may take the form of either specialized fibers that are grouped together in a sense organ (e.g., the eye or nose) or grouped together within the trunk of the nerve to form ganglia. The fibers enter the brain to coalesce to form the nuclei of termination. Lesions that affect the peripheral portion or trunks of the cranial nerves are called infranuclear lesions. Lesions that affect the nuclei of the cranial nerves are called nuclear lesions. Lesions that affect the central connections of the cranial nerves are called supranuclear lesions.

TABLE 1–1 The Cranial Nerves

- 1st—Olfactory
- 2nd—Optic
- 3rd—Oculomotor
- 4th—Trochlear
- 5th—Trigeminal
- 6th—Abducens
- 7th—Facial
- 8th—Acoustic/auditory/vestibulocochlear
- 9th—Glossopharyngeal
- 10th—Vagus
- 11th—Spinal accessory
- 12th—Hypoglossal

When evaluating a patient presenting with a cranial nerve abnormality, it is also helpful for the clinician to remember that the first two cranial nerves, the olfactory and the optic, are intimately associated with the quite specialized anatomic structures of the nose and eye and are subject to myriad diseases that may present as a cranial nerve lesion. The remaining 10 cranial nerves are much more analogous in structure and function to the spinal nerves and thus more subject to entrapment and/or compression from extrinsic processes such as a tumor, an aneurysm, or an aberrant blood vessel rather than primary disease processes.

SUGGESTED READINGS

Campbell W: DeJong's The Neurological Examination, ed 6. Philadelphia, Lippincott Williams and Wilkins, 2005.

Goetz CG: Textbook of Clinical Neurology, ed 2. Philadelphia, Saunders, 2003.

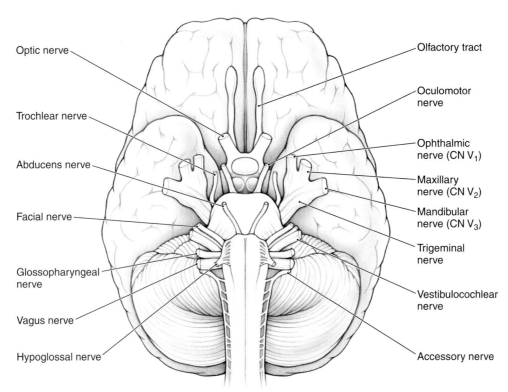

Optic nerve

Trochlear nerve

Abducens nerve

Facial nerve

Glossopharyngeal
nerve

Vagus nerve

Hypoglossal nerve

Olfactory tract

Oculomotor
nerve

Ophthalmic
nerve (CN V$_1$)

Maxillary
nerve (CN V$_2$)

Mandibular
nerve (CN V$_3$)

Trigeminal
nerve

Vestibulocochlear
nerve

Accessory nerve

FIGURE 1–1 The superficial origin of the cranial nerves.

CHAPTER 2

The Olfactory Nerve—Cranial Nerve I

The first cranial nerve is known as the olfactory nerve and is denoted by the Roman numeral I. It is composed of special afferent nerve fibers that are responsible for our sense of smell. The olfactory nerve and associated structures include the chemoreceptors known as the olfactory receptor cells, which are located in the epithelium covering the roof, septum, and superior conchae of the nasal cavity (Fig. 2-1). Inhaled substances dissolve in the moist atmosphere of the nasal cavity and stimulate its chemoreceptors. If a firing threshold is reached, these chemoreceptors initiate action potentials that fire in proportion to the intensity of the stimulus. These stimuli are transmitted via fibers of the olfactory nerve that traverse the cribriform plate to impinge on the olfactory bulb, which contains the cell bodies of the secondary sensory neurons that make up the olfactory tract.

The olfactory tract projects into the cerebral cortex to areas known as the lateral, intermediate, and medial olfactory areas. The lateral olfactory area is most important to humans' sense of smell, with the intermediate area less so. The medial olfactory area, via its interconnections with the limbic system, serves to help mediate humans' emotional response to smell. Collectively, the olfactory receptor cells, epithelium, and bulb tracts and areas are known as the rhinencephalon (Fig. 2-2).

All three olfactory areas interact with a number of autonomic centers via a network of interconnected fibers. The medial forebrain bundle carries information from all three olfactory areas to the hypothalamus, while the stria terminalis carries olfactory information from the amygdala to the preoptic region of the cerebral cortex. The stria medullaris carries olfactory information to the

TABLE 2–1 How to Test Function of the Olfactory Nerve

1. Ascertain that the nasal passages are open.
2. Have the patient close his or her eyes.
3. Occlude one nostril.
4. Place a vial of nonirritating test substance (e.g., fresh ground coffee or oil of lemon) near to open nostril
   Note: Avoid irritating substances such as oil of peppermint that may stimulate the peripheral endings of the trigeminal nerve of the nasal mucosa.
5. Have the patient inhale forcibly.
6. Ascertain whether the patient can perceive an odor.
   Note: The ability to identify what the odor is requires higher cerebral function, and it is the perception of odor or lack thereof rather than its identification that is important.
7. Repeat the above process with the ipsilateral nostril.

TABLE 2–2 Causes of Anosmia

- Congenital
- Upper respiratory tract infections
- Nasal sprays containing zinc
- Facial and nasal trauma
- Prolonged exposure to tobacco smoke
- Enlarged adenoids
- Nasal polyps
- Paranasal sinusitis
- Head trauma damaging the cribriform plate or olfactory areas of the cerebral cortex
- Cerebrovascular accident
- Tumors involving the
  Paranasal sinuses
  Pituitary gland
  Cranial vault, including gliomas, meningiomas, and neuroblastomas

habenular nucleus, which along with the hypothalamus interfaces with a number of cranial nerves to mediate humans' visceral responses associated with smell. Examples of such visceral responses include the dorsal motor nuclei of the vagus nerve (10th cranial nerve), which can modulate nausea and vomiting and changes in gastrointestinal motility, as well as the superior and inferior salivatory nuclei, which modulate salivation.

Abnormalities of the olfactory nerve may result in a condition known as anosmia, or the inability to smell. A simple approach to the testing of smell is outlined in Table 2-1. Anosmia can be permanent or temporary like that occurring with bad allergies or colds. It may be congenital or acquired; the most common causes of anosmia are listed in Table 2-2. Although anosmia might seem at first glance to be of little consequence, the lack of smell is associated with significant morbidity and mortality due to impairment of the extremely important warning function that olfaction plays in activities of daily living. The ingestion of spoiled foods, the inability to smell toxic gases such as the mercapten in natural gas, or the inability to smell the smoke of a house fire are just a few examples of how the inability to smell can harm.

SUGGESTED READINGS

Campbell W: DeJong's The Neurological Examination, ed 6. Philadelphia, Lippincott Williams and Wilkins, 2005.
Goetz CG: Textbook of Clinical Neurology, ed 2. Philadelphia, WB Saunders, 2003.

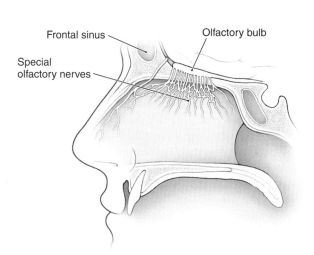

FIGURE 2–1 The olfactory epithelium.

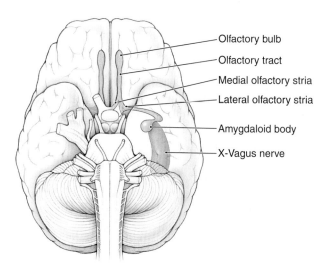

FIGURE 2–2 The olfactory bulb, tract, and areas.

CHAPTER 3

The Optic Nerve—Cranial Nerve II

Functional Anatomy of the Optic Nerve

The second cranial nerve is known as the optic nerve and is denoted by the Roman numeral II. Its special afferent sensory fibers carry visual information from the retina to the cerebral cortex for processing and interpretation. In order to best understand abnormalities of vision, it is helpful for the clinician to think about these abnormalities in context of the functional anatomy of the optic nerve. Light enters the eye in the form of photons, which pass through the cornea, aqueous humor, pupil, lens, and vitreous humor to reach the retina (Fig. 3-1). Special photoreceptor cells known as the rods and cones, which are located in the deep layers of the retina, begin the conversion of the photons into electrical signals. As these photoreceptor cells are stimulated, they become hyperpolarized and produce either depolarization (stimulation) or hyperpolarization (inhibition) of the bipolar cells, which are the primary sensory neurons of the visual pathway.

The bipolar cells synapse with and either stimulate or inhibit the ganglion cells that are the secondary sensory neurons of the visual pathway. The axons of the ganglion cells converge at the optic disc near the center of the retina. These axons then exit the posterior aspect of the eye as the optic nerve (cranial nerve II) (Fig. 3-2). Exiting the orbit via the optic canal, the optic nerve enters the middle cranial fossa to join the ipsilateral optic nerve to form the optic chiasm. Fibers from each optic nerve cross the midline to exit the chiasm together as the opposite optic tract (Fig. 3-3).

The optic tracts containing fibers from both optic nerves travel posteriorly passing around the cerebral peduncles of the midbrain. Most of the fibers of the optic tracts synapse with the tertiary sensory neurons of the lateral geniculate nucleus within their contralateral thalamus (see Fig. 3-3). A few optic tract fibers travel to the pretectal region of the midbrain and provide necessary information for the pupillary light reflex. Via the optic radiations, the tertiary sensory neurons of the lateral geniculate nuclei project to the primary visual cortex, which is located in the occipital lobe (Fig. 3-3).

The Visual Field Pathways

The entire area that is seen by the eye when it is focused on a central point is called the visual field of that eye. It must be remembered that the photons entering the cornea converge and pass through the narrow pupil with the entire visual field being projected on the retina in a reversed and upside down orientation (Fig. 3-4). This means that the upper half of the retina is stimulated with photons from the lower half of the visual field and the lower half of the retina is stimulated with photons from the upper half of the visual field. Furthermore, the right half of the retina receives stimuli from the left visual field and the left half of the retina receives stimuli from the right half of the visual field.

Given the consistent way that the ganglion cells from the retina group together to form the optic nerve and carry information to the primary visual cortex, the clinician may find it useful to divide the visual field of each eye into four quadrants: (1) the nasal hemiretina, which lies medial to the fovea; (2) the temporal hemiretina, which lies lateral to the fovea; (3) the superior hemiretina, which lies superior to the fovea; and (4) the inferior hemiretina, which lies inferior to the fovea (see Fig. 3-4). The axons of the ganglion cells of the nasal hemiretina decussate at the optic chiasm and travel on to project onto the contralateral lateral geniculate nucleus and midbrain. The axons of the ganglion cells of the temporal hemiretina remain ipsilateral through their course and project onto the ipsilateral lateral geniculate nucleus and midbrain (Fig. 3-4). The axons of the ganglion cells of the superior hemiretina carrying images from the inferior visual field project via the parietal lobe portion of the optic radiations to the portion of the primary visual cortex located above the calcarine fissure (Figs. 3-4 and 3-5). The axons of the ganglion cells of the inferior hemiretina carrying images from the superior visual field project via the temporal lobe portion of the optic radiations to the portion of the primary visual cortex located below the calcarine fissure (Figs. 3-4 and 3-5). Axons of the ganglion cells from the center of the retina or fovea project onto the tip of the occipital pole. Armed with the above knowledge of the functional anatomy of the visual pathway and the optic nerve, based on the patient's symptoms and visual abnormalities, the clinician can reliably predict what portion of the visual pathway is affected.

Clinical Evaluation of the Optic Nerve and Visual Pathway

Evaluation of optic nerve function also by necessity includes evaluation of retinal function. The clinician examines each of the patient's eyes individually and begins the examination with an assessment of visual acuity. Distant vision is tested using a standard Snellen test chart, and near vision is tested by having the patient read the smallest type possible from a Jaeger reading test card placed 14 inches from the eye being tested. Color blindness, which occurs in approximately 3% to 4% of males and 0.3% of women, can be tested by having the patient read isochromatic plates such as the Ishihara plates, with an inability to read the embedded numbers in the presence of normal visual acuity highly suggestive of color blindness.

The next step in evaluation of the optic nerve and associated structures of the visual pathway is examination of the visual fields. Although there is intrapatient variation in visual fields due to the patient's facial characteristics and shape of the globe and orbit, the following general observations can be made. In health, a person is able to see laterally approximately 90 to 100 degrees and medially approximately 60 degrees. The patient can see upward approximately 50 to 60 degrees and downward 60 to 70 degrees with the eye fixed in the midline. The easiest test for evaluation for significant visual field loss is the confrontation test. The confrontation test is performed with the clinician using his or her own visual fields as a control. To perform the confrontation test for visual fields, the examiner and patient both cover opposite eyes, and with the examiner standing approximately 3 feet in front of the patient, the examiner slowly brings his or her finger into each quadrant of the visual field. The patient is instructed to inform the examiner the second the examiner's finger is seen, with the examiner comparing his or her own response with that of the patient's (Fig. 3-6). While beyond the scope of this review, the clinician should be aware that specific patterns of visual field loss are associated with specific clinical abnormalities of the optic nerve and visual pathways, such as homonymous hemianopia, which is often associated with occipital lobe neoplasms or stroke; bitemporal hemianopia, which is often associated with pituitary adenomas; and so on.

Fundoscopic examination of the retina and the optic disc is an essential part of the evaluation of the optic nerve. The optic disc, which is located just medial and slightly above the center of the fundus, should appear oval in shape and pale pink in color. The margin of the optic disc should be clearly defined with the margins slightly elevated (Fig. 3-7). A pale or poorly defined optic disc is highly suggestive of pathology of the optic nerve, as is a swollen head of the optic nerve, which is called papilledema. Papilledema is pathognomonic for increased intracranial pressure (Fig. 3-8). It should be

TABLE 3–1 Common Diseases that Result in Visual Impairment

Systemic Diseases

- Diabetes mellitus
- Hypertension
- Vitamin A deficiency
- Vitamin B_{12} deficiency
- Lead poisoning
- Migraine with aura
- Graves' disease
- Sarcoidosis
- Collagen vascular diseases
- Atherosclerosis and stroke
- Sickle cell disease
- Multiple sclerosis
- Refsum's disease
- Tay-Sachs disease

Infection

- HIV-associated infections including cytomegalovirus
- Trachoma
- Bacterial infections including gonococcal infections
- Parasitic infections including onchocerciasis
- Spirochete infections including syphilis
- Viral infections
- Leprosy

Eye Diseases

- Macular degeneration
- Glaucoma
- Cataracts
- Retinitis pigmentosa
- Rod and cone dystrophy
- Best disease, also known as vitelliform macular dystrophy

Trauma

- Burns
- Projectile injuries
- Side effects of medications
- Bungee cord and rubber band injuries
- Fish hook injuries
- Firework injuries
- Sports injuries
- Complications of eye surgery

Neoplasms

- Optic gliomas
- Melanoma
- Pituitary adenoma

noted that optic neuritis associated with multiple sclerosis may resemble papilledema and confuse the diagnosis.

Abnormalities of the retinal vessels seen on fundoscopic examination may also provide the clinician with useful diagnostic information. Occlusion of the central retinal artery can result in sudden visual loss and is associated with a pale, edematous optic disc and thin arteries, which can only be followed outward a short distance from the disc. Atherosclerosis can be identified by noting a silver wire appearance of the retinal arteries. Systemic hypertension can result in arterial narrowing and cotton wool patches that appear stuck onto the retina. Common abnormalities of the optic nerve and visual pathways are listed in Table 3-1.

SUGGESTED READINGS

Campbell W: DeJong's The Neurological Examination, ed 6. Philadelphia, Lippincott Williams and Wilkins, 2005.

Goetz CG: Textbook of Clinical Neurology, ed 2. Philadelphia, Saunders, 2003.

Waldman SD: Migraine headache. In: Atlas of Common Pain Syndromes, ed 2. Philadelphia, Saunders, 2008.

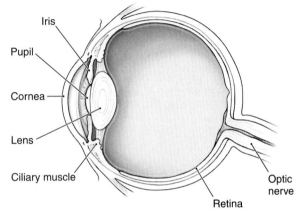

FIGURE 3–1 The path of light though the eye.

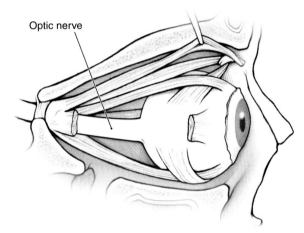

FIGURE 3–2 The optic nerve.

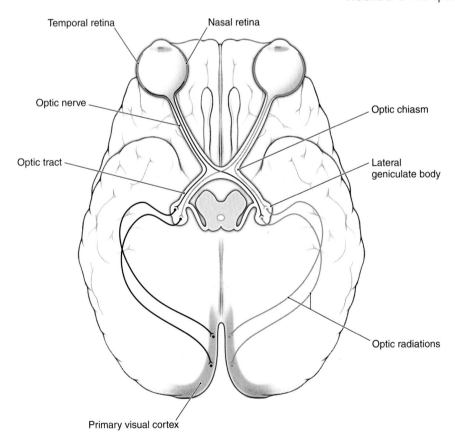

FIGURE 3–3 The visual pathway.

Visual field pathway

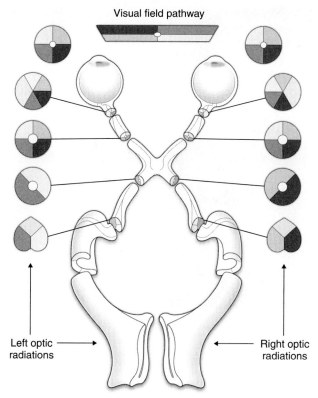

Left optic radiations

Right optic radiations

FIGURE 3–4 Visual field pathways.

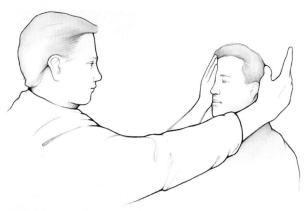

FIGURE 3–6 Confrontation method of visual field testing.

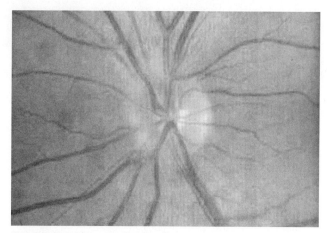

FIGURE 3–7 The normal optic disc.

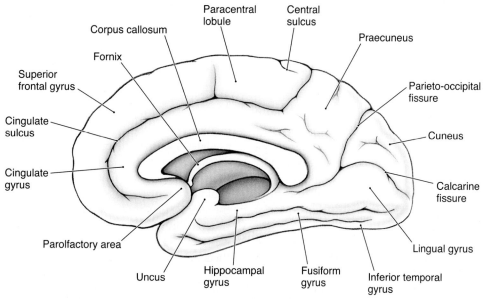

FIGURE 3–5 The relationship of the calcarine fissure to the cerebral hemisphere.

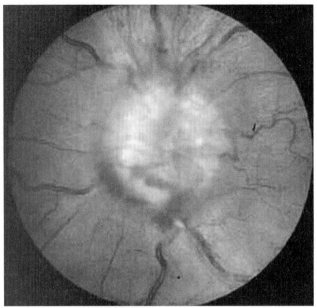

FIGURE 3–8 Papilledema.

CHAPTER 4

The Oculomotor Nerve—Cranial Nerve III

The oculomotor nerve is the third cranial nerve and is denoted by the Roman numeral III. It is made up of both general somatic efferent and general visceral efferent fibers, which serve two distinct functions. The general somatic efferent fibers of the oculomotor nerve provide motor innervation to four of the six extraocular muscles: (1) the ipsilateral inferior rectus muscle, (2) the ipsilateral inferior oblique muscle, (3) the ipsilateral medial rectus muscle, and (4) the contralateral superior rectus muscle (Fig. 4-1). The superior oblique muscles are innervated by the trochlear nerve (cranial nerve IV), and the lateral rectus muscles are innervated by the abducens nerve (cranial nerve VI) (see Chapters 5 and 7). The actions of the six extraocular muscles are summarized in Table 4-1. The general somatic efferent fibers of the oculomotor nerve also provide motor innervation to levator palpebrae superioris muscles bilaterally, which elevate the upper eyelids (Fig. 4-2).

The general somatic efferent fibers of the oculomotor nerve that provide motor innervation to four of the six extraocular muscles originate from the oculomotor nucleus located near the midline just ventral to the cerebral aqueduct in the rostral midbrain at the level of the superior colliculus (Fig. 4-3). The oculomotor nucleus is bordered medially by the Edinger-Westphal nucleus (see later). Efferent general somatic fibers exit the oculomotor nucleus and pass ventrally in the tegmentum of the midbrain, passing through the red nucleus and medial portion of the cerebral peduncle to emerge in the interpeduncular fossa at the junction of the midbrain and pons.

Exiting the brainstem, the oculomotor nerve (cranial nerve III) passes between the posterior cerebral and superior cerebellar arteries and then passes through the dura mater to enter the cavernous sinus. The nerve runs along the lateral wall of the cavernous sinus just superior to the trochlear nerve (cranial nerve IV) and enters the orbit via the superior orbital fissure. After entering the orbit, the oculomotor nerve passes through the tendinous ring of the extraocular muscles and then divides into the superior and inferior divisions. The superior division travels superiorly just lateral to the optic nerve to innervate both the superior rectus and levator palpebrae superioris muscles. The inferior division of oculomotor nerve divides into three branches to innervate the medial rectus, inferior rectus, and inferior oblique muscles (Fig. 4-4).

TABLE 4–1 Actions of the Extraocular Muscles

Muscle	Innervation	Primary Action	Secondary Action	Tertiary Action
Superior rectus	CN III	Elevation	Intorsion	Adduction
Medial rectus	CN III	Adduction	...	...
Inferior rectus	CN III	Depression	Extorsion	Adduction
Inferior oblique	CN III	Extorsion	Elevation	Abduction
Superior oblique	CN IV	Intorsion	Depression	Abduction
Lateral rectus	CN VI	Abduction	...	...

CN, cranial nerve.

The general visceral efferent motor fibers of the oculomotor nerve mediate the eye's accommodation and pupillary light reflexes by providing parasympathetic innervation of the constrictor pupillae and ciliary muscles of the eye (see Fig. 4-2). After entering the orbit, preganglionic parasympathetic fibers leave the inferior division of the oculomotor nerve to synapse in the ciliary ganglion, which lies deep to the superior rectus muscle near the tendinous ring of the extraocular muscles (see Fig. 4-2). Postganglionic fibers exit the ciliary ganglion via the short ciliary nerves, which enter the posterior aspect of the globe at a point near the spot where the optic nerve exits the eye. Traveling anteriorly between the choroid and the sclera, these postganglionic fibers innervate the ciliary muscles, which alter the shape of the lens, as well as the constrictor muscle of the iris, which constricts the aperture of the iris (see Fig. 4-2).

Disorders of the oculomotor nerve can be caused by central lesions that affect the oculomotor or Edinger-Westphal nuclei such as stroke or space-occupying lesions such as tumor, abscess, or aneurysm. Increased intracranial pressure due to subdural hematoma, sagittal sinus thrombosis, or abscess can compromise the nuclei and/or the efferent fibers of the oculomotor nerve as they exit the brainstem and travel toward the orbit with resultant abnormal nerve function. Traction on the oculomotor nerve due to loss of cerebrospinal fluid has also been implicated in cranial nerve III palsy. Small vessel disease due to diabetes or vasculitis associated with temporal arteritis may cause ischemia and even infarction of the oculomotor nerve with resultant pathologic symptoms.

In almost all disorders of the oculomotor nerve, symptoms will take the form of either a palsy of the extraocular muscles presenting as diplopia, strabismus, or an inability to look upward or downward or by a ptosis of the eyelids. Compromise of the visceral fibers of the oculomotor nerve can result in anisocoria, the loss of the direct or consensual light reflex, and/or the loss of accommodation. Examples of these abnormalities include the Argyll Robertson pupil most frequently associated with syphilis, Adie's pupil, and the Marcus Gunn pupil.

SUGGESTED READINGS

Campbell W: DeJong's The Neurological Examination, ed 6. Philadelphia, Lippincott Williams and Wilkins, 2005.

Goetz CG: Textbook of Clinical Neurology, ed 2. Philadelphia, Saunders, 2003.

Waldman SD: Post-dural puncture headache. In: Atlas of Uncommon Pain Syndromes, ed 2. Philadelphia, Saunders, 2008.

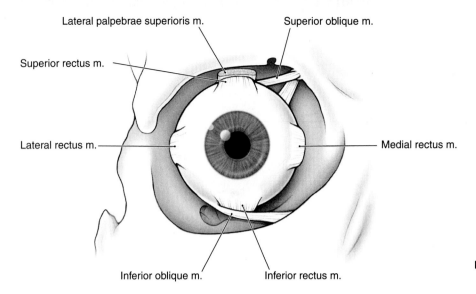

FIGURE 4–1 The extraocular muscles.

Labels: Lateral palpebrae superioris m., Superior oblique m., Superior rectus m., Lateral rectus m., Medial rectus m., Inferior oblique m., Inferior rectus m.

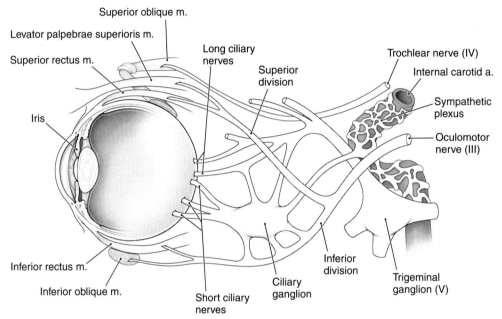

FIGURE 4–2 The oculomotor nerve.

Labels: Superior oblique m., Levator palpebrae superioris m., Superior rectus m., Long ciliary nerves, Superior division, Trochlear nerve (IV), Internal carotid a., Sympathetic plexus, Oculomotor nerve (III), Iris, Inferior rectus m., Inferior oblique m., Short ciliary nerves, Ciliary ganglion, Inferior division, Trigeminal ganglion (V)

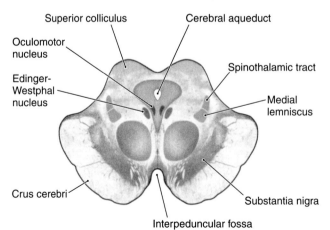

FIGURE 4–3 The oculomotor and Edinger-Westphal nuclei.

Labels: Superior colliculus, Cerebral aqueduct, Oculomotor nucleus, Spinothalamic tract, Edinger-Westphal nucleus, Medial lemniscus, Crus cerebri, Substantia nigra, Interpeduncular fossa

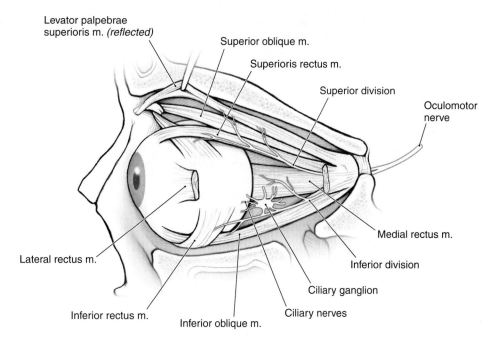

Levator palpebrae
superioris m. *(reflected)*

Superior oblique m.

Superioris rectus m.

Superior division

Oculomotor
nerve

Medial rectus m.

Inferior division

Ciliary ganglion

Ciliary nerves

Inferior oblique m.

Inferior rectus m.

Lateral rectus m.

FIGURE 4–4 The path of the oculomotor nerve within the orbit.

CHAPTER 5

The Trochlear Nerve—Cranial Nerve IV

The trochlear nerve (cranial nerve IV) is composed of somatic general efferent motor fibers and is denoted by the Roman numeral IV. It innervates the superior oblique extraocular muscle of the contralateral orbit (Fig. 5-1). Contraction of the superior oblique extraocular muscle intorts (rotates inward), depresses, and abducts the globe. As outlined in Chapter 4, the superior oblique extraocular muscles work in concert with the five other extraocular muscles to allow the eye to perform its essential functions of tracking and fixation on objects.

The fibers of the trochlear nerve originate from the trochlear nucleus, which is just ventral to the cerebral aqueduct in the tegmentum of the midbrain at the level of the inferior colliculus. As the trochlear nerve leaves the trochlear nucleus, it travels dorsally, wrapping itself around the cerebral aqueduct to then decussate in the superior medullary velum. The decussated fibers of the trochlear nerve then exit the dorsal surface of the brainstem just below the contralateral inferior colliculus, where they then curve around the brainstem, leaving the subarachnoid space along with the oculomotor nerve (cranial nerve III) between the superior cerebellar

and posterior cerebral arteries (Fig. 5-2). The trochlear nerve then enters the cavernous sinus and runs anteriorly along the lateral wall of the sinus with the oculomotor (cranial nerve III), trigeminal (cranial nerve V), and abducens (cranial nerve VI) nerves.

Exiting the cavernous sinus, the trochlear nerve enters the orbit via the superior orbital fissure. Unlike the oculomotor nerve, the trochlear nerve does not pass through the tendinous ring of the extraocular muscles but passes just above the ring (Fig. 5-3). The trochlear nerve then crosses medially along the roof of the orbit above the levator palpebrae and superior rectus muscles to innervate the superior oblique muscle (see Fig. 5-1).

Disorders of the trochlear nerve can be caused by central lesions that affect the trochlear nucleus such as stroke or space-occupying lesions such as tumor, abscess, or aneurysm. Increased intracranial pressure due to subdural hematoma, sagittal sinus thrombosis, or abscess can compromise the nucleus and/or the efferent fibers of the trochlear nerve as they exit the brainstem and travel toward the orbit with resultant abnormal nerve function. Traction on the trochlear nerve due to loss of cerebrospinal fluid has also been implicated in cranial nerve IV palsy. Small vessel disease due to diabetes or vasculitis associated with temporal arteritis may cause ischemia and even infarction of the trochlear nerve with resultant pathologic symptoms.

In almost all disorders of the trochlear nerve, symptoms will take the form of a palsy of the superior oblique muscle, most commonly presenting as the inability to look inward and downward. Often, the patient will complain of the difficulty in walking down stairs due to the inability to depress the affected eye or eyes. On physical examination, the clinician may note extorsion (outward rotation) of the affected eye due to the unopposed action of the inferior oblique muscle (Fig. 5-4, *A*). In an effort to compensate, the patient may deviate his or her face forward and downward with the chin rotated toward the affected side in order to look downward (Figure 5-4, *B*).

SUGGESTED READINGS

Campbell W: DeJong's The Neurological Examination, ed 6. Philadelphia, Lippincott Williams and Wilkins, 2005.

Goetz CG: Textbook of Clinical Neurology, ed 2. Philadelphia, Saunders, 2003.

Waldman SD: Post-dural puncture headache. In: Atlas of Uncommon Pain Syndromes, ed 2. Philadelphia, Saunders, 2008.

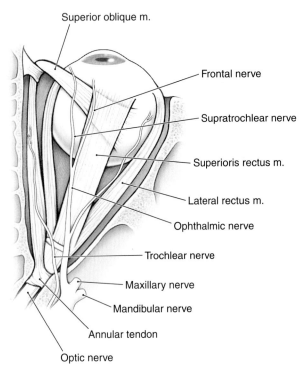

FIGURE 5–1 The relationship of the trochlear nerve and the superior oblique extraocular muscle.

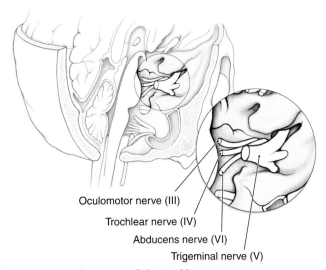

FIGURE 5–2 The course of the trochlear nerve.

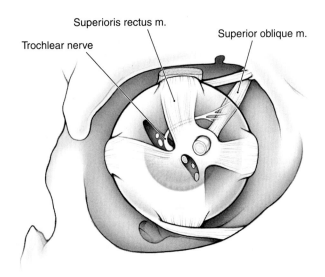

FIGURE 5–3 The relationship of the terminal trochlear nerve to the orbit and tendinous ring of the extraocular muscles.

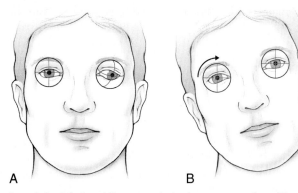

FIGURE 5–4 A, The unopposed action of the inferior oblique muscle in the presence of trochlear nerve palsy results in extorsion of the globe and associated weak downward gaze. **B,** To compensate for the unopposed action of the inferior oblique muscle in the presence of trochlear palsy, the patient deviates his face forward and downward with the chin rotated toward the affected side.

CHAPTER 6

The Trigeminal Nerve—Cranial Nerve V

The trigeminal nerve is the fifth cranial nerve and is denoted by the Roman numeral V. The trigeminal nerve has three divisions and provides sensory innervation for the forehead and eye (ophthalmic V_1), cheek (maxillary V_2), and lower face and jaw (mandibular V_3), as well as motor innervation for the muscles of mastication (Fig. 6-1). The fibers of the trigeminal nerve arise in the trigeminal nerve nucleus, which is the largest of the cranial nerve nuclei. Extending from the midbrain to the upper cervical spinal cord, the trigeminal nerve nucleus is divided into three parts: (1) the mesencephalic trigeminal nucleus, which receives proprioceptive and mechanoreceptor fibers from the mandible and teeth; (2) the main trigeminal nucleus, which receives the majority of the touch and position fibers; and (3) the spinal trigeminal nucleus, which receives pain and temperature fibers.

The sensory fibers of the trigeminal nerve exit the brainstem at the level of the mid-pons with a smaller motor root emerging from the mid-pons at the same level. These roots pass in a forward and lateral direction in the posterior cranial fossa across the border of the petrous bone. They then enter a recess called Meckel's cave, which is formed by an invagination of the surrounding dura mater into the middle cranial fossa. The dural pouch that lies just behind the ganglion is called the trigeminal cistern and contains cerebrospinal fluid.

The gasserian ganglion is canoe shaped, with the three sensory divisions: (1) the ophthalmic division (V_1), which exits the cranium via the superior orbital fissure; (2) the maxillary division (V_2), which exits the cranium via the foramen rotundum into the pterygopalatine fossa where it travels anteriorly to enter the infraorbital canal to exit through the infraorbital foramen; and the mandibular division (V_3), which exits the cranium via the foramen ovale anterior convex aspect of the ganglion (Fig. 6-2). A small motor root joins the mandibular division as it exits the cranial cavity via the foramen ovale.

Three major branches emerge from the trigeminal ganglion (Fig. 6-3). Each branch innervates a different dermatome. Each branch exits the cranium through a different site. The first division (V_1; ophthalmic nerve) exits the cranium through the superior orbital fissure, entering the orbit to innervate the globe and skin in the area above the eye and forehead.

The second division, V_2, maxillary nerve, exits through a round hole, the foramen rotundum, into a space posterior to the orbit, the pterygopalatine fossa. It then reenters a canal running inferior to the orbit, the infraorbital canal, and exits through a small hole, the infraorbital foramen, to innervate the skin below the eye and above the mouth. The third division, V_3, mandibular nerve, exits the cranium through an oval hole, the foramen ovale. Sensory fibers of the third division either travel directly to their target tissues or reenter the mental canal to innervate the teeth with the terminal branches of this division exiting anteriorly via the mental foramen to provide sensory cutaneous innervation to the skin overlying the mandible.

Disorders of the trigeminal nerve generally take the form of trigeminal neuralgia. Trigeminal neuralgia occurs in many patients because of tortuous blood vessels that compress the trigeminal root as it exits the brainstem. Acoustic neuromas, cholesteatomas, aneurysms, angiomas, and bony abnormalities of the skull may also lead to the compression of nerve. The severity of pain produced by trigeminal neuralgia can only be rivaled by that of cluster headache. Uncontrolled pain has been associated with suicide and therefore should be treated as an emergency. Attacks can be triggered by daily activities involving contact with the face such as brushing the teeth, shaving, or washing. Pain can be controlled with medication in most patients. About 2% to 3% of those patients experiencing trigeminal neuralgia also have multiple sclerosis. Trigeminal neuralgia is also called tic douloureux.

SUGGESTED READINGS

Campbell W: DeJong's The Neurological Examination, ed 6. Philadelphia, Lippincott Williams and Wilkins, 2005.

Goetz CG: Textbook of Clinical Neurology, ed 2. Philadelphia, Saunders, 2003.

Waldman SD: Trigeminal neuralgia. In: Atlas of Common Pain Syndromes, ed 2. Philadelphia, Saunders, 2008.

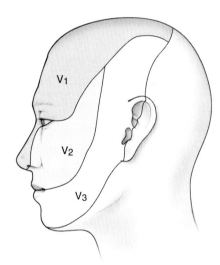

FIGURE 6–1 The sensory divisions of the trigeminal nerve.

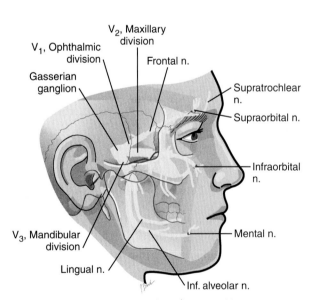

FIGURE 6–2 The gasserian ganglion. (From Waldman SD: Atlas of Interventional Pain Management, ed 2. Philadelphia, WB Saunders, 2005.)

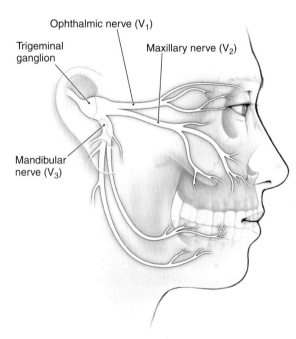

FIGURE 6–3 The peripheral anatomy of the trigeminal nerve.

CHAPTER 7

The Abducens Nerve—Cranial Nerve VI

The abducens nerve is the sixth cranial nerve and is denoted by the Roman numeral VI. The abducens nerve is composed of somatic general efferent motor fibers. It innervates the lateral rectus extraocular muscle of the ipsilateral orbit (Fig. 7-1). Contraction of the lateral rectus extraocular muscle abducts the globe. As outlined in Chapter 4, the lateral rectus extraocular muscle works in concert with the five other extraocular muscles to allow the eye to perform its essential functions of tracking and fixation of objects.

The fibers of the abducens nerve originate from the abducens nucleus, which is located just ventral to the fourth ventricle in the caudal pons at the level of the facial colliculus. As the abducens nerve leaves the abducens nucleus, it travels ventrally, exiting the brainstem at the border of the pons and medullary pyramids. The abducens nerve then courses superiorly adjacent to the ventral surface of the pons where, upon reaching the apex of the petrous portion of the temporal bone, the nerve abruptly turns anteriorly to enter the cavernous sinus (Fig. 7-2). After entering the cavernous sinus, the abducens nerve runs anteriorly along the lateral wall of the sinus with the oculomotor (cranial nerve III), trochlear (cranial nerve IV), and trigeminal (cranial nerve V) nerves. Exiting the cavernous sinus, the abducens nerve enters the orbit via the superior orbital fissure and passes through the tendinous ring of the extraocular muscles to innervate the lateral rectus muscle (Fig. 7-3).

Disorders of the abducens nerve can be caused by central lesions that affect the abducens nucleus such as stroke (especially of the pons) or space-occupying lesions such as tumor, abscess, or aneurysm. Increased intracranial pressure due to subdural hematoma, sagittal sinus thrombosis, or abscess can compromise the nucleus and/or the efferent fibers of the abducens nerve as they exit the brainstem and travel toward the orbit with resultant abnormal nerve function. Traction on the abducens nerve due to loss of cerebrospinal fluid has also been implicated in cranial nerve VI palsy. Small vessel disease due to diabetes or vasculitis associated with temporal arteritis may cause ischemia and even infarction of the abducens nerve with resultant pathologic symptoms. Statistically, microvascular disease associated with diabetes is far and away the most common cause of isolated abducens (cranial nerve VI) palsy (Fig. 7-4).

In almost all disorders of the abducens nerve, symptoms will take the form of a palsy of the lateral rectus muscle most commonly presenting as the inability of the patient to fixate on an object placed laterally to the affected side. Clinically, the patient will be unable to abduct the eye on the affected side past the midline gaze combined with the inability to adduct the eye opposite the lesion past midline gaze.

From the cavernous sinus, the abducens nerve enters the orbit through the superior orbital fissure.

Cranial nerve VI passes through the tendinous ring of the extraocular muscles and innervates the lateral rectus muscle on its deep surface.

SUGGESTED READINGS

Campbell W: DeJong's The Neurological Examination, ed 6. Philadelphia, Lippincott Williams and Wilkins, 2005.

Goetz CG: Textbook of Clinical Neurology, ed 2. Philadelphia, Saunders, 2003.

Waldman SD: Post-dural puncture headache. In: Atlas of Uncommon Pain Syndromes, ed 2. Philadelphia, Saunders, 2008.

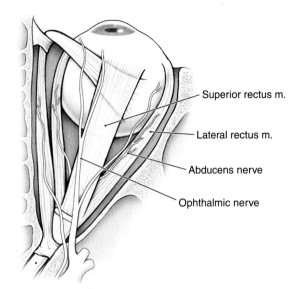

FIGURE 7–1 The relationship of the abducens nerve and the lateral rectus muscle.

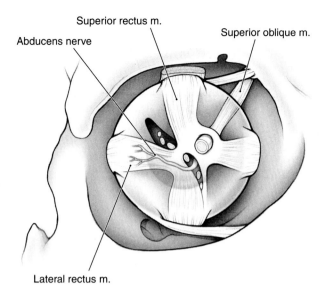

FIGURE 7–3 The innervation of the lateral rectus muscle.

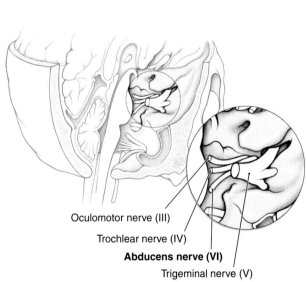

Oculomotor nerve (III)

Trochlear nerve (IV)

Abducens nerve (VI)

Trigeminal nerve (V)

FIGURE 7–2 The course of the abducens nerve.

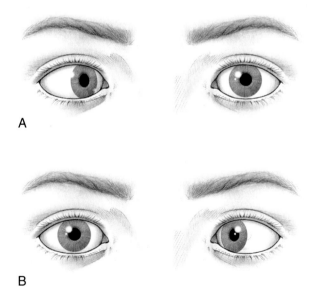

FIGURE 7–4 Right abducens palsy. **A,** With right abducens palsy, the affected (right) eye is adducted at rest. **B,** With right abducens palsy, the affected (right) eye cannot abduct.

CHAPTER 8

The Facial Nerve—Cranial Nerve VII

The facial nerve is the seventh cranial nerve and is denoted by the Roman numeral VII. The facial nerve is made up of four types of fibers, each with its own unique function (Fig. 8-1). The first and most important type of fiber is the branchial motor special efferent component (Fig. 8-2). Making up the largest portion of facial nerve fibers, the branchial motor component provides voluntary control of the muscles of facial expression, including buccinator, occipitalis, and platysma muscles, as well as the posterior belly of the digastric, stylohyoid, and stapedius muscles.

The second functional component of the facial nerve is the visceral motor component, which is made up of general visceral efferent fibers (see Fig. 8-1). The visceral motor component provides parasympathetic innervation of the mucous membranes of nasopharynx, hard and soft palate, and the lacrimal, submandibular, and sublingual glands (Fig. 8-3).

The third functional component of the facial nerve is the special sensory component, which is made up of special afferent fibers (see Fig. 8-1). The special sensory component provides taste sensation for the anterior two thirds of tongue as well as the hard and soft palates (Fig. 8-4).

The fourth functional component of the facial nerve is the general sensory component which is made up of general somatic afferent fibers (see Fig. 8-1). The general sensory component of the facial nerve provides sensory innervation for the skin of the concha of the auricle and for a small area behind the ear (Fig. 8-5). The visceral motor, special sensory, and general sensory components are covered in a clearly defined fascial sheath separate from the branchial motor special efferent fibers and collectively are known as the nervus intermedius.

The most common disorder of the facial nerve encountered in clinical practice is Bell's palsy. Presenting as sudden paralysis of the muscles of facial expression, this disorder is quite distressing to the patient (Fig. 8-6). The signs and symptoms of Bell's palsy in addition to the facial paralysis are listed in Table 8-1. The intensity of symptoms associated with Bell's palsy

TABLE 8–1 Signs and Symptoms of Bell's Palsy

- Sudden onset of unilateral facial paralysis or weakness
- Facial ptosis and difficulty forming facial expressions
- Inability to fully close eye and protect cornea
- Pain behind or in front of the ear on the affected side
- Hyperacusia (hypersensitivity to loud sounds)on the affected side
- Pain, usually in the ear on the affected side
- Headache
- Loss of taste in the anterior two thirds of the tongue
- Increased saliva production with associated drooling

can range from mild to severe with an onset to peak of 48 hours. While the exact etiology of Bell's palsy remains elusive, it is believed that the most likely cause of this cranial nerve palsy is nerve inflammation, swelling, and ischemia due to viral infection. The herpes simplex virus has been most commonly implicated in this disorder, and there is anecdotal evidence that the addition of acyclovir to a short course of oral prednisone will shorten the course of the disease and improve the outcome. However, the most important therapeutic intervention in the patient suffering from Bell's palsy is to protect the cornea of the affected eye by using lubricating eye drops and an eye patch, especially during sleep, to avoid corneal damage. Improvement after the onset of symptoms of Bell's palsy is gradual and recovery times vary from patient to patient. Most patients begin to get better within 2 weeks after the initial onset of symptoms, and most recover completely, with normal function returning within 3 to 6 months. In rare cases, the symptoms may persist longer or may become permanent.

SUGGESTED READINGS

Campbell W: DeJong's The Neurological Examination, ed 6. Philadelphia, Lippincott Williams and Wilkins, 2005.
Goetz CG: Textbook of Clinical Neurology, ed 2. Philadelphia, Saunders, 2003.

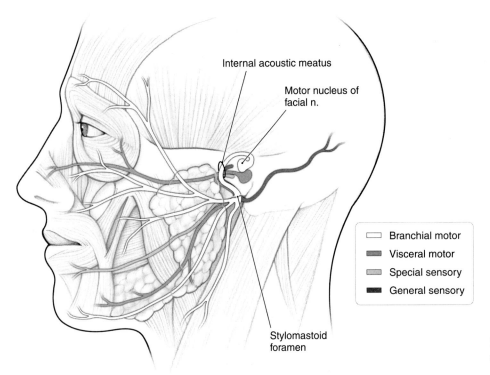

FIGURE 8–1 The four functional components of the facial nerve.

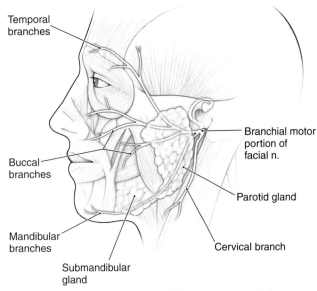

FIGURE 8–2 The branchial motor fiber component of the facial nerve.

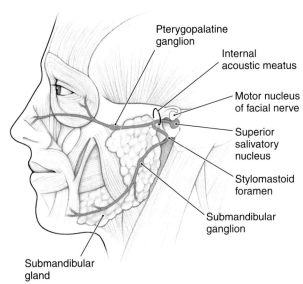

FIGURE 8–3 The visceral motor fiber component of the facial nerve.

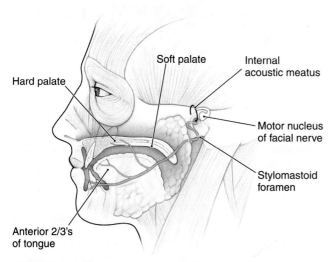

FIGURE 8–4 The special visceral sensory component of the facial nerve.

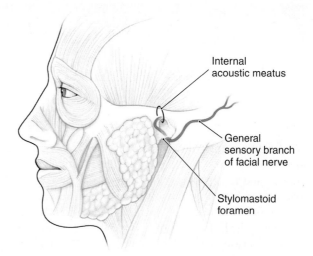

FIGURE 8–5 The general sensory fiber component of the facial nerve.

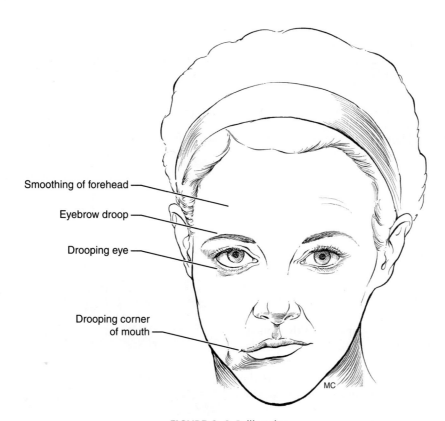

FIGURE 8–6 Bell's palsy.

CHAPTER 9

The Vestibulocochlear Nerve—Cranial Nerve VIII

The eighth cranial nerve is known by several names—the acoustic, the auditory, and the vestibulocochlear nerve—and is denoted by the Roman numeral VIII. The nerve is, in fact, not a single nerve but is made up of two distinct fiber bundles, the cochlear and vestibular nerves, each of which has its own special functions, special peripheral receptors, and central pathways and endpoints. For ease in understanding, each will be discussed separately.

The Cochlear Nerve

The cochlear nerve is primarily responsible for transmitting the electrical impulses generated for hearing and localization of sound. The nerve has its origin in the bipolar cells of the spiral ganglion of the cochlea, which is located adjacent to the inner margin of the bony spiral lamina. The peripheral fibers pass to the organ of Corti, which in essence serves as a microphone in that it converts sound waves into electrical action potentials that will travel up the auditory pathway to ultimately end at the auditory cortex (Fig. 9-1). The central fibers pass inferiorly through the foramina of the tractus spiralis foraminosus or through the foramen centrale into the outer aspect of the internal auditory meatus (Fig. 9-2). The cochlear nerve then passes along the internal auditory meatus with the vestibular nerve. The cochlear nerve then passes through the subarachnoid space at a level just above the flocculus to terminate in the cochlear nucleus.

From the cochlear nucleus, action potentials that began at the organ of Corti travel upward through the trapezoidal body and cross to the contralateral side to synapse within the superior olivary nuclei (Fig. 9-3). Using input from both ears, superior olivary nucleus is one of the key nuclei for localizing sound. Continuing up the auditory pathway, part of the fibers continue in a superior direction to the inferior colliculus while the remaining fibers synapse at the lateral lemniscal nuclei before decussating and continuing upward to the contralateral inferior colliculus (see Fig. 9-3). From the inferior colliculus, the auditory pathway either crosses to the contralateral inferior colliculus or continues on to the medial geniculate body, which is situated on the ventral posterior portion of the thalamus. From the medial geniculate body, signals continue up the auditory pathway to the auditory cortex.

The Vestibular Nerve

The vestibular nerve is primarily responsible for carrying impulses involved in maintaining equilibrium. It arises in the primary vestibular bipolar neurons whose cell bodies make up the Scarpa ganglion in the internal auditory canal (see Fig. 9-2). Each of the bipolar neurons consists of a superior and inferior cell group related to superior and inferior divisions of the vestibular nerve trunk.

The superior division of the vestibular nerve innervates the cristae of the superior and lateral canals, the anterosuperior part of the macula of the saccule, and the macula of the utricle. The inferior division of the vestibular nerve innervates the crista of the posterior canal and the main portion of the macula of the saccule. At a point just medial to the vestibular ganglion, the nerve fibers of both divisions of the vestibular nerve merge into a single trunk, which then enters the brainstem (Fig. 9-4). Most of the afferent fibers then terminate in one of the four ventricular nuclei, which contain the cell bodies of the

TABLE 9–1 Common Disorders of the Vestibulocochlear Nerve

Disorders of Hearing

- Cerebropontine angle tumors
- Acoustic neuromas
- Infection
- Drug-induced ototoxicity
- Aging
- Exposure to loud noises
- Genetic
- Stroke

Disorders of Equilibrium

- Meniere's disease
- Otitis media
- Labyrinthitis
- Stroke

Disorders of Otoliths

- Drug induced

second-order neurons of the vestibular nerve. These nuclei are located on the floor of the fourth ventricle. Some vestibular nuclei receive only primary vestibular afferents, but most receive afferents from the cerebellum, reticular formation, spinal cord, and contralateral vestibular nuclei. From the vestibular nuclei, fibers travel to the spinal cord, the extraocular nuclei, and the cerebellum to aid in the maintenance of balance. The terminal projections of the vestibular pathway in humans are not fully defined, but fibers appear to extend to the temporal lobe near the auditory cortex as well as to the insula.

Clinically, disorders of the acoustic nerve most often take the form of disorders of hearing, balance, or both. Examples of some of the more common diseases responsible for disorders of the acoustic nerve are listed in Table 9-1.

SUGGESTED READINGS

Campbell W: DeJong's The Neurological Examination, ed 6. Philadelphia, Lippincott Williams and Wilkins, 2005.

Goetz CG: Textbook of Clinical Neurology, ed 2. Philadelphia, Saunders, 2003.

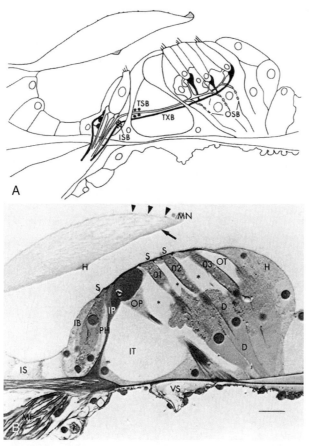

FIGURE 9–1 The organ of Corti. **A,** Line drawing. Filled fibers represent efferents, and nonfilled fibers represent afferents. Note inner spiral bundle (ISB), tunnel spiral bundle (TSB), tunnel crossing bundle (TXB), and outer spiral bundle (OSB). **B,** Photomicrograph showing radial section of organ of Corti containing Hensen's cells (H), outer tunnel of Corti (OT), Deiters' cells (D), spaces of Nuel *(asterisks)*, three outer hair cell rows (03, 02, 01), outer pillar cells (OP), inner tunnel of Corti (IG), inner pillar cells (IP), inner hair cells (I), hair cell stereocilia (S), inner phalangeal cells (PH), and inner border cells (IB). Also shown are inner sulcus cells (IS), myelinated nerve fibers (MF) of spiral lamina, vas spirale (VS), tectorial membrane with Hensen's stripe (H), Hardesty's membrane *(arrow)*, marginal net (MN), and cover net *(arrowheads)*. (From Cummings CW, et al. [eds]: Otolaryngology: Head and Neck Surgery, ed 4. Philadelphia, Mosby, 2005.)

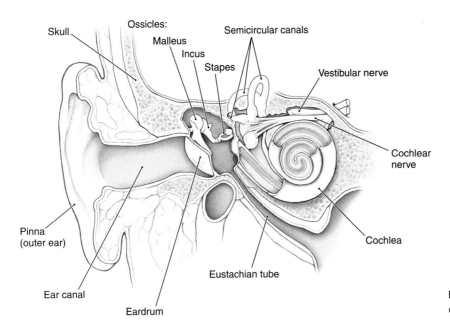

FIGURE 9–2 The paths of the peripheral cochlear and vestibular nerves.

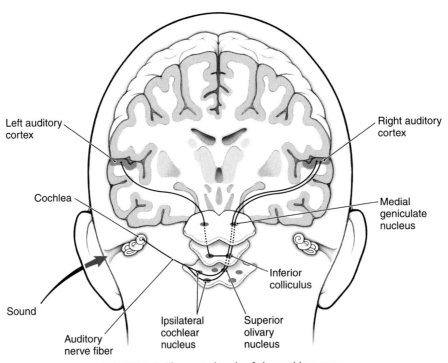

FIGURE 9–3 The central path of the cochlear nerve.

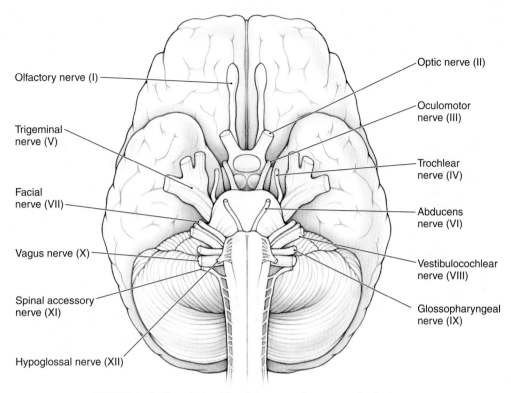

Olfactory nerve (I)

Trigeminal nerve (V)

Facial nerve (VII)

Vagus nerve (X)

Spinal accessory nerve (XI)

Hypoglossal nerve (XII)

Optic nerve (II)

Oculomotor nerve (III)

Trochlear nerve (IV)

Abducens nerve (VI)

Vestibulocochlear nerve (VIII)

Glossopharyngeal nerve (IX)

FIGURE 9–4 The relationship of the acoustic nerve at the brainstem.

CHAPTER 10

The Glossopharyngeal Nerve—Cranial Nerve IX

The glossopharyngeal nerve is the ninth cranial nerve and is denoted by the Roman numeral IX. The glossopharyngeal nerve is made up of five types of fibers, each with a unique function. The first type, the branchial motor special efferent fibers, provide innervation of the stylopharyngeus muscle, which allows voluntary elevation of the pharynx during swallowing and speech.

The second type, the visceral motor general efferent fibers, provide parasympathetic innervation of the smooth muscle and glands of the pharynx, the larynx, and the viscera of the thorax and abdomen. The third fiber type is the visceral sensory general afferent, which carries efferent baroreceptor information from the carotid sinus and chemoreceptors from the carotid body necessary to maintain homeostasis.

The fourth type of fiber comprising the glossopharyngeal nerve is the general sensory somatic afferent fibers, which provide cutaneous sensory information from the external ear, the internal surface of the tympanic membrane, the upper pharynx, and the posterior third of the tongue. The fifth type, the special sensory afferent fibers, provide the sensation of taste from the posterior third of the tongue.

To best understand the anatomy of the glossopharyngeal nerve, the specific anatomy of each type of fibers and their associated functions will be examined individually. The branchial motor special efferent fibers originate from the nucleus ambiguus in the reticular formation of the medulla and then pass anteriorly and laterally to exit the medulla, along with the other fiber components of the glossopharyngeal nerve between the olive and the inferior cerebellar peduncle (Fig. 10-1). These components join together to exit the base of the skull via the jugular foramen. The branchial motor special efferent fibers then pass inferiorly deep to the styloid process to innervate the posterior border of the stylopharyngeus muscle to provide for voluntary control of this muscle during swallowing and speech (Fig. 10-2).

The visceral motor general efferent preganglionic fibers originate in the inferior salivatory nucleus of the rostral medulla and travel anteriorly and laterally to exit the brainstem between the olive and the inferior cerebellar peduncle along with the other fibers of the glossopharyngeal nerve. Exiting from the lateral aspect of the medulla, the visceral motor fibers join the other components of the glossopharyngeal nerve to enter the jugular foramen. Inside the jugular foramen, there are two glossopharyngeal ganglia, which contain the nerve cell bodies that mediate general, visceral, and special sensation for the glossopharyngeal nerve. The visceral motor fibers pass through both ganglia without synapsing and exit the inferior ganglion along with other general sensory fibers of the glossopharyngeal nerve as the tympanic nerve. Before exiting the jugular foramen, the tympanic nerve enters the petrous portion of the temporal bone and passes superiorly via the inferior tympanic canaliculus into the tympanic cavity, where it forms a plexus of the surface of the middle ear to provide sensation. Visceral motor fibers pass through this plexus and coalesce to become the lesser petrosal nerve, which travels back through the temporal bone to emerge into the middle cranial fossa. The lesser petrosal nerve then passes anteriorly to exit the base of the skull through the foramen ovale along with the third (mandibular) division of the trigeminal nerve. The lesser petrosal nerve then synapses in the otic ganglion, which is situated immediately below the foramen ovale.

Postganglionic fibers from the otic ganglion travel along with the auriculotemporal branch of third division of the trigeminal nerve to enter the substance of the parotid gland. These fibers carry impulses from the higher centers to cause the parotid gland to increase or decrease secretions in response to such stimuli as the smell of food or fear.

The visceral sensory general afferent fibers of the glossopharyngeal nerve innervate the baroreceptors of the carotid sinus and chemoreceptors of the carotid body (Fig. 10-3). From the carotid body and sinus, these sensory fibers ascend and join the other components of glossopharyngeal nerve at the inferior hypoglossal ganglion that contains the cell bodies of these neurons. The nerve fibers leave the ganglion and travel superiorly to enter the base of the skull at the jugular foramen. Exiting the jugular foramen, the visceral sensory general afferent fibers enter the lateral medulla between the olive and the

inferior cerebellar peduncle and descend in the tractus solitarius to synapse in the caudal nucleus solitarius. From the nucleus solitarius, interconnections are made with multiple areas in the reticular formation and the hypothalamus to mediate cardiovascular and respiratory reflex responses to changes in blood pressure, and serum concentrations of carbon dioxide and oxygen necessary to maintain homeostasis.

The general sensory somatic afferent fibers carry pain, temperature, and touch information from the skin of the external ear, internal surface of the tympanic membrane, the walls of the upper pharynx, and the posterior third of the tongue. Sensory fibers from the skin of the external ear initially travel with the auricular branch of the vagus nerve with those fibers innervating the middle ear combining as part of the tympanic nerve. Pain, temperature, and touch information from the upper pharynx and posterior third of the tongue ascend via the pharyngeal branches of the glossopharyngeal nerve. The cell bodies for these peripheral portions of the glossopharyngeal nerve are located in the superior or inferior glossopharyngeal ganglia that reside within the jugular foramen. Leaving the glossopharyngeal ganglia, these general sensory neurons then pass superiorly through the jugular foramen to enter the brainstem at the level of the medulla where they descend in the spinal trigeminal tract and synapse in the caudal spinal nucleus of the trigeminal nerve. Ascending secondary neurons originating from the spinal nucleus of the trigeminal nerve project to the contralateral ventral posteromedial nucleus of the thalamus via the ventral trigeminothalamic tract. Tertiary neurons from the ventral posteromedial nucleus of the thalamus project via the posterior limb of the internal capsule to the sensory cortex of the post-central gyrus.

The special sensory afferent fibers have their origin in the posterior third of the tongue and ascend via the pharyngeal branches of the glossopharyngeal nerve to the inferior glossopharyngeal ganglion that contains the cell bodies of these primary neurons. The central processes of these neurons leave the inferior ganglion and pass superiorly through the jugular foramen to enter the brainstem at the level of the rostral medulla between the olive and inferior cerebellar peduncle. At this point, these special sensory afferent fibers ascend in the tractus solitarius and synapse in the caudal nucleus solitarius. Special sensory afferent taste fibers from the facial and vagus cranial nerves also ascend and synapse at this location. Secondary special sensory afferent neurons originating in the nucleus solitarius project bilaterally and travel superiorly via the central tegmental tract to the ventral posteromedial nuclei of the thalamus. Tertiary special sensory afferent neurons from the ventral posteromedial nuclei of the thalamus then project via the posterior limb of the internal capsule to the gustatory cortex of the parietal lobe.

Clinically, the most common painful condition involving the glossopharyngeal nerve is glossopharyngeal neuralgia. Glossopharyngeal neuralgia is a rare condition characterized by paroxysms of pain in the sensory division of the ninth cranial nerve. Clinically, the pain of glossopharyngeal neuralgia resembles that of trigeminal neuralgia, but the incidence of this painful condition is significantly less. The pain of glossopharyngeal neuralgia is rarely complicated by associated cardiac dysrhythmias and asystole, which is thought to be due to an overflow phenomenon from the glossopharyngeal to the vagus nerve at the point at which they exit the jugular foramen in proximity to one another (Fig. 10-4).

SUGGESTED READINGS

Campbell W: DeJong's The Neurological Examination, ed 6. Philadelphia, Lippincott Williams and Wilkins, 2005.

Goetz CG: Textbook of Clinical Neurology, ed 2. Philadelphia, Saunders, 2003.

Waldman SD: Glossopharyngeal neuralgia. In: Atlas of Uncommon Pain Syndromes, ed 2. Philadelphia, Saunders, 2008.

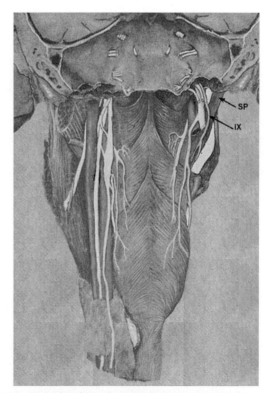

FIGURE 10–2 The glossopharyngeal nerve as it exits the jugular foramen along with the vagus and spinal accessory nerves. Note the branch of the glossopharyngeal nerve (IX) to the stylopharyngeus muscle (SP).

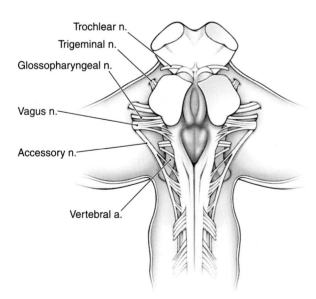

FIGURE 10–1 The path of the glossopharyngeal nerve as it exits the brainstem.

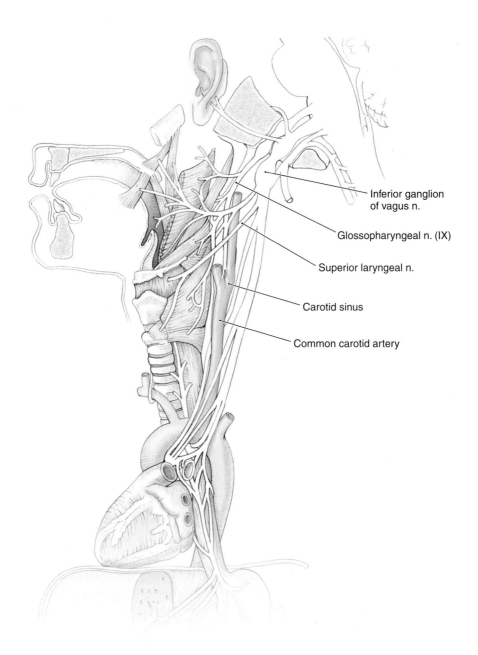

Inferior ganglion
of vagus n.

Glossopharyngeal n. (IX)

Superior laryngeal n.

Carotid sinus

Common carotid artery

FIGURE 10–3 The relationship of the glossopharyngeal nerve and the carotid sinus and body.

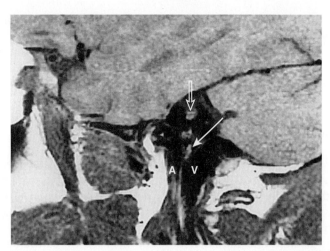

FIGURE 10–4 Sagittal T1-weighted image through the jugular foramen. The jugular vein (V) is located posterior to the internal carotid artery (A). The glossopharyngeal and vagus nerves are visible between the two structures *(solid arrows)*. The internal auditory canal and vestibulocochlear nerve complex is visible superiorly. (From Edelman RR, Hesselink JR, Zlatkin M, et al. [eds]: Clinical Magnetic Resonance Imaging, Vol 2, ed 3. Philadelphia, Saunders, 2007.)

CHAPTER 11

The Vagus Nerve—Cranial Nerve X

The vagus nerve is the tenth cranial nerve and is denoted by the Roman numeral X. The vagus nerve is made up of five types of fibers, each with its own unique function (Fig. 11-1). The first type of fiber is the special visceral efferent fibers, which provide innervation of the striated muscle of the pharynx; the striated muscles of the larynx with the exception of the stylopharyngeus muscle, which is innervated by the glossopharyngeal nerve, and the tensor veli palatini muscle, which is innervated by the trigeminal nerve; and the palatoglossus muscle of the tongue with the rest of the muscles of the tongue are innervated by cranial nerve XII.

The second type of fiber comprising the vagus nerve is the general visceral efferent fibers, which provide parasympathetic innervation of the smooth muscle and glands of the pharynx, the larynx, and the viscera of the thorax and abdomen. The third fiber type is the general visceral afferent fibers, which provide visceral sensory information from the larynx, esophagus, trachea, and abdominal and thoracic viscera, as well as from the stretch receptors of the aortic arch and chemoreceptors of the aortic bodies.

The fourth type of fiber comprising the vagus nerve is the general somatic afferent fibers, which provide cutaneous sensory information from the posterior skin of the ear, the external surface of the tympanic membrane, the pharynx, and the external auditory meatus. The fifth type of nerve fiber is the special visceral afferent fibers, which provide the sensation of taste from taste buds located on the root of the tongue and on the epiglottis.

To best understand the anatomy of the vagus nerve, the specific anatomy of each type of fiber and its associated functions will be examined individually. The special efferent fibers originate from the nucleus ambiguus, which is located in the reticular formation of the medulla. These motor fibers leave the nucleus ambiguus and pass anteriorly and laterally to exit the medulla posterior to the olive as a series of 8 to 12 small rootlike structures. These rootlike structures pass along with fibers of the spinal accessory nerve into the jugular foramen of the skull. The remaining fiber types of the vagus nerve also enter the jugular foramen and give rise to the superior and inferior vagal ganglia, which lie within the jugular foramen. The special visceral afferent fibers rejoin the rest of the vagus nerve fibers at a point just below the inferior vagal ganglion.

Exiting inferiorly through the jugular foramen, the vagus nerve travels between the internal jugular vein and internal carotid artery within the carotid sheath, giving off three major branches containing special visceral efferent fibers: (1) the pharyngeal branch, (2) the superior laryngeal nerve, and (3) the recurrent laryngeal nerve (Fig. 11-2). The pharyngeal branch provides the primary motor innervation to the pharynx including the levator palatini muscle, the salpingopharyngeus muscle, the superior, middle, and inferior constrictor muscles, the palatopharyngeus muscle, as well as the palatoglossus muscle of the tongue.

Branching from the main trunk of the vagus nerve just below the pharyngeal nerve, the superior laryngeal nerve travels inferiorly just adjacent to the pharynx and divides into internal and external laryngeal nerves. The external laryngeal nerve supplies fibers to innervate the inferior constrictor muscle of the pharynx, as well as providing motor innervation to the cricothyroid muscle, which helps control the movements of the vocal cords. The internal laryngeal nerve serves as the primary sensory nerve of the larynx.

The recurrent laryngeal nerve provides motor innervation to the intrinsic muscles of the larynx, which provide the majority of movement of the vocal cords (see Fig. 11-2). The paths of the left and right recurrent laryngeal nerves vary slightly with the left recurrent laryngeal nerve dividing from the main vagus nerve at the level of the aortic arch. The left recurrent laryngeal nerve then dips posteriorly around the aortic arch to ascend through the superior mediastinum to enter the groove between the esophagus and trachea. The right recurrent laryngeal nerve divides from the main vagus nerve at the level of the right subclavian artery to enter the superior mediastinum. The right recurrent laryngeal nerve then dips posteriorly around the subclavian artery to ascend in the groove between the esophagus and trachea.

The general visceral efferent fibers provide parasympathetic innervation of the smooth muscle and glands of the pharynx, the larynx, and the viscera of the thorax and abdomen. Stimulation of these fibers results in contraction of the smooth muscles as well as increased secretions from the glands that these general visceral efferent fibers innervate. Stimulation of these fibers also slows the cardiac rate, causes bronchoconstriction and increased bronchiolar secretions, and increases motility of the gastrointestinal tract with increased gastrointestinal secretions.

The general visceral efferent fibers of the vagus nerve originate in the dorsal motor nucleus of the vagus, which is located in the floor of the fourth ventricle in the rostral medulla as well as in the central gray matter of the caudal medulla. These fibers travel inferiorly via the spinal trigeminal tract to exit the lateral medulla, where they join other fibers of the vagus nerve to exit the base of the skull through the jugular foramen. The general visceral efferent fibers travel with the rest of the vagus nerve

inferiorly between the internal jugular vein and internal carotid artery within the carotid sheath. Branches of these fibers provide innervation to the secretomotor glands of the larynx and pharynx. As these fibers travel into the thorax, they arborize into plexuses that surround the major vasculature and the esophagus. These fibers then recoalesce to provide preganglionic parasympathetic innervation to the stomach, intestines, and organs of the abdomen (Fig. 11-3).

The general visceral afferent fibers of the vagus nerve provide sensory information from the larynx, esophagus, trachea, and abdominal and thoracic viscera, as well as the stretch receptors of the aortic arch and chemoreceptors of the aortic bodies. These general visceral afferent fibers then surround the abdominal viscera and coalesce to join the gastric nerves, which travel superiorly through the esophageal hiatus of the diaphragm to merge with the esophageal plexus. These fibers combine with general visceral afferent fibers from the heart and lungs and then join the ascending fibers in the esophageal plexus, which converge to form the left and right vagus nerves, which ascend within the carotid sheath between the internal jugular vein and internal carotid artery.

Within the jugular foramen, these fibers enter the inferior vagal ganglion and then exit the foramen to travel superiorly to enter the medulla. The fibers then descend in the tractus solitarius to synapse in the caudal nucleus solitarius from where they project to multiple areas of the reticular formation where autonomic control of the cardiovascular, respiratory, and gastrointestinal functions take place via the general visceral efferent fibers of the vagus nerve.

The general somatic afferent fibers provide cutaneous sensory information from the posterior skin of the ear, the external surface of the tympanic membrane, the pharynx, and the external auditory meatus. These sensory fibers from the external ear, external auditory canal, and external surface of the tympanic membrane are carried via the auricular branch of vagus nerve and travel into the jugular foramen to enter the superior vagal ganglion.

General somatic information from the larynx and pharynx travels in the recurrent laryngeal and internal laryngeal nerves, which coalesce and ascend into the jugular foramen with the vagus nerve to enter the superior vagal ganglion. The central processes of these general sensory afferent fibers leave the jugular foramen and travel superiorly to enter the medulla, where they exit the vagal ganglia and pass through the jugular foramen to enter the brainstem at the level of the medulla, where they descend in the spinal trigeminal tract and synapse in the spinal nucleus of the trigeminal nerve. Ascending secondary neurons from the spinal nucleus of the trigeminal nerve project to the contralateral ventral posteromedial nucleus of the thalamus via the ventral trigeminothalamic tract. Tertiary neurons from the thalamus project via the posterior limb of the internal capsule to the sensory cortex of the post-central gyrus.

Clinically, disorders of the vagus nerve can be subtle, but depending on where the nerve is compromised, certain physical findings should lead the clinician to think about disorders involving the vagus nerve. The most obvious physical findings associated with compromise of the vagus nerve include hoarseness secondary to the paralysis of the intrinsic muscles of the larynx on the affected side and/or difficulty in swallowing due to the inability to elevate the soft palate on the affected side as a result of paralysis of the levator veli palatini muscle.

The clinician may note that the uvula may deviate to the side opposite the nerve compromise due to the unopposed action of the intact levator veli palatini muscle. Surgical trauma or compression of the recurrent laryngeal nerve by tumor or adenopathy can result in paralysis of the intrinsic muscles of the larynx controlling the vocal cord on the affected side.

SUGGESTED READINGS

Campbell W: DeJong's The Neurological Examination, ed 6. Philadelphia, Lippincott Williams and Wilkins, 2005.

Goetz CG: Textbook of Clinical Neurology, ed 2. Philadelphia, Saunders, 2003.

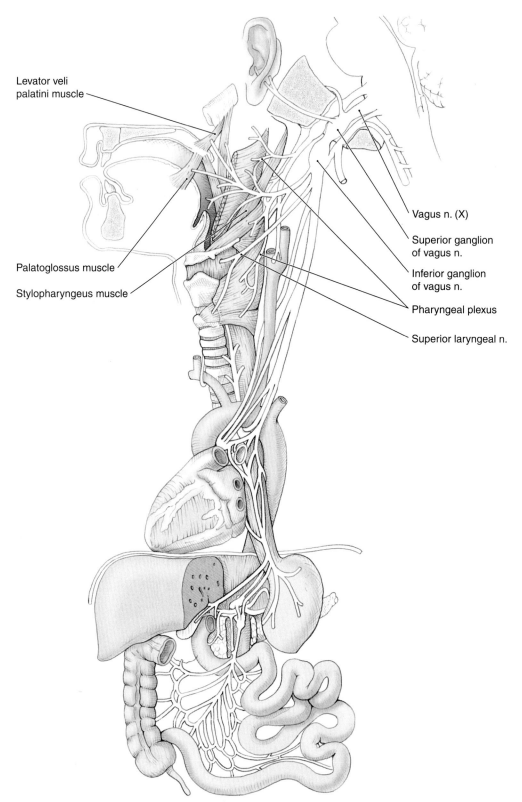

Levator veli
palatini muscle

Palatoglossus muscle

Stylopharyngeus muscle

Vagus n. (X)

Superior ganglion
of vagus n.

Inferior ganglion
of vagus n.

Pharyngeal plexus

Superior laryngeal n.

FIGURE 11–1 The anatomy of the vagus nerve.

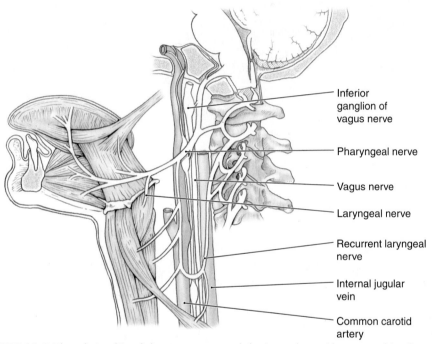

Inferior ganglion of vagus nerve

Pharyngeal nerve

Vagus nerve

Laryngeal nerve

Recurrent laryngeal nerve

Internal jugular vein

Common carotid artery

FIGURE 11–2 The relationship of the vagus nerve and the internal carotid artery and jugular vein.

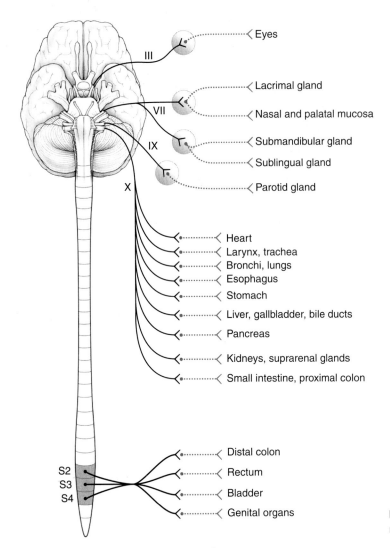

III

VII

IX

X

Eyes

Lacrimal gland

Nasal and palatal mucosa

Submandibular gland

Sublingual gland

Parotid gland

Heart

Larynx, trachea

Bronchi, lungs

Esophagus

Stomach

Liver, gallbladder, bile ducts

Pancreas

Kidneys, suprarenal glands

Small intestine, proximal colon

Distal colon

Rectum

Bladder

Genital organs

S2
S3
S4

FIGURE 11–3 The visceral innervation by the vagus nerve is far reaching.

CHAPTER 12

The Spinal Accessory Nerve—Cranial Nerve XI

The spinal accessory nerve is the eleventh cranial nerve and is denoted by the Roman numeral XI. The spinal accessory nerve consists of both a cranial root and a spinal root, which are made up of branchial special visceral efferent fibers. These fibers have their origin in the caudal nucleus ambiguus and pass anteriorly and laterally to exit the medulla between the olive and inferior cerebellar peduncle just below the exiting fibers of cranial nerve X (Fig. 12-1). The smaller cranial root fibers of the spinal accessory nerve briefly join with the larger spinal root fibers of the spinal accessory nerve and then enter the jugular foramen together. Within the foramen, the cranial root fibers split from the spinal root fibers and join the vagus nerve to exit the skull through the foramen together along with the glossopharyngeal nerve (Fig. 12-2). The fibers of the cranial portion of the spinal accessory nerve follow the extracranial course of the vagus nerve to help provide motor innervation to the larynx and pharynx.

The fibers of the spinal root of the spinal accessory nerve have their origin not in the medulla like the cranial portion of the spinal accessory nerve but in the lateral portion of the ventral grey matter of the upper five or six segments of the cervical spinal cord. These motor fibers travel laterally and exit the cervical spinal cord between the dorsal and ventral spinal nerve roots. After exiting the cervical spinal cord, the fibers of the spinal root of the spinal accessory nerves pass inferiorly to enter the posterior fossa, where they join with the cranial root fibers of the spinal accessory nerve to pass through the jugular foramen where the cranial root fibers again separate from the spinal root fibers to join the vagus nerve.

The fibers of the spinal root of the spinal accessory nerve exit the jugular foramen medial to the styloid process and travel in a downward and posterior trajectory to enter the upper portion of the sternocleidomastoid muscle on its deep surface, where some of the fibers innervate the muscle and other fibers pass through the posterior triangle of the neck to innervate the trapezius muscle (Fig. 12-3).

Clinically, disorders affecting the spinal accessory nerve manifest as weakness or paralysis of the sternocleidomastoid and/or trapezius muscles. Damage to the spinal root of cranial nerve XI is a lower motor neuron lesion and results in weakness or flaccid paralysis of the sternocleidomastoid and/or trapezius muscles. The strength of the sternocleidomastoid muscle can best be tested by having the patient turn the head while the examiner applies resistance to the patient's mandible on the affected side (Fig. 12-4). Weakness of the trapezius muscle will result in a drop shoulder characterized by downward displacement and lateral rotation of the scapula on the affected side (Fig. 12-5).

SUGGESTED READINGS

Campbell W: DeJong's The Neurological Examination, ed 6. Philadelphia, Lippincott Williams and Wilkins, 2005.

Goetz CG: Textbook of Clinical Neurology, ed 2. Philadelphia, Saunders, 2003.

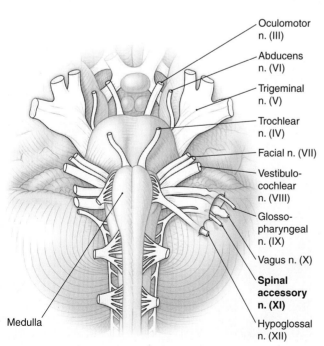

FIGURE 12–1 The spinal accessory nerve exits the medulla just below the fibers of the vagus nerve.

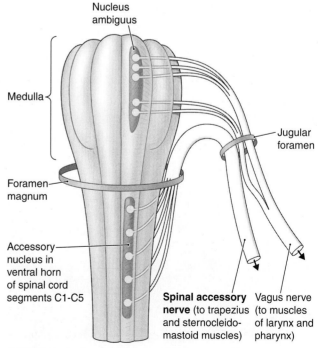

FIGURE 12–2 The spinal accessory nerve exits the jugular foramen along with the vagus and glossopharyngeal nerves.

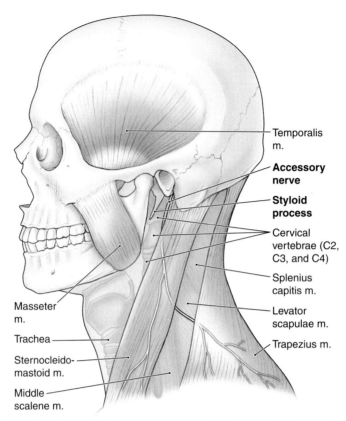

Temporalis m.

Accessory nerve

Styloid process

Cervical vertebrae (C2, C3, and C4)

Splenius capitis m.

Levator scapulae m.

Trapezius m.

Masseter m.

Trachea

Sternocleido-mastoid m.

Middle scalene m.

FIGURE 12–3 The relationship of the spinal accessory nerve and the sternocleidomastoid and trapezius muscles.

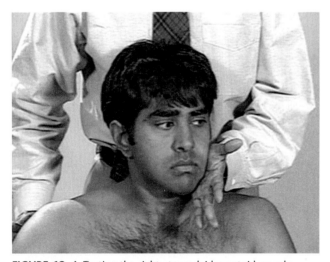

FIGURE 12–4 Testing the right sternocleidomastoid muscle against resistance.

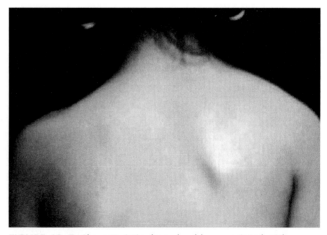

FIGURE 12–5 Characteristic drop shoulder associated with weakness of the trapezius muscle.

CHAPTER 13

The Hypoglossal Nerve—Cranial Nerve XII

The hypoglossal nerve is the twelfth cranial nerve and is denoted by the Roman numeral XII. It is made up of only general somatic efferent motor fibers and provides innervation for all of the intrinsic and three of the four extrinsic muscles of the tongue. The fibers of the hypoglossal nerve originate from the hypoglossal nucleus, which is located in the tegmentum of the medulla. General somatic efferent motor fibers leave the hypoglossal nucleus and travel ventrally to exit the brainstem as a series of rootlets at the ventrolateral sulcus, which is located between the pyramid and the olive (Fig. 13-1). These rootlets coalesce to the hypoglossal nerve, which exits the posterior cranial fossa via the hypoglossal foramen where it lies medial to the glossopharyngeal, vagus, and spinal accessory nerves that exited the cranial vault via the jugular foramen. Passing lateral and downward with these cranial nerves in between the internal carotid artery and internal jugular vein, the hypoglossal nerve then turns anteriorly passing just lateral to the bifurcation of the common carotid artery to run along the lateral surface of the hyoglossus muscle (Fig. 13-2). The fibers of the hypoglossal nerve then divide to provide motor innervation to all of the intrinsic and three of the extrinsic muscles of the tongue, the genioglossus, styloglossus, and hyoglossus, with the palatoglossus muscle innervated by the vagus nerve (see Fig. 13-2).

Clinically, weakness of the hypoglossal nerve manifests as tongue deviation to the affected side due to the unopposed action of the muscles innervated by the hypoglossal nerve on the contralateral side. With time, atrophy of the affected side of the tongue may also be identified (Fig. 13-3). To evaluate hypoglossal nerve function, the examiner asks the patient to protrude his or her tongue in the midline (Fig. 13-4). The examiner then places a tongue blade against the side of the tongue and has the patient press against the blade.

SUGGESTED READINGS

Campbell W: DeJong's The Neurological Examination, ed 6. Philadelphia, Lippincott Williams and Wilkins, 2005.

Goetz CG: Textbook of Clinical Neurology, ed 2. Philadelphia, Saunders, 2003.

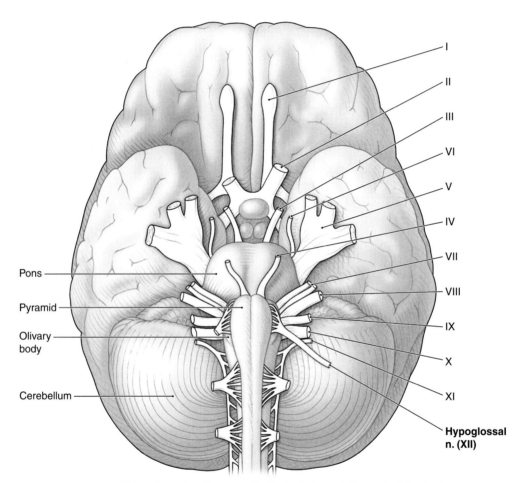

I
II
III
VI
V
IV
VII
VIII
IX
X
XI
Hypoglossal n. (XII)

Pons
Pyramid
Olivary body
Cerebellum

FIGURE 13–1 The hypoglossal nerve exits the brainstem at the ventrolateral sulcus.

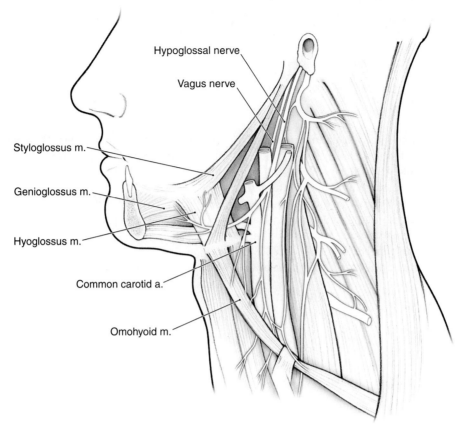

FIGURE 13–2 The extracranial path of the hypoglossal nerve.

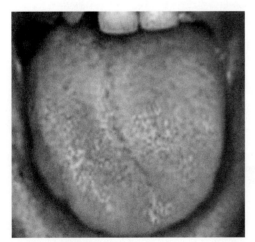

FIGURE 13–3 Hypoglossal nerve palsy with characteristic tongue deviation to the affected side.

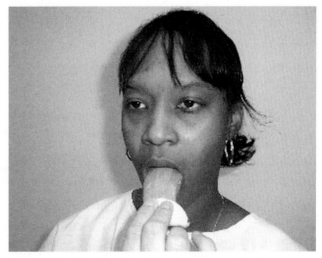

FIGURE 13–4 Examination of hypoglossal nerve function.

CHAPTER 14

The Sphenopalatine Ganglion

The sphenopalatine ganglion (pterygopalatine, nasal, or Meckel's ganglion) is located in the pterygopalatine fossa, posterior to the middle nasal turbinate (Fig. 14-1). It is covered by a 1- to 1.5-mm layer of connective tissue and mucous membrane. This 5-mm triangular structure sends major branches to the gasserian ganglion, trigeminal nerves, carotid plexus, facial nerve, and superior cervical ganglion. The sphenopalatine ganglion can be blocked by topical application of local anesthetic via the transnasal approach or by injection via the lateral approach or through the greater palatine foramen.

SUGGESTED READINGS

Netter FH: Nerves of the nasal cavity. In: Atlas of Human Anatomy, ed 4. Philadelphia, Saunders, 2006.

Waldman SD: Cluster headache. In: Atlas of Common Pain Syndromes, ed 2. Philadelphia, Saunders, 2008.

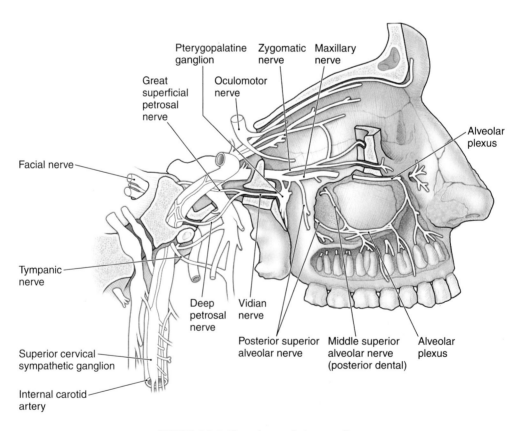

FIGURE 14–1 The sphenopalatine ganglion.

CHAPTER 15

The Greater and Lesser Occipital Nerves

The greater occipital nerve arises from fibers of the dorsal primary ramus of the second cervical nerve and, to a lesser extent, from fibers from the third cervical nerve. The greater occipital nerve pierces the fascia just below the superior nuchal ridge along with the occipital artery. It supplies the medial portion of the posterior scalp as far anterior as the vertex (Fig. 15-1).

The lesser occipital nerve arises from the ventral primary rami of the second and third cervical nerves. The lesser occipital nerve passes superiorly along the posterior border of the sternocleidomastoid muscle, dividing into cutaneous branches that innervate the lateral portion of the posterior scalp and the cranial surface of the pinna of the ear (see Fig. 15-1). The greater and lesser occipital nerves have been implicated as the nerves subserving the pain of the headache syndrome occipital neuralgia. The pain of occipital neuralgia is characterized as persistent pain at the base of the skull with occasional sudden shocklike paresthesias in the distribution of the greater and lesser occipital nerves (see Fig. 15-1).

SUGGESTED READINGS

Campbell W: DeJong's The Neurological Examination, ed 6. Philadelphia, Lippincott Williams and Wilkins, 2005.

Goetz CG: Textbook of Clinical Neurology, ed 2. Philadelphia, Saunders, 2003.

Waldman SD: Occipital neuralgia. In: Atlas of Common Pain Syndromes, ed 2. Philadelphia, Saunders, 2008.

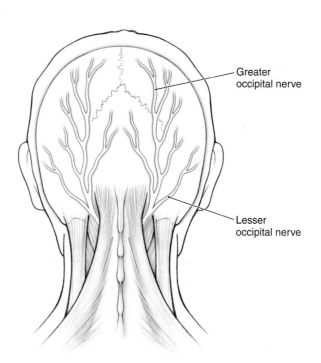

Greater occipital nerve

Lesser occipital nerve

FIGURE 15–1 The pain of occipital neuralgia is characterized as persistent pain at the base of the skull with occasional sudden shocklike paresthesias.

CHAPTER 16

The Temporomandibular Joint

The temporomandibular joint is a true joint that has both gliding and hinge movement. It is the most used joint in the body. The temporomandibular joint represents the articulation between the squamous portion of the temporal bone and the condyle of the mandible (Fig. 16-1). The condyle of the mandible is elliptically shaped with its long axis oriented in the mediolateral plane. The articular surface of the temporal bone is composed of the concave articular fossa and the convex articular eminence (Fig. 16-2).

Separating the articular surface of the temporal bone and the condyle of the mandible is the meniscus, which is a fibrous, saddle-shaped structure whose attachments serve to divide the joint into an anterior and a posterior portion (Fig. 16-3). Anteriorly, a thick band attaches the meniscus to the anterior joint, and posteriorly, the meniscus attaches to the thick posterior band that attaches the meniscus to the posterior joint. The posterior joint contains a vascular supply and is innervated with sensory fibers. The portion of the meniscus that is between the anterior and posterior band is the intermediate zone.

To open the mouth, two distinct movements of the components of the temporomandibular joint must occur: (1) rotation and (2) translation. When the mouth is closed, the thick posterior band of the meniscus lies immediately above the mandibular condyle. As the mouth is opened, the mandibular condyle translates forward with the thinner intermediate zone of the meniscus becoming the articulating surface between the condyle and the articular eminence. When the mouth is fully open, the condyle may lie partially or completely beneath the anterior band of the meniscus.

In temporomandibular joint dysfunction, the posterior band of the meniscus is anteriorly displaced in front of the condyle. As the meniscus translates anteriorly, the posterior band remains in front of the condyle and the bilaminar zone of the meniscus becomes stretched and weakened. If the displaced posterior band reduces or returns to its normal position when the condyle reaches a certain point in translation, the patient will experience a pop that, due to the sensory innervation of the posterior band, may be painful. If the posterior band does not reduce with full translation of the mandibular condyle, the patient may experience a painful grinding sensation. Over time, if this condition persists, the bilaminar zone of the meniscus may become perforated or torn resulting in further deterioration of temporomandibular joint function.

SUGGESTED READINGS

Netter FH: Muscles involved in mastication. In: Atlas of Human Anatomy, ed 4. Philadelphia, Saunders, 2006.

Waldman SD: Trigeminal neuralgia. In: Atlas of Common Pain Syndromes, ed 2. Philadelphia, Saunders, 2008.

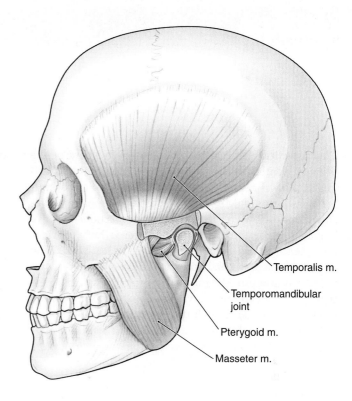

FIGURE 16–1 The anatomy of the temporomandibular joint.

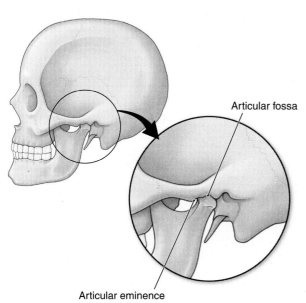

FIGURE 16–2 Relationship of the articular surface of the temporomandibular joint.

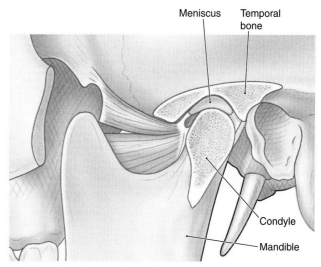

FIGURE 16–3 The meniscus of the temporomandibular joint.

CHAPTER 17

The Superficial Cervical Plexus

The superficial cervical plexus arises from fibers of the primary ventral rami of the first, second, third, and fourth cervical nerves. Each nerve divides into an ascending and a descending branch providing fibers to the nerves above and below, respectively. This collection of nerve branches makes up the cervical plexus, which provides both sensory and motor innervation (Fig. 17-1). The most important motor branch is the phrenic nerve, with the plexus also providing motor fibers to the spinal accessory nerve and to the paravertebral and deep muscles of the neck. Each nerve, with the exception of the first cervical nerve, provides significant cutaneous sensory innervation. These nerves converge at the midpoint of the sternocleidomastoid muscle at its posterior margin to provide sensory innervation to the skin of the lower mandible, neck, and supraclavicular fossa. Terminal sensory fibers of the superficial cervical plexus contribute to nerves including the greater auricular and lesser occipital nerves.

SUGGESTED READINGS

Netter FH: Cutaneous nerves of the head and neck. In: Atlas of Human Anatomy, ed 4. Philadelphia, Saunders, 2006.

Waldman SD: Superficial cervical plexus block. In: Atlas of Interventional Pain Management, ed 2. Philadelphia, Saunders, 2004.

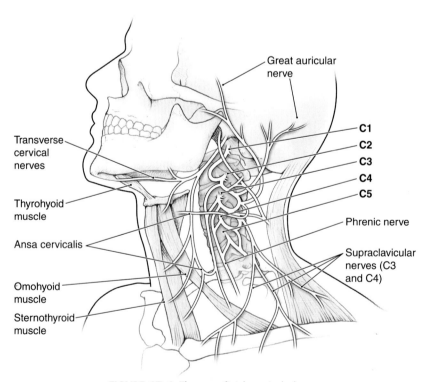

FIGURE 17–1 The superficial cervical plexus.

CHAPTER **18**

The Deep Cervical Plexus

The deep cervical plexus arises from fibers of the primary ventral rami of the first, second, third, and fourth cervical nerves. Each nerve divides into an ascending and descending branch providing fibers to the nerves above and below, respectively. This collection of nerve branches makes up the deep cervical plexus, which provides both sensory and motor innervation (Fig. 18-1). The most important motor branch of the cervical plexus is the phrenic nerve. The plexus also provides motor fibers to the spinal accessory nerve and to the paravertebral and deep muscles of the neck. Each nerve, with the exception of the first cervical nerve, provides significant cutaneous sensory innervation. Terminal sensory fibers of the deep cervical plexus contribute fibers to the greater auricular and lesser occipital nerves.

SUGGESTED READINGS

Netter FH: Nerves of the head and neck. In: Atlas of Human Anatomy, ed 4. Philadelphia, Saunders, 2006.

Waldman SD: Deep cervical plexus block. In: Atlas of Interventional Pain Management, ed 2. Philadelphia, Saunders, 2004.

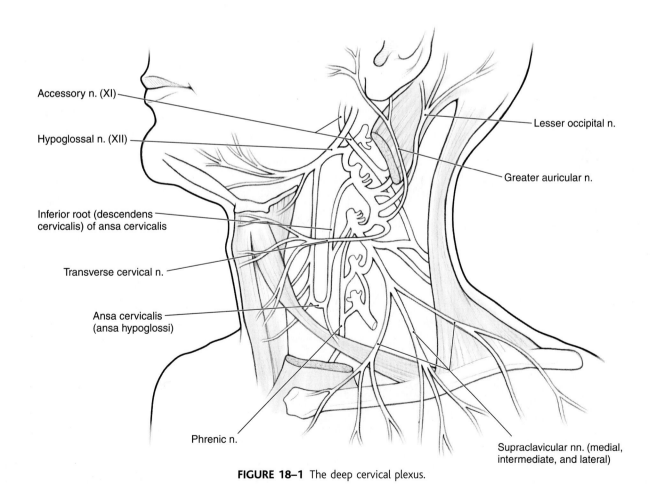

FIGURE 18–1 The deep cervical plexus.

CHAPTER 19

The Stellate Ganglion

The stellate ganglion refers to the ganglion formed by the fusion of the inferior cervical and the first thoracic ganglia as they meet anterior to the vertebral body of C7 (Fig. 19-1). The structures anterior to the ganglion include the skin and subcutaneous tissue, the sternocleidomastoid, and the carotid sheath. The dome of the lung lies anterior and inferior to the ganglion. The prevertebral fascia, vertebral body of C7, esophagus, and thoracic duct lie medially. Structures posterior to the ganglion include the longus colli muscle, anterior scalene muscle, vertebral artery, brachial plexus sheath, and neck of the first rib.

SUGGESTED READINGS

Netter FH: Nerves of the head and neck. In: Atlas of Human Anatomy, ed 4. Philadelphia, Saunders, 2006.

Waldman SD: Stellate ganglion block. In: Atlas of Interventional Pain Management, ed 2. Philadelphia, Saunders, 2004.

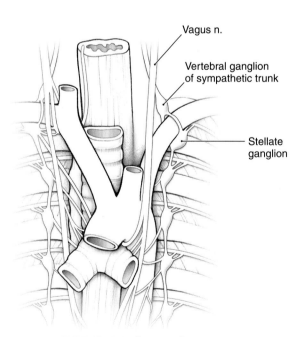

Vagus n.

Vertebral ganglion of sympathetic trunk

Stellate ganglion

FIGURE 19–1 Stellate ganglion anatomy.

The Cervical Vertebrae

The Vertebrae of the Cervical Spine

To fully understand the functional anatomy of the cervical spine and the impact its unique characteristics make in the evolution of the myriad painful conditions that have the cervical spine as their nidus, one must first recognize that unlike the thoracic and lumbar spine, whose functional units are quite similar, the cervical spine must be thought of as being composed of two distinct and dissimilar functional units. The first type of functional unit consists of the atlanto-occipital and the atlantoaxial units (Figs. 20-1 and 20-2). While these units serve to help provide structural static support for the head, they are uniquely adapted to their primary function of facilitating focused movement of the head to allow the optimal functioning of the eyes, ears, nose, and throat. The uppermost two functional units are susceptible to trauma and the inflammatory arthritides as well as the degenerative changes that occur as a result of the aging process.

The second type of functional unit that makes up the cervical spine is very similar to the functional units of the thoracic and lumbar spine and serves primarily as a structural support for the head and secondarily to aid in the positioning of the sense organs located in the head (Figs. 20-3 and 20-4). It is this second type of functional unit that is composed of the lower five cervical vertebrae and their corresponding intervertebral discs that is responsible for the majority of painful conditions encountered in clinical practice (Fig. 20-5).

The Mobility of the Cervical Spine

The cervical spine has the greatest range of motion of the entire spinal column and allows movement in all planes. Its greatest movement occurs from the atlanto-occipital joint to the third cervical vertebra. Movement of the cervical spine occurs as a synchronized effort of the entire cervical spine and its associated musculature, with the upper two cervical segments providing the greatest contribution to rotation, flexion, extension, and lateral bending. During flexion of the cervical spine, the spinal canal is lengthened, the intervertebral foramina become larger, and the anterior portion of the intervertebral disc

becomes compressed (see Fig. 20-5, *B*). During extension of the cervical spine, the spinal canal becomes shortened, the intervertebral foramina become smaller, and the posterior portion of the anterior disc becomes compressed (Fig. 20-5, *C*). With lateral bending and/or rotation, the contralateral intervertebral foramina become larger while the ipsilateral intervertebral foramina become smaller. In health, none of these changes in size results in functional disability or pain; however, in disease, these movements may result in nerve impingement with its attendant pain and functional disability.

The Cervical Vertebral Canal

The bony cervical vertebral canal serves as a protective conduit for the spinal cord and as an exit point of the cervical nerve roots. Because of the bulging of the cervical neuromeres as well as the other fibers that must traverse the cervical vertebral canal to reach the lower portions of the body, the cervical spinal cord occupies a significantly greater proportion of the space available in the spinal canal relative to the space occupied by the thoracic and lumbar spinal cord. This decreased space results in less shock-absorbing effect of the spinal fluid during trauma and also results in compression of the cervical spinal cord with attendant myelopathy when bone or intervertebral disc compromises the spinal canal. Such encroachment of the cervical cord by degenerative changes and/or disc herniation can occur over a period of time, and the resultant loss of neurologic function due to myelopathy can be subtle—as a result, a delay in diagnosis is not uncommon.

The cervical vertebral canal is funnel shaped with its largest diameter at the atlantoaxial space progressing to its narrowest point at the C5-6 interspace. It is not surprising that this narrow point serves as the nidus of many painful conditions of the cervical spine. The shape of the cervical vertebral canal in humans is triangular but is subject to much anatomic variability among patients. Those patients with a more trifoil shape generally are more susceptible to cervical radiculopathy in the face of any pathologic process that narrows the cervical vertebral canal or negatively impacts the normal range of motion of the cervical spine.

The Cervical Nerves and Their Relationship with the Cervical Vertebrae

The cervical nerve roots are each composed of fibers from a dorsal root that carries primarily sensory information and a ventral root that carries primarily motor information. As the dorsal and ventral contributions to the cervical nerve roots move away from the cervical spinal cord, they coalesce into a single anatomic structure that becomes the individual cervical nerve roots. As these coalescing nerve fibers pass through the intervertebral foramen, they give off small branches with the anterior portion of the nerve providing innervation to the anterior pseudo-joint of Luschka and the annulus of the disc and the posterior portion of the nerve providing innervation to the zygapophyseal joints of each adjacent vertebra between which the nerve root is exiting through. These nerve fibers are thought to carry pain impulses from these anatomic structures and support the notion of the intervertebral disc and zygapophyseal joint as distinct pain generators separate and apart from the more conventional view of the compressed spinal nerve root as the sole source of pain emanating from the cervical spine. As the nerve fibers exit the intervertebral foramen, they fully coalesce into a single nerve root and travel forward and downward into the protective gutter made up of the transverse process of the vertebral body to provide innervation to the head, neck, and upper extremities (Fig. 20-6).

Implications for the Clinician

The bony cervical spine is a truly amazing anatomic element in terms of both its structure and function. Although vitally important to humans' day-to-day safety and survival, with the exception of cervicogenic and tension-type headache, the two uppermost segments of the cervical spine are not the source of the majority of painful conditions involving the cervical spine commonly encountered in clinical practice. However, the lower five segments provide an ample opportunity for the evolution of myriad common painful complaints, most notably cervical radiculopathy and cervicalgia including cervical facet syndrome.

SUGGESTED READINGS

Netter FH: Cervical vertebrae: Atlas and axis. In: Atlas of Human Anatomy, ed 4. Philadelphia, Saunders, 2006.

Netter FH: Cervical vertebrae: Uncovertebral joints. In: Atlas of Human Anatomy, ed 4. Philadelphia, Saunders, 2006.

Waldman SD: Thoracic outlet syndrome. In: Atlas of Uncommon Pain Syndromes, ed 2. Philadelphia, Saunders, 2008.

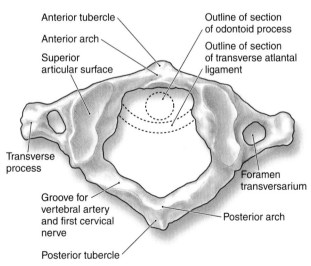

FIGURE 20–1 Atlas—the first cervical vertebra.

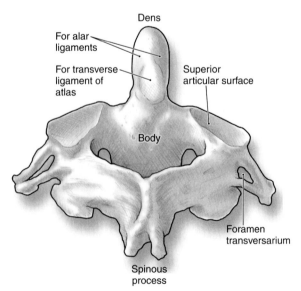

FIGURE 20–2 Axis—the second cervical vertebra.

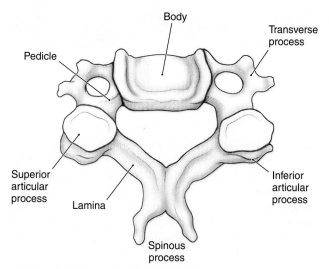

FIGURE 20–3 Superior view of a typical cervical vertebra.

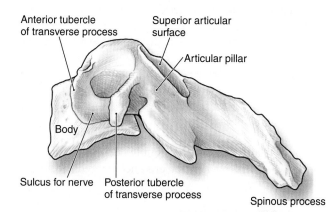

FIGURE 20-4 Lateral view of a typical cervical vertebra.

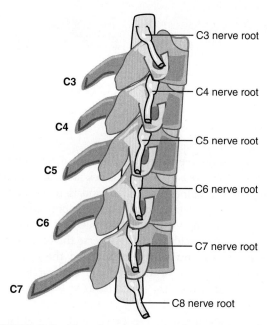

FIGURE 20–6 Position of cervical nerves relative to cervical vertebrae. (From Waldman SD: Physical Diagnosis of Pain: An Atlas of Signs and Symptoms. Philadelphia, Saunders, 2006, p 4.)

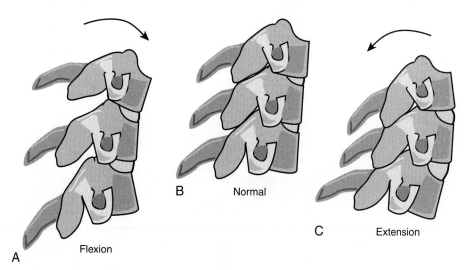

FIGURE 20–5 Functional units of the cervical spine in (**A**), flexed, (**B**), normal, and (**C**), extended positions. (From Waldman SD: Physical Diagnosis of Pain: An Atlas of Signs and Symptoms. Philadelphia, Saunders, 2006, p 3.)

CHAPTER 21

Functional Anatomy of the Cervical Intervertebral Disc

The cervical intervertebral disc has two major functions: the first is to serve as the major shock-absorbing structure of the cervical spine, and the second is to facilitate the synchronized movement of the cervical spine while at the same time helping to prevent impingement of the neural structures and vasculature that traverse the cervical spine. Both the shock-absorbing function and the movement/ protective function of the cervical intervertebral disc are functions of the disc structure, as well as of the laws of physics that affect it.

To understand how the cervical intervertebral disc functions in health and becomes dysfunctional in disease, it is useful to think of the disc as a closed fluid-filled container. The outside of the container is made up of a top and bottom called the endplates, which are composed of relatively inflexible hyaline cartilage. The sides of the cervical intervertebral disc are made up of a woven criss-crossing matrix of fibroelastic fibers that tightly attaches to the top and bottom endplates. This woven matrix of fibers is called the annulus, and it completely surrounds the sides of the disc (Fig. 21-1). The interlaced structure of the annulus results in an enclosing mesh that is extremely strong yet at the same time very flexible, which facilitates the compression of the disc during the wide range of motion of the cervical spine (Fig. 21-2).

Inside of this container consisting of the top and bottom endplates and surrounding annulus is the water-containing mucopolysaccharide gel-like substance called the nucleus pulposus (see Fig. 21-1). The nucleus is incompressible and transmits any pressure placed on one portion of the disc to the surrounding nucleus.

In health, the water-filled gel creates a positive intradiscal pressure, which forces apart the adjacent vertebra and helps protect the spinal cord and exiting nerve roots. When the cervical spine moves, the incompressible nature of the nucleus pulposus maintains a constant intradiscal pressure while some fibers of the disc relax and others contract.

As the cervical intervertebral disc ages, it becomes less vascular and loses its ability to absorb water into the disc. This results in degradation of the disc's shock-absorbing and motion-facilitating functions. This problem is made worse by degeneration of the annulus, which allows portions of the disc wall to bulge, distorting the ability of the nucleus pulposus to evenly distribute the forces placed on it throughout the entire disc. This exacerbates disc dysfunction and can contribute to further disc deterioration, which may ultimately lead to actual complete disruption of the annulus and extrusion of the nucleus (Fig. 21-3). It is the deterioration of the disc that is responsible for many of the painful conditions emanating from the cervical spine that are encountered in clinical practice.

SUGGESTED READINGS

Manchukanti L, Singh V, Boswell MV: Cervical radiculopathy. In: Pain Management. Philadelphia, Saunders, 2007.

Sial KA, Simopoulos TT, Bajwa ZH, et al: Cervical facet syndrome. In: Pain Management. Philadelphia, Saunders, 2007.

Waldman SD: Functional anatomy of the cervical spine. In: Physical Diagnosis of Pain: An Atlas of Signs and Symptoms. Philadelphia, Saunders, 2006.

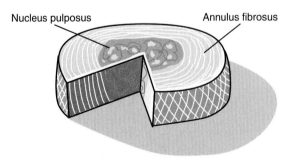

Nucleus pulposus   Annulus fibrosus

FIGURE 21–1 The cervical intervertebral disc can be thought of as a closed, fluid-filled container. (From Waldman SD: Physical Diagnosis of Pain: An Atlas of Signs and Symptoms. Philadelphia, Saunders, 2006, p 5.)

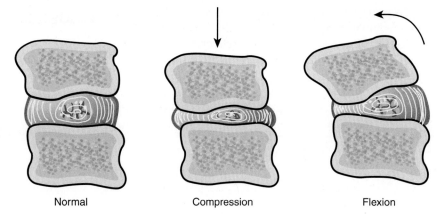

FIGURE 21–2 The cervical intervertebral disc is a strong yet flexible structure, shown here in the range of motion of the cervical spine. (From Waldman SD: Physical Diagnosis of Pain: An Atlas of Signs and Symptoms. Philadelphia, Saunders, 2006, p 6.)

Normal · Compression · Flexion

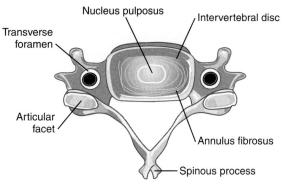

FIGURE 21–3 Normal cervical disc. (From Waldman SD: Physical Diagnosis of Pain: An Atlas of Signs and Symptoms. Philadelphia, Saunders, 2006, p 7.)

CHAPTER 22

The Cervical Dermatomes

In humans, the innervation of the skin, muscles, and deep structures is determined embryologically at an early stage of fetal development, and there is amazingly little intersubject variability. Each segment of the spinal cord and its corresponding spinal nerves have a consistent segmental relationship that allows the clinician to ascertain the probable spinal level of dysfunction based on the pattern of pain, muscle weakness, and deep tendon reflex changes.

Figure 22-1 is a dermatome chart that the clinician will find useful in determining the specific spinal level subserving a patient's pain. In general, the cervical spinal segments move down the upper extremity from cephalad to caudad on the lateral border of the upper extremity and from caudad to cephalad on the medial border.

In general, in humans, the more proximal the muscle, the more cephalad is the spinal segment, with the ventral muscles innervated by higher spinal segments than the corresponding dorsal muscles. It should be remembered that pain perceived in the region of a given muscle or joint may not be coming from the muscle or joint but simply be referred by problems at the same cervical spinal segment that innervates the muscles.

Furthermore, the clinician needs to be aware that the relative consistent pattern of dermatomal and myotomal distribution breaks down when the pain is perceived in the deep structures of the upper extremity (e.g., the joints and tendinous insertions). With pain in these regions, the clinician should refer to the sclerotomal chart in Figure 22-2. This is particularly important if a neurodestructive procedure at the spinal cord level is being considered, as the sclerotomal level of the nerves subserving the pain may be several segments higher or lower than the dermatomal or myotomal levels the clinician would expect.

SUGGESTED READINGS

Campbell W: DeJong's The Neurological Examination, ed 6. Philadelphia, Lippincott Williams and Wilkins, 2005.

Goetz CG: Textbook of Clinical Neurology, ed 2. Philadelphia, Saunders, 2003.

Waldman SD: The cervical dermatomes. In: Physical Diagnosis of Pain: An Atlas of Signs and Symptoms. Philadelphia, Saunders, 2006.

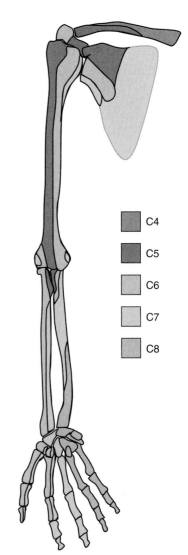

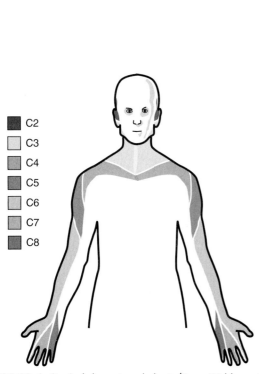

FIGURE 22–1 Cervical dermatomal chart. (From Waldman SD: Physical Diagnosis of Pain: An Atlas of Signs and Symptoms. Philadelphia, Saunders, 2006, p 20.)

FIGURE 22–2 Cervical sclerotomal chart. (From Waldman SD: Physical Diagnosis of Pain: An Atlas of Signs and Symptoms. Philadelphia, Saunders, 2006, p 21.)

The Meninges

Surrounding the central nervous system, the meninges, along with the bony skull, spine, and cerebrospinal fluid, function as the primary protectors of the central nervous system. The meninges are composed of three distinct layers: (1) the dura mater, (2) the arachnoid mater, and the pia mater (Fig. 23-1). The most superficial of the meninges, the dura mater is separated from the arachnoid by a potential space known as the subdural space. Between the arachnoid mater and the pia mater lies the subarachnoidal space, which contains the cerebrospinal fluid and cerebral arteries. The pia mater is adherent to the brain and spinal cord.

The dura mater is a thick, fibrous dual-layer membrane consisting of an outer periosteal layer and an inner meningeal layer. These layers are normally fused but can separate to form large venous channels known as the dural sinuses. The dura mater contains larger blood vessels that divide and subdivide into the minute capillaries of the pia mater. The dura mater can be thought of as an envelope surrounding the arachnoid mater. The dura mater aids in the support of the dural sinuses as well as dividing and covering a variety of central nervous system structures including the falx cerebri. The dura mater receives sensory innervation from the trigeminal nerve in the anterior and middle fossa and from branches of the olfactory, oculomotor, vagus, and hypoglossal cranial nerves.

The middle layer of the meninges is a thin, delicate spider web–appearing membrane known as the arachnoid mater. Unlike the pia mater, the arachnoid mater does not follow the convoluted surface of the brain and looks like a loose-fitting sac with many small filaments called arachnoid trabeculae that pass from the arachnoid through the subarachnoid space to merge with the tissue of the pia mater. These arachnoid trabeculae help keep the contents of the central nervous system stabilized and aid in the cushioning function of the meninges. The arachnoid mater is covered with flat mesothelial cells, which in health are impermeable to the spinal fluid it contains within the subarachnoid space. The subarachnoid space widens at the cisterna magna, which is located between the medulla and cerebellum and a number of other cisterns located throughout the central nervous system. Small granulations of the arachnoid extend into the sagittal sinus and venous lacunae and serve as one-way valves to absorb excess cerebrospinal fluid (Fig. 23-2).

Closely adherent to the brain and spinal cord, the pia mater is the innermost layer of meninges. A very delicate membrane, the pia mater invests all of the gyri and sulci of the brain as well as covering the spinal cord. The pia mater is responsible for providing mechanical support for the blood vessels that pass from the arachnoid mater via the subarachnoid space. A perivascular space known as the Virchow-Robin space is the point at which these blood vessels pass through the pia and provide the blood supply to the brain and spinal cord via a vast network of capillaries. Like the arachnoid mater, the pia mater is covered with a layer of flat cells that is impervious to fluid.

SUGGESTED READING

Netter FH: Meninges and superficial cerebral veins. In: Atlas of Human Anatomy, ed 4. Philadelphia, Saunders, 2006.

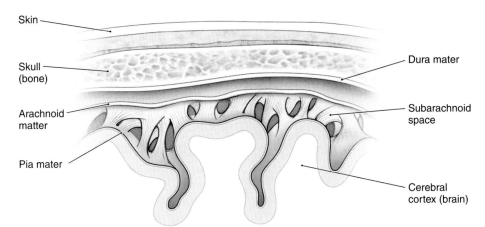

FIGURE 23–1 Relationship of the skull and meninges.

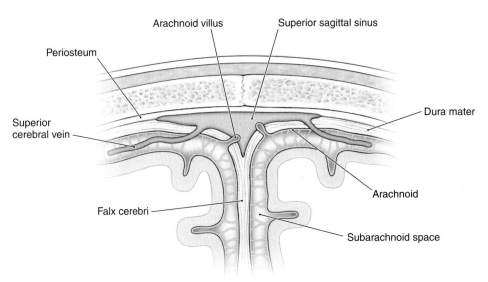

FIGURE 23–2 The subarachnoid villi.

CHAPTER 24

The Cervical Epidural Space

The superior boundary of the cervical epidural space is the fusion of the periosteal and spinal layers of dura at the foramen magnum. It should be recognized that these structures will allow drugs injected into the cervical epidural space to travel beyond their confines if the volume of injectate is large enough. This fact probably explained many of the early problems associated with the use of

cervical epidural nerve block for surgical anesthesia when the large volumes of local anesthetics in vogue at the time were injected.

The epidural space continues inferiorly to the sacrococcygeal membrane. The cervical epidural space is bounded anteriorly by the posterior longitudinal ligament and posteriorly by the vertebral laminae and the ligamentum flavum (Fig. 24-1). It should be noted that the ligamentum flavum is relatively thin in the cervical region, thickening as it continues inferiorly to the lumbar spine. This fact has direct clinical implications in that the loss of resistance when performing cervical epidural nerve block is more subtle than when performing the loss-of-resistance technique in the lumbar or lower thoracic region.

The vertebral pedicles and intervertebral foramina form the lateral limits of the epidural space (Fig. 24-2). The degenerative changes and narrowing of the intervertebral foramina associated with aging may be marked in the cervical region. This results in a decreased leakage of local anesthetic out of the foramina accounting in part for the decreased local anesthetic dosage requirements in the elderly when performing cervical epidural nerve block.

The distance between the ligamentum flavum and dura is greatest at the L2 innerspace, measuring 5 to 6 mm in the adult. Because of the enlargement of the cervical spinal cord corresponding to the neuromeres serving the upper extremities, this distance is decreased to 1.5 to 2.0 mm at the seventh cervical vertebra (Fig. 24-3, *A*). It should be noted that flexion of the neck moves this cervical enlargement superiorly, resulting in a widening of the epidural space to 3.0 to 4.0 mm at the C7–T1 interspace (Fig. 24-3, *B*). This fact has important clinical implications if cervical epidural block is performed in the lateral or prone positions.

Contents of the Epidural Space

FAT

The epidural space is filled with fatty areolar tissue. The amount of epidural fat varies in direct proportion to the amount of fat stored elsewhere in the body. The epidural fat is relatively vascular and appears to change to a denser consistency with aging. This change in consistency may account for the significant variations in required drug dosage in adults, especially when utilizing the caudal approach to the epidural space. The epidural fat appears to perform two functions: (1) it serves as a shock absorber for the other contents of the epidural space as well as the dura and the contents of the dural sac, and (2) it serves as a depot for drugs injected into the cervical epidural space. This second function has direct clinical implications when choosing opioids for cervical epidural administration.

EPIDURAL VEINS

The epidural veins are concentrated primarily in the anterolateral portion of the epidural space. These veins are valveless and hence transmit both the intrathoracic and intra-abdominal pressures. As pressures in either of these body cavities increase due to Valsalva or compression of the inferior vena cava by the gravid uterus or tumor mass, the epidural veins distend and decrease the volume of the epidural space. This decrease in volume can directly affect the volume of drug needed to obtain a given level of neural blockade. Because this venous plexus serves the entire spinal column, it acts as a ready conduit for the spread of hematogenous infection.

EPIDURAL ARTERIES

The arteries that supply the bony and ligamentous confines of the cervical epidural space as well as the cervical spinal cord enter the cervical epidural space via two routes: (1) the intervertebral foramina and (2) direct anastomoses from the intracranial portions of the vertebral arteries. There are significant anastomoses between the epidural arteries. The epidural arteries lie primarily in the lateral portions of the epidural space. Trauma to the epidural arteries can result in epidural hematoma formation and/or compromise of the blood supply of the spinal cord itself.

LYMPHATICS

The lymphatics of the epidural space are concentrated in the region of the dural roots, where they remove foreign material from the subarachnoid and epidural space.

Structures Encountered During Midline Insertion of a Needle into the Cervical Epidural Space

After traversing the skin and subcutaneous tissues, the styleted epidural needle will impinge on the supraspinous ligament that runs vertically between the apices of the spinous processes (Fig. 24-4, *A*). The supraspinous ligament offers some resistance to the advancing needle. This ligament is dense enough to hold a needle in position even when the needle is released.

The interspinous ligament that runs obliquely between the spinous processes is next encountered, offering additional resistance to needle advancement (Fig. 24-4, *B*). As the interspinous ligament is contiguous with the ligamentum flavum, the pain management specialist may perceive a "false" loss of resistance when the needle tip enters the space between the interspinous ligament and the ligamentum flavum. This phenomenon is more pronounced in the cervical region than in the lumbar due to the less well-defined ligaments.

A significant increase in resistance to needle advancement signals that the needle tip is impinging on the dense ligamentum flavum. Because the ligament is made up almost entirely of elastin fibers, there is a continued increase in resistance as the needle traverses the ligamentum flavum due to the drag of the ligament on the needle (Fig. 24-4, *C*). A sudden loss of resistance occurs as the needle tip enters the epidural space (Fig. 24-4, *D*). There should be essentially no resistance to drugs injected into the normal epidural space.

SUGGESTED READINGS

Waldman SD: Cervical epidural block: Translaminar approach. In: Atlas of Interventional Pain Management, ed 2. Philadelphia, Saunders, 2004.

Waldman SD: Cervical epidural nerve block. In: Interventional Pain Management, ed 2. Philadelphia, Saunders, 2001.

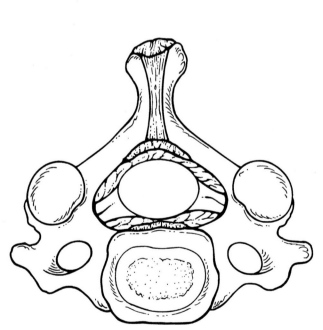

FIGURE 24–1 The cervical epidural space. (From Waldman SD: Interventional Pain Management, ed 2. Philadelphia, Saunders, 2001, p 374.)

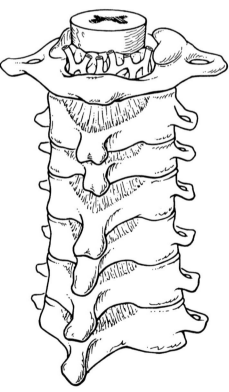

FIGURE 24–2 The vertebral pedicles and intervertebral foramina form the lateral limits of the epidural space. (From Waldman SD: Interventional Pain Management, ed 2. Philadelphia, Saunders, 2001, p 375.)

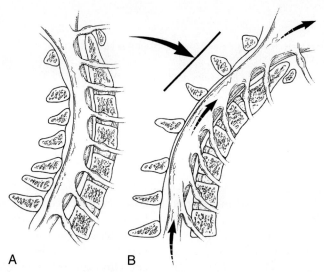

FIGURE 24–3 The distance between the ligamentum flavum and dura is greatest at the L2 innerspace, measuring 5 to 6 mm in the adult. This distance is decreased to 1.5 to 2.0 mm at the seventh cervical vertebra (**A**) and then widens to 3.0 to 4.0 mm at the C7–T1 interspace (**B**). (From Waldman SD: Interventional Pain Management, ed 2. Philadelphia, Saunders, 2001, p 375.)

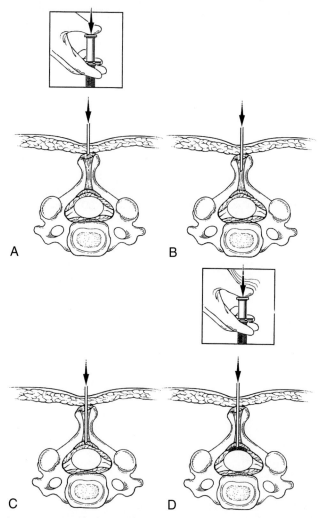

FIGURE 24–4 A, The supraspinous ligament is the first point of resistance to the advancing needle. **B,** The interspinous ligament offers additional resistance to needle advancement. **C,** Needle in ligamentum flavum. **D,** Needle through ligamentum flavum with "animated" loss of resistance. (From Waldman SD: Interventional Pain Management, ed 2. Philadelphia, Saunders, 2001, p 376.)

CHAPTER 25

The Cervical Facet Joints

The cervical facet joints are diarthrodial-type joints that are formed by the articulations of the superior and inferior articular facets of adjacent vertebrae (Fig. 25-1). The cervical facet joints are inclined at 45 degrees from the horizontal plane and angled 85 degrees from the sagittal plane. Except for the atlanto-occipital and atlantoaxial joints, the remaining cervical facet joints are true joints in that they are lined with synovium and possess a true joint capsule. Relative to the joint capsules of other areas of the spine, the joint capsules of the cervical facet joints are relatively lax to allow for the sliding/gliding motion of the joints. This capsule is richly innervated by type I, II, and III mechanoreceptors and free nerve endings and supports the notion of the facet joint as a pain generator. This innervation is also important for proprioception and is a part of the protective muscular reflexes that protect the joint during its range of motion.

The cervical facet joint is susceptible to arthritic changes and trauma caused by acceleration-deceleration injuries. Such damage to the joint results in pain secondary to synovial joint inflammation and adhesions.

The atlantoaxial and the occipitoatlantal joints are innervated by the ventral rami of the first and second cervical spinal nerves. The C2-3 facet joint is innervated by two branches of the dorsal ramus of the third cervical spinal nerve with the remaining cervical facets, C3-4 to C7-T1, supplied by the dorsal rami medial branches that arise one level cephalad and caudad to the joint. Each facet joint receives innervation from two spinal levels. This fact has clinical import in that it provides an explanation for the ill-defined nature of facet-mediated pain and also explains why the dorsal nerve from the vertebra above the offending level must often also be blocked to provide complete pain relief.

Each joint receives fibers from the dorsal ramus at the same level as the vertebra as well as fibers from the dorsal ramus of the vertebra above. At each level, the dorsal ramus provides a medial branch that wraps around the convexity of the articular pillar of its respective vertebra (Fig. 25-2). This location is constant for the C4-7 nerves and allows a simplified approach for treatment of cervical facet syndrome.

SUGGESTED READINGS

Netter FH: Cervical vertebrae: Atlas and axis. In: Atlas of Human Anatomy, ed 4. Philadelphia, Saunders, 2006.

Netter FH: Cervical vertebrae: Uncovertebral joints. In: Atlas of Human Anatomy, ed 4. Philadelphia, Saunders, 2006.

Waldman SD: Cervical facet block: Medial branch approach. In: Atlas of Interventional Pain Management, ed 2. Philadelphia, Saunders, 2004.

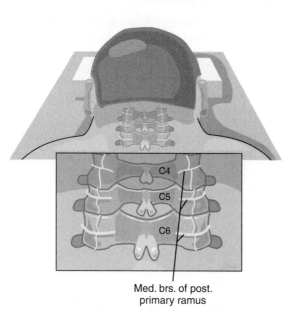

FIGURE 25–1 The cervical facet joints. (From Waldman SD: Atlas of Interventional Pain Management, ed 2. Philadelphia, Saunders, 2004, p 117.)

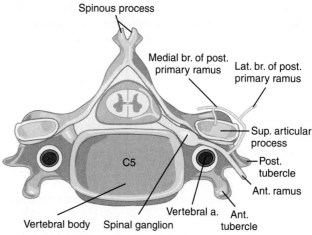

FIGURE 25–2 Innervation of the cervical facet joint. (From Waldman SD: Atlas of Interventional Pain Management, ed 2. Philadelphia, Saunders, 2004, p 117.)

CHAPTER **26**

The Ligaments of the Cervical Spine

A complex system of ligaments serves to stabilize and protect the cervical spine. As with the upper cervical bony vertebrae, the ligaments stabilizing the upper cervical vertebrae are also specialized to better serve their function. The transverse ligament serves to tightly secure the odontoid process (dens) of axis (C2) against the anterior arch of atlas (C1). This ligament arises from the tubercles of atlas and allows for stable rotation of atlas on the odontoid process as well as serving as a major stabilizer of the cervical spine during flexion, extension, and lateral bending (Fig. 26-1).

The alar ligament serves as one of the most important stabilizers of the cervical spine by limiting both axial rotation and lateral bending while still allowing some degree of flexion and extension. The alar ligaments extend from the lateral aspects of the dens to the ipsilateral medial occipital condyles as well as to the ipsilateral atlas. If the alar ligaments are damaged, hypermobility

of the joint can result in significant functional disability and pain symptomatology (Fig. 26-2).

The anterior atlanto-occipital ligament is a strong, dense ligament that is further strengthened in the midline by a central rounded cord-like structure (Fig. 26-3). This important ligament passes inferiorly from the anterior margin of the foramen magnum to the anterior arch of atlas and then continues on as the anterior longitudinal ligament (Fig. 26-4). Arising from the tectorial membrane, the posterior longitudinal ligament also stabilizes the cervical spine by limiting excessive flexion and mobility of the spine (see Fig. 26-4).

Also helping to stabilize the cervical spine are the supraspinous and interspinous ligaments and the ligamentum flavum. The ligamentum nuchae is a dense fibrous band that extends from the occipital protuberance to the spinous process of the seventh cervical vertebra. It continues caudally running along the tips of the spinous processes as the supraspinous ligament (see Fig. 26-4). The interspinous ligament runs between the spinous processes and aids in limiting flexion and anterior slippage of vertebrae onto one another (see Fig. 26-4). The ligamentum flavum, an important landmark in the loss of resistance epidural space identification technique extends from the anterior surface of the cephalad vertebra to the posterior surface of the caudad vertebra as well as connecting to the ventral aspect of the facet joint capsules (see Fig. 26-4).

SUGGESTED READINGS

Netter FH: Cervical vertebrae: Atlas and axis. In: Atlas of Human Anatomy, ed 4. Philadelphia, Saunders, 2006.

Netter FH: Cervical vertebrae: Uncovertebral joints. In: Atlas of Human Anatomy, ed 4. Philadelphia, Saunders, 2006.

Waldman SD: Cervical facet block: Medial branch approach. In: Atlas of Interventional Pain Management, ed 2. Philadelphia, Saunders, 2004.

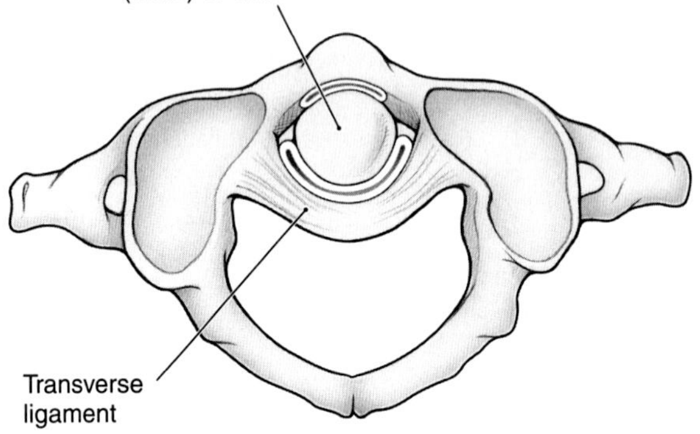

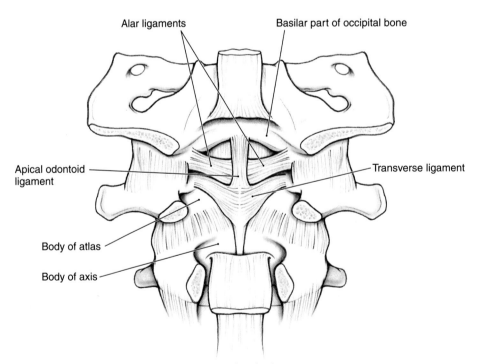

FIGURE 26–1 The transverse ligament of atlas.

FIGURE 26–2 The alar ligaments.

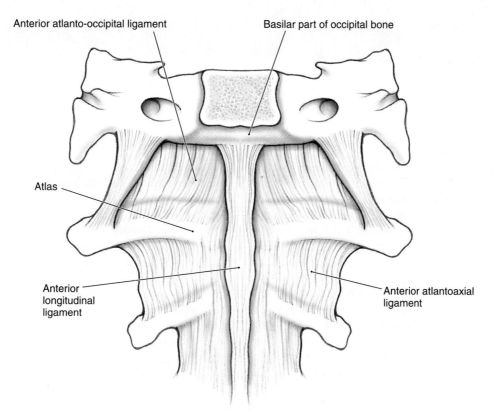

FIGURE 26–3 The anterior longitudinal ligament.

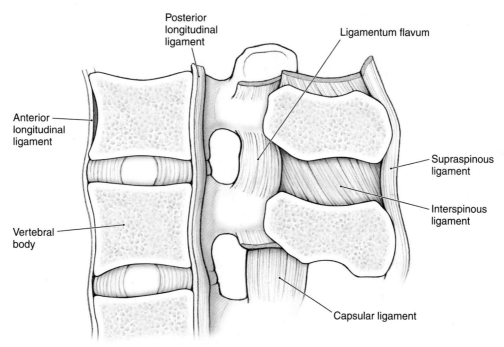

FIGURE 26–4 The interspinous ligaments.

CHAPTER 27

Functional Anatomy of the Thoracic Vertebrae

The 12 thoracic vertebrae can be thought of from a structural viewpoint as having three separate shapes with the smaller upper four thoracic vertebrae sharing characteristics in common with the cervical vertebra (i.e., vertically oriented articular facets and posteriorly directed spinous processes), the larger lower four thoracic vertebrae sharing characteristics in common with the lumbar vertebrae (i.e., large bodies, heavy transverse and spinous processes, and more lateral projecting articular facets) (Fig. 27-1). The middle four thoracic vertebrae share characteristics with both the cervical and lumbar regions (i.e., obliquely downward-oriented articular processes and elongated, delicate, and inferiorly inclined spinous processes).

Although there is significant intrapatient variability regarding the characteristics of the thoracic vertebrae, some generalizations can be made. In most patients, a distinguishing characteristic of the first 10 thoracic vertebrae is the presence of articular facets for the ribs. Each of these vertebrae contains two pairs of these costal demifacets on its body and one on each transverse process (Fig. 27-2). Typical ribs articulate with the inferior demifacet and transverse process of a thoracic vertebra and the superior demifacet of the vertebra below it.

The 11th and 12th thoracic vertebrae lack a superior costal demifacet. The 11th and 12th ribs only articulate with the 11th and 12th thoracic vertebrae, respectively (Fig. 27-3).

The upper thoracic vertebral interspaces from T1 to T2 and the lower thoracic vertebral interspaces from T10 to T12 are functionally equivalent insofar as the technique of epidural block is concerned (see Fig. 27-1). The technique of performing epidural block at the level of the upper and the lower thoracic vertebral interspaces is analogous to lumbar epidural block. The thoracic vertebral interspaces between T3 and T9 are functionally unique because of the acute downward angle of the spinous processes. Blockade of these middle thoracic interspaces requires use of the paramedian approach to the thoracic epidural space.

SUGGESTED READINGS

Netter FH: Thoracic vertebrae: Atlas and axis. In: Atlas of Human Anatomy, ed 4. Philadelphia, Saunders, 2006.

Waldman SD: Thoracic epidural block: The translaminar approach. In: Atlas of Interventional Pain Management, ed 2. Philadelphia, Saunders, 2004.

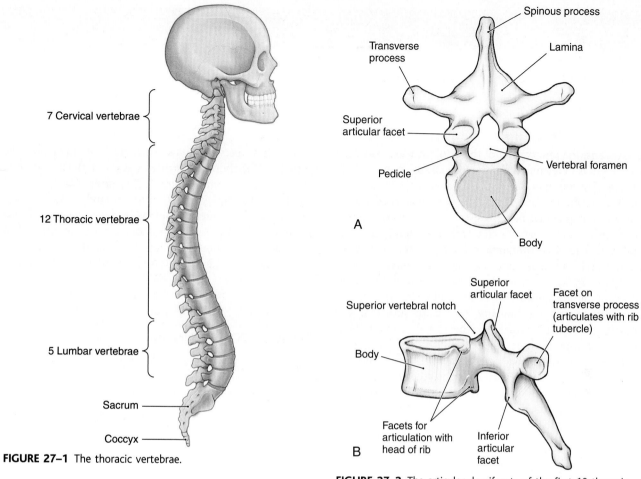

FIGURE 27–1 The thoracic vertebrae.

FIGURE 27–2 The articular demifacets of the first 10 thoracic vertebrae.

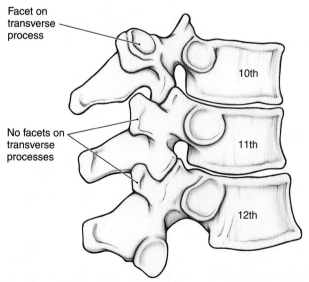

FIGURE 27–3 Unique characteristics of the facets of the atypical thoracic vertebrae (after H. Grey).

CHAPTER 28

The Thoracic Dermatomes

In humans, the innervation of the skin, muscles, and deep structures is determined embryologically at an early stage of fetal development, and there is amazingly little inter-subject variability. Each segment of the spinal cord and its corresponding spinal nerves have a consistent segmental relationship that allows the clinician to ascertain the probable spinal level of dysfunction based on the pattern of pain, muscle weakness, and deep tendon reflex changes.

Figure 28-1 is a dermatome chart that is useful in determining the specific spinal level subserving a patient's pain. In general, in humans, the more proximal the muscle, the more cephalad is the spinal segment with the ventral muscles innervated by higher spinal segments than the corresponding dorsal muscles. It should be remembered that pain perceived in the region of a given muscle or joint may not be coming from the muscle or joint but may simply be referred by problems at the same cervical spinal segment that innervates the muscles. The thoracic dermatomes cover the axillary and thoracic region, with T3 to T12 covering the thorax and trunk to the hip girdle. Important landmarks that are useful to the clinician include the fact that in most patients, the nipples are situated in the middle of T4 dermatome, the umbilicus is located at the T10 dermatome, and the T12 dermatome is located at the level of the iliac crests.

SUGGESTED READINGS

Campbell W: DeJong's The Neurological Examination, ed 6. Philadelphia, Lippincott Williams and Wilkins, 2005.

Goetz CG: Textbook of Clinical Neurology, ed 2. Philadelphia, Saunders, 2003.

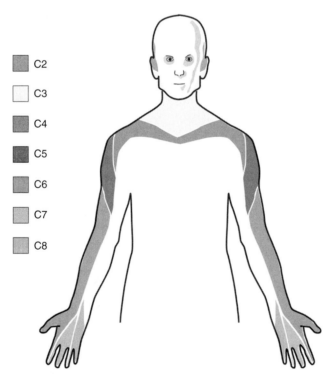

- C2
- C3
- C4
- C5
- C6
- C7
- C8

FIGURE 28–1 Thoracic dermatomal chart. (From Waldman SD: Physical Diagnosis of Pain: An Atlas of Signs and Symptoms. Philadelphia, Saunders, 2006, p 20.)

CHAPTER 29

Functional Anatomy of the Lumbar Spine

The Bony Elements

The lumbar spine is composed of five vertebrae numbered from cephalad to caudad L1 to L5. The primary functions of the lumbar vertebrae are to bear the weight of the upper body and to allow for coordinated movement of the low back and pelvis in flexion, extension, and lateral bending. Like the rest of the spine, the lumbar vertebrae serve a secondary protective role by enclosing the cauda equina and related structures in a bony canal. Unlike the specialized upper lumbar vertebrae, which are dissimilar from their lower counterparts, the lumbar vertebrae are structurally similar.

Each vertebra is made up of an anterior weight-bearing vertebral body and a posterior neural arch (Fig. 29-1). The posterior neural arch has three specialized processes that allow attachment of the muscles of posture and a variety of ligaments. These processes are the spinous process that lies in the midline posteriorly and the two transverse processes that lie laterally. The area of the neural arch between the spinous process and the transverse process is called the lamina. The area between the transverse process and the vertebral body is called the pedicle.

Movement

Movement of adjacent lumbar vertebrae is allowed by three joints. The first is composed of the inferior and superior endplates of the vertebral bodies and their interposed intervertebral disc (Fig. 29-2). The second and third are the two facet joints that are also known as zygapophyseal joints, which are made up of the inferior articular process of the superior adjacent vertebrae and the ipsilateral superior articular process of the inferior adjacent vertebrae (Fig. 29-3). This configuration allows flexion, extension, and a limited degree of lateral bending while at the same time contributing significantly to the lateral stability of the lumbar spine.

The Intervertebral Disc

The lumbar intervertebral disc has two major functions: (1) the first is to serve as the major shock-absorbing structure of the lumbar spine, and (2) the second is to facilitate the synchronized movement of the lumbar spine while at the same time helping to prevent impingement of the neural structures and associated structures that traverse the lumbar spine. Both the shock-absorbing function and the movement/protective function of the lumbar intervertebral disc are a function of the disc's structure as well as of the laws of physics that affect it (see later).

To understand how the lumbar intervertebral disc functions in health and becomes dysfunctional in disease, it is useful to think of the disc as a closed fluid-filled container. The outside of the container is made up of a top and bottom called the endplates, which are composed of relatively inflexible hyaline cartilage. The sides of the lumbar intervertebral disc are made up of a woven crisscrossing matrix of fibroelastic fibers that tightly attaches to the top and bottom endplates. This woven matrix of fibers is called the annulus, and it completely surrounds the sides of the disc. The interlaced structure of the annulus results in an enclosing mesh that is extremely strong yet at the same time very flexible, which facilitates the compression of the disc during the wide range of motion of the lumbar spine.

Inside of this container consisting of the top and bottom endplates and surrounding annulus is the water-containing mucopolysaccharide gel-like substance called the nucleus pulposus. The nucleus is incompressible and transmits any pressure placed on one portion of the disc to the surrounding nucleus. In health, the water-filled gel creates a positive intradiscal pressure that forces apart the adjacent vertebra and helps protect the spinal cord and exiting nerve roots. When the lumbar spine moves, the incompressible nature of the nucleus pulposus maintains a constant intradiscal pressure, while some fibers of the disc relax and others contract.

As the lumbar intervertebral disc ages, it becomes less vascular and loses its ability to absorb water into the disc. This results in a degradation of the disc's shock-absorbing and motion-facilitating functions. This problem is made worse by degeneration of the annulus, which allows portions of the disc wall to bulge, distorting the ability of the nucleus pulposus to evenly distribute the forces placed on it throughout the entire disc. This exacerbates the disc dysfunction and can contribute to further disc deterioration, which may ultimately lead to actual complete disruption of the annulus and extrusion of the nucleus. It is the deterioration of the disc that is responsible for many of the painful conditions emanating from the lumbar spine that are encountered in clinical practice.

SUGGESTED READINGS

Netter FH: The lumbar spine. In: Atlas of Human Anatomy, ed 4. Philadelphia, Saunders, 2006.

Waldman SD: Functional anatomy of the lumbar spine. In: Physical Diagnosis of Pain: An Atlas of Signs and Symptoms. Philadelphia, Saunders, 2006.

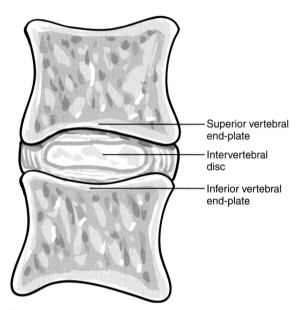

FIGURE 29–2 The processes of the posterior neural arch. (From Waldman SD: Physical Diagnosis of Pain: An Atlas of Signs and Symptoms. Philadelphia, Saunders, 2006, p 221.)

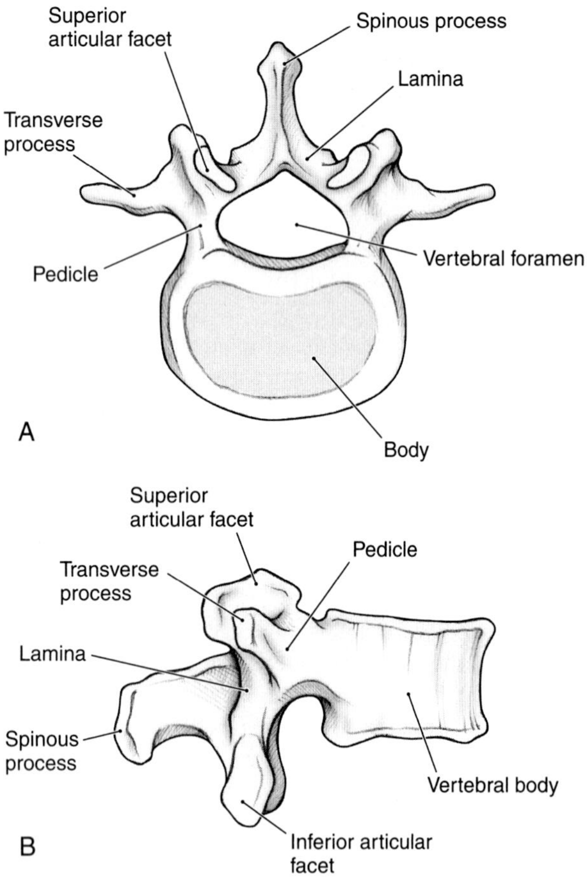

FIGURE 29–1 Anatomy of the lumbar vertebra.

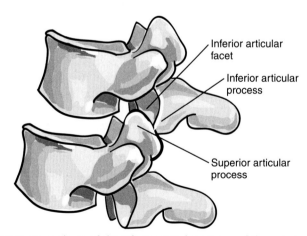

FIGURE 29–3 The zygapophyseal joints are made up of the inferior articular process of the superior adjacent vertebra and the ipsilateral superior articular process of the inferior adjacent vertebra. (From Waldman SD: Physical Diagnosis of Pain: An Atlas of Signs and Symptoms. Philadelphia, Saunders, 2006, p 221.)

CHAPTER **30**

Functional Anatomy of the Lumbar Intervertebral Disc

The Normal Intervertebral Disc

The normal disc consists of the central gel-like nucleus pulposus that is surrounded concentrically by a dense fibroelastic ring called the annulus. The top and bottom of the disc are contained by a cartilaginous endplate that is adjacent to the vertebral body. On magnetic resonance imaging, the normal lumbar disc appears symmetric with low signal intensity on T1-weighted images and high signal intensity throughout the disc on T2-weighted images. In health, the margins of the lumbar disc do not extend beyond the margins of the adjacent vertebral bodies (Fig. 30-1).

The Degenerated Disc

As the disc ages, both the nucleus and annulus undergo structural and biochemical changes that affect both the disc's appearance on magnetic resonance imaging and the disc's ability to function properly. While this degenerative process is a normal part of aging, it can be accelerated by trauma to the lumbar spine, infection, and smoking. If the degenerative process is severe enough, many, but not all, patients will experience clinical symptoms.

As the degenerative process occurs, the nucleus pulposus begins to lose its ability to maintain an adequate level of hydration as well as its ability to maintain a proper mixture of proteoglycans necessary to keep the gel-like consistency of the nuclear material. Degenerative clefts develop within the nuclear matrix, and portions of the nucleus become replaced with collagen, which leads to a further degradation of the shock-absorbing abilities and flexibility of the disc. As this process continues, the laws of physics (primarily Pascal's law), which allow the disc to maintain an adequate intradiscal pressure to push the adjacent vertebrae apart, no longer apply, leading to a further deterioration of function with the onset of clinical symptoms.

In addition to degenerative changes affecting the nucleus pulposus, the degenerative process affects the annulus as well. As the annulus ages, the complex interwoven mesh of fibroelastic fibers begins to break down with small tears occurring within the mesh. As these tears occur, the exposed collagen fibers stimulate the ingrowth of richly innervated granulation tissue, which may account for discogenic pain. These tears can be easily demonstrated on magnetic resonance imaging as linear structures of high signal intensity on T2-weighted images that correlate with positive results when provocative discography is performed on the affected disc (Fig. 30-2). When identified as the source of pain on discography, these annular tears can be treated with intradiscal electrothermal annuloplasty with good results.

The Diffusely Bulging Disc

As the degenerative process continues, further breakdown and tearing of the annular fibers and continued loss of hydration of the nucleus pulposus lead to a loss of intradiscal pressure with resultant disc space narrowing, which may lead to an exacerbation of clinical symptoms. As the disc space gradually narrows due to decreased intradiscal pressure, the anterior and posterior longitudinal ligaments grow less taut and allow the discs to bulge beyond the margins of the vertebral body (Fig. 30-3, *A* and *B*). This may cause impingement of bone or disc on nerve, adding impingement-induced pain to the pain emanating from the disc annulus itself. These findings are clearly demonstrated on magnetic resonance imaging and should alert the clinician to the possibility of multifactorial sources of the patient's pain symptoms and functional disability.

The Focal Disc Protrusion

As the disc annulus and nucleus pulposus continue to degenerate, the ability of the annulus to completely contain and compress the nucleus pulposus is lost, and with it the incompressible nature of the nucleus pulposus is also lost. This leads to focal areas of annular wall weakness, which allow the nucleus pulposus to protrude into the spinal canal or against pain-sensitive structures (Fig. 30-3, *C*). Such protrusions are focal in nature and are easily seen on both T1- and T2-weighted magnetic resonance images. These focal disc protrusions may be either relatively asymptomatic if the focal bulge does not impinge on any pain-sensitive structures or may be highly symptomatic, presenting clinically as pure discogenic pain or as radicular pain if the focal protrusion extends into a neural foramen or the spinal canal.

The Focal Disc Extrusion

Focal disc extrusion is frequently symptomatic due to the fact that the disc material frequently migrates cranially or caudally, resulting in impingement of exiting nerve roots and the creation of an intense inflammatory reaction as the nuclear material irritates the nerve root. This chemical irritation is thought to be responsible for the intense pain experienced by many patients with focal disc extrusion and may be seen on magnetic resonance imaging as high-intensity signals on T2-weighted images. Although more pronounced than a focal disc protrusion, focal disc extrusion is similar in that the extruded disc material remains contiguous with the parent disc material (Fig. 30-3, *D*).

The Sequestered Disc

When a portion of the nuclear material detaches itself from its parent disc material and migrates, the disc

fragment is called a sequestered disc (Fig. 30-3, *E*). Sequestered disc fragments frequently migrate in a cranial or caudal direction and become impacted beneath a nerve root or between the posterior longitudinal ligament and the bony spine. Sequestered disc fragments can cause significant clinical pain symptoms and often require surgical intervention. Sequestered disc fragments will often enhance on post contrast–enhanced T1-weighted images and demonstrate a peripheral rim of high-intensity signal due to the inflammatory reaction the nuclear material elicits on T2-weighted images. Failure to identify and remove sequestered disc fragments often leads to a poor surgical result.

SUGGESTED READINGS

Netter FH: The lumbar spine. In: Atlas of Human Anatomy, ed 4. Philadelphia, Saunders, 2006.

Waldman SD: Functional anatomy of the lumbar spine. In: Physical Diagnosis of Pain: An Atlas of Signs and Symptoms. Philadelphia, Saunders, 2006.

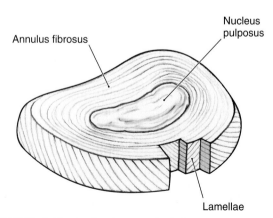

FIGURE 30–1 The lumbar intervertebral disc.

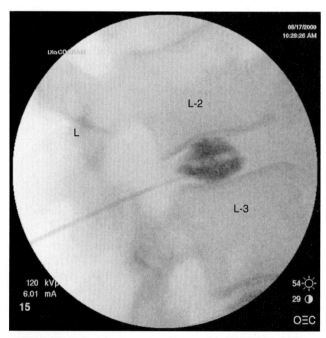

FIGURE 30–2 Annular tears are seen on this T2-weighted MR image as linear structures of high signal intensity. (From Waldman SD: Atlas of Interventional Pain Management, ed 2. Philadelphia, Saunders, 2004, p 565.)

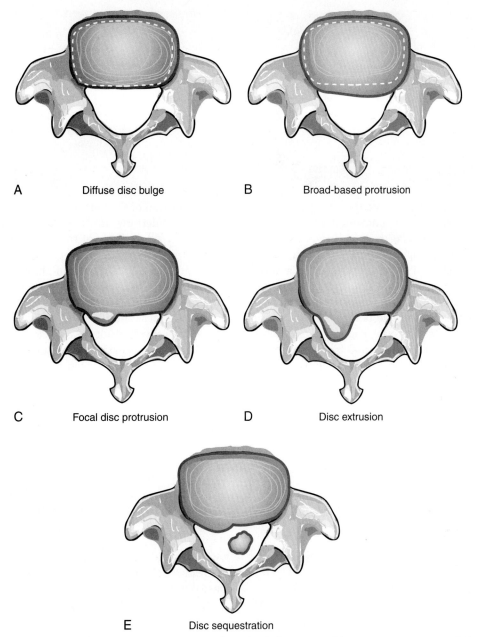

FIGURE 30–3 Various types of lumbar disc degeneration. **A,** Diffuse disc bulge. **B,** Broad-based protrusion. **C,** Focal disc protrusion. **D,** Disc extrusion. **E,** Disc sequestration. (From Waldman SD: Physical Diagnosis of Pain: An Atlas of Signs and Symptoms. Philadelphia, Saunders, 2006, p 226.)

CHAPTER 31

Functional Anatomy of the Sacrum

Sacrum

The triangular sacrum consists of the five fused sacral vertebrae, which are dorsally convex (Fig. 31-1). The sacrum inserts in a wedgelike manner between the two iliac bones, articulating superiorly with the fifth lumbar vertebra and caudad with the coccyx. On the anterior concave surface, there are four pairs of unsealed anterior sacral foramina that allow passage of the anterior rami of the upper four sacral nerves. The posterior sacral foramina are smaller than their anterior counterparts. Leakage of drugs injected into the sacral canal is effectively prevented by the sacrospinal and multifidus muscles. The vestigial remnants of the inferior articular processes project downward on each side of the sacral hiatus. These bony projections are called the sacral cornua and represent important clinical landmarks when performing caudal epidural nerve block.

Although there are gender- and race-determined differences in the shape of the sacrum, they are of little importance relative to the ultimate ability to successfully perform caudal epidural nerve block on a given patient.

Coccyx

The triangular coccyx is made up of three to five rudimentary vertebrae. Its superior surface articulates with the inferior articular surface of the sacrum. The tip of the coccyx is an important clinical landmark when performing caudal epidural nerve block.

Sacral Hiatus

The sacral hiatus is formed by the incomplete midline fusion of the posterior elements of the lower portion of the S4 and the entire S5 vertebrae (see Fig. 31-1). This U-shaped space is covered posteriorly by the sacrococcygeal ligament, which is also an important clinical landmark when performing caudal epidural nerve block. Penetration of the sacrococcygeal ligament provides direct access to the epidural space of the sacral canal.

Sacral Canal

A continuation of the lumbar spinal canal, the sacral canal continues inferiorly to terminate at the sacral hiatus (Fig. 31-2). The volume of the sacral canal with all of its contents removed averages approximately 34 mL in dried bone specimens. It should be emphasized that much smaller volumes of local anesthetic (i.e., 5 to 10 mL) are used in day-to-day pain management practice. The use of large volumes of local anesthetic, especially in the area of pain management, will result in an unacceptable level of local anesthetic–induced side effects, such as incontinence and urinary retention, and should be avoided.

CONTENTS OF THE SACRAL CANAL

The sacral canal contains the inferior termination of the dural sac, which ends between S1 and S3 (Fig. 31-3). The five sacral nerve roots and the coccygeal nerve all traverse the canal, as does the terminal filament of the spinal cord, the filum terminale. The anterior and posterior rami of the S1-4 nerve roots exit from their respective anterior and posterior sacral foramina. The S5 roots and coccygeal nerves leave the sacral canal via the sacral hiatus. These nerves provide sensory and motor innervation to their respective dermatomes and myotomes. They also provide partial innervation to several pelvic organs, including the uterus, fallopian tubes, bladder, and prostate.

The sacral canal also contains the epidural venous plexus, which generally ends at S4 but may continue inferiorly. Most of these vessels are concentrated in the anterior portion of the canal. Both the dural sac and epidural vessels are susceptible to trauma by advancing needles or catheters cephalad into the sacral canal. The remainder of the sacral canal is filled with fat, which is subject to an age-related increase in its density. Some investigators believe this change is responsible for the increased incidence of "spotty" caudal epidural nerve blocks in adults.

SUGGESTED READINGS

Netter FH: The sacrum. In: Atlas of Human Anatomy, ed 4. Philadelphia, Saunders, 2006.

Waldman SD: Caudal epidural nerve block. In: Interventional Pain Management, ed 2. Philadelphia, Saunders, 2001.

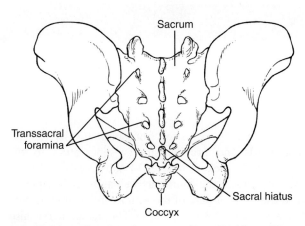

FIGURE 31–1 The triangular sacrum. (From Waldman SD: Interventional Pain Management, ed 2. Philadelphia, Saunders, 2001, p 520.)

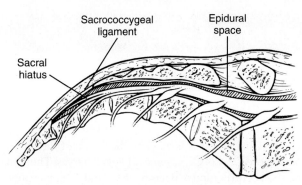

FIGURE 31–2 The sacral canal. (From Waldman SD: Interventional Pain Management, ed 2. Philadelphia, Saunders, 2001, p 521.)

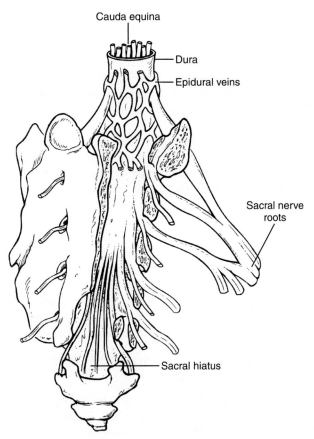

FIGURE 31–3 Contents of the sacral canal. (From Waldman SD: Interventional Pain Management, ed 2. Philadelphia, Saunders, 2001, p 521.)

CHAPTER 32

The Brachial Plexus

The brachial plexus is formed by the fusion of the anterior rami of the C5, C6, C7, C8, and T1 spinal nerves. There may also be a contribution of fibers from C4 and T2 spinal nerves. The plexus provides both motor and sensory innervation. It provides motor innervation to all of the muscles of the upper extremity except the levator scapulae and trapezius muscles. It supplies all of the cutaneous sensory innervation to the upper extremity except for part of the axilla that is innervated by the intercostobrachial nerve and the dorsal scapular area that is supplied by cutaneous branches of dorsal rami (Fig. 32-1). The brachial plexus communicates with the sympathetic trunk by gray rami communicantes that arise from the middle and inferior cervical sympathetic ganglia and the first thoracic sympathetic ganglion.

Structurally, the anatomy of the brachial plexus is best understood by dividing the subdivisions of the plexus into roots, trunks, divisions, cords, and terminal branches. Each subdivision of the brachial plexus will be discussed individually (Fig. 32-2).

The roots of the brachial plexus are composed of the anterior or ventral rami of spinal nerves C5 to T1. After these roots exit their respective intravertebral foramen, they unite to form three trunks. The ventral rami of C5 and C6 unite to form the upper trunk, the ventral ramus of C7 continues as the middle trunk, and the ventral rami of C8 and T1 unite to form the lower trunk.

Each trunk subdivides into an anterior and a posterior division, with the anterior division supplying the flexor muscles of the upper extremity and the posterior division supplying the extensor muscles of the upper extremity. The anterior divisions of the upper and middle trunks combine to form the lateral cord. The anterior division of the lower trunk forms the medial cord. All three posterior divisions from each of the three cords unite to form the posterior cord, with all of the cords named according to the position relative to the axillary artery (Fig. 32-3).

The terminal branches of the brachial plexus are composed of both motor and sensory fibers (Fig. 32-4). The musculocutaneous nerve arises from the lateral cord and provides motor innervation to the flexor compartment of the upper extremity and sensory innervation to the radial aspect of the forearm. The ulnar nerve arises from the medial cord and provides motor innervation to the intrinsic muscles of the hand and sensory innervation to the ulnar aspect of the little finger, the ulnar aspect of the ring finger, and the ulnar aspect of the dorsum of the hand.

The median nerve arises from both the lateral and medial cords and provides motor innervation to the majority of the flexor muscles of the forearm and the thenar muscles of the thumb as well as sensory innervation to the radial aspect of the thumb, index, middle, and radial aspect of the ring finger. The radial nerve also arises from the posterior cord of the brachial plexus and provides motor innervation to the extensor muscles of the elbow, wrist, and fingers as well as sensory innervation to the skin on the dorsum of the hand on the radial side. The axillary nerve also arises from the posterior cord and provides motor innervation to the deltoid and teres major muscles as well as sensory innervation to the shoulder joint and the cutaneous sensory innervation to the lower deltoid muscle.

The branches of the brachial plexus are nerves that arise from the brachial plexus but contain only sensory or motor fibers. These branches include the dorsal scapular nerve, which arises from the root of C5 and provides motor innervation to the rhomboideus major and rhomboideus minor muscles. The long thoracic nerve of Bell arises from the C5-7 roots and provides motor innervation to the serratus anterior muscle. Arising from the upper trunk, the subclavius nerve provides motor innervation to the subclavius muscle, and the suprascapular nerve provides motor innervation to the supraspinatus and infraspinatus muscles. From the lateral cord, the lateral pectoral nerve provides motor innervation to the clavicular head of the pectoralis major muscle. From the medial cord, the medial pectoral nerve provides motor innervation to the sternocostal head of the pectoralis major muscle as well as to the pectoralis minor muscle.

Cutaneous branches of the brachial plexus include the medial brachial cutaneous nerve, which carries sensory information from the distal medial aspect of the lower extremity as well as from the ulnar aspect of the forearm. Clinically, lesions affecting any subdivision of the brachial plexus can produce motor and/or sensory deficits depending on the portion of the plexus affected.

SUGGESTED READINGS

Campbell W: DeJong's The Neurological Examination, ed 6. Philadelphia, Lippincott Williams and Wilkins, 2005.

Goetz CG: Textbook of Clinical Neurology, ed 2. Philadelphia, Saunders, 2003.

Netter FH: The brachial plexus. In: Atlas of Human Anatomy, ed 4. Philadelphia, Saunders, 2006.

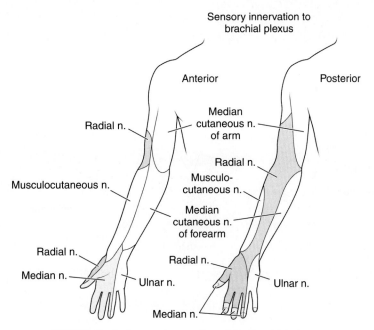

FIGURE 32–1 Sensory innervation of the brachial plexus.

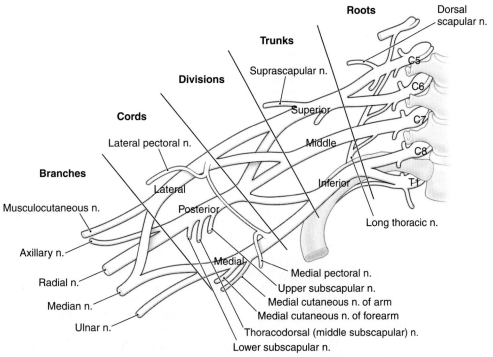

FIGURE 32–2 Subdivision of the brachial plexus.

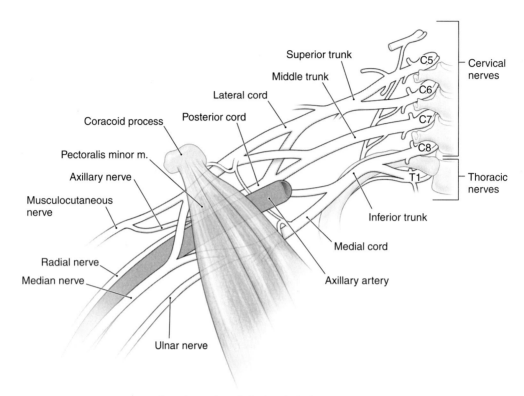

FIGURE 32–3 The relationship of the brachial plexus and the axillary artery.

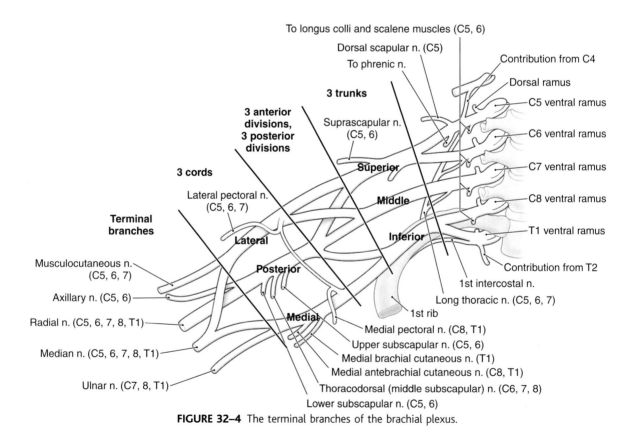

FIGURE 32–4 The terminal branches of the brachial plexus.

CHAPTER 33

The Musculocutaneous Nerve

Arising from the lateral cord of the brachial plexus at the level of the inferior border of the pectoralis major muscle, the musculocutaneous nerve provides motor innervation to the flexor compartment of the upper extremity and sensory innervation to the radial aspect of the forearm (Fig. 33-1). The musculocutaneous nerve passes through the coracobrachialis muscle, providing motor innervation. The nerve then passes at an oblique angle between the brachialis muscle and biceps brachii muscle to provide their motor innervation with the nerve ending up on the lateral side of the upper extremity. Just above the elbow and lateral to the tendon of the biceps brachii muscle, the nerve pierces the deep fascia to continue inferiorly as the lateral antebrachial cutaneous nerve.

Injuries to the musculocutaneous nerve can take the form of either entrapment of the nerve as it passes between the biceps aponeurosis and the fascia of the brachialis muscle or stretch injuries secondary to shoulder dislocations. Rarely, transection of the nerve by stab wounds or surgical trauma can occur. Clinically, injuries that are isolated to the nerve and that do not involve the brachial plexus will present as painless weakness of elbow flexion and supination combined with a localized sensory deficit on the radial side of the forearm.

SUGGESTED READINGS

Campbell W: DeJong's The Neurological Examination, ed 6. Philadelphia, Lippincott Williams and Wilkins, 2005.
Goetz CG: Textbook of Clinical Neurology, ed 2. Philadelphia, Saunders, 2003.
Netter FH: The brachial artery in situ. In: Atlas of Human Anatomy, ed 4. Philadelphia, Saunders, 2006.

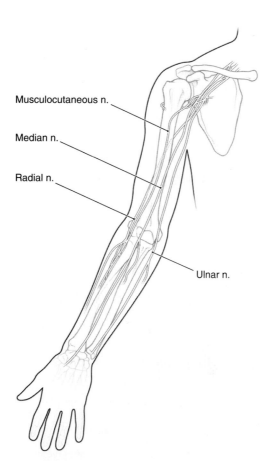

Musculocutaneous n.

Median n.

Radial n.

Ulnar n.

FIGURE 33–1 The musculocutaneous nerve.

CHAPTER 34

The Ulnar Nerve

The ulnar nerve arises from the medial cord of the brachial plexus (see Fig. 32-1). It is made up of fibers from C6-T1 spinal roots. The nerve lies anterior and inferior to the axillary artery in the 3:00 o'clock–to–6:00 o'clock quadrant. Exiting the axilla, the ulnar nerve descends into the upper arm along with the brachial artery. At the middle of the upper arm, the nerve courses medially to pass between the olecranon process and medial epicondyle of the humerus (see Fig. 33-1). The nerve then passes between the heads of the flexor carpi ulnaris muscle continuing downward, moving radially along with the ulnar artery. At a point approximately 1 inch proximal to the crease of the wrist, the ulnar nerve divides into the dorsal and palmar branches. The dorsal branch provides sensation to the ulnar aspect of the dorsum of the hand and the dorsal aspect of the little finger and the ulnar half of the ring finger (Fig. 34-1). The palmar branch provides sensory innervation to the ulnar aspect of the palm of the hand and the palmar aspect of the little finger and the ulnar half of the ring finger (see Fig. 34-1). Clinically, the most common site of entrapment of the ulnar nerve is at the elbow and is known as tardy ulnar palsy.

SUGGESTED READINGS

Campbell W: DeJong's The Neurological Examination, ed 6. Philadelphia, Lippincott Williams and Wilkins, 2005.

Goetz CG: Textbook of Clinical Neurology, ed 2. Philadelphia, Saunders, 2003.

Netter FH: The brachial artery in situ. In: Atlas of Human Anatomy, ed 4. Philadelphia, Saunders, 2006.

Waldman SD: Ulnar nerve block at the elbow. In: Atlas of Interventional Pain Management, ed 2. Philadelphia, Saunders, 2004.

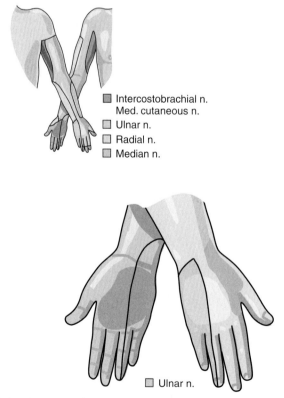

Intercostobrachial n.
Med. cutaneous n.
Ulnar n.
Radial n.
Median n.

Ulnar n.

FIGURE 34–1 Sensory distribution of the ulnar nerve. (From Waldman SD: Ulnar nerve block at the elbow. In: Atlas of Interventional Pain Management, ed 2. Philadelphia, Saunders, 2004, p 186.)

The Median Nerve

The median nerve arises from the lateral and medial cords of the brachial plexus and is made up of fibers from C5-T1 spinal roots (see Fig. 32-1). The nerve lies anterior and superior to the axillary artery. Exiting the axilla, the median nerve descends into the upper arm along with the brachial artery. At the level of the elbow, the brachial artery is just medial to the biceps muscle. At this level, the median nerve lies just medial to the brachial artery (see Fig. 33-1). As the median nerve proceeds downward into the forearm, it gives off numerous branches that provide motor innervation to the flexor muscles of the forearm. These branches are susceptible to nerve entrapment by aberrant ligaments, muscle hypertrophy, and direct trauma. The nerve approaches the wrist overlying the radius. It lies deep to and between the tendons of the palmaris longus muscle and the flexor carpi radialis muscle at the wrist. The median nerve then passes beneath the flexor retinaculum and through the carpal tunnel, with the nerve's terminal branches providing sensory innervation to a portion of the palmar surface of the hand as well as to the palmar surface of the thumb, index and middle fingers, and the radial portion of the ring finger (Fig. 35-1). The median nerve also provides sensory innervation to the distal dorsal surface of the index and middle fingers and the radial portion of the ring finger. Clinically, the median nerve is most commonly entrapped at the wrist, resulting in carpal tunnel syndrome.

SUGGESTED READINGS

Campbell W: DeJong's The Neurological Examination, ed 6. Philadelphia, Lippincott Williams and Wilkins, 2005.

Goetz CG: Textbook of Clinical Neurology, ed 2. Philadelphia, Saunders, 2003.

Netter FH: The brachial artery in situ. In: Atlas of Human Anatomy, ed 4. Philadelphia, Saunders, 2006.

Waldman SD: Median nerve block at the wrist. In: Atlas of Interventional Pain Management, ed 2. Philadelphia, Saunders, 2004.

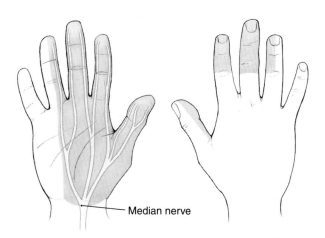

Median nerve

FIGURE 35–1 The sensory distribution of the median nerve.

CHAPTER 36

The Radial Nerve

The radial nerve arises from the posterior cord of the brachial plexus and is made up of fibers from C5-T1 spinal roots (see Fig. 32-1). The nerve lies posterior and inferior to the axillary artery in the 6:00 o'clock–to–9:00 o'clock quadrant. Exiting the axilla, the radial nerve passes between the medial and long heads of the triceps muscle. As the nerve curves across the posterior aspect of the humerus, it supplies a motor branch to the triceps. Continuing its downward path, it gives off a number of sensory branches to the upper arm (Fig. 36-1).

At a point between the lateral epicondyle of the humerus and the musculospiral groove, the radial nerve divides into its two terminal branches. The superficial branch continues down the arm along with the radial artery and provides sensory innervation to the dorsum of the wrist and the dorsal aspects of a portion of the thumb and index and middle fingers (Fig. 36-2). The deep branch provides the majority of the motor innervation to the extensors of the forearm. Clinically, radial nerve entrapment occurs much less commonly than entrapment of the median and ulnar nerves. Damage to the radial nerve as it curves around the shaft of the humerus at the time of humeral fractures is a common cause of radial nerve palsy. This injury is characterized by palsy or paralysis of all extensors of the wrist and digits, as well as of the forearm supinators. Numbness occurs over the dorsoradial aspect of the hand and the dorsal aspect of the radial 3½ digits.

SUGGESTED READINGS

Campbell W: DeJong's The Neurological Examination, ed 6. Philadelphia, Lippincott Williams and Wilkins, 2005.

Goetz CG: Textbook of Clinical Neurology, ed 2. Philadelphia, Saunders, 2003.

Netter FH: The brachial artery in situ. In: Atlas of Human Anatomy, ed 4. Philadelphia, Saunders, 2006.

Waldman SD: Radial nerve block at the wrist. In: Atlas of Interventional Pain Management, ed 2. Philadelphia, Saunders, 2004.

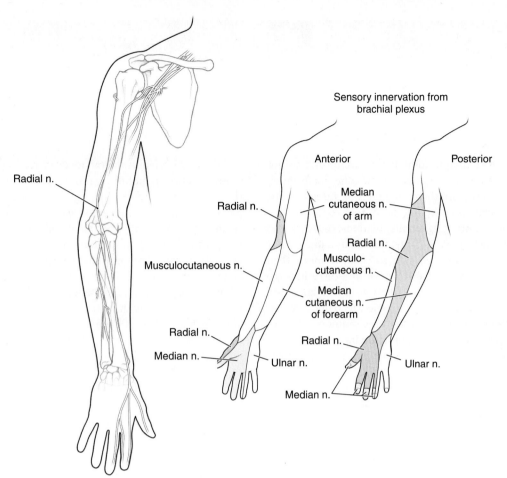

FIGURE 36–1 The radial nerve.

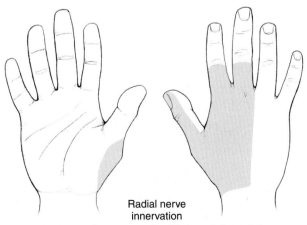

Radial nerve
innervation

FIGURE 36–2 The sensory distribution of the radial nerve.

CHAPTER 37

Functional Anatomy of the Shoulder Joint

The shoulder is a unique joint for a variety of reasons. Unlike the knee and the hip with their inherent primary stability that results from their solid bony architecture, the shoulder is a relatively unstable joint held together by a complex combination of ligaments, tendons, muscles, and unique soft tissues—most notably, the labrum and rotator cuff. What the shoulder lacks in stability, it more than makes up for in its extensive range of motion. Although not a true weight-bearing joint like the hip or knee, the shoulder joint is subjected to extreme mechanical forces due to its extensive range of motion. Common activities such as lifting objects overhead or throwing serve to magnify these mechanical load factors and make the joint susceptible to repetitive motion injuries.

In order to make the most of the information gleaned from the physical examination of the shoulder, one must fully understand the functional anatomy of the shoulder. To fully understand the functional anatomy of the shoulder, one must recognize that the shoulder joint cannot be thought of as a single joint like the knee but rather as four separate joints working in concert to function as one (Fig. 37-1). These four joints are:

- The sternoclavicular joint
- The acromioclavicular joint
- The glenohumeral joint
- The scapulothoracic joint

While the glenohumeral joint is responsible for the main functional mobility of the shoulder joint, each of the other joints works synergistically with its counterparts to allow for the extensive and extremely varied range of motion of the shoulder joint. This unique range of motion of the shoulder joint is further enhanced by the unusual physical characteristics of the humeral head and the glenoid fossa. While the articular surfaces of most joints are well matched in terms of their complementary shape with one another (e.g., the acetabulum and the femoral head), the large, rounded humeral head is amazingly mismatched to the much smaller and shallower, ovoid-shaped glenoid fossa (Fig. 37-2). While this mismatch allows for the unique range of motion of the shoulder joint, it also contributes to the relative instability of the joint and is in large part responsible for the shoulder joint's propensity for injury. To this end, the shoulder joint is the most commonly dislocated large joint in the body!

SUGGESTED READINGS

Netter FH: Shoulder (glenohumeral joint). In: Atlas of Human Anatomy, ed 4. Philadelphia, Saunders, 2006.

Waldman SD: Clinical correlates: Functional anatomy of the shoulder. In: Physical Diagnosis of Pain: An Atlas of Signs and Symptoms. Philadelphia, Saunders, 2006.

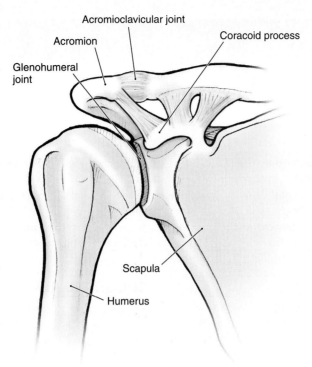

FIGURE 37–1 The shoulder joint.

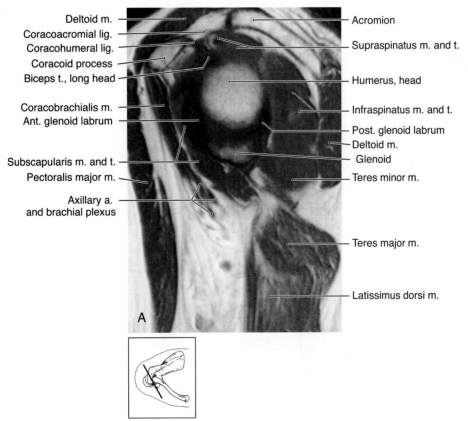

FIGURE 37–2 Sagittal view of the shoulder. (From Kang HS, Ahn JM, Resnik D: MRI of the Extremities: An Anatomic Atlas, ed. 2. Philadelphia, Saunders, 2002, pp 32 and 33.)

CHAPTER **38**

The Acromioclavicular Joint

The acromioclavicular joint is formed by distal end of the clavicle and the anterior and medial aspect of the acromion (Fig. 38-1). The strength of the joint is in large part due to the dense coracoclavicular ligament, which attaches the bottom of the distal end of the clavicle to the coracoid process. A small indentation can be felt where the clavicle abuts the acromion. The joint is completely surrounded by an articular capsule. The superior portion of the joint is covered by the superior acromioclavicular ligament, which attaches the distal clavicle to the upper surface of the acromion. The inferior portion of the joint is covered by the inferior acromioclavicular ligament, which attaches the inferior portion of the distal clavicle to the acromion. Both of these ligaments further add to the joint's stability.

The acromioclavicular joint may or may not contain an articular disc. The volume of the acromioclavicular joint space is small and care must be taken not to disrupt the joint by forcefully injecting large volumes of local anesthetic and steroid into the intra-articular space when performing this injection technique.

SUGGESTED READINGS

Netter FH: Shoulder (acromioclavicular joint). In: Atlas of Human Anatomy, ed 4. Philadelphia, Saunders, 2006.
Waldman SD: Clinical correlates: Functional anatomy of the shoulder. In: Physical Diagnosis of Pain: An Atlas of Signs and Symptoms. Philadelphia, Saunders, 2006.

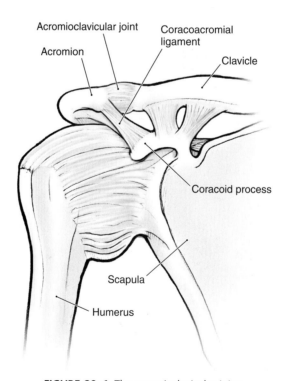

FIGURE 38–1 The acromioclavicular joint.

CHAPTER 39

The Subdeltoid Bursa

The acromial arch covers the superior aspect of the shoulder joint and articulates with the clavicle at the acromioclavicular joint. The acromioclavicular joint is formed by the distal end of the clavicle and the anterior and medial aspect of the acromion. The strength of the joint is due to the dense coracoclavicular ligament, which attaches the bottom of the distal end of the clavicle to the coracoid process. The superior portion of the joint is covered by the superior acromioclavicular ligament, which attaches the distal clavicle to the upper surface of the acromion. The inferior portion of the joint is covered by the inferior acromioclavicular ligament, which attaches the inferior portion of the distal clavicle to the acromion. The subdeltoid bursa lies primarily under the acromion extending laterally between the deltoid muscle and joint capsule (Fig. 39-1). The subdeltoid bursa is subject to the development of bursitis secondary to overuse or misuse of the shoulder.

SUGGESTED READING

Waldman SD: Subdeltoid bursitis. In: Atlas of Common Pain Syndromes, ed 2. Philadelphia, Saunders, 2008.

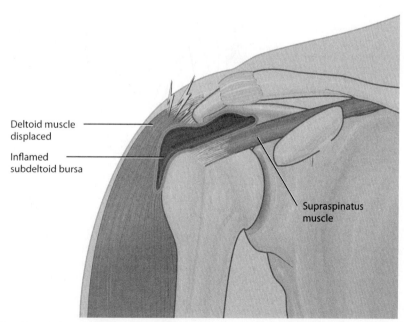

FIGURE 39–1 The subdeltoid bursa. (From Waldman SD: Atlas of Pain Management Injection Techniques. Philadelphia, Saunders, 2000, p 61.)

CHAPTER 40

The Biceps Tendon

The biceps tendon, along with conjoined tendons of the rotator cuff, aids in the stability of the shoulder joint. The biceps muscle, which is innervated by the musculocutaneous nerve, supinates the forearm and flexes the elbow joint. The biceps muscle has a long and a short head (Fig. 40-1). The long head has its origin in the supraglenoid tubercle of the scapula, and the short head has its origin from the tip of the coracoid process of the scapula. The long head exits the shoulder joint via the bicipital groove, where it is susceptible to tendinitis. The long head is joined by the short head in the middle portion of the upper arm. The insertion of the biceps muscle is into the posterior potion of the radial tuberosity. The biceps muscle and tendons are susceptible to trauma and to wear and tear from overuse and misuse. If the damage becomes severe enough, the tendon of the long head of the biceps can rupture, leaving the patient with a telltale "Popeye" biceps.

SUGGESTED READINGS

Netter FH: Muscle of the rotator cuff. In: Atlas of Human Anatomy, ed 4. Philadelphia, Saunders, 2006.
Waldman SD: Bicipital tendinitis. In: Atlas of Common Pain Syndromes, ed 2. Philadelphia, Saunders, 2008.

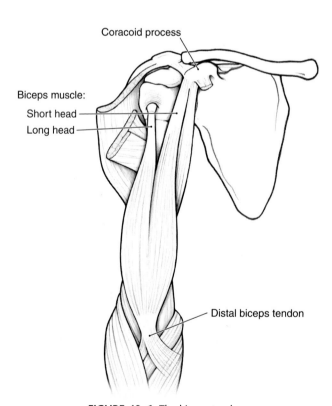

FIGURE 40–1 The biceps tendon.

Functional Anatomy of the Rotator Cuff

To fully understand the role of the rotator cuff in health and disease, the clinician must first appreciate that the rotator cuff must be thought of as a functional musculotendinous unit rather than as four discrete muscles. Although it is true that the supraspinatus, infraspinatus, teres minor, and subscapularis muscles contribute to the rotator cuff, it is not only the muscles but also their fascia and, most important, their tendons that comprise the functional unit we call the rotator cuff (Fig. 41-1).

Arising from the superior aspect of the scapula, the supraspinatus muscle and its covering fascia wrap themselves around the superior humeral head and terminate as a strong tendon that inserts into the uppermost facet of the greater tuberosity of the humerus. The infraspinatus muscle arises from the inferior aspect of the scapula, and its muscle fibers and fascia transform and merge into a dense tendon that passes behind the capsule of the glenohumeral joint to insert into the middle facet of the greater tuberosity of the humerus. The teres minor muscle arises from the mediolateral portion of the scapula and the fascia of the infraspinatus muscle, and its muscle fibers and fascia transform into a tendon that passes behind and below the glenohumeral capsule to insert into the inferior facet of the greater tuberosity of the humerus. The subscapularis muscle arises from the medial portion of the anterior surface of the scapula, and as its muscle fibers transform into a tendon, they extend laterally to attach to the lesser tubercle of the humerus.

One of the primary functions of the musculotendinous units that comprise the rotator cuff is to provide stabilization of the glenohumeral joint during shoulder motion, as well as to strengthen the relatively weak glenohumeral joint capsule. The supraspinatus and infraspinatus musculotendinous unit help to reinforce the superior aspect of the glenohumeral joint capsule; the teres minor musculotendinous unit, the posterior aspect of the joint capsule; and the subscapularis musculotendinous unit, the anterior portion of the joint capsule. The rotator cuff also serves as an important initiator of abduction of the upper extremity. In addition to these functions, the rotator cuff helps to stabilize the shoulder by counterbalancing the inherent upward force of the deltoid muscle during shoulder motion.

When thinking about the role of the rotator cuff in shoulder motion, it is useful to think of all of the muscles and their associated fascia and tendons actively working as a single unit. They work in concert to maintain the stability of the shoulder joint throughout a wide and varied range of motion. The rotator cuff accomplishes this amazing task by allowing each component muscle to smoothly and subtly vary the strength and velocity of contraction and relaxation as the shoulder moves through its range of motion. It is also important to recognize that the rotator cuff does not function as an isolated structure but works together with the other muscles and structures of the shoulder, including the deltoid muscle, the long head of the biceps muscle, and the coracohumeral and glenohumeral ligaments, to allow a complex and unique range of motion of the shoulder relative to the other joints of the body.

Given the complex interaction of these musculotendinous units with each other, as well as their interaction with their surrounding structures, it should not be surprising that disease of one structure can severely affect the function of the other interdependent structures. Due to the tenuous nature of the blood supply to the tendons of the rotator cuff, these structures are particularly vulnerable to damage. Weakening of the tendons due to ischemic changes and chronic inflammation can first lead to rotator cuff tendinopathy and, if left untreated, ultimately to rotator cuff tear.

SUGGESTED READINGS

Netter FH: Muscles of the rotator cuff. In: Atlas of Human Anatomy, ed 4. Philadelphia, Saunders, 2006.

Waldman SD: Rotator cuff tear. In: Atlas of Common Pain Syndromes, ed 2. Philadelphia, Saunders, 2008.

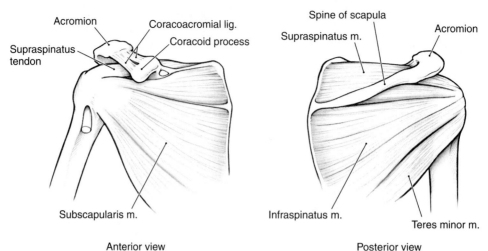

FIGURE 41–1 The muscles and tendons of the rotator cuff.

CHAPTER 42

The Supraspinatus Muscle

The supraspinatus muscle is the most important muscle of the rotator cuff. It provides joint stability and with the deltoid muscle adducts the arm at the shoulder by fixing the head of the humerus firmly against the glenoid fossa. The supraspinatus muscle is innervated by the suprascapular nerve. The supraspinatus muscle has its origin from the supraspinous fossa of the scapula and inserts into the upper facet of the greater tuberosity of the humerus (Fig. 42-1). The muscle passes across the superior aspect of the shoulder joint with the inferior portion of the tendon intimately involved with the joint capsule. The supraspinatus muscle and tendons are susceptible to trauma and to wear and tear from overuse and misuse.

SUGGESTED READING

Netter FH: Muscles of the rotator cuff. In: Atlas of Human Anatomy, ed 4. Philadelphia, Saunders, 2006.

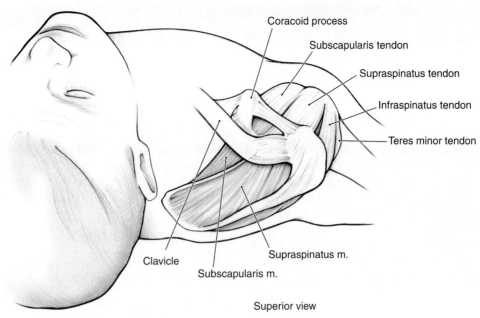

Coracoid process

Subscapularis tendon

Supraspinatus tendon

Infraspinatus tendon

Teres minor tendon

Clavicle

Subscapularis m.

Supraspinatus m.

Superior view

FIGURE 42–1 The supraspinatus muscle.

CHAPTER 43

The Infraspinatus Muscle

The infraspinatus muscle is part of the rotator cuff. It provides shoulder joint stability and along with the teres minor muscle externally rotates the arm at the shoulder. The infraspinatus muscle is innervated by the suprascapular nerve. The infraspinatus muscle has its origin in the infraspinous fossa of the scapula and inserts into the middle facet of the greater tuberosity of the humerus (see Fig. 42-1). It is at this insertion that infraspinatus tendinitis most commonly occurs.

The infraspinatus muscle and tendons are susceptible to trauma and to wear and tear from overuse and misuse.

SUGGESTED READING

Netter FH: Muscles of the rotator cuff. In: Atlas of Human Anatomy, ed 4. Philadelphia, Saunders, 2006.

CHAPTER 44

The Subscapularis Muscle

The subscapularis muscle is part of the rotator cuff. It provides shoulder joint stability along with the supraspinatus, infraspinatus, and teres minor muscles. The subscapularis muscle medially rotates the arm at the shoulder. The subscapularis muscle is innervated by branches of the posterior cord of the brachial plexus, the upper and lower subscapular nerves. The subscapularis muscle has its origin in the subscapular fossa of the anterior scapula and inserts into the lesser tuberosity of the humerus.

It is at this insertion that subscapularis tendinitis most commonly occurs (Fig. 44-1). The subscapularis muscle and tendons are susceptible to trauma and to wear and tear from overuse and misuse.

SUGGESTED READING

Netter FH: Muscles of the rotator cuff. In: Atlas of Human Anatomy, ed 4. Philadelphia, Saunders, 2006.

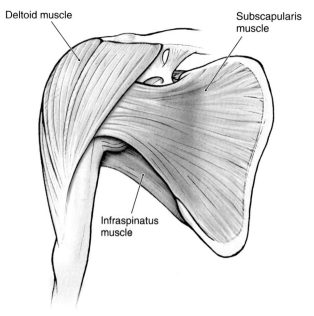

FIGURE 44–1 The subscapularis muscle.

The Subcoracoid Bursa

The coracoid process of the scapula projects upward and forward above the glenoid fossa (Fig. 45-1). The coracoid process provides attachment for the coracoclavicular ligament as well as the short head of the biceps. The long head of the biceps has its origin just inferior to the coracoid process in the supraglenoid tubercle of the scapula. The long head exits the shoulder joint via the bicipital groove where it is susceptible to tendinitis. The long head is joined by the short head in the middle portion of the upper arm. The insertion of the biceps muscle is into the posterior portion of the radial tuberosity.

The subcoracoid bursa lies between the joint capsule and the coracoid process. It is susceptible to irritation by pressure from the coracoid process against the head of the humerus during extreme arm movement or when previous damage to the musculotendinous unit of the shoulder allows abnormal movement of the head of the humerus in the glenoid fossa.

SUGGESTED READING

Waldman SD: Subcoracoid bursitis. In: Atlas of Pain Management Injection Techniques, ed 2. Philadelphia, Saunders, 2007.

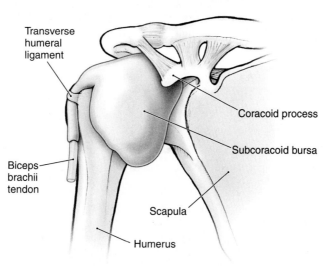

Transverse humeral ligament

Coracoid process

Subcoracoid bursa

Biceps brachii tendon

Scapula

Humerus

FIGURE 45–1 The subcoracoid bursa.

CHAPTER 46

Functional Anatomy of the Elbow Joint

The proper functioning of the elbow is essential for humans to successfully carry out their activities of daily living. With elbow dysfunction, bathing, getting dressed, and even using the toilet become problematic. Although conventionally thought of as a hinge joint analogous to the knee, in fact the elbow's unique compound range of motion is due to the interplay between the hinge-type function and the rotational pronation and supination that allow precise position of the hand with its highly mobile fingers and opposing thumb. The three bones that constitute the joint—the humerus, the ulna, and the radius—each has specialized ends to facilitate the elbow's function and strength (Fig. 46-1).

From a functional anatomy viewpoint, the elbow has three areas that are involved in the vast majority of elbow disorders: (1) the humeral-radial interface, (2) the humeral-ulnar interface, and (3) the radial-ulnar interface. The humeral-ulnar interface is composed of the area surrounding and including the trochlea of the humerus and the trochlear notch, coronoid process, and olecranon of the ulna (Fig. 46-2). The humeral-radial interface is composed of the area surrounding and including the capitulum of the humerus and the radial head (Fig. 46-3). The radial-ulnar interface is composed of the area surrounding and including the head of the radius and the radial notch of the ulna (Fig. 46-4).

The humeral-radial interface and the humeral-ulnar interface allow for the elbow's hinge-type movement. These articular interfaces and the joint's surrounding ligaments contribute to the stability of the elbow in flexion and, to a lesser extent, extension. In health, this hinge portion of the elbow can traverse approximately 150 degrees. Due to the shape of the humeral trochlea and the ulnar trochlear notch, the arm moves into a valgus position of the forearm in extension. This valgus position is called the carrying angle and is 10 to 15 degrees in men and up to 18 degrees in women. When the arm flexes, it moves into a more varus position, which functionally puts the hand in closer proximity to the mouth to aid in feeding. Flexion of the arm at the elbow is carried out primarily by the biceps and brachialis muscles with extension carried out primarily by the opposing triceps muscle. The insertion points of the muscles are common sites of elbow pain and dysfunction.

In addition to the bony architecture and surrounding ligaments, the elbow is richly endowed with bursae to facilitate the joint's varied movements. These bursae are extremely susceptible to overuse, inflammation, and even infection and are also common sites of elbow pain and dysfunction. Most notably, the olecranon and cubital bursae are commonly affected. When these bursae become inflamed, they can impinge and irritate their associated tendons and tendinous insertions with resultant tendinitis and occasionally nerve entrapment.

SUGGESTED READINGS

Netter FH: Bones of the elbow. In: Atlas of Human Anatomy, ed 4. Philadelphia, Saunders, 2006.

Waldman SD: Clinical correlates: Functional anatomy of the shoulder. In: Physical Diagnosis of Pain: An Atlas of Signs and Symptoms. Philadelphia, Saunders, 2006.

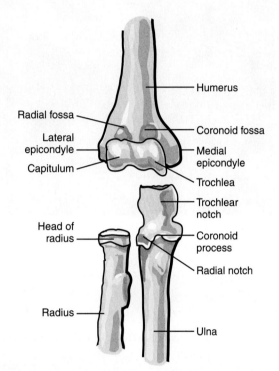

FIGURE 46–1 Bony anatomy of the elbow joint. (From Waldman SD: Physical Diagnosis of Pain: An Atlas of Signs and Symptoms. Philadelphia, Saunders, 2006, p 114.)

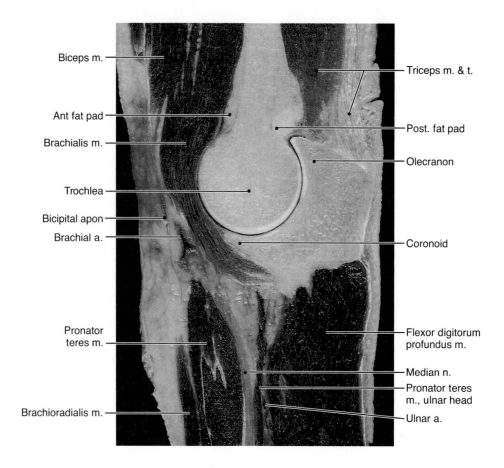

Biceps m.

Ant fat pad

Brachialis m.

Trochlea

Bicipital apon

Brachial a.

Pronator teres m.

Brachioradialis m.

Triceps m. & t.

Post. fat pad

Olecranon

Coronoid

Flexor digitorum profundus m.

Median n.

Pronator teres m., ulnar head

Ulnar a.

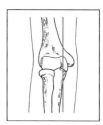

FIGURE 46–2 Humeral-ulnar interface. (From Kang HS, Ahn JM, Resnik D: MRI of the Extremities: An Anatomic Atlas. Philadelphia, Saunders, 2002, p 113.)

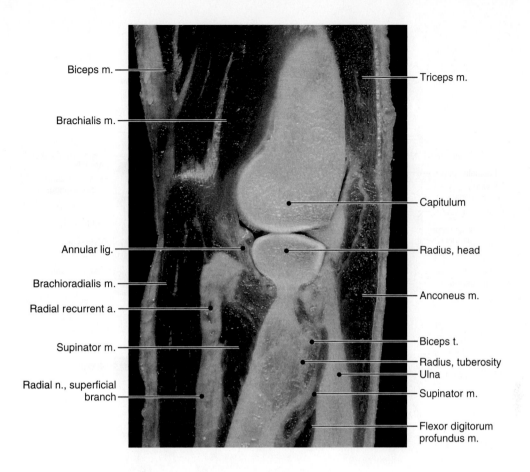

Biceps m.

Brachialis m.

Annular lig.

Brachioradialis m.

Radial recurrent a.

Supinator m.

Radial n., superficial branch

Triceps m.

Capitulum

Radius, head

Anconeus m.

Biceps t.

Radius, tuberosity

Ulna

Supinator m.

Flexor digitorum profundus m.

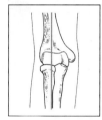

FIGURE 46–3 Humeral-radial interface. (From Kang HS, Ahn JM, Resnik D: MRI of the Extremities: An Anatomic Atlas. Philadelphia, Saunders, 2002, p 123.)

Elbow, transverse

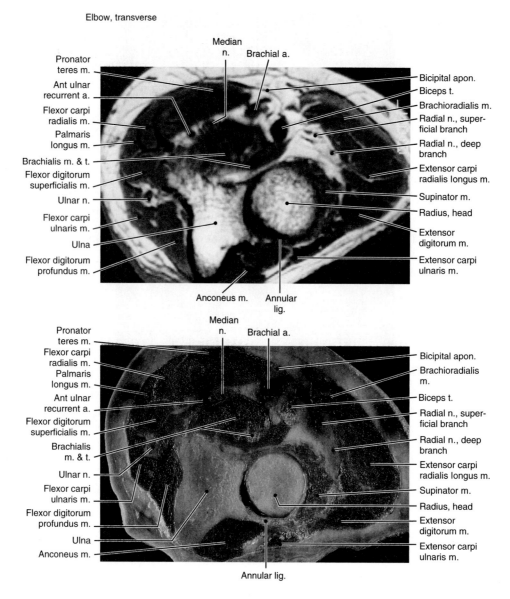

Median n.
Brachial a.

Pronator teres m.
Ant ulnar recurrent a.
Flexor carpi radialis m.
Palmaris longus m.
Brachialis m. & t.
Flexor digitorum superficialis m.
Ulnar n.
Flexor carpi ulnaris m.
Ulna
Flexor digitorum profundus m.

Bicipital apon.
Biceps t.
Brachioradialis m.
Radial n., superficial branch
Radial n., deep branch
Extensor carpi radialis longus m.
Supinator m.
Radius, head
Extensor digitorum m.
Extensor carpi ulnaris m.

Anconeus m.
Annular lig.

Median n.
Brachial a.

Pronator teres m.
Flexor carpi radialis m.
Palmaris longus m.
Ant ulnar recurrent a.
Flexor digitorum superficialis m.
Brachialis m. & t.
Ulnar n.
Flexor carpi ulnaris m.
Flexor digitorum profundus m.
Ulna
Anconeus m.

Bicipital apon.
Brachioradialis m.
Biceps t.
Radial n., superficial branch
Radial n., deep branch
Extensor carpi radialis longus m.
Supinator m.
Radius, head
Extensor digitorum m.
Extensor carpi ulnaris m.

Annular lig.

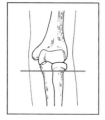

FIGURE 46–4 Radial-ulnar interface. (From Kang HS, Ahn JM, Resnik D: MRI of the Extremities: An Anatomic Atlas. Philadelphia, Saunders, 2002, p 104.)

The Olecranon Bursa

The elbow joint is a synovial hinge-type joint that serves as the articulation between the humerus, radius, and ulna. The joint's primary function is to position the wrist to optimize hand function. The joint allows flexion and extension at the elbow as well as pronation and supination of the forearm. The joint is lined with synovium. The entire joint is covered by a dense capsule that thickens medially to form the ulnar collateral ligament and medially to form the radial collateral ligaments. These dense ligaments coupled with the elbow joint's deep bony socket make this joint extremely stable and relatively resistant to subluxation and dislocation. The anterior and posterior joint capsule is less dense and may become distended if there is a joint effusion. The olecranon bursa lies in the posterior aspect of the elbow joint between the olecranon process of the ulna and the overlying skin (Fig. 47-1). The olecranon bursa may become inflamed as a result of direct trauma or overuse of the joint.

The elbow joint is innervated primarily by the musculocutaneous and radial nerves with the ulnar and median nerves providing varying degrees of innervation. At the middle of the upper arm, the ulnar nerve courses medially to pass between the olecranon process and medial epicondyle of the humerus. The nerve is susceptible to entrapment and trauma at this point. At the elbow, the median nerve lies just medial to the brachial artery and is occasionally damaged during brachial artery cannulation for blood gases.

SUGGESTED READING

Waldman SD: Subdeltoid bursitis. In: Atlas of Common Pain Syndromes, ed 2. Philadelphia, Saunders, 2008.

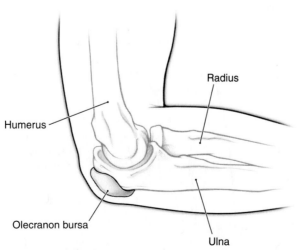

FIGURE 47–1 The olecranon bursa.

CHAPTER **48**

The Radial Nerve at the Elbow

The radial nerve is made up of fibers from C5-T1 spinal roots. The nerve lies posterior and inferior to the axillary artery. Exiting the axilla, the radial nerve passes between the medial and long heads of the triceps muscle. As the nerve curves across the posterior aspect of the humerus, it supplies a motor branch to the triceps. Continuing its downward path, it gives off a number of sensory branches to the upper arm. At a point between the lateral epicondyle of the humerus and the musculospiral groove, the radial nerve divides into its two terminal branches (Fig. 48-1). The superficial branch continues down the arm along with the radial artery and provides sensory innervation to the dorsum of the wrist and the dorsal aspects of a portion of the thumb, index, and middle finger. The deep posterior interosseous branch provides the majority of the motor innervation to the extensors of the forearm.

SUGGESTED READINGS

Tsai P, Steinberg DR: Median and radial nerve compression about the elbow. J Bone Joint Surg Am 90A:420-428, 2008.

Waldman SD: Radial nerve block at the elbow. In Waldman SD: Atlas of Interventional Pain Management, ed 2. Philadelphia, Saunders, 2004.

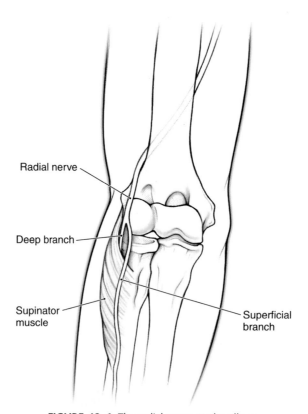

FIGURE 48–1 The radial nerve at the elbow.

The Cubital Tunnel

The ulnar nerve is made up of fibers from C6-T1 spinal roots. The nerve lies anterior and inferior to the axillary artery in the 3 o'clock–to–6 o'clock quadrant. Exiting the axilla, the ulnar nerve descends into the upper arm along with the brachial artery. At the middle of the upper arm, the nerve courses medially to pass between the olecranon process and medial epicondyle of the humerus. This passage is known as the cubital tunnel (Fig. 49-1). It is at this point that the entrapment of the ulnar nerve responsible for cubital tunnel syndrome occurs. The nerve then enters the cubital tunnel and passes between the heads of the flexor carpi ulnaris muscle, continuing downward and moving radially along with the ulnar artery. At a point approximately 1 inch proximal to the crease of the wrist, the ulnar divides into the dorsal and palmar branches. The dorsal branch provides sensation to the ulnar aspect of the dorsum of the hand and the dorsal aspect of the little and the ulnar half of the ring finger. The palmar branch provides sensory innervation to the ulnar aspect of the palm of the hand and the palmar aspect of the little and the ulnar half of the ring finger.

SUGGESTED READING

Waldman SD: Cubital tunnel syndrome. In: Atlas of Pain Management Injection Techniques, ed 2. Philadelphia, Saunders, 2007.

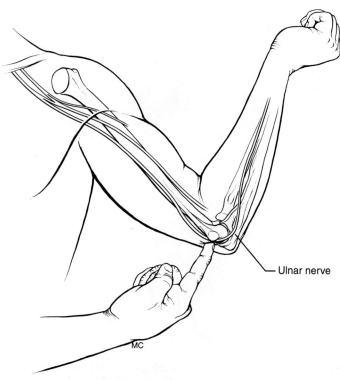

FIGURE 49–1 The cubital tunnel.

CHAPTER 50

The Anterior Interosseous Nerve

The median nerve is made up of fibers from C5-T1 spinal roots. The nerve lies anterior and superior to the axillary artery. Exiting the axilla, the median nerve descends into the upper arm along with the brachial artery. At the level of the elbow, the brachial artery is just medial to the biceps muscle. At this level, the median nerve lies just medial to the brachial artery. As the median nerve proceeds downward into the forearm, it gives off numerous branches, which provide motor innervation to the flexor muscles of the forearm including the anterior interosseous nerve (Fig. 50-1). These branches are susceptible to nerve entrapment by aberrant ligaments, muscle hypertrophy, and direct trauma. In the case of the anterior interosseous nerve, this can take the form of anterior interosseous syndrome. The nerve approaches the wrist overlying the radius. It lies deep to and between the tendons of the palmaris longus muscle and the flexor carpi radialis muscle at the wrist. The terminal branches of the median nerve provide sensory innervation to a portion of the palmar surface of the hand as well as the palmar surface of the thumb, index, middle, and the radial portion of the ring finger. The median nerve also provides sensory innervation to the distal dorsal surface of the index and middle finger and the radial portion of the ring finger.

SUGGESTED READING

Waldman SD: Anterior interosseous syndrome. In: Atlas of Pain Management Injection Techniques, ed 2. Philadelphia, Saunders, 2007.

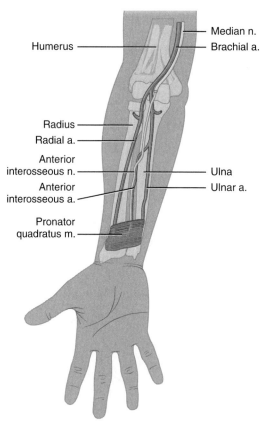

FIGURE 50–1 The anterior interosseous nerve. (From Waldman SD: Atlas of Pain Management Injection Techniques, ed 2. Philadelphia, Saunders, 2007, p 193.)

The Lateral Antebrachial Cutaneous Nerve

The lateral antebrachial cutaneous nerve is a continuation of the musculocutaneous nerve. The musculocutaneous nerve passes through the fascia lateral to the biceps tendon before it continues into the forearm as the lateral antebrachial cutaneous nerve (Fig. 51-1). The nerve is susceptible to entrapment at this point. The lateral antebrachial cutaneous nerve passes behind the cephalic vein where it divides into a volar branch, which continues along the radial border of the forearm where it provides sensory innervation to the skin over the lateral half of the volar surface of the forearm. It passes anterior to the radial artery at the wrist to provide sensation to the base of the thumb. The dorsal branch provides sensation to the dorsal lateral surface of the forearm.

SUGGESTED READING

Waldman SD: Lateral antebrachial cutaneous nerve entrapment syndrome. In: Atlas of Pain Management Injection Techniques, ed 2. Philadelphia, Saunders, 2007.

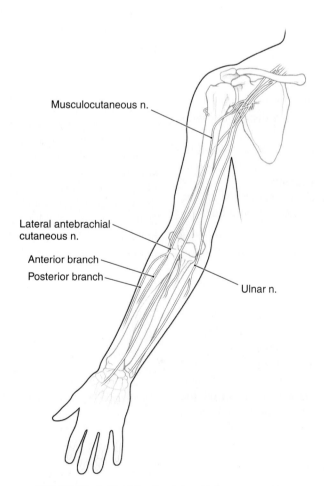

FIGURE 51–1 The lateral antebrachial cutaneous nerve.

CHAPTER 52

Functional Anatomy of the Wrist

In humans, the wrist functions to transfer the forces and motions of the hand to the forearm and proximal upper extremity. The wrist allows movement in three planes:

1. Flexion/extension
2. Radial/ulnar deviation
3. Pronation/supination

To understand the functional anatomy of the wrist, it is important for the clinician to understand that the wrist is not a single joint but in fact is a complex of five separate joints or compartments that work in concert to allow humans to carry out their activities of daily living (Fig. 52-1). These five joints are:

1. The distal radioulnar joint, which is composed of the distal radius and ulna and their interosseous membrane
2. The radiocarpal joint, which is composed of the distal radius and the proximal surfaces of the scaphoid and lunate bones
3. The ulnar carpal joint, which is composed of the distal ulna and the triangular fibroelastic cartilage whose function is to connect the distal ulna with the lunate and triquetrum
4. The proximal carpal joints, which connect the scaphoid, lunate, and triquetrum via the dorsal, palmar, and interosseous ligaments
5. The midcarpal joints, which are composed of the capitate, hamate, trapezium, and trapezoid bones

The interaction of the many osseous elements that make up the wrist is made possible by a complex collection of ligamentous structures and a unique structure called the triangular fibroelastic cartilage (TFC). Although a comprehensive review of the ligaments of the wrist is beyond the scope and purpose of this chapter, it is helpful for the clinician to understand the basic anatomy. In general, the ligaments can be thought of as being intrinsic to the wrist (i.e., having their origin and insertion on the carpal bones) or extrinsic to the wrist (i.e., having their origin on the distal radius or ulna and insertion on the carpal bones). All of the ligaments of the wrist have in common a close proximity to the bones of the wrist,

which increases their ability to transfer force to the forearm and proximal upper extremity. This lack of interposing muscle and/or soft tissue also makes the ligamentous structures of the wrist—the nerves, blood vessels, and bones beneath them—more susceptible to injury.

Located primarily between the distal ulna and the lunate and triquetrum, the triangular fibroelastic cartilage is a unique structure that in ways functions in a manner analogous to an intervertebral disc and in ways more like a ligament (Fig. 52-2). The TFC is made up of very strong fibroelastic fibers, and it acts like an intervertebral disc in that it serves as the primary shock absorber of the wrist and acts like a ligament in that it serves as the primarily stabilizer for the distal radioulnar joint. The TFC is susceptible to trauma and, due to its poor vascular supply, often heals poorly following injury or surgical interventions, especially on its radial surface.

The musculotendinous units that are responsible for wrist movement find their origins at the elbow and insert on the metacarpals. They can be grouped as flexors, extensors, and deviators. The primary wrist flexors are the flexor carpi radialis and the flexor carpi ulnaris. The primary wrist extensors are the extensor carpi radialis longus and the extensor carpi radialis brevis. The primary radial deviator is the abductor pollicis longus, and the primary ulnar deviator is the extensor carpi ulnaris. The flexor tendons are held in place by the flexor retinaculum, which extends laterally from the trapezium and scaphoid to the pisiform and hook of the hamate bone. By preventing bowing of the flexor tendons under load, it is estimated that the flexor retinaculum increases the force of the flexor tendons fivefold.

SUGGESTED READINGS

Netter FH: Bones of the wrist. In: Atlas of Human Anatomy, ed 4. Philadelphia, Saunders, 2006.

Netter FH: Ligaments of the wrist. In: Atlas of Human Anatomy, ed 4. Philadelphia, Saunders, 2006.

Waldman SD: Functional anatomy of the wrist. In: Physical Diagnosis of Pain: An Atlas of Signs and Symptoms. Philadelphia, Saunders, 2006.

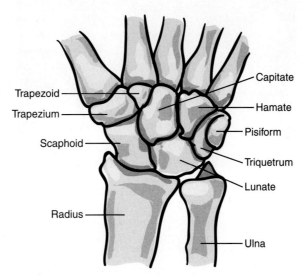

FIGURE 52–1 Bony anatomy of the wrist. (From Waldman SD: Physical Diagnosis of Pain: An Atlas of Signs and Symptoms. Philadelphia, Saunders, 2006, p 154.)

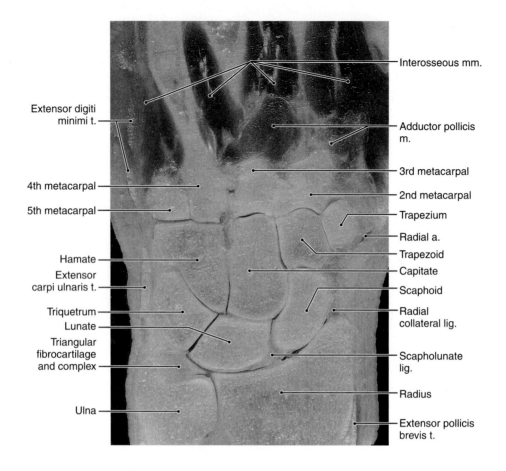

Interosseous mm.

Extensor digiti
minimi t.

Adductor pollicis
m.

3rd metacarpal

4th metacarpal

2nd metacarpal

5th metacarpal

Trapezium

Radial a.

Hamate

Trapezoid

Extensor
carpi ulnaris t.

Capitate

Scaphoid

Triquetrum

Radial
collateral lig.

Lunate

Triangular
fibrocartilage
and complex

Scapholunate
lig.

Radius

Ulna

Extensor pollicis
brevis t.

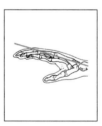

FIGURE 52–2 The triangular fibroelastic cartilage. (From Kang HS, Ahn JM, Resnik D: MRI of the Extremities: An Anatomic Atlas. Philadelphia, Saunders, 2002, p 163.)

The Carpal Tunnel

The median nerve is made up of fibers from C5-T1 spinal roots. The nerve lies anterior and superior to the axillary artery in the 12:00 o'clock–to–3:00 o'clock quadrant. Exiting the axilla, the median nerve descends into the upper arm along with the brachial artery. At the level of the elbow, the brachial artery is just medial to the biceps muscle. At this level, the median nerve lies just medial to the brachial artery. As the median nerve proceeds downward into the forearm, it gives off numerous branches that provide motor innervation to the flexor muscles of the forearm. These branches are susceptible to nerve entrapment by aberrant ligaments, muscle hypertrophy, and direct trauma. The nerve approaches the wrist overlying the radius. It lies deep to and between the tendons of the palmaris longus muscle and the flexor carpi radialis muscle at the wrist.

The median nerve then passes beneath the flexor retinaculum and through the carpal tunnel with the nerve's terminal branches providing sensory innervation to a portion of the palmar surface of the hand as well as the palmar surface of the thumb, index, middle, and radial portion of the ring finger (Fig. 53-1). The median nerve also provides sensory innervation to the distal dorsal surface of the index and middle finger and the radial portion of the ring finger. The carpal tunnel is bounded on three sides by the carpal bones and is covered by the transverse carpal ligament. In addition to the median nerve, it contains a number of flexor tendon sheaths, blood vessels, and lymphatics. Compression of the median nerve as it passes through the carpal tunnel is known as carpal tunnel syndrome.

SUGGESTED READING

Waldman SD: Carpal tunnel syndrome. In: Atlas of Pain Management Injection Techniques, ed 2. Philadelphia, Saunders, 2007.

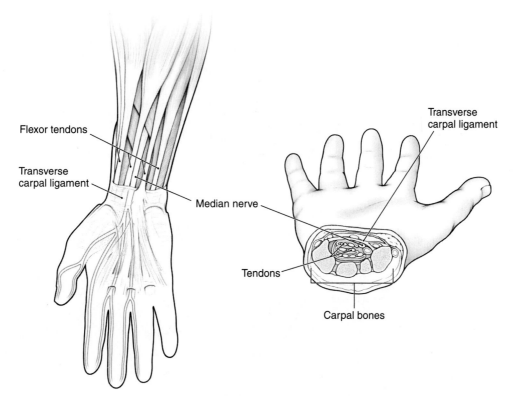

FIGURE 53–1 The carpal tunnel.

CHAPTER 54

The Ulnar Tunnel

The ulnar canal, also known as Guyon's canal, is the space between the pisiform and hamate bones of the wrist through which the ulnar nerve and artery pass (Fig. 54-1). It is at this point that the ulnar nerve is subject to compression in a manner analogous to the median nerve in carpal tunnel syndrome. Ulnar tunnel syndrome is caused by compression of the ulnar nerve as it passes through Guyon's canal at the wrist. The most common causes of compression of the ulnar nerve at this anatomic location include space-occupying lesions, including ganglion cysts and ulnar artery aneurysms, fractures of the distal ulna and carpals, and repetitive motion injuries that compromise the ulnar nerve as it passes through this closed space. This entrapment neuropathy presents most commonly as a pure motor neuropathy without pain.

SUGGESTED READING

Waldman SD: Ulnar tunnel syndrome. In: Atlas of Pain Management Injection Techniques, ed 2. Philadelphia, Saunders, 2007.

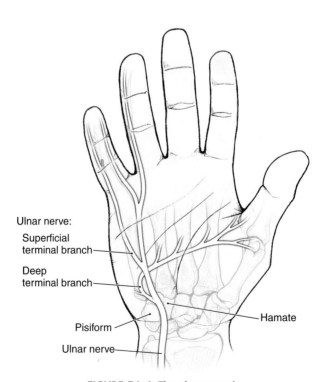

FIGURE 54–1 The ulnar tunnel.

CHAPTER 55

The Carpometacarpal Joint

The carpometacarpal joint is a synovial, saddle-shaped joint that serves as the articulation between the trapezium and the base of the first metacarpal (Fig. 55-1). The joint's primary function is to optimize the pinch function of the hand. The joint allows flexion, extension, abduction, adduction, and a small amount of rotation. The joint is lined with synovium, and the resultant synovial space allows intra-articular injection. It is covered by a relatively weak capsule that surrounds the entire joint and is susceptible to trauma if the joint is subluxed.

The carpometacarpal joint may also become inflamed as a result of direct trauma or overuse of the joint.

SUGGESTED READINGS

Netter FH: Bones of the hand. In: Atlas of Human Anatomy, ed 4. Philadelphia, Saunders, 2006.

Waldman SD: Injection of the carpometacarpal joint of the thumb. In: Atlas of Pain Management Injection Techniques, ed 2. Philadelphia, Saunders, 2007.

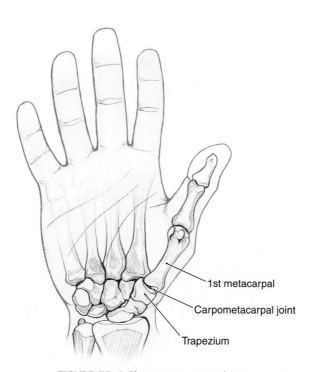

1st metacarpal

Carpometacarpal joint

Trapezium

FIGURE 55–1 The carpometacarpal joint.

CHAPTER 56

The Carpometacarpal Joints of the Fingers

The carpometacarpal joints of the fingers are synovial plane joints that serve as the articulation between the carpals and the metacarpals and also allow articulation of the bases of the metacarpal bones with one another (Fig. 56-1). Movement of the joints is limited to a slight gliding motion, with the carpometacarpal joint of the little finger possessing the greatest range of motion. The joint's primary function is to optimize the grip function of the hand. In most patients, there is a common joint space. The joint is strengthened by anterior, posterior, and interosseous ligaments.

SUGGESTED READINGS

Netter FH: Bones of the hand. In: Atlas of Human Anatomy, ed 4. Philadelphia, Saunders, 2006.

Waldman SD: Injection of the carpometacarpal joint of the fingers. In: Atlas of Pain Management Injection Techniques, ed 2. Philadelphia, Saunders, 2007.

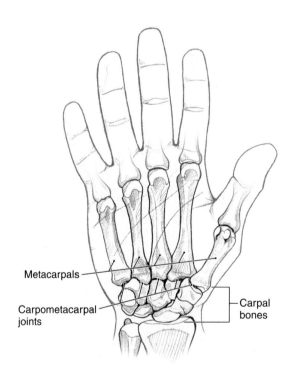

Metacarpals

Carpometacarpal joints

Carpal bones

FIGURE 56–1 The carpometacarpal joints of the finger.

CHAPTER 57

The Metacarpophalangeal Joints

The metacarpophalangeal joint is a synovial, ellipsoid-shaped joint that serves as the articulation between the base of the proximal phalanges and the head of its respective metacarpal (Fig. 57-1). The joint's primary role is to optimize the gripping function of the hand. The joint allows flexion, extension, abduction, and adduction. The joint is lined with synovium, and the resultant synovial space allows intra-articular injection. It is covered by a capsule that surrounds the entire joint and is susceptible to trauma if the joint is subluxed. Ligaments help strengthen the joints; the palmar ligaments are particularly strong.

SUGGESTED READINGS

Netter FH: Bones of the hand. In: Atlas of Human Anatomy, ed 4. Philadelphia, Saunders, 2006.
Waldman SD: Injection of the metacarpophalangeal joints of the fingers. In: Atlas of Pain Management Injection Techniques, ed 2. Philadelphia, Saunders, 2007.

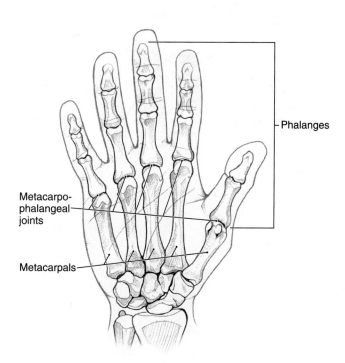

FIGURE 57–1 The metacarpophalangeal joints.

CHAPTER 58

The Interphalangeal Joints

The interphalangeal joints are synovial hinge-shaped joints that serve as the articulation between the phalanges (Fig. 58-1). The interphalangeal joint's primary role is to optimize the gripping function of the hand. The joint allows flexion and extension. The joint is lined with synovium, and the resultant synovial space allows intra-articular injection. It is covered by a capsule that surrounds the entire joint and is susceptible to trauma if the joint is subluxed. Volar and collateral ligaments help strengthen the joint; the palmar ligaments are particularly strong.

SUGGESTED READINGS

Netter FH: Bones of the hand. In: Atlas of Human Anatomy, ed 4. Philadelphia, Saunders, 2006.

Waldman SD: Injection of the interphalangeal joints of the fingers. In: Atlas of Pain Management Injection Techniques, ed 2. Philadelphia, Saunders, 2007.

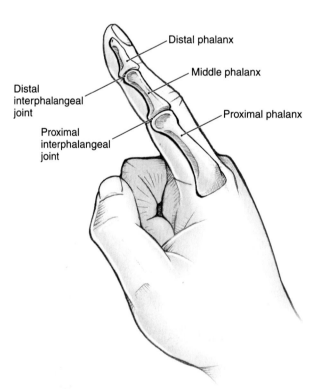

FIGURE 58–1 The interphalangeal joints.

The Intercostal Nerves

The intercostal nerves arise from the anterior division of the thoracic paravertebral nerve. A typical intercostal nerve has four major branches (Fig. 59-1). The first branch is the unmyelinated postganglionic fibers of the gray rami communicantes, which interface with the sympathetic chain. The second branch is the posterior cutaneous branch, which innervates the muscles and skin of the paraspinal area. The third branch is the lateral cutaneous division, which arises in the anterior axillary line. The lateral cutaneous division provides the majority of the cutaneous innervation of the chest and abdominal wall. The fourth branch is the anterior cutaneous branch supplying innervation to the midline of the chest and abdominal wall (Fig. 59-2). Occasionally, the terminal branches of a given intercostal nerve may actually cross the midline to provide sensory innervation to the contralateral chest and abdominal wall. The 12th nerve is called the subcostal nerve and is unique in that it gives off a branch to the first lumbar nerve, thus contributing to the lumbar plexus.

SUGGESTED READINGS

Netter FH: Typical thoracic spinal nerve. In: Atlas of Human Anatomy, ed 4. Philadelphia, Saunders, 2006.
Waldman SD: Intercostal nerve block. In: Atlas of Interventional Pain Management, ed 2. Philadelphia, Saunders, 2004.

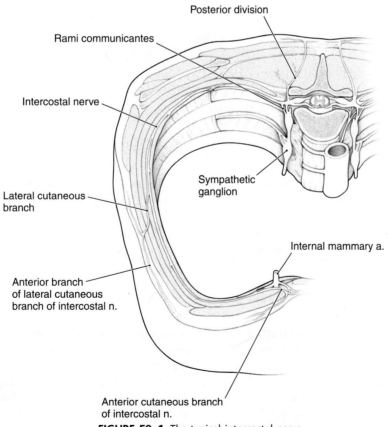

FIGURE 59–1 The typical intercostal nerve.

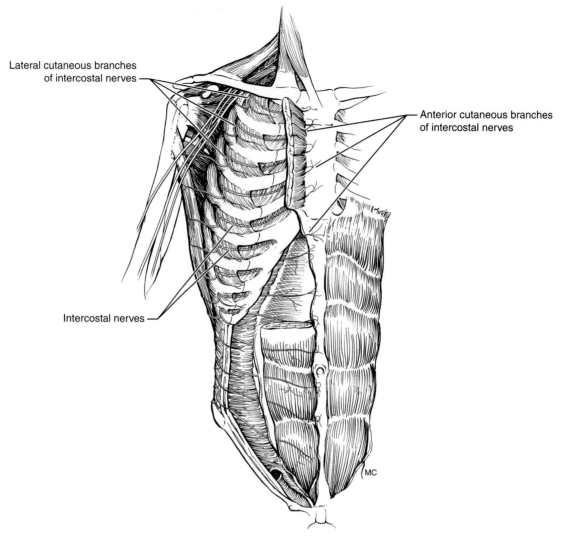

Lateral cutaneous branches
of intercostal nerves

Anterior cutaneous branches
of intercostal nerves

Intercostal nerves

MC

FIGURE 59–2 The branches of the intercostal nerve.

CHAPTER **60**

The Thoracic Sympathetic Chain and Ganglia

The preganglionic fibers of the thoracic sympathetics exit the intervertebral foramen along with the respective thoracic paravertebral nerves (Fig. 60-1). After exiting the intervertebral foramen, the thoracic paravertebral nerve gives off a recurrent branch that loops back through the foramen to provide innervation to the spinal ligaments, meninges, and its respective vertebra. The thoracic paravertebral nerve also interfaces with the thoracic sympathetic chain via the myelinated preganglionic fibers of the white rami communicantes as well as the unmyelinated postganglionic fibers of the gray rami communicantes (Fig. 60-2). At the level of the thoracic sympathetic ganglia, preganglionic and postganglionic fibers synapse. Additionally, some of the postganglionic fibers return to their respective somatic nerves via the gray rami communicantes. These fibers provide sympathetic innervation to the vasculature, sweat glands, and pilomotor muscles of the skin. Other thoracic sympathetic postganglionic fibers travel to the cardiac plexus and course up and down the sympathetic trunk to terminate in distant ganglia.

The first thoracic ganglion is fused with the lower cervical ganglion to help make up the stellate ganglion. As the chain moves caudad, it changes its position with the upper thoracic ganglia just beneath the rib and the lower thoracic ganglia moving more anterior to rest along the posterolateral surface of the vertebral body. The pleural space lies lateral and anterior to the thoracic

sympathetic chain. Given the proximity of the thoracic somatic nerves to the thoracic sympathetic chain, the potential exists for both neural pathways to be blocked when performing blockade of the thoracic sympathetic ganglion.

SUGGESTED READINGS

Netter FH: Typical thoracic spinal nerve. In: Atlas of Human Anatomy, ed 4. Philadelphia, Saunders, 2006.

Waldman SD: Thoracic sympathetic ganglion block. In: Atlas of Interventional Pain Management, ed 2. Philadelphia, Saunders, 2004.

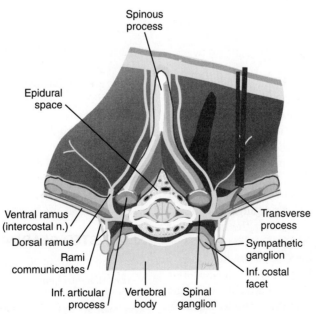

FIGURE 60–1 The thoracic sympathetic chain. (From Waldman SD: Atlas of Interventional Pain Management, ed 2. Philadelphia, Saunders, 2004, p 240.)

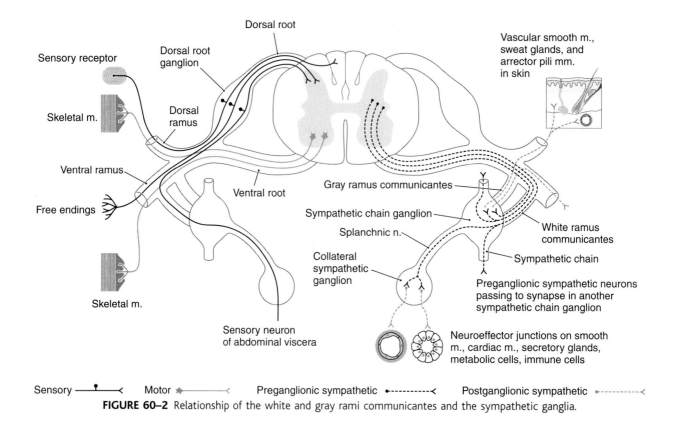

Sensory ————•——< Motor ★————< Preganglionic sympathetic •----------< Postganglionic sympathetic •----------<

FIGURE 60–2 Relationship of the white and gray rami communicantes and the sympathetic ganglia.

CHAPTER 61

The Splanchnic Nerves

The sympathetic innervation of the abdominal viscera originates in the anterolateral horn of the spinal cord. Preganglionic fibers from T5-12 exit the spinal cord in conjunction with the ventral roots to join the white communicating rami on their way to the sympathetic chain. Rather than synapsing with the sympathetic chain, these preganglionic fibers pass through it to ultimately synapse on the celiac ganglia. The greater, lesser, and least splanchnic nerves provide the major preganglionic contribution to the celiac plexus and transmit the majority of nociceptive information from the viscera. The splanchnic nerves are contained in a narrow compartment made up by the vertebral body and the pleura laterally, the posterior mediastinum ventrally, and the pleural attachment to the vertebra dorsally. This compartment is bounded caudally by the crura of the diaphragm. The volume of this compartment is approximately 10 mL on each side.

The greater splanchnic nerve has its origin from the T5-10 spinal roots (Fig. 61-1). The nerve travels along the thoracic paravertebral border through the crus of the diaphragm into the abdominal cavity, ending on the celiac ganglion of its respective side. The lesser splanchnic nerve arises from the T10-11 roots and passes with the greater nerve to end at the celiac ganglion. The least splanchnic nerve arises from the T11-12 spinal roots and passes through the diaphragm to the celiac ganglion.

SUGGESTED READINGS

Netter FH: Sympathetic nervous system: General topography. In: Atlas of Human Anatomy, ed 4. Philadelphia, Saunders, 2006.

Waldman SD: Splanchnic nerve block: Classic two-needle technique. In: Atlas of Interventional Pain Management, ed 2. Philadelphia, Saunders, 2004.

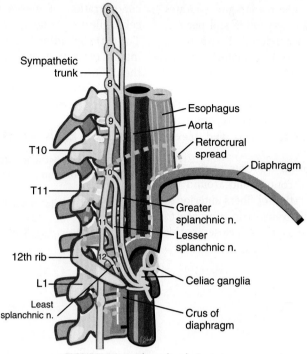

Sympathetic
trunk

Esophagus

Aorta

Retrocrural
spread

Diaphragm

T10

T11

Greater
splanchnic n.

Lesser
splanchnic n.

12th rib

L1

Celiac ganglia

Least
splanchnic n.

Crus of
diaphragm

FIGURE 61–1 The splanchnic nerves.

CHAPTER 62

The Celiac Plexus

The sympathetic innervation of the abdominal viscera originates in the anterolateral horn of the spinal cord. Preganglionic fibers from T5-12 exit the spinal cord in conjunction with the ventral roots to join the white communicating rami on their way to the sympathetic chain. Rather than synapsing with the sympathetic chain, these preganglionic fibers pass through it to ultimately synapse on the celiac ganglia. The greater, lesser, and least splanchnic nerves provide the major preganglionic contribution to the celiac plexus. The greater splanchnic nerve has its origin from the T5-10 spinal roots (Fig. 62-1). The nerve travels along the thoracic paravertebral border through the crus of the diaphragm into the abdominal cavity, ending on the celiac ganglion of its respective side. The lesser splanchnic nerve arises from the T10-11 roots and passes with the greater nerve to end at the celiac ganglion. The least splanchnic nerve arises from the T11-12 spinal roots and passes through the diaphragm to the celiac ganglion.

Interpatient anatomic variability of the celiac ganglia is significant, but the following generalizations can be drawn from anatomic studies of the celiac ganglia. The number of ganglia vary from one to five and range in diameter from 0.5 to 4.5 cm. The ganglia lie anterior and anterolateral to the aorta. The ganglia located on the left are uniformly more inferior than their right-sided counterparts by as much as a vertebral level, but both groups of ganglia lie below the level of the celiac artery. The ganglia usually lie approximately at the level of the first lumbar vertebra.

Postganglionic fibers radiate from the celiac ganglia to follow the course of the blood vessels to innervate the abdominal viscera (Fig. 62-2). These organs include much of the distal esophagus, stomach, duodenum, small intestine, ascending and proximal transverse colon, adrenal glands, pancreas, spleen, liver, and biliary system. It is these postganglionic fibers, the fibers arising from the preganglionic splanchnic nerves, and the celiac ganglion that make up the celiac plexus. The diaphragm separates the thorax from the abdominal cavity while still permitting the passage of the thoracoabdominal structures, including the aorta, vena cava, and splanchnic nerves. The diaphragmatic crura are bilateral structures that arise from the anterolateral surfaces of the upper two or three lumbar vertebrae and discs. The crura of the diaphragm serve as a barrier to effectively separate the splanchnic nerves from the celiac ganglia and plexus below.

The celiac plexus is anterior to the crus of the diaphragm. The plexus extends in front of and around the aorta, with the greatest concentration of fibers anterior to the aorta. With the single-needle transaortic approach to celiac plexus block, the needle is placed close to this concentration of plexus fibers. The relationship of the celiac plexus to the surrounding structures is as follows: The aorta lies anterior and slightly to the left of the anterior margin of the vertebral body. The inferior vena cava lies to the right, with the kidneys posterolateral to the great vessels. The pancreas lies anterior to the celiac plexus. All of these structures lie within the retroperitoneal space.

SUGGESTED READINGS

Netter FH: Sympathetic nervous system: General topography. In: Atlas of Human Anatomy, ed 4. Philadelphia, Saunders, 2006.

Waldman SD: Celiac nerve block: Classic two-needle retrocrural technique. In: Atlas of Interventional Pain Management, ed 2. Philadelphia, Saunders, 2004.

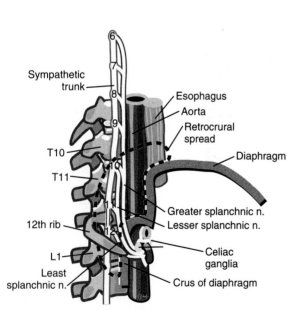

FIGURE 62–1 The celiac plexus. (From Waldman SD: Atlas of Interventional Pain Management, ed 2. Philadelphia, Saunders, 2004, p 268.)

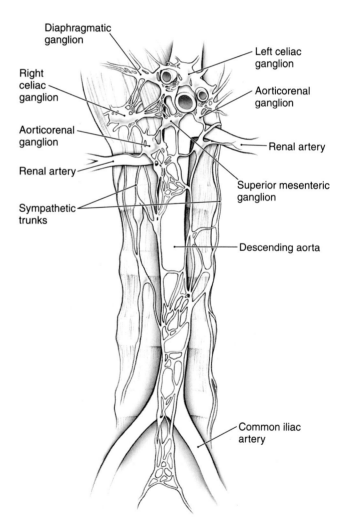

FIGURE 62–2 Relationship of the arteries, viscera, and sympathetic nerves.

CHAPTER 63

The Lumbar Sympathetic Nerves and Ganglia

The preganglionic fibers of the lumbar sympathetic nerves exit the intervertebral foramina along with the lumbar paravertebral nerves. After exiting the intervertebral foramen, the lumbar paravertebral nerve gives off a recurrent branch that loops back through the foramen to provide innervation to the spinal ligaments, meninges, and its respective vertebra. The upper lumbar paravertebral nerve also interfaces with the lumbar sympathetic chain via the myelinated preganglionic fibers of the white rami communicantes. All five of the lumbar nerves interface with the unmyelinated postganglionic fibers of the gray rami communicantes. At the level of the lumbar sympathetic ganglia, preganglionic and postganglionic fibers synapse (Fig. 63-1). Additionally, some of the postganglionic fibers return to their respective somatic nerves via the gray rami communicantes. Other lumbar sympathetic postganglionic fibers travel to the aortic and hypogastric plexus and course up and down the sympathetic trunk to terminate in distant ganglia.

In many patients, the first and second lumbar ganglia are fused. These ganglia and the remainder of the lumbar chain and ganglia lie at the anterolateral margin of the lumbar vertebral bodies. The peritoneal cavity lies lateral and anterior to the lumbar sympathetic chain. Given the proximity of the lumbar somatic nerves to the lumbar sympathetic chain, the potential exists for both neural pathways to be blocked when performing blockade of the lumbar sympathetic ganglion.

SUGGESTED READINGS

Netter FH: Autonomic nerves and ganglia of abdomen. In: Atlas of Human Anatomy, ed 4. Philadelphia, Saunders, 2006.

Waldman SD: Lumbar sympathetic nerve block. In: Atlas of Interventional Pain Management, ed 2. Philadelphia, Saunders, 2004.

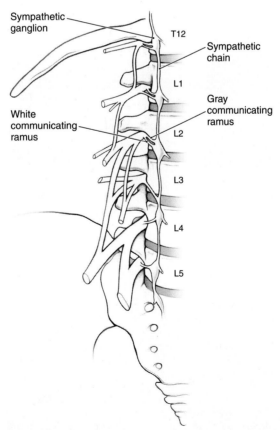

FIGURE 63–1 The lumbar sympathetic nerves and ganglia.

CHAPTER 64

The Lumbar Plexus

The lumbar plexus lies within the substance of the psoas muscle (Fig. 64-1). The plexus is made up of the ventral roots of the first four lumbar nerves and, in some patients, a contribution from the 12th thoracic nerve. The nerves lie in front of the transverse processes of their respective vertebrae; as they course inferolaterally, they divide into a number of peripheral nerves. The ilioinguinal and iliohypogastric nerves are branches of the L1 nerves, with an occasional contribution of fibers from T12. The genitofemoral nerve is made up of fibers from L1 and L2. The lateral femoral cutaneous nerve is derived from fibers of L2 and L3. The obturator nerve receives fibers from L2-4, and the femoral nerve is made up of fibers from L2-4. The pain management specialist should be aware of the considerable interpatient variability in terms of the actual spinal nerves that provide fibers to make up these peripheral branches. This variability means that differential neural blockade on an anatomic basis must be interpreted with caution.

The rationale behind lumbar plexus block using the psoas compartment technique is to block the nerves that compose the lumbar plexus because they lie enclosed by the vertebral bodies medially, the quadratus lumborum laterally, and the psoas major muscle ventrally. Solutions injected in this "compartment" flow caudally and cranially to bathe the lumbar nerve roots just as they enter the psoas muscle.

SUGGESTED READINGS

Netter FH: Lumbar plexus in situ. In: Atlas of Human Anatomy, ed 4. Philadelphia, Saunders, 2006.

Waldman SD: Lumbar plexus block. In: Atlas of Interventional Pain Management, ed 2. Philadelphia, Saunders, 2004.

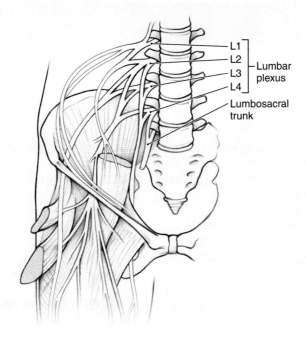

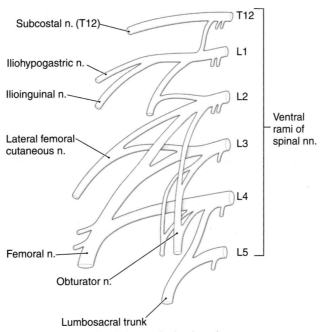

FIGURE 64–1 The lumbar plexus.

CHAPTER 65

The Sciatic Nerve

The sciatic nerve innervates the distal lower extremity and foot with the exception of the medial aspect of the calf and foot, which are subserved by the saphenous nerve (Fig. 65-1). The largest nerve in the body, the sciatic nerve is derived from the L4, L5, and S1-3 nerve roots. The roots fuse together in front of the anterior surface of the lateral sacrum on the anterior surface of the piriform muscle. The nerve travels inferiorly and leaves the pelvis just below the piriform muscle via the sciatic notch. The sciatic nerve lies anterior to the gluteus maximus muscle and, at this muscle's lower border, lies halfway between the greater trochanter and the ischial tuberosity. The sciatic nerve courses downward past the lesser trochanter to lie posterior and medial to the femur (Fig. 65-2). In the mid-thigh, the nerve gives off branches to the hamstring muscles and the adductor magnus muscle. In most patients, the nerve divides to form the tibial and common peroneal nerves in the upper portion of the popliteal fossa, although these nerves sometimes remain separate through their entire course. The tibial nerve continues downward to innervate the distal lower extremity, whereas the common peroneal nerve travels laterally to innervate a portion of the knee joint and, via its lateral cutaneous branch, provides sensory innervation to the back and lateral side of the upper calf.

SUGGESTED READINGS

Netter FH: Nerves of hip and buttock. In: Atlas of Human Anatomy, ed 4. Philadelphia, Saunders, 2006.

Waldman SD: Sciatic nerve block: The anterior approach. In: Atlas of Interventional Pain Management, ed 2. Philadelphia, Saunders, 2004.

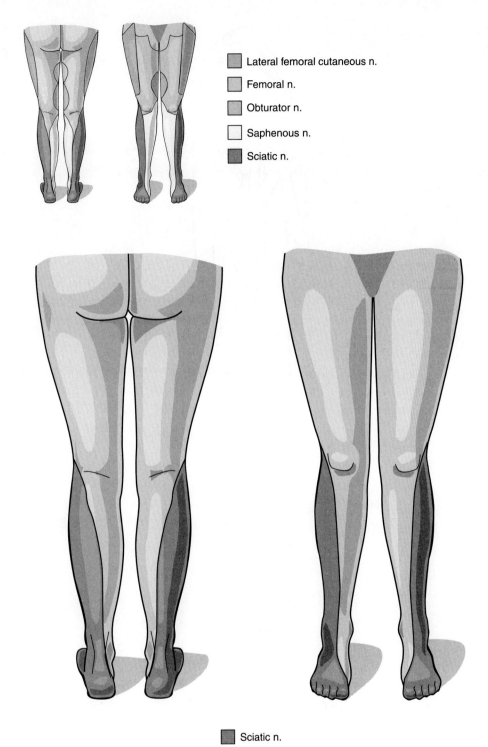

Lateral femoral cutaneous n.

Femoral n.

Obturator n.

Saphenous n.

Sciatic n.

Sciatic n.

FIGURE 65–1 The sciatic nerve. (From Waldman SD: Atlas of Interventional Pain Management, ed 2. Philadelphia, Saunders, 2004, p 467.)

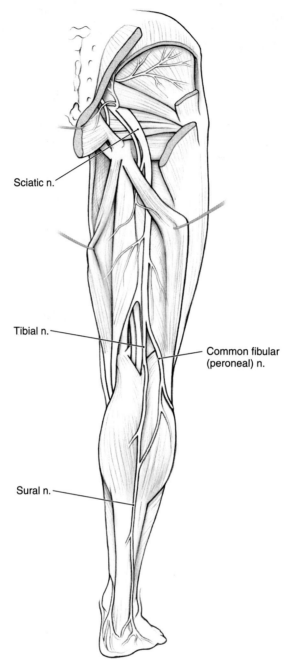

FIGURE 65–2 The courses of the sciatic nerve.

The Femoral Nerve

The femoral nerve innervates the anterior portion of the thigh and medial calf. The femoral nerve is derived from the posterior branches of the L2, L3, and L4 nerve roots. The roots fuse together in the psoas muscle and descend laterally between the psoas and iliacus muscles to enter the iliac fossa. The femoral nerve gives off motor fibers to the iliac muscle and then passes beneath the inguinal ligament to enter the thigh (Fig. 66-1). The femoral nerve is just lateral to the femoral artery as it passes beneath the inguinal ligament and is enclosed with the femoral artery and vein within the femoral sheath. The nerve gives off motor fibers to the sartorius, quadriceps femoris, and pectineus muscles. It also provides sensory fibers to the knee joint as well as the skin overlying the anterior thigh (Fig. 66-2). The nerve is easily blocked as it passes through the femoral triangle.

SUGGESTED READINGS

Netter FH: Arteries and nerves of thigh: Anterior view. In: Atlas of Human Anatomy, ed 4. Philadelphia, Saunders, 2006.
Waldman SD: Femoral nerve block. In: Atlas of Interventional Pain Management, ed 2. Philadelphia, Saunders, 2004.

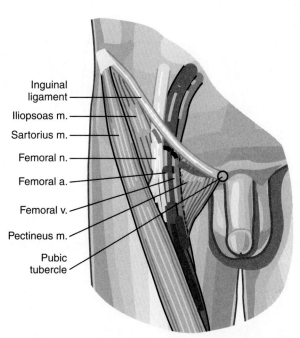

Inguinal ligament
Iliopsoas m.
Sartorius m.
Femoral n.
Femoral a.
Femoral v.
Pectineus m.
Pubic tubercle

FIGURE 66–1 The femoral nerve. (From Waldman SD: Femoral nerve block. In: Atlas of Interventional Pain Management, ed 2. Philadelphia, Saunders, 2004, p 452.)

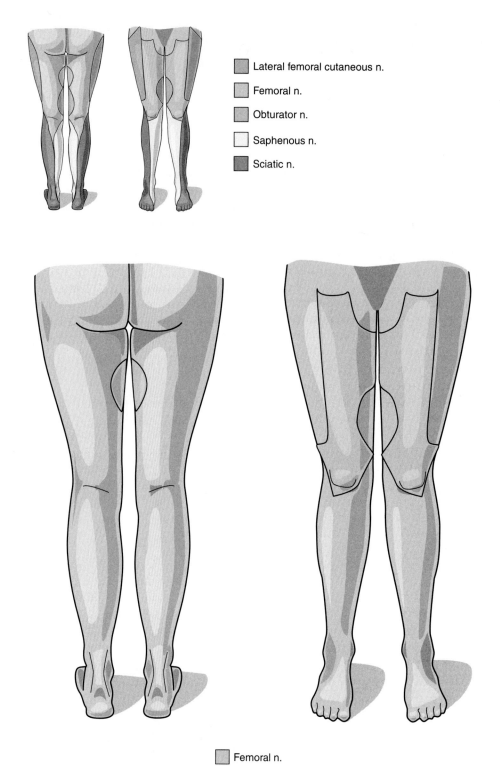

FIGURE 66–2 Sensory distribution of the femoral nerve. (From Waldman SD: Femoral nerve block. In: Atlas of Interventional Pain Management, ed 2. Philadelphia, Saunders, 2004, p 450.)

CHAPTER 67

The Lateral Femoral Cutaneous Nerve

The lateral femoral cutaneous nerve is formed from the posterior divisions of the L2 and L3 nerves. The nerve leaves the psoas muscle and courses laterally and inferiorly to pass just beneath the ilioinguinal nerve at the level of the anterior superior iliac spine. The nerve passes under the inguinal ligament and then travels beneath the fascia lata, where it divides into an anterior and a posterior branch (Fig. 67-1). The anterior branch provides limited cutaneous sensory innervation over the anterolateral thigh (Fig. 67-2). The posterior branch provides cutaneous sensory innervation to the lateral thigh from just above the greater trochanter to the knee. Entrapment of the lateral femoral cutaneous nerve is known as meralgia paresthetica.

SUGGESTED READINGS

Netter FH: Arteries and nerves of thigh: Anterior view. In: Atlas of Human Anatomy, ed 4. Philadelphia, Saunders, 2006.

Waldman SD: Lateral femoral cutaneous nerve block: The anterior approach. In: Atlas of Interventional Pain Management, ed 2. Philadelphia, Saunders, 2004.

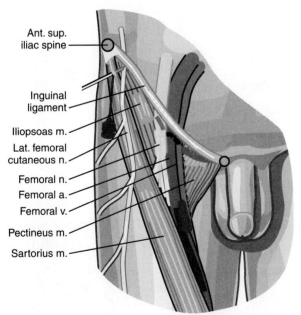

FIGURE 67–1 Lateral femoral cutaneous nerve. (From Waldman SD: Lateral femoral cutaneous nerve block. In: Atlas of Interventional Pain Management, ed 2. Philadelphia, Saunders, 2004, p 457.)

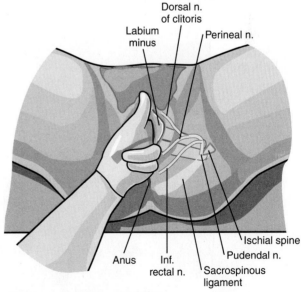

FIGURE 67–2 Sensory distribution of the lateral femoral cutaneous nerve. (From Waldman SD: Lateral femoral cutaneous nerve block. In: Atlas of Interventional Pain Management, ed 2. Philadelphia, Saunders, 2004, p 455.)

CHAPTER **68**

The Ilioinguinal Nerve

The ilioinguinal nerve is a branch of the L1 nerve root with a contribution from T12 in some patients. The nerve follows a curvilinear course that takes it from its origin in the L1 and occasionally T12 somatic nerves to inside the concavity of the ilium. The ilioinguinal nerve continues anteriorly to perforate the transverse abdominis muscle at the level of the anterior superior iliac spine (Fig. 68-1). The nerve may interconnect with the iliohypogastric nerve as it continues to pass along its course medially and inferiorly, where it accompanies the spermatic cord through the inguinal ring and into the inguinal canal. The distribution of the sensory innervation of the ilioinguinal nerves varies from patient to patient because there may be considerable overlap with the iliohypogastric nerve. In general, the ilioinguinal nerve provides sensory innervation to the upper portion of the skin of the inner thigh and the root of the penis and upper scrotum in men or the mons pubis and lateral labia in women (Fig. 68-2). Entrapment of the ilioinguinal nerve is known as ilioinguinal neuralgia.

SUGGESTED READINGS

Netter FH: Arteries and nerves of thigh: Anterior view. In: Atlas of Human Anatomy, ed 4. Philadelphia, Saunders, 2006.
Waldman SD: Ilioinguinal nerve block. In: Atlas of Interventional Pain Management, ed 2. Philadelphia, Saunders, 2004.

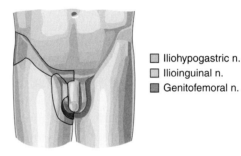

☐ Iliohypogastric n.
☐ Ilioinguinal n.
☐ Genitofemoral n.

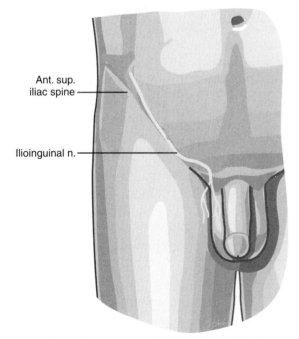

Ant. sup. iliac spine

Ilioinguinal n.

FIGURE 68–1 Ilioinguinal nerve. (From Waldman SD: Ilioinguinal nerve block. In: Atlas of Interventional Pain Management, ed 2. Philadelphia, Saunders, 2004, p 297.)

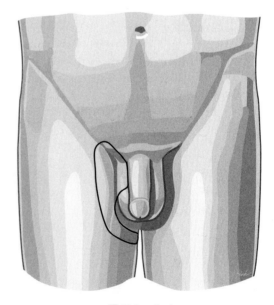

☐ Ilioinguinal n.

FIGURE 68–2 Sensory distribution of the ilioinguinal nerve. (From Waldman SD: Ilioinguinal nerve block. In: Atlas of Interventional Pain Management, ed 2. Philadelphia, Saunders, 2004, p 295.)

The Iliohypogastric Nerve

The iliohypogastric nerve is a branch of the L1 nerve root with a contribution from T12 in some patients. The nerve follows a curvilinear course that takes it from its origin in the L1 and occasionally T12 somatic nerves to inside the concavity of the ilium. The iliohypogastric nerve continues anteriorly to perforate the transverse abdominis muscle to lie between it and the external oblique muscle (Fig. 69-1). At this point, the iliohypogastric nerve divides into an anterior and a lateral branch. The lateral branch provides cutaneous sensory innervation to the posterolateral gluteal region. The anterior branch pierces the external oblique muscle just beyond the anterior superior iliac spine to provide cutaneous sensory innervation to the abdominal skin above the pubis (Fig. 69-2). The nerve may interconnect with the ilioinguinal nerve along its course, resulting in variation of the distribution of the sensory innervation of the iliohypogastric and ilioinguinal nerves. Entrapment of the iliohypogastric nerve is known as iliohypogastric neuralgia.

SUGGESTED READINGS

Netter FH: Arteries and nerves of thigh: Anterior view. In: Atlas of Human Anatomy, ed 4. Philadelphia, Saunders, 2006.

Waldman SD: Iliohypogastric nerve block. In: Atlas of Interventional Pain Management, ed 2. Philadelphia, Saunders, 2004.

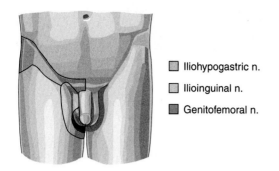

☐ Iliohypogastric n.

☐ Ilioinguinal n.

☐ Genitofemoral n.

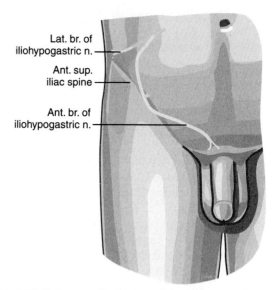

Lat. br. of
iliohypogastric n. —

Ant. sup.
iliac spine —

Ant. br. of
iliohypogastric n. —

FIGURE 69–2 Sensory distribution of the iliohypogastric nerve. (From Waldman SD: Iliohypogastric nerve block. In: Atlas of Interventional Pain Management, ed 2. Philadelphia, Saunders, 2004, p 299.)

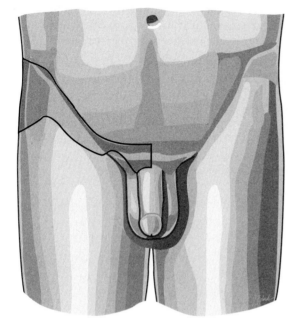

☐ Iliohypogastric n.

FIGURE 69–1 Iliohypogastric nerve. (From Waldman SD: Iliohypogastric nerve block. In: Atlas of Interventional Pain Management, ed 2. Philadelphia, Saunders, 2004, p 301.)

CHAPTER **70**

The Genitofemoral Nerve

The genitofemoral nerve is a branch of the L1 nerve root with a contribution from T12 in some patients. The nerve follows a curvilinear course that takes it from its origin in the L1 and occasionally T12 and L2 somatic nerves to inside the concavity of the ilium. The genitofemoral nerve descends obliquely in an anterior course through the psoas major muscle to emerge on the abdominal surface opposite L3 or L4 (Fig. 70-1). The nerve descends subperitoneally behind the ureter and divides into a genital and femoral branch just above the inguinal ligament. In males, the genital branch travels through the inguinal canal passing inside the deep inguinal ring to innervate the cremaster muscle and skin of the scrotum (Fig. 70-2). In females, the genital branch follows the course of the round ligament and provides innervation to the ipsilateral mons pubis and labia majora. In males and females, the femoral branch descends lateral to the external iliac artery to pass behind the inguinal ligament. The nerve enters the femoral sheath lateral to the femoral artery to innervate the skin of the anterior superior femoral triangle.

SUGGESTED READINGS

Netter FH: Arteries and nerves of thigh: Anterior view. In: Atlas of Human Anatomy, ed 4. Philadelphia, Saunders, 2006.
Waldman SD: Genitofemoral nerve block. In: Atlas of Interventional Pain Management, ed 2. Philadelphia, Saunders, 2004.

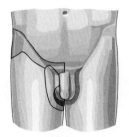

☐ Iliohypogastric n.
☐ Ilioinguinal n.
■ Genitofemoral n.

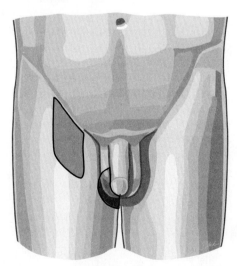

■ Genitofemoral n.

FIGURE 70–1 Genitofemoral nerve. (From Waldman SD: Genitofemoral nerve block. In: Atlas of Interventional Pain Management, ed 2. Philadelphia, Saunders, 2004, p 305.)

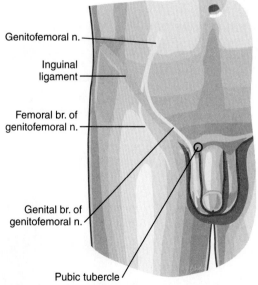

Genitofemoral n.

Inguinal ligament

Femoral br. of genitofemoral n.

Genital br. of genitofemoral n.

Pubic tubercle

FIGURE 70–2 Sensory distribution of the genitofemoral nerve. (From Waldman SD: Genitofemoral nerve block. In: Atlas of Interventional Pain Management, ed 2. Philadelphia, Saunders, 2004, p 303.)

CHAPTER **71**

The Obturator Nerve

The obturator nerve provides the majority of innervation to the hip joint. It is derived from the posterior divisions of the L2, L3, and L4 nerves. The nerve leaves the medial border psoas muscle and courses inferiorly to pass the pelvis, where it joins the obturator vessels to travel via the obturator canal to enter the thigh (Fig. 71-1). The nerve then divides into an anterior and posterior branch. The anterior branch supplies an articular branch to provide sensory innervation to the hip joint, motor branches to the superficial hip adductors, and a cutaneous branch to the medial aspect of the distal thigh (Fig. 71-2).

The posterior branch provides motor innervation to the deep hip adductors and an articular branch to the posterior knee joint.

SUGGESTED READINGS

Netter FH: Arteries and nerves of thigh: Anterior view. In: Atlas of Human Anatomy, ed 4. Philadelphia, Saunders, 2006.

Waldman SD: Obturator nerve block. In: Atlas of Interventional Pain Management, ed 2. Philadelphia, Saunders, 2004.

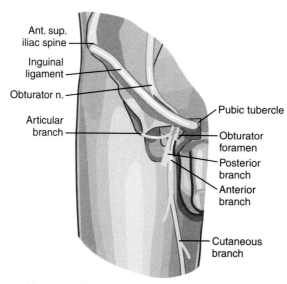

FIGURE 71–1 Obturator nerve. (From Waldman SD: Obturator nerve block. In: Atlas of Interventional Pain Management, ed 2. Philadelphia, Saunders, 2004, p 461.)

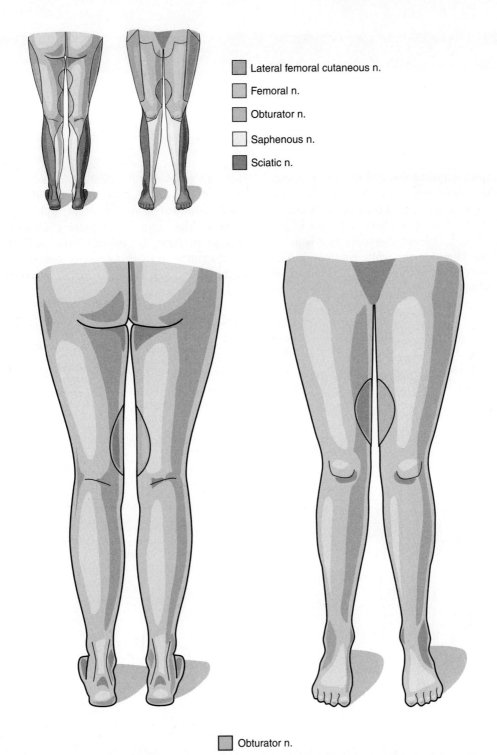

Lateral femoral cutaneous n.

Femoral n.

Obturator n.

Saphenous n.

Sciatic n.

Obturator n.

FIGURE 71–2 Sensory distribution of the obturator nerve. (From Waldman SD: Obturator nerve block: The anterior approach. In: Atlas of Interventional Pain Management, ed 2. Philadelphia, Saunders, 2004, p 459.)

CHAPTER 72

The Hypogastric Plexus and Nerves

The hypogastric plexus can be thought of as a continuation of the lumbar sympathetic chain. The preganglionic fibers of the hypogastric plexus find their origin primarily in the lower thoracic and upper lumbar region of the spinal cord. These preganglionic fibers interface with the lumbar sympathetic chain via the white communicantes. Postganglionic fibers exit the lumbar sympathetic chain and, together with fibers from the parasympathetic sacral ganglion, make up the superior hypogastric plexus (Fig. 72-1).

The superior hypogastric plexus lies in front of L4 as a coalescence of fibers. As these fibers descend, at a level of L5, they begin to divide into the hypogastric nerves following in close proximity the iliac vessels. As the hypogastric nerves continue their lateral and inferior course, they are accessible for neural blockade as they pass in front of the L5-S1 interspace. The hypogastric nerves pass downward from this point, following the concave curve of the sacrum and passing on each side of the rectum to form the inferior hypogastric plexus. These nerves continue their downward course along each side of the bladder to provide innervation to the pelvic viscera and vasculature (Fig. 72-2).

SUGGESTED READINGS

Netter FH: Nerves of large intestine. In: Atlas of Human Anatomy, ed 4. Philadelphia, Saunders, 2006.
Waldman SD: Hypogastric plexus block. In: Atlas of Interventional Pain Management, ed 2. Philadelphia, Saunders, 2004.

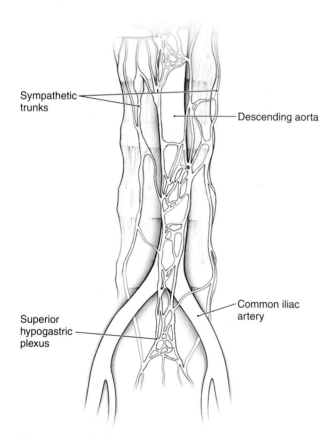

FIGURE 72–1 The hypogastric plexus.

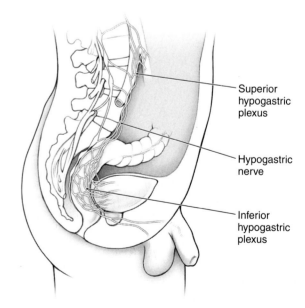

FIGURE 72–2 Sensory distribution of the hypogastric plexus.

CHAPTER **73**

The Ganglion of Impar

The lumbar sympathetic chains continue their inferior path into the pelvis traveling in front of the sacrum. Each pelvic portion of the sympathetic chain is made up of four or five ganglia that are connected together with interganglionic cords with the terminal ganglia serving as a terminal coalescence known as the ganglion of Impar (also known as the ganglion of Walther). The ganglion of Impar lies in front of the coccyx just below the sacrococcygeal junction and is amenable to blockade at this level (Fig. 73-1). The ganglion receives fibers from the lumbar and sacral portions of the sympathetic and parasympathetic nervous systems and provides sympathetic innervation to portions of the pelvic viscera and genitalia.

SUGGESTED READINGS

Netter FH: Nerves of large intestine. In: Atlas of Human Anatomy, ed 4. Philadelphia, Saunders, 2006.

Waldman SD: Ganglion of Walther (Impar) block. In: Atlas of Interventional Pain Management, ed 2. Philadelphia, Saunders, 2004.

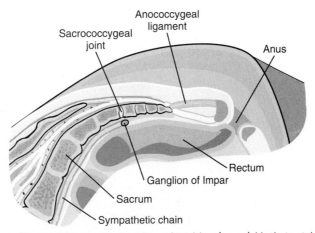

FIGURE 73–1 The ganglion of Impar. (From Waldman SD: Ganglion of Walther (Impar) block. In: Atlas of Interventional Pain Management, ed 2. Philadelphia, Saunders, 2004, p 421.)

CHAPTER 74

The Tibial Nerve

The tibial nerve is one of the two major continuations of the sciatic nerve, the other being the common peroneal nerve. The tibial nerve provides sensory innervation to the posterior portion of the calf, the heel, and the medial plantar surface (Fig. 74-1). The tibial nerve splits from the sciatic nerve at the superior margin of the popliteal fossa and descends in a slightly medial course through the popliteal fossa (Fig. 74-2). The tibial nerve block at the knee lies just beneath the popliteal fascia and is readily accessible for neural blockade. The tibial nerve continues its downward course, running between the two heads of the gastrocnemius muscle, passing deep to the soleus muscle. The nerve courses medially between the Achilles tendon and the medial malleolus, where it divides into the medial and lateral plantar nerves, providing sensory innervation to the heel and medial plantar surface (see Fig. 74-1; Fig. 74-3). The tibial nerve is occasionally subject to compression at this point and is known as posterior tarsal tunnel syndrome.

SUGGESTED READINGS

Netter FH: Arteries and nerves of thigh: Posterior views. In: Atlas of Human Anatomy, ed 4. Philadelphia, Saunders, 2006.

Waldman SD: Tibial nerve block at the knee. In: Atlas of Interventional Pain Management, ed 2. Philadelphia, Saunders, 2004.

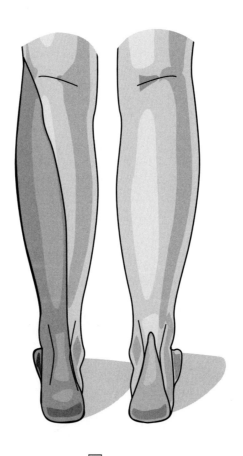

☐ Tibial n.

■ Sciatic n.

FIGURE 74–1 Sensory distribution of the tibial nerve. (From Waldman SD: Tibial nerve block at the knee. In: Atlas of Interventional Pain Management, ed 2. Philadelphia, Saunders, 2004, p 478.)

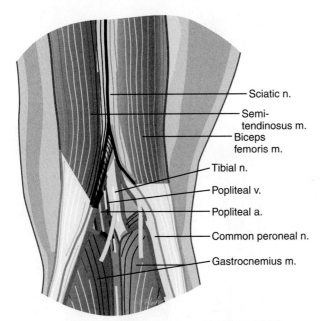

Sciatic n.

Semi-
tendinosus m.

Biceps
femoris m.

Tibial n.

Popliteal v.

Popliteal a.

Common peroneal n.

Gastrocnemius m.

FIGURE 74–2 The tibial nerve. (From Waldman SD: Tibial nerve block at the knee. In: Atlas of Interventional Pain Management, ed 2. Philadelphia, Saunders, 2004, p 480.)

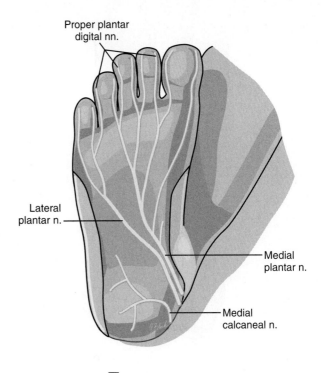

Proper plantar
digital nn.

Lateral
plantar n.

Medial
plantar n.

Medial
calcaneal n.

☐ Tibial n.

FIGURE 74–3 Sensory distribution of the medial and lateral plantar nerves. (From Waldman SD: Tibial nerve block at the knee. In: Atlas of Interventional Pain Management, ed 2. Philadelphia, Saunders, 2004, p 480.)

CHAPTER 75

The Common Peroneal Nerve

The common peroneal nerve is one of the two major continuations of the sciatic nerve, the other being the tibial nerve. The common peroneal nerve provides sensory innervation to the inferior portion of the knee joint and the posterior and lateral skin of the upper calf (Fig. 75-1). The common peroneal nerve is derived from the posterior branches of the L4, the L5, and the S1 and S2 nerve roots. The nerve splits from the sciatic nerve at the superior margin of the popliteal fossa and descends laterally behind the head of the fibula (Fig. 75-2). The common peroneal nerve is subject to compression at this point by such circumstances as improperly applied casts and tourniquets. The nerve is also subject to compression as it continues its lateral course, winding around the fibula through the fibular tunnel, which is made up of the posterior border of the tendinous insertion of the peroneus longus muscle and the fibula itself. Just distal to the fibular tunnel the nerve divides into its two terminal branches, the superficial and the deep peroneal nerves. Each of these branches is subject to trauma and may be blocked individually as a diagnostic and therapeutic maneuver.

SUGGESTED READINGS

Netter FH: Arteries and nerves of thigh: Posterior views. In: Atlas of Human Anatomy, ed 4. Philadelphia, Saunders, 2006.

Waldman SD: Common peroneal nerve block at the knee. In: Atlas of Interventional Pain Management, ed 2. Philadelphia, Saunders, 2004.

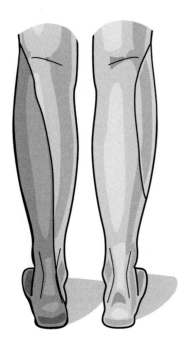
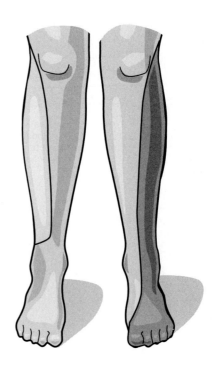

☐ Common peroneal n.

■ Sciatic n.

FIGURE 75–1 Sensory distribution of the common peroneal nerve. (From Waldman SD: Common peroneal nerve block at the knee. In: Atlas of Interventional Pain Management, ed 2. Philadelphia, Saunders, 2004, p 496.)

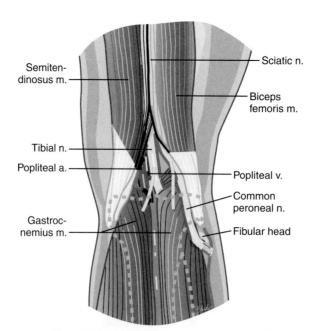

FIGURE 75–2 The common peroneal nerve. (From Waldman SD: Common peroneal nerve block at the knee. In: Atlas of Interventional Pain Management, ed 2. Philadelphia, Saunders, 2004, p 497.)

CHAPTER 76

Functional Anatomy of the Hip

The hip is a ball-and-socket–type joint that is composed of the femoral head and the cup-shaped acetabulum (Fig. 76-1). The femoral head is completely covered with hyaline cartilage except for a central area called the fovea, which is the point of attachment for the ligamentum teres. In contradistinction to its homologue, the glenoid fossa of the shoulder, which is very shallow, the acetabulum, which is composed of the confluence of the ilium, ischium, and pubic bones, is much deeper. This deeper, cup-shaped configuration of the acetabulum adds much stability to the hip joint compared with the shoulder, whose stability is due primarily to the ligaments and labrum. The cup of the acetabulum is endowed with a horseshoe-shaped articular cartilage with the open portion of the horseshoe allowing passage of the ligamentum teres (Fig. 76-2). Within the ligamentum teres is the central branch of the obturator artery, which provides blood supply to fovea of the femoral head. This blood supply is very susceptible to disruption from trauma and, if compromised, may cause avascular osteonecrosis of the femoral head (Fig. 76-3).

The femoral head is connected to the femoral shaft by the neck of the femur, which in health forms an angle of 125 to 140 degrees with the femoral shaft and serves to align the femoral head in the coronal plane with the femoral condyles in the standing adult. There are two major bony outcroppings at the junction of the femoral neck and shaft of the femur—the greater trochanter and the lesser trochanter. The greater trochanter on the lateral femoral neck serves as the attachment point for the gluteal muscles, and the medially situated lesser trochanter serves as the attachment point for the hip adductors (see Fig. 76-3).

The hip joint is further strengthened by a fibrous articular capsule and a trio of ligaments—the iliofemoral, ischiofemoral, and pubofemoral ligaments. The iliofemoral ligament provides support anteriorly, with the ischiofemoral and pubofemoral ligaments providing the majority of posterior support.

The muscles of the hip provide movement in three planes: (1) flexion and extension, (2) adduction and abduction, and (3) internal and external rotation. Flexion of the hip is provided primarily by the iliopsoas muscle, with extension provided primarily by the gluteus maximus and hamstrings. Abduction of the hip is primarily provided by the gluteus medius and gluteus medius muscles, with adduction provided primarily by the adductor brevis and longus muscles. External rotation is provided primarily by the obturator, quadratus femoris, and gemelli muscles, with internal rotation provided by the tensor fascia lata, gluteus medius, and gluteus minimus muscles. Movement of these muscles is facilitated by a number of bursae, which are subject to inflammation and can serve as a nidus of hip dysfunction and pain.

SUGGESTED READINGS

Netter FH: Femur. In: Atlas of Human Anatomy, ed 4. Philadelphia, Saunders, 2006.

Waldman SD: Clinical correlates: Functional anatomy of the hip. In: Physical Diagnosis of Pain: An Atlas of Signs and Symptoms. Philadelphia, Saunders, 2006.

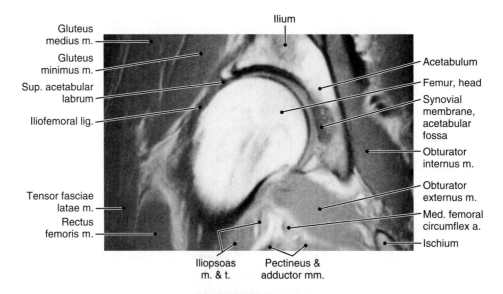

Gluteus medius m.
Gluteus minimus m.
Sup. acetabular labrum
Iliofemoral lig.
Tensor fasciae latae m.
Rectus femoris m.
Ilium
Acetabulum
Femur, head
Synovial membrane, acetabular fossa
Obturator internus m.
Obturator externus m.
Med. femoral circumflex a.
Ischium
Iliopsoas m. & t.
Pectineus & adductor mm.

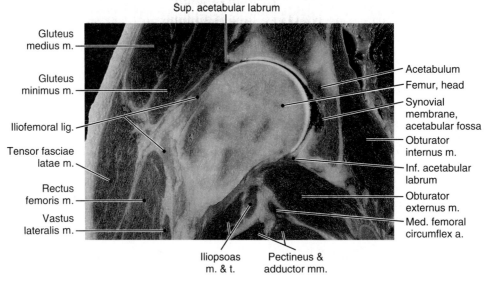

Sup. acetabular labrum
Gluteus medius m.
Gluteus minimus m.
Iliofemoral lig.
Tensor fasciae latae m.
Rectus femoris m.
Vastus lateralis m.
Acetabulum
Femur, head
Synovial membrane, acetabular fossa
Obturator internus m.
Inf. acetabular labrum
Obturator externus m.
Med. femoral circumflex a.
Iliopsoas m. & t.
Pectineus & adductor mm.

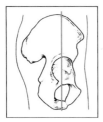

FIGURE 76–1 Hip, coronal view. (From Kang HS, Ahn JM, Resnik D: MRI of the Extremities: An Anatomic Atlas, ed 2. Philadelphia, Saunders, 2002, p 226.)

Hip, transverse

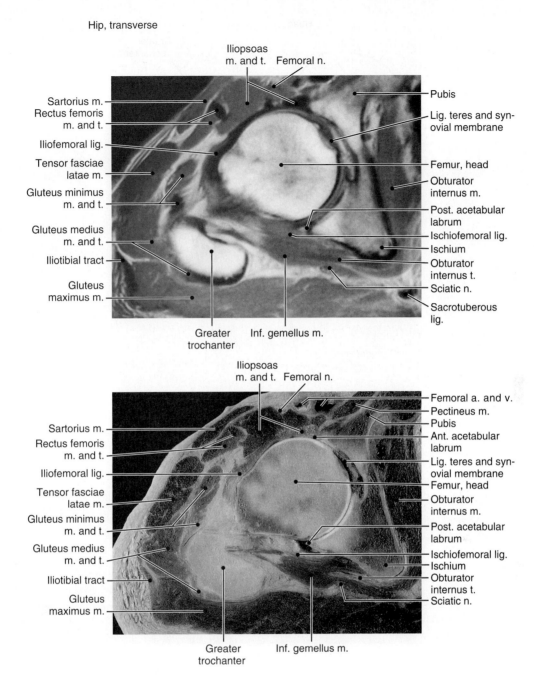

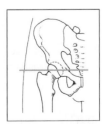

FIGURE 76–2 Hip, transverse view. (From Kang HS, Ahn JM, Resnik D: MRI of the Extremities: An Anatomic Atlas, ed 2. Philadelphia, Saunders, 2002, p 240.)

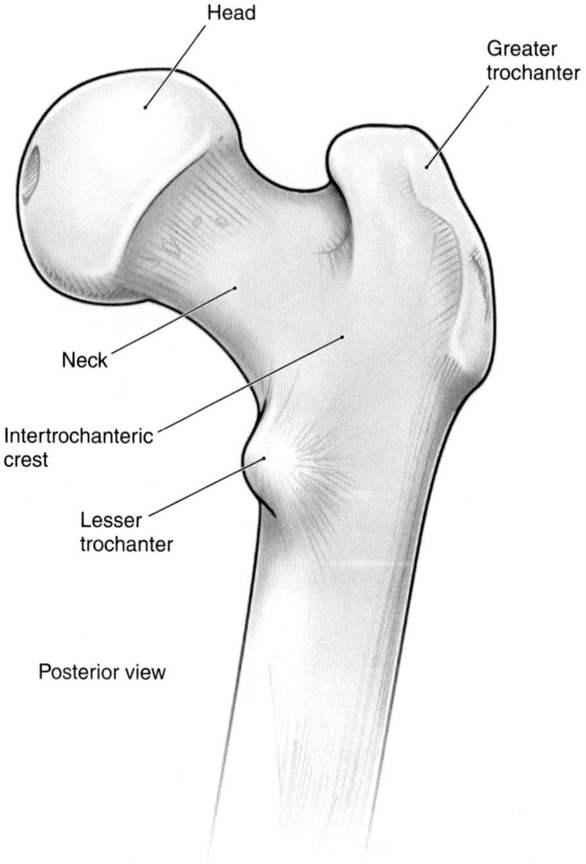

FIGURE 76–3 The proximal femur.

CHAPTER 77

The Ischial Bursa

The ischial bursa lies between the gluteus maximus muscle and the ischial tuberosity (Fig. 77-1). The action of the gluteus maximus muscle includes the flexion of trunk on thigh when maintaining a sitting position when riding a horse. This action can irritate the ischial bursa, as can repeated pressure against the bursa forcing it against the ischial tuberosity. The hamstring muscles find a common origin at the ischial tuberosity and can be irritated from overuse or misuse. The action of the hamstrings includes flexion of the lower extremity at the knee. Running on soft or uneven surfaces can cause a tendinitis at the origin of the hamstring muscles.

SUGGESTED READING

Waldman SD. Ischial bursitis pain. In: Atlas of Pain Management Injection Techniques, ed 2. Philadelphia, Saunders, 2007.

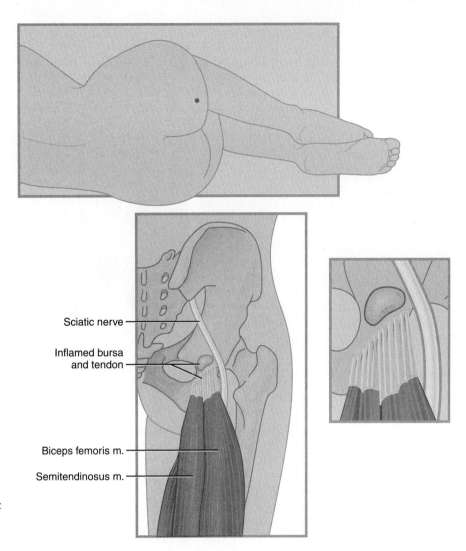

FIGURE 77–1 The ischial bursa. (From Waldman SD: Atlas of Pain Management Injection Techniques, ed 2. Philadelphia, Saunders, 2007, p 347.)

Sciatic nerve

Inflamed bursa and tendon

Biceps femoris m.

Semitendinosus m.

CHAPTER 78

The Gluteal Bursa

The gluteal bursae lie between the gluteal maximus, medius, and minimus muscles as well as between these muscles and the underlying bone (Fig. 78-1). These bursae may exist as a single bursal sac or in some patients may exist as a multisegmented series of sacs which may be loculated in nature. There is significant intrapatient variability in the size, number, and location of the gluteal bursae. The action of the gluteus maximus muscle includes the flexion of trunk on thigh when maintaining a sitting position when riding a horse. This action can irritate the gluteal bursae, as can repeated trauma from repetitive activity, including running.

SUGGESTED READING

Waldman SD: Gluteal bursitis pain. In: Atlas of Pain Management Injection Techniques, ed 2. Philadelphia, Saunders, 2007.

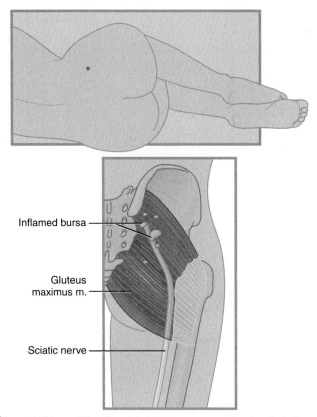

FIGURE 78–1 The gluteal bursa. (From Waldman SD: Atlas of Pain Management Injection Techniques, ed 2. Philadelphia, Saunders, 2007, p 351.)

Inflamed bursa

Gluteus maximus m.

Sciatic nerve

CHAPTER 79

The Trochanteric Bursa

The trochanteric bursa lies between the greater trochanter and the tendon of the gluteus medius and the iliotibial tract (Fig. 79-1). The gluteus medius muscle has its origin from the outer surface of the ilium, and its fibers pass downward and laterally to attach on the lateral surface of the greater trochanter. The gluteus medius locks the pelvis in place when walking and running. This action can irritate the trochanteric bursa, as can repeated trauma from repetitive activity, including jogging on soft or uneven surfaces or overuse of exercise equipment for lower extremity strengthening. The gluteus medius muscle is innervated by the superior gluteal nerve.

SUGGESTED READING

Waldman SD: Trochanteric bursitis pain. In: Waldman SD: Atlas of Pain Management Injection Techniques, ed 2. Philadelphia, Saunders, 2007.

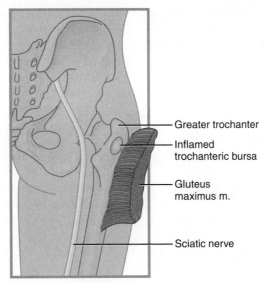

FIGURE 79–1 The trochanteric bursa. (From Waldman SD: Atlas of Pain Management Injection Techniques, ed 2. Philadelphia, Saunders, 2007, p 365.)

CHAPTER 80

Functional Anatomy of the Sacroiliac Joint

The axial spine rests on the sacrum, a triangular fusion of vertebrae arranged in a kyphotic curve and ending with the attached coccyx in the upper buttock. Iliac wings (innominate bones) attach on either side, forming a bowl with a high back and a shallow front. Three joints result from this union: the pubic symphysis in the anterior midline and the left and right sacroiliac joints in the back (Fig. 80-1). Multiple ligaments and fascia attach across these joint spaces, limiting motion and providing stability (Figs. 80-2 and 80-3). The hip joints are formed by the femoral heads and the acetabular sockets deep within the innominate bones. The hips create a direct link between the lower extremities and the spine, to relay ground reaction forces from weight bearing and motion. A physiologic balance between lumbar lordosis and sacral curvature exists both at rest and in motion. Changes in pelvic tilt and lumbar lordosis occur in the anteroposterior (AP) plane, relying on attached muscles and fascia, but do not have a significant effect on the sacroiliac joints owing to a self-bracing mechanism. The sacrum positioned between the innominate bones functions as a keystone in an arch, allowing only cephalocaudad (CC) and AP motion.

Innervation is varied and extensive owing to the size of this joint, which includes outflow from anterior and posterior rami of L3-S1.

The sacroiliac is a synovial (diarthrodial) joint that is more mobile in youth than later in life. The upper two thirds of the joint becomes more fibrotic in adulthood. The female pelvis is also more mobile to accommodate pregnancy and parturition. Ligament and muscle attachments help to maintain stability of the pelvic ring latissimus, allowing movement within limits. Further motion is also limited by the irregular shape of the joint articulation, in which ridges and grooves increase resistance friction and add to the keystone arch structure. Prolonged loading (such as standing or sitting for long periods) and alterations of the sacral base (leg asymmetry or ligamentous injury) are associated with joint hypermobility and resultant low back pain.

Multiple muscle attachments cross the sacroiliac joints and contribute to pelvic stability and force transfer. The thoracolumbar fascia includes attachments to the 12th rib, lumbar spinous and lateral processes, and pelvic brim. Fascial and muscle attachments expand to include erector spinae, internal obliques, serratus posterior inferior, sacrotuberous ligament, dorsal sacroiliac ligament, iliolumbar ligament, posterior iliac spine, and sacral crest. Major muscles attached to the sacroiliac include the gluteus maximus, gluteus medius, latissimus dorsi, multifidus, biceps femoris, psoas, piriformis, obliquus, and transversus abdominis. The purpose of these muscles is not for motion but to confer stability for loading and unloading forces produced by walking and running.

Motion

Ligaments also limit mobility of the sacroiliac joint and functionally comprise the distal two thirds of the joint. Motion is described in three dimensions: AP, CC, and left-right (LR). The major ligaments and their actions are listed next (see Figs. 80-2 and 80-3).

1. The interosseous ligament resists joint separation and motion in the cephalad or AP directions.
2. Dorsal sacroiliac ligament covers and assists the interosseous ligament.
3. The anterior sacroiliac ligament, a thickening of the anterior inferior joint capsule, resists CC and LR motion.
4. The sacrospinous ligament resists rotational motion of the pelvis around the axial spine.
5. The iliolumbar ligaments resist motion between the distal lumbar segments, and the sacrum and help to stabilize the sacral position between the iliac wings.
6. The sacrotuberous ligament resists flexion of the iliacs on the axial spine.
7. The pubic symphysis resists AP motion of the innominates, shear, and LR forces.

Next, actual movement of the pelvis and sacroiliac joints and their functions are reviewed. We have already established that ground reaction forces from weight bearing pass through the legs and pelvis to the spine. The point in the body where these forces are in balance is termed the *center of gravity* and has been determined to be about 2 cm below the navel. Gravity can also be considered a force line that produces different effects on the pelvic girdle as it shifts from anterior to posterior relative to the center of the acetabular fossae. Body posture and positioning, muscle strength, and weight distribution determine alterations in the force lines. An anterior force line produces anterior (downward) rotation of the pelvis, decreasing tension in the sacrotuberous ligament and maintaining tension in the posterior interosseous ligaments. As the line of gravity moves posterior to the acetabula, the pelvis rotates posterior (i.e., the anterior rim tilts upward), and the sacrotuberous and posterior interosseous ligaments tighten. This is easier to visualize if we imagine a line between the femoral heads on which the pelvis rotates. The vertical distance of motion is about 2.5 cm in each direction at L3. The pelvis also rotates in relation to the spine during walking. As the legs alternately move forward, the pelvic innominate bones rotate forward and toward midline, but the spine and sacrum counterrotate, although to a lesser degree. The sacroiliac joint lies between these moving planes and forces—central to vertical, horizontal, and rotational activity. Hula and belly dancers have perfected rhythmic pelvic motion, much to the delight of their audiences.

Dysfunction of the joint without direct trauma commonly arises from an imbalance in the anterior pelvis without adequate stabilization of posterior (sacrotuberous and interosseous) ligaments. Lifting or bending while leaning forward produces anterior pelvic tilt that slightly separates the innominates from the sacrum, making unilateral AP shift more likely, especially if proper ergonomic technique is not used. The net effect of such a unilateral anterior rotation on the ipsilateral side would be to raise the pelvic brim and posterior superior iliac spine (PSIS) and cause "apparent" leg lengthening in supine positions and shortening in long sitting. (By *apparent* is meant that the affected leg is not necessarily longer, but appears to be so, owing to its attachment to the hip socket, which is rotated forward, or caudad, in a supine position. Long sitting in this situation positions the acetabulum posterior to the sacroiliac joint, resulting in apparent shortening.) Bilateral anterior sacroiliac rotation would not produce leg length asymmetry but would stretch the iliopsoas, simulating tight and tender hip flexors. Posterior unilateral rotation would produce ipsilateral PSIS and brim drop as well as a shortening of the supine leg and lengthening with long sitting.

Pain Generators

The net effect of this type of sustained unilateral force is to create an imbalance of attached myofascial insertions. Pain may result from periosteal irritation or circulatory congestion on the shortened side and loss of strength and tenderness on the elongated side. The joint line is stressed by the combined muscle and ligament pull, resisting resolution and normal positioning.

The sacroiliac joint line is densely innervated by several levels of spinal nerves (L3-S1) and may produce lumbar disc–like symptoms when stimulated. Muscle insertions near the area, such as the gluteus maximus and hamstrings, refer pain to the hip and ischial area, respectively, when stressed. The most commonly described symptom appears to be aching or hypersensitivity along the joint line to the ipsilateral hip and trochanter (Fig. 80-4).

Other pains, reported less frequently, occur about 2 inches lateral to the umbilicus on a line between the navel and anterior superior iliac spine (ASIS) or referred into the groins and testicles. Sitting can be painful when anterior rotation of the pelvis changes the relationship of acetabulum to femoral head. Because the ischial tuberosity cannot move while the subject is seated, balanced support for the pelvic "bowl" is lost, an effect aggravated by the tendency to sit lopsided. The resultant forces produce AP or LR torque on the sacroiliac joint. Standing decreases this pain because the femoral heads are repositioned and can in this fashion buttress the pelvis. Sciatic nerve stretch may also be relieved by allowing the pelvis to rotate, thereby shifting weight to the opposite leg.

SUGGESTED READINGS

Netter FH: Pelvic diaphragm: Male. In: Atlas of Human Anatomy, ed 4. Philadelphia, Saunders, 2006.
Simon S: Sacroiliac joint pain and related disorders. In Waldman SD (ed): Pain Management. Philadelphia, Saunders, 2007.

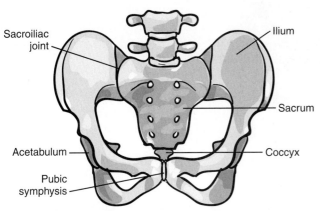

FIGURE 80–1 Anatomy of the bony pelvis. (From Waldman SD. Sacroiliac joint: Pain and related disorders. In: Pain Management. Philadelphia, Saunders, 2007, p 811.)

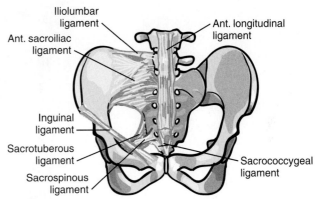

FIGURE 80–2 The anterior ligaments of the pelvis. (From Waldman SD. Sacroiliac joint: Pain and related disorders. In: Pain Management. Philadelphia, Saunders, 2007, p 811.)

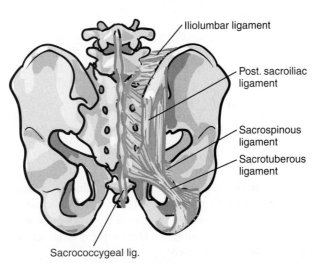

FIGURE 80–3 The posterior ligaments of the pelvis. (From Waldman SD. Sacroiliac joint: Pain and related disorders. In: Pain Management. Philadelphia, Saunders, 2007, p 812.)

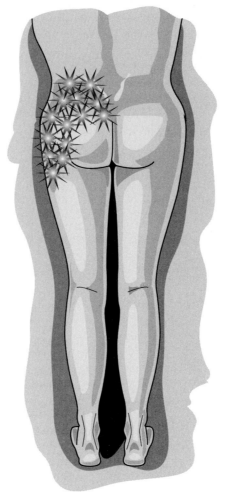

FIGURE 80–4 Distribution of pain emanating from the sacroiliac joint. (From Waldman SD. Sacroiliac joint: Pain and related disorders. In: Pain Management. Philadelphia, Saunders, 2007, p 813.)

CHAPTER 81

Functional Anatomy of the Knee

The knee is the largest joint in the body in terms of articular surface and joint volume. It is capable of amazingly complex movements that encompass highly coordinated flexion and extension. The knee joint is best thought of as a cam that is capable of locking in a stable position. Even the most simple movements of the knee involve an elegantly coordinated rolling and gliding movement of the femur on the tibia. Due to the complex nature of these movements, the knee is extremely susceptible to functional abnormalities with relatively minor alterations in the anatomy from arthritis or damage to the cartilage or ligaments.

While both clinician and lay person think of the knee joint as a single joint, from the viewpoint of understanding the functional anatomy, it is more helpful to think of the knee as two separate, but interrelated, joints: the femoral-tibial and the femoral-patellar joints (Fig. 81-1). Both joints share a common synovial cavity, and dysfunction of one joint can easily affect the function of the other.

The femoral-tibial joint is made up of the articulation of the femur and the tibia. Interposed between the two bones are two fibrocartilaginous structures known as the medial and lateral menisci (Fig. 81-2). The menisci serve to help transmit the forces placed on the femur across the joint onto the tibia. The menisci possess the property of plasticity in that they are able to change their shape in response to the variable forces placed on the joint through its complex range of motion. The medial and lateral menisci are relatively avascular and receive the bulk of their nourishment from the synovial fluid, which means that there is little potential for healing when these important structures are traumatized.

The femoral-patellar joint's primary function is to use the patella, which is a large sesamoid bone embedded in the quadriceps tendon, to improve the mechanical advantage of the quadriceps muscle. The medial and lateral articular surfaces of the sesamoid interface with the articular groove of the femur (Fig. 81-3). In extension, only the superior pole of the patella is in contact with the articular surface of the femur. As the knee flexes, the patella is drawn superiorly into the trochlear groove of the femur.

The majority of the knee joint's stability comes from the ligaments and muscles surrounding it, with little contribution from the bony elements. The main ligaments of the knee are the anterior and posterior cruciate ligaments, which provide much of the anteroposterior stability of the knee, and the medial and lateral collateral ligaments, which provide much of the valgus and varus stability (Fig. 81-4). All of these ligaments also help prevent excessive rotation of the tibia in either direction. There are also a number of secondary ligaments, which add further stability to this inherently unstable joint.

The main extensor of the knee is the quadriceps muscle, which attaches to the patella via the quadriceps tendon. Fibrotendinous expansions of the vastus medialis and vastus lateralis insert into the sides of the patella and are subject to strain and sprain. The hamstrings are the main flexors of the knee along with help from the gastrocnemius, sartorius, and gracilis muscles. Medial rotation of the flexed knee is via the medial hamstring muscle, and lateral rotation of the knee is controlled by the biceps femoris muscle.

The knee is well endowed with a variety of bursae to facilitate movement. Bursae are formed from synovial sacs whose purpose it is to allow easy sliding of muscles and tendons across one another at areas of repeated movement. These synovial sacs are lined with a synovial membrane that is invested with a network of blood vessels that secrete synovial fluid. Inflammation of the bursa results in an increase in the production of synovial fluid with swelling of the bursal sac. With overuse or misuse, these bursae may become inflamed, enlarged, and, on rare occasions, infected. Given that the knee shares a common synovial cavity, inflammation of one bursa can cause significant dysfunction and pain of the entire knee.

SUGGESTED READINGS

Netter FH: Knee: Medial and lateral views. In: Atlas of Human Anatomy, ed 4. Philadelphia, Saunders, 2006.

Waldman SD: Functional anatomy of the knee. In: Physical Diagnosis of Pain: An Atlas of Signs and Symptoms. Philadelphia, Saunders, 2006.

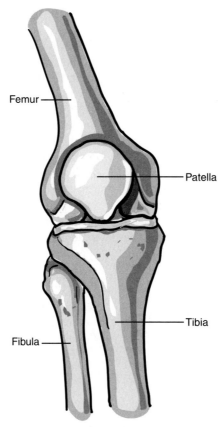

FIGURE 81–1 Functional anatomy of the knee is easier to understand if it is viewed as two separate but interrelated joints: the femoral-tibial and the femoral-patellar joints. (From Waldman SD: Physical Diagnosis of Pain: An Atlas of Signs and Symptoms. Philadelphia, Saunders, 2006, p 322.)

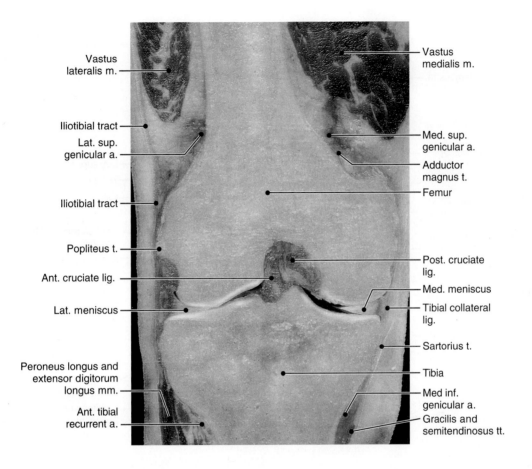

Vastus lateralis m.

Iliotibial tract

Lat. sup. genicular a.

Iliotibial tract

Popliteus t.

Ant. cruciate lig.

Lat. meniscus

Peroneus longus and extensor digitorum longus mm.

Ant. tibial recurrent a.

Vastus medialis m.

Med. sup. genicular a.

Adductor magnus t.

Femur

Post. cruciate lig.

Med. meniscus

Tibial collateral lig.

Sartorius t.

Tibia

Med inf. genicular a.

Gracilis and semitendinosus tt.

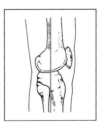

FIGURE 81–2 Coronal view of the knee. (From Kang HS, Ahn JM, Resnik D: MRI of the Extremities: An Anatomic Atlas, ed. 2. Philadelphia, Saunders, 2002, p 301.)

Rectus
femoris m.

Prefemoral
fat body

Quadriceps t.

Suprapatellar
bursa

Suprapatellar
fat body

Patella

Transverse lig.

Lat. inf. genicular a.

Infrapatellar
fat body

Patellar lig.

Tibia

Tibial n.

Lat. sup. genicular a.

Tibial n.

Femur

Oblique popliteal lig.
and joint capsule

Ant. cruciate lig.

Post.
meniscofemoral lig.
of Wrisberg

Post. cruciate lig.

Gastrocnemius,
lat. head and plantaris
mm.

Popliteal
v. and tibial n.

Popliteus m.

Soleus m.

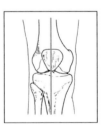

FIGURE 81–3 Sagittal view of the knee. (From Kang HS, Ahn JM, Resnik D: MRI of the Extremities: An Anatomic Atlas, ed. 2. Philadelphia, Saunders, 2002, p 341.)

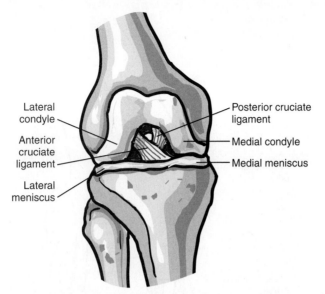

FIGURE 81–4 The main ligaments of the knee. (From Waldman SD: Physical Diagnosis of Pain: An Atlas of Signs and Symptoms. Philadelphia, Saunders, 2006, p 325.)

CHAPTER 82

The Suprapatellar Bursa

The suprapatellar bursa extends superiorly from beneath the patella under the quadriceps femoris muscle and its tendon (Fig. 82-1). The bursa is held in place by a small portion of the vastus intermedius muscle called the articularis genus muscle. Both the quadriceps tendon and the suprapatellar bursa are subject to the development of inflammation following overuse, misuse, or direct trauma. The quadriceps tendon is made up of fibers from the four muscles that comprise the quadriceps muscle: the vastus lateralis, the vastus intermedius, the vastus medialis, and the rectus femoris. These muscles are the primary extensors of the lower extremity at the knee. The tendons of these muscles converge and unite to form a single exceedingly strong tendon. The patella functions as a sesamoid bone within the quadriceps tendon with fibers of the tendon expanding around the patella forming the medial and lateral patellar retinacula, which help strengthen the knee joint. These fibers are called expansions and are subject to strain, and the tendon proper is subject to the development of tendinitis. The suprapatellar, infrapatellar, and prepatellar bursae may also concurrently become inflamed with dysfunction of the quadriceps tendon.

SUGGESTED READINGS

Netter FH: Knee: Medial and lateral views. In: Atlas of Human Anatomy, ed 4. Philadelphia, Saunders, 2006.

Waldman SD: Functional anatomy of the knee. In: Physical Diagnosis of Pain: An Atlas of Signs and Symptoms. Philadelphia, Saunders, 2006.

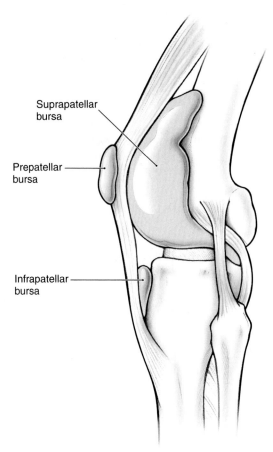

Suprapatellar bursa

Prepatellar bursa

Infrapatellar bursa

FIGURE 82–1 The suprapatellar bursa.

CHAPTER 83

The Prepatellar Bursa

The prepatellar bursa lies between the subcutaneous tissues and the patella (Fig. 83-1). The bursa is held in place by the ligamentum patellae. Both the quadriceps tendon and the prepatellar bursa are subject to the development of inflammation following overuse, misuse, or direct trauma. The quadriceps tendon is made up of fibers from the four muscles that comprise the quadriceps muscle: the vastus lateralis, the vastus intermedius, the vastus medialis, and the rectus femoris. These muscles are the primary extensors of the lower extremity at the knee. The tendons of these muscles converge and unite to form a single exceedingly strong tendon. The patella functions as a sesamoid bone within the quadriceps tendon with fibers of the tendon expanding around the patella forming the medial and lateral patellar retinacula, which help strengthen the knee joint. These fibers are called expansions and are subject to strain, and the tendon proper is subject to the development of tendinitis. The suprapatellar, infrapatellar, and prepatellar bursa may also concurrently become inflamed with dysfunction of the quadriceps tendon.

SUGGESTED READINGS

Netter FH: Knee: Medial and lateral views. In: Atlas of Human Anatomy, ed 4. Philadelphia, Saunders, 2006.
Waldman SD: Functional anatomy of the knee. In: Physical Diagnosis of Pain: An Atlas of Signs and Symptoms. Philadelphia, Saunders, 2006.

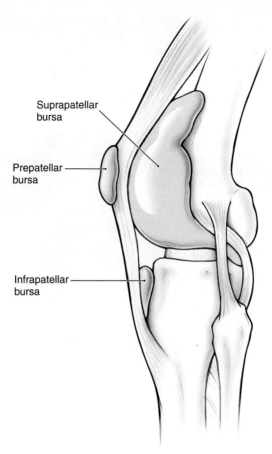

Suprapatellar bursa

Prepatellar bursa

Infrapatellar bursa

FIGURE 83–1 The prepatellar bursa.

The Superficial Infrapatellar Bursa

The superficial infrapatellar bursa lies between the subcutaneous tissues and the ligamentum patellae (Fig. 84-1). The bursa is held in place by the ligamentum patellae. Both the ligamentum patellae and the superficial infrapatellar bursa are subject to the development of inflammation following overuse, misuse, or direct trauma. The ligamentum patellae is attached above to the lower patella and below to the tibia. The fibers that make up the ligamentum patellae are continuations of the tendon of the quadriceps femoris muscle. The quadriceps tendon is made up of fibers from the four muscles that comprise the quadriceps muscle: the vastus lateralis, the vastus intermedius, the vastus medialis, and the rectus femoris. These muscles are the primary extensors of the lower extremity at the knee. The tendons of these muscles converge and unite to form a single exceedingly strong tendon. The patella functions as a sesamoid bone within the quadriceps tendon with fibers of the tendon expanding around the patella forming the medial and lateral patellar retinacula, which help strengthen the knee joint. These fibers are called expansions and are subject to strain, and the tendon proper is subject to the development of tendinitis.

SUGGESTED READINGS

Netter FH: Knee: Medial and lateral views. In: Atlas of Human Anatomy, ed 4. Philadelphia, Saunders, 2006.

Waldman SD: Functional anatomy of the knee. In: Physical Diagnosis of Pain: An Atlas of Signs and Symptoms. Philadelphia, Saunders, 2006.

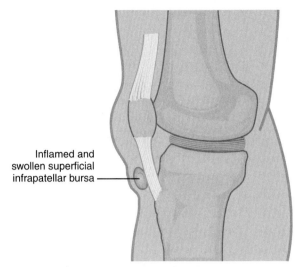

Inflamed and
swollen superficial
infrapatellar bursa —

FIGURE 84–1 The superficial infrapatellar bursa. (From Waldman SD: Atlas of Pain Management Injection Techniques. Philadelphia, Saunders, 2007, p 459.)

CHAPTER 85

The Deep Infrapatellar Bursa

The deep infrapatellar bursa lies between the ligamentum patellae and the tibia (Fig. 85-1). The bursa is held in place by the ligamentum patellae. Both the ligamentum patellae and the deep infrapatellar bursa are subject to the development of inflammation following overuse, misuse, or direct trauma. The ligamentum patellae is attached above to the lower patella and below to the tibia. The fibers that make up the ligamentum patellae are continuations of the tendon of the quadriceps femoris muscle. The quadriceps tendon is made up of fibers from the four muscles that comprise the quadriceps muscle: the vastus lateralis, the vastus intermedius, the vastus medialis, and the rectus femoris. These muscles are the primary extensors of the lower extremity at the knee. The tendons of these muscles converge and unite to form a single exceedingly strong tendon. The patella functions as a sesamoid bone within the quadriceps tendon with fibers of the tendon expanding around the patella forming the medial and lateral patellar retinacula, which help strengthen the knee joint. These fibers are called expansions and are subject to strain, and the tendon proper is subject to the development of tendinitis.

SUGGESTED READINGS

Netter FH: Knee: Medial and lateral views. In: Atlas of Human Anatomy, ed 4. Philadelphia, Saunders, 2006.

Waldman SD: Functional anatomy of the knee. In: Physical Diagnosis of Pain: An Atlas of Signs and Symptoms. Philadelphia, Saunders, 2006.

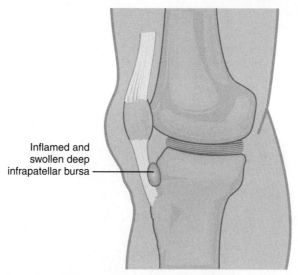

FIGURE 85–1 The deep infrapatellar bursa. (From Waldman SD: Atlas of Pain Management Injection Techniques. Philadelphia, Saunders, 2007, p 463.)

Inflamed and swollen deep infrapatellar bursa

CHAPTER 86

The Pes Anserine Bursa

The pes anserine bursa lies between the combined tendinous insertion of the sartorius, gracilis, and semitendinosus muscles and the medial tibia (Fig. 86-1). The bursa is subject to the development of inflammation following overuse, misuse, or direct trauma. The medial collateral ligament is often also involved if the medial knee has been subjected to trauma. The medial collateral ligament is a broad, flat, bandlike ligament that runs from the medial condyle of the femur to the medial aspect of the shaft of the tibia where it attaches just above the groove of the semimembranosus muscle. It also attaches to the edge of

the medial semilunar cartilage. The medial collateral ligament is crossed at its lower part by the tendons of the sartorius, gracilis, and semitendinosus muscles.

SUGGESTED READINGS

Netter FH: Knee: Medial and lateral views. In: Atlas of Human Anatomy, ed 4. Philadelphia, Saunders, 2006.

Waldman SD: Functional anatomy of the knee. In: Physical Diagnosis of Pain: An Atlas of Signs and Symptoms. Philadelphia, Saunders, 2006.

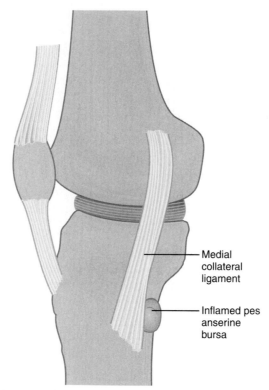

FIGURE 86–1 The pes anserine bursa. (From Waldman SD: Atlas of Pain Management Injection Techniques, ed 2. Philadelphia, Saunders, 2007, p 468.)

CHAPTER 87

The Iliotibial Band Bursa

The iliotibial band bursa lies between the iliotibial band and the lateral condyle of the femur. The iliotibial band is an extension of the fascia lata which inserts at the lateral condyle of the tibia. The iliotibial band can rub backwards and forwards over the lateral epicondyle of the femur and irritate the iliotibial bursa beneath it (Fig. 87-1). The iliotibial bursa is subject to the development of inflammation following overuse, misuse or direct trauma.

SUGGESTED READING

Waldman SD: Iliotibial band bursitis pain. In: Atlas of Pain Management Injection Techniques, ed 2. Philadelphia, Saunders, 2007.

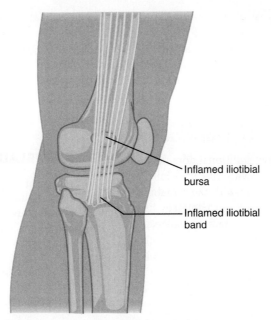

Inflamed iliotibial
bursa

Inflamed iliotibial
band

FIGURE 87–1 The iliotibial band bursa. (From Waldman SD: Atlas of Pain Management Injection Techniques. Philadelphia, Saunders, 2007, p 471.)

Functional Anatomy of the Ankle and Foot

To best understand the functional anatomy of the ankle and foot, the clinician is best served by viewing the ankle as being composed of three distinct functional units: (1) the hindfoot, which is made up of the calcaneus and talus; (2) the midfoot, which is made up of the five tarsal bones; and (3) the forefoot, which is made up of the metatarsals and phalanges (Fig. 88-1). While these units are functionally distinct, normal walking requires a highly and subtly coordinated interaction between them.

The Hindfoot

The distal joint between the tibia and fibula allows very little movement with the hinge joint formed by the distal ends of the tibia and fibula and the talus providing dorsiflexion and plantar flexion needed for ambulation. The medial and lateral malleoli extend along the sides of the talus to form a mortise that provides stability and prevents ankle rotation (Fig. 88-2). This joint is further

strengthened by the deltoid ligament medially and the anterior talofibular, posterior talofibular, and calcaneofibular ligaments laterally. These ligaments are subject to strain and sprain and are often the source of ankle pain and dysfunction following seemingly minor trauma.

The talocalcaneal joint, which lies between the talus and calcaneus, allows for additional range of motion of the ankle joint and makes up for the limitations of motion placed on the joint by the mortise structure of the talus and medial and lateral malleoli by permitting approximately 30 degrees of foot inversion and 15 to 20 degrees of foot eversion, which allows walking on uneven surfaces.

The Midfoot

The midtarsal joints are made up of the calcaneocuboid and talonavicular joints. These joints contribute to further range of motion by allowing 20 degrees of adduction of the foot and approximately 10 degrees of abduction of the foot. These movements add to the flexibility of the foot and are thought to aid in climbing, and they are aided by the gliding motions of the intertarsal joints between the navicular, cuneiform, and cuboid bones.

The Forefoot

The metatarsophalangeal joints allow additional dorsiflexion and plantar flexion of the foot with the first joint allowing 80 to 90 degrees of dorsiflexion with the remaining metatarsophalangeal joints allowing approximately 40 degrees of dorsiflexion. The first metatarsophalangeal joint allows about 40 to 50 degrees of plantar flexion with the remaining joints allowing 35 to 40 degrees of plantar flexion.

The interphalangeal joints are made up of proximal and distal units. The proximal interphalangeal joints do not extend but allow approximately 50 degrees of plantar flexion. The distal interphalangeal joints allow approximately 25 degrees of dorsiflexion and 40 to 50 degrees of plantar flexion.

SUGGESTED READINGS

Netter FH: Bones of the foot. In: Atlas of Human Anatomy, ed 4. Philadelphia, Saunders, 2006.

Netter FH: Ligaments and tendons of the ankle. In: Atlas of Human Anatomy, ed 4. Philadelphia, Saunders, 2006.

Waldman SD: Functional anatomy of the ankle and foot. In: Physical Diagnosis of Pain: An Atlas of Signs and Symptoms. Philadelphia, Saunders, 2006.

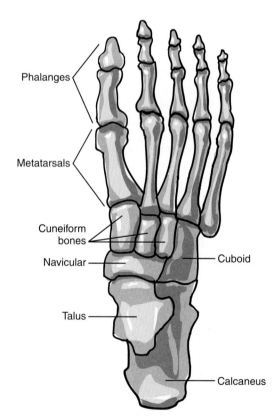

FIGURE 88–1 The foot and ankle. (From Waldman SD: Physical Diagnosis of Pain: An Atlas of Signs and Symptoms. Philadelphia, Saunders, 2006, p 360.)

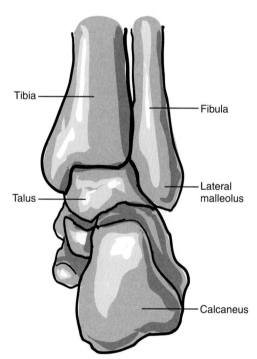

FIGURE 88–2 The hindfoot. (From Waldman SD: Physical Diagnosis of Pain: An Atlas of Signs and Symptoms. Philadelphia, Saunders, 2006, p 361.)

CHAPTER **89**

The Deltoid Ligament

The ankle is a hinge-type articulation between the distal tibia, the two malleoli, and the talus. The articular surface is covered with hyaline cartilage, which is susceptible to arthritis. The joint is surrounded by a dense capsule, which helps strengthen the ankle. The joint capsule is lined with a synovial membrane, which attaches to the articular cartilage. The ankle joint is innervated by the deep peroneal and tibial nerves.

The major ligaments of the ankle joint include the deltoid, anterior talofibular, calcaneofibular, and posterior talofibular ligaments, which provide the majority of strength to the ankle joint. The deltoid ligament is exceptionally strong and is not as subject to strain as the anterior talofibular ligament. The deltoid ligament has two layers (Fig. 89-1). Both attach above to the medial malleolus. A deep layer attaches below to the medial body of the talus with the superficial fibers attaching to the medial talus and the sustentaculum tali of the calcaneus and the navicular tuberosity.

SUGGESTED READINGS

Netter FH: Bones of the foot. In: Atlas of Human Anatomy, ed 4. Philadelphia, Saunders, 2006.

Netter FH: Ligaments and tendons of the ankle. In: Atlas of Human Anatomy, ed 4. Philadelphia, Saunders, 2006.

Waldman SD: Functional anatomy of the ankle and foot. In: Physical Diagnosis of Pain: An Atlas of Signs and Symptoms. Philadelphia, Saunders, 2006.

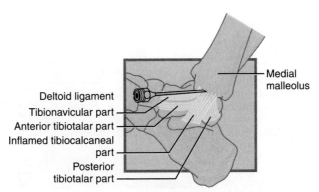

FIGURE 89–1 The deltoid ligament. (From Waldman SD: Atlas of Pain Management Injection Techniques. Philadelphia, Saunders, 2007, p 512.)

CHAPTER 90

The Anterior Talofibular Ligament

The ankle is a hinge-type articulation between the distal tibia, the two malleoli and the talus. The articular surface is covered with hyaline cartilage which is susceptible to arthritis. The joint is surrounded by a dense capsule which helps strengthen the ankle. The joint capsule is lined with a synovial membrane which attaches to the articular cartilage. The ankle joint is innervated by the deep peroneal and tibial nerves.

The major ligaments of the ankle joint include the talofibular, anterior talofibular, calcaneofibular, and posterior talofibular ligaments which provide the majority of strength to the ankle joint. The talofibular ligament is not as strong as the deltoid ligament and is susceptible to strain. The anterior talofibular ligament runs from the anterior border of the lateral malleolus to the lateral surface of the talus (Fig. 90-1).

SUGGESTED READINGS

Netter FH: Bones of the foot. In: Atlas of Human Anatomy, ed 4. Philadelphia, Saunders, 2006.

Netter FH: Ligaments and tendons of the ankle. In: Atlas of Human Anatomy, ed 4. Philadelphia, Saunders, 2006.

Waldman SD: Functional anatomy of the ankle and foot. In: Physical Diagnosis of Pain: An Atlas of Signs and Symptoms. Philadelphia, Saunders, 2006.

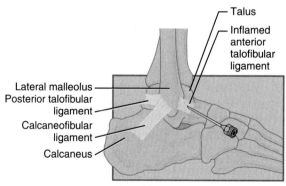

FIGURE 90–1 The anterior talofibular ligament. (From Waldman SD: Atlas of Pain Management Injection Techniques. Philadelphia, Saunders, 2007, p 518.)

CHAPTER 91

The Anterior Tarsal Tunnel

The common peroneal nerve is one of the two major continuations of the sciatic nerve, the other being the tibial nerve. The common peroneal nerve provides sensory innervation to the inferior portion of the knee joint and the posterior and lateral skin of the upper calf. The common peroneal nerve is derived from the posterior branches of the L4 and L5 and the S1 and S2 nerve roots. The nerve splits from the sciatic nerve at the superior margin of the popliteal fossa and descends laterally behind the head of the fibula. The common peroneal nerve is subject to compression at this point by improperly applied casts, tourniquets, etc. The nerve is also subject to compression as it continues its lateral course winding around the fibula through the fibular tunnel, which is made up of the posterior border of the tendinous insertion of the peroneus longus muscle and the fibula itself. Just distal to the fibular tunnel, the nerve divides into its two terminal branches, the superficial and the deep peroneal nerves. Each of these branches is subject to trauma and may be blocked individually as a diagnostic and therapeutic maneuver.

The deep branch continues down the leg in conjunction with the tibial artery and vein to provide sensory innervation to the web space of the first and second toes and adjacent dorsum of the foot (Fig. 91-1). Although this distribution of sensory fibers is small, this area is often the site of Morton's neuroma surgery and thus important to the regional anesthesiologist. The deep peroneal nerve provides motor innervation to all of the toe extensors. The deep peroneal nerve passes beneath the dense superficial fascia of the ankle, where it is subject to entrapment.

SUGGESTED READINGS

Netter FH: Bones of the foot. In: Atlas of Human Anatomy, ed 4. Philadelphia, Saunders, 2006.

Netter FH: Ligaments and tendons of the ankle. In: Atlas of Human Anatomy, ed 4. Philadelphia, Saunders, 2006.

Waldman SD: Functional anatomy of the ankle and foot. In: Physical Diagnosis of Pain: An Atlas of Signs and Symptoms. Philadelphia, Saunders, 2006.

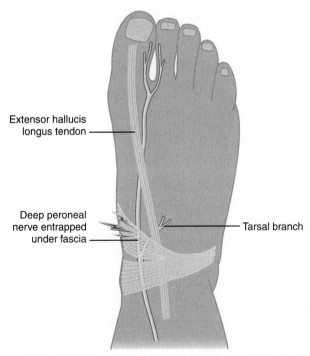

Extensor hallucis longus tendon

Deep peroneal nerve entrapped under fascia

Tarsal branch

FIGURE 91–1 The anterior tarsal tunnel. (From Waldman SD: Atlas of Pain Management Injection Techniques. Philadelphia, Saunders, 2007, p 521.)

CHAPTER 92

The Posterior Tarsal Tunnel

The tibial nerve is one of the two major continuations of the sciatic nerve, the other being the common peroneal nerve. The tibial nerve provides sensory innervation to the posterior portion of the calf, the heel, and medial plantar surface. The tibial nerve splits from the sciatic nerve at the superior margin of the popliteal fossa and descends in a slightly medial course through the popliteal fossa. The tibial nerve at the ankle lies just beneath the popliteal fascia and is readily accessible for neural blockade. The tibial nerve continues its downward course, running between the two heads of the gastrocnemius muscle passing deep to the soleus muscle. The nerve courses medially between the Achilles tendon and the medial malleolus, where it divides into the medial and lateral plantar nerves, providing sensory innervation to the heel and medial plantar surface (Fig. 92-1). The tibial nerve is subject to compression at this point as the nerve passes through the posterior tarsal tunnel. The posterior tarsal tunnel is made up of the flexor retinaculum, the bones of the ankle, and the lacunate ligament. In addition to the posterior tibial nerve, the tunnel contains the posterior tibial artery and a number of flexor tendons.

SUGGESTED READINGS

Netter FH: Bones of the foot. In: Atlas of Human Anatomy, ed 4. Philadelphia, Saunders, 2006.

Netter FH: Ligaments and tendons of the ankle. In: Atlas of Human Anatomy, ed 4. Philadelphia, Saunders, 2006.

Waldman SD: Functional anatomy of the ankle and foot. In: Physical Diagnosis of Pain: An Atlas of Signs and Symptoms. Philadelphia, Saunders, 2006.

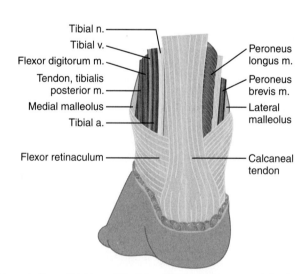

FIGURE 92–1 The posterior tarsal tunnel. (From Waldman SD: Atlas of Pain Management Injection Techniques. Philadelphia, Saunders, 2007, p 525.)

The Achilles Tendon

The Achilles tendon is the thickest and strongest tendon in the body, yet also very susceptible to rupture. The common tendon of the gastrocnemius muscle, the Achilles tendon begins at mid-calf and continues downward to attach to the posterior calcaneus, where it may become inflamed (Fig. 93-1). The Achilles tendon narrows during this downward course, becoming most narrow approximately 5 cm above its calcaneal insertion. It is this narrowmost point at which tendinitis may also occur. A bursa is located between the Achilles tendon and the base of the tibia and the upper posterior calcaneus.

This bursa may also become inflamed as a result of coexistent Achilles tendinitis and confuse the clinical picture.

SUGGESTED READINGS

Netter FH: Bones of the foot. In: Atlas of Human Anatomy, ed 4. Philadelphia, Saunders, 2006.

Netter FH: Ligaments and tendons of the ankle. In: Atlas of Human Anatomy, ed 4. Philadelphia, Saunders, 2006.

Waldman SD: Functional anatomy of the ankle and foot. In: Physical Diagnosis of Pain: An Atlas of Signs and Symptoms. Philadelphia, Saunders, 2006.

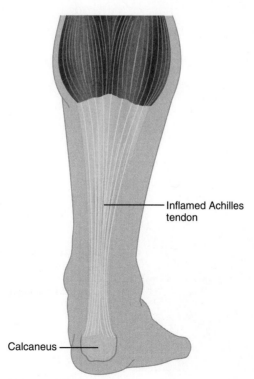

Inflamed Achilles tendon

Calcaneus

FIGURE 93–1 The Achilles tendon. (From Waldman SD: Atlas of Pain Management Injection Techniques. Philadelphia, Saunders, 2007, p 533.)

CHAPTER 94

The Achilles Bursa

The Achilles bursa lies between the Achilles tendon and the base of the tibia and the posterior calcaneus (Fig. 94-1). The bursa is subject to the development of inflammation following overuse, misuse, or direct trauma. The Achilles tendon is the thickest and strongest tendon in the body, yet it is also very susceptible to rupture. The common tendon of the gastrocnemius muscle, the Achilles tendon begins at mid-calf and continues downward to attach to the posterior calcaneus, where it may become inflamed (see Fig. 94-1). The Achilles tendon narrows during this downward course, becoming most narrow approximately 5 cm above its calcaneal insertion. It is this narrowmost point at which tendinitis may also occur. Tendinitis, especially at the calcaneal insertion, may mimic Achilles bursitis and may make diagnosis difficult.

SUGGESTED READINGS

Netter FH: Bones of the foot. In: Atlas of Human Anatomy, ed 4. Philadelphia, Saunders, 2006.

Netter FH: Ligaments and tendons of the ankle. In: Atlas of Human Anatomy, ed 4. Philadelphia, Saunders, 2006.

Waldman SD: Functional anatomy of the ankle and foot. In: Physical Diagnosis of Pain: An Atlas of Signs and Symptoms. Philadelphia, Saunders, 2006.

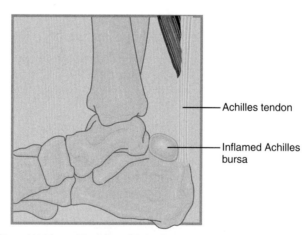

FIGURE 94–1 The Achilles bursa. (From Waldman SD: Atlas of Pain Management Injection Techniques, ed 2. Philadelphia, Saunders, 2007, p 536.)

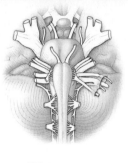

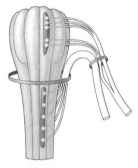

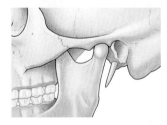

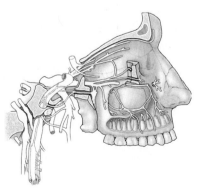

Neuroanatomy

CHAPTER 95

The Spinal Cord—Gross Anatomy

The central nervous system is composed of the brain and the spinal cord, which function both in concert and independently to control and integrate myriad functions necessary for humans to exist. It is important for the clinician to recognize that the spinal cord does much more than serve as a conduit for information to the brain; it also functions independently to process and modulate huge amounts of data every second of the day. Dysfunction of these independent functions can lead to significant morbidity and if the dysfunction is severe enough, as in the case of spinal cord injury, significantly contribute to the mortality of the individual unfortunate enough to suffer from this problem.

The length of the average adult spinal cord in health is approximately 18 inches. There is a shallow longitudinal indentation along the length of the dorsal surface of the spinal cord that is called the posterior median sulcus and a corresponding deeper longitudinal indentation along the length of the ventral surface of the spinal cord that is called the anterior median fissure (Fig. 95-1). Enlargement of the spinal cord occurs in both the cervical and lumbar regions as the result of increased gray matter involved with the interneurons responsible for integrating and relaying sensory and motor information from the extremities (Fig. 95-2). The cervical enlargement contains interneurons for the nerves that supply the upper extremities and pectoral girdle as well as fibers from regions inferior to the cervical region, such as thoracic, lumbar, and sacral. The lumbar enlargement contains interneurons for the nerves that supply the lower extremities and pelvis as well as fibers from the more inferior sacral region.

Inferior to the lumbar enlargement, the spinal cord narrows as the sacral spinal cord contains only tracts that begin or end in the pelvic region. The end of the spinal cord tapers to a point called the conus medullaris at the level of the first lumbar vertebra. The distal spinal cord is tethered distally by the filum terminale, which is a fibrous ligamentous structure that attaches to the conus medullaris proximally and passes inferiorly to attach to the second or third sacral segment as part of the coccygeal ligament.

SUGGESTED READING

Netter FH: Spinal cord and ventral rami in situ. In: Atlas of Human Anatomy, ed 4. Philadelphia, Saunders, 2006.

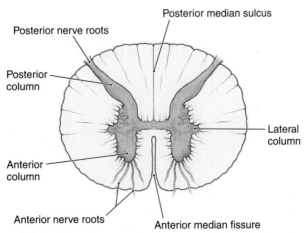

FIGURE 95–1 Cross-sectional anatomy of the spinal cord.

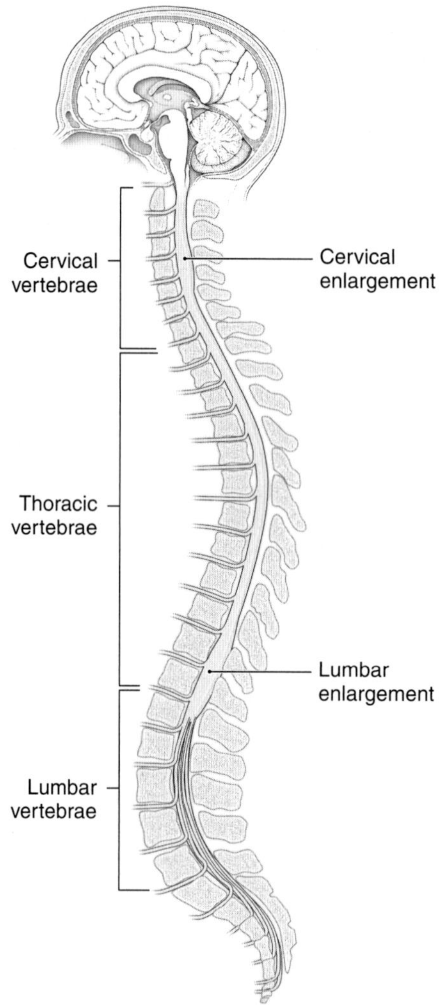

FIGURE 95–2 The cervical and lumbar enlargements.

CHAPTER 96

The Spinal Cord—Cross-Sectional Anatomy

The spinal cord is divided into 31 anatomic segments with each segment being identified by a letter and number. In the nomenclature schema, C stands for cervical, T for thoracic, L for lumbar, and S for sacral, with the associated number designating the specific spinal segment (e.g., L3, S1, etc.). Each spinal segment has a corresponding pair of dorsal root ganglia that contain the nerve cell bodies of the sensory neurons (Fig. 96-1). These ganglia lie between the

pedicles belonging to the vertebrae just above and just below the ganglia. Attached to each of the dorsal sensory ganglia is a dorsal nerve root that contains the axons of the sensory neurons arising from the dorsal root ganglia. The dorsal sensory nerve root joins the ventral motor nerve roots to coalesce to form a spinal nerve root and exit between its adjacent vertebrae via the intervertebral foramina (see later) (see Fig. 96-1).

Anterior to the dorsal root, the ventral nerve root exits the spinal cord carrying axons of both somatic and visceral neurons. Just distal to the dorsal root ganglion, the dorsal sensory nerve root and ventral nerve roots coalesce to form a single spinal nerve. This single spinal nerve root is a mixed nerve containing both motor and sensory fibers and exits between its adjacent vertebrae via the intervertebral foramina (see Fig. 96-1). The spinal nerve roots continue on to innervate their respective dermatomes, myotomes, and sclerotomes.

SUGGESTED READINGS

Netter FH: Spinal membranes and nerve roots. In: Atlas of Human Anatomy, ed 4. Philadelphia, Saunders, 2006.

Netter FH: Spinal nerve origin: Cross section. In: Atlas of Human Anatomy, ed 4. Philadelphia, Saunders, 2006.

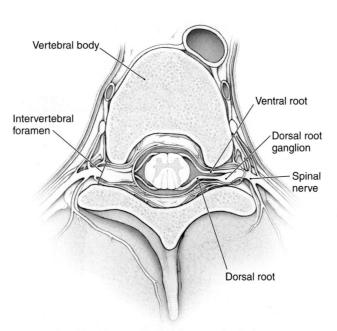

FIGURE 96–1 Cross section of a typical spinal segment.

CHAPTER 97

Organization of the Spinal Cord

A clear understanding of the organization of the spinal cord is necessary if the clinician is to understand how pain impulses are modulated and transmitted in health and disease. Functionally, the spinal cord is divided in half by the anterior median fissure and the posterior median sulcus. Centrally, there is an H-shaped structure made up primarily of gray matter consisting of nerve cell bodies and glial cells (Fig. 97-1). This gray matter is pierced in its middle by the central canal. Projecting outward from the gray matter toward the points at which the dorsal and ventral roots exit the spinal cord are the horns of the gray matter. Surrounding the gray matter is the white matter, which contains the myelinated and unmyelinated axons, which are organized into tracts and columns (see later).

The cell bodies of the gray matter of the spinal cord are organized into nuclei, each of which has specific functions, with the sensory nuclei grouped together in the dorsal portion of the spinal cord to receive and relay peripheral sensory information via the dorsal roots and the motor nuclei grouped together in the ventral portion of the spinal cord to relay motor commands via the ventral roots to the periphery (Fig. 97-2). The concept that dorsal roots carry sensory information and the ventral roots carry motor information is known as the Bell-Magendie law. It should be noted that there are special areas of the gray matter called commissures that contain axons that cross from one side of the spinal cord to the other.

Just as the gray matter is highly organized into nuclei with each nucleus responsible for a specific anatomic area, the white matter is likewise organized into columns or funiculi that contain tracts or fasciculi whose homogeneous axons convey motor or sensory information to and from a specific anatomic area. In general, all of the axons within a tract carry information in the same direction, with the ascending tracts of white matter carrying information toward the brainstem and brain and the descending white matter tracts carrying motor commands from the higher centers into the spinal cord. Like the gray matter, there are commissural tracts within the white matter that carry sensory or motor information between spinal segments.

SUGGESTED READINGS

Netter FH: Spinal membranes and nerve roots. In: Atlas of Human Anatomy, ed 4. Philadelphia, Saunders, 2006.
Netter FH: Spinal nerve origin: Cross section. In: Atlas of Human Anatomy, ed 4. Philadelphia, Saunders, 2006.

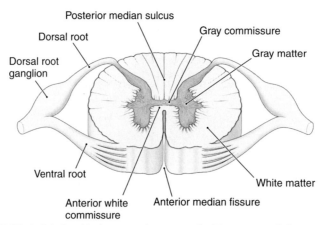

FIGURE 97–1 Relationship between the gray and white matter of the spinal cord.

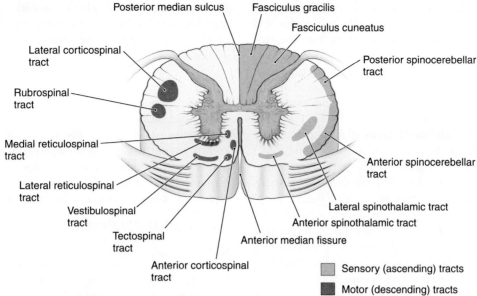

FIGURE 97–2 Organization of the nuclei and tracts of the spinal cord.

The Spinal Nerves—Organizational and Anatomic Considerations

Just distal to the dorsal root ganglion, the dorsal sensory nerve root and ventral nerve roots coalesce to form a single spinal nerve. This single spinal nerve root is a mixed nerve containing both motor and sensory fibers, and it exits between its adjacent vertebrae via the intervertebral foramina. There are 31 pairs of spinal nerves and each can be identified by a nomenclature schema. In this nomenclature schema, C stands for cervical, T for thoracic, L for lumbar, and S for sacral, with the associated number designating the specific spinal segment (e.g., L3, S1, etc.) (Fig. 98-1).

The first pair of spinal nerves is designated C1, and they exit between the skull and the first cervical vertebra. The second pair of cervical spinal nerves exit between the first and second cervical vertebrae and are designated the C2 spinal nerves. This nomenclature system continues throughout the cervical spine with the last pair of cervical nerves exiting between the seventh cervical vertebra and the first thoracic vertebra. These last cervical nerves are designated C8 to take into account that the first cervical nerve exits between the skull and

the first cervical vertebra and that there are only seven cervical vertebrae. Thus, there are seven cervical vertebrae and eight cervical spinal nerves.

The remaining spinal nerves caudad to the first thoracic vertebra take their names from the vertebra just superior—for example, the first thoracic spinal nerve T1 exits just beneath the first thoracic vertebra, the second thoracic spinal nerve T2 exits just beneath the second thoracic vertebra, and so on.

Each spinal nerve is covered by connective tissue, which is arranged in three distinct concentric layers. These layers are (1) the outermost epineurium, (2) the central perineurium, and (3) the innermost endoneurium (Fig. 98-2). The epineurium is made up of a dense network of collagen fibers that form a tough sheath that protects the integrity of the nerve. At the level of the intervertebral foramen, the epineurium of each spinal nerve becomes invested into the dura mater of the spinal cord. The perineurium serves to divide the spinal nerve into a series of compartments that are known as fascicles. These fascicles contain discrete bundles of axons. The perineurium also supports the arteries and veins that serve the axons contained in the fascicles. Surrounding the individual axons is the delicate connective tissue known as the endoneurium. Small capillaries branch off of vessels in the perineurium to provide oxygen and nutrients to the individual axons and associated Schwann cells of the nerve.

As mentioned, each spinal nerve is formed from the coalescence of fibers from the dorsal and ventral nerve roots as these fibers pass through the intervertebral foramen (Fig. 98-3). As the spinal nerve passes distally, it divides into several branches, each with a specific function. In the thoracic and upper lumbar segments, the first branch of each spinal nerve is made up of myelinated fibers known as the white ramus, which carries visceral motor fibers to the nearby autonomic ganglia associated with the sympathetic chain. Two groups of unmyelinated postganglion fibers exit the ganglion, with one group

forming the gray rami, which innervate smooth muscles and glands in the trunk and extremities. These fibers that provide innervation to the smooth muscles and glands in the trunk and extremities rejoin the spinal nerves, while the preganglionic and postganglionic fibers that innervate the viscera do not rejoin the spinal nerves but form discrete autonomic nerves (e.g., the splanchnic nerves that serve the organs of the abdominal and pelvic cavities). Collectively, the white and gray rami are known as the rami communicantes or communicating branches. The dorsal ramus of each spinal nerve is responsible for providing sensory data from a specific area of the body known as a dermatome (Fig. 98-4).

SUGGESTED READINGS

Netter FH: Spinal membranes and nerve roots. In: Atlas of Human Anatomy, ed 4. Philadelphia, Saunders, 2006.
Netter FH: Spinal nerve origin: Cross section. In: Atlas of Human Anatomy, ed 4. Philadelphia, Saunders, 2006.

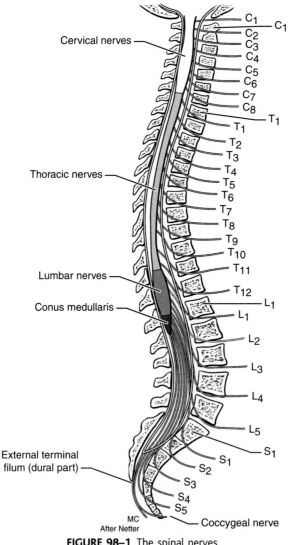

FIGURE 98–1 The spinal nerves.

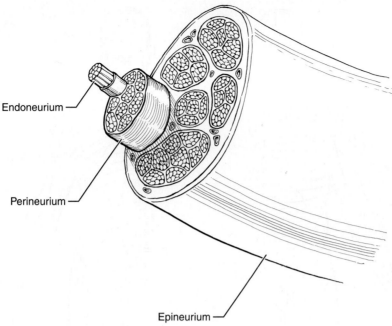

Endoneurium

Perineurium

Epineurium

FIGURE 98–2 The connective tissue of the typical spinal nerve.

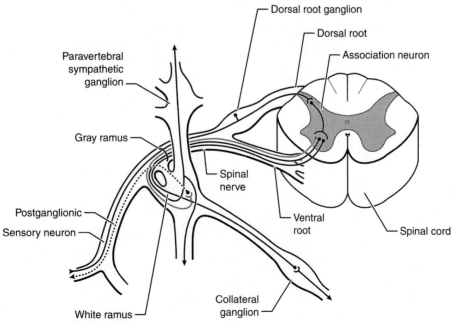

Dorsal root ganglion

Dorsal root

Association neuron

Paravertebral sympathetic ganglion

Gray ramus

Spinal nerve

Postganglionic

Sensory neuron

Ventral root

Spinal cord

White ramus

Collateral ganglion

FIGURE 98–3 The peripheral distribution of the typical spinal nerve.

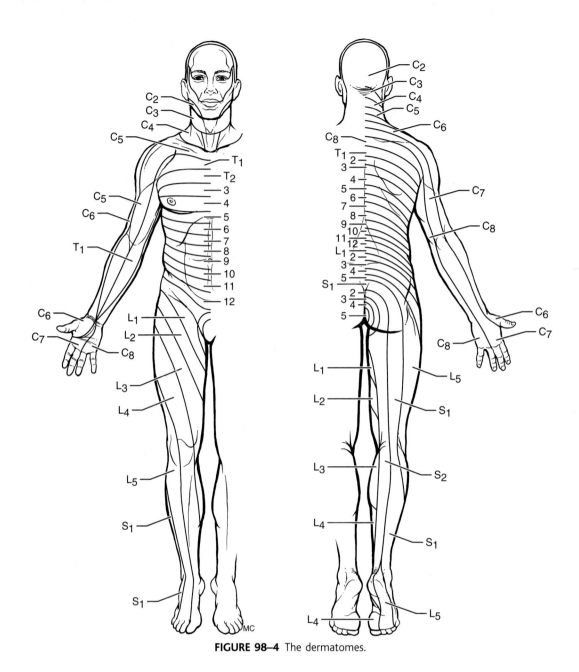

FIGURE 98–4 The dermatomes.

The Spinal Reflex Arc

Reflexes are immediate involuntary motor responses to a specific stimulus that are designed to help maintain homeostasis across a wide range of conditions. Although reflexes can be modulated at the spinal cord level as well as from descending input from the higher centers, in general a specific reflex shows amazingly little variability with the same stimulus producing essentially the same response. The pathway that subserves a specific reflex is known as the reflex arc. The steps of a typical reflex are summarized in Table 99-1.

The gray matter of the spinal cord is involved in a variety of reflexes ranging from the simple monosynaptic stretch reflex to complex polysynaptic reflexes that are modulated by descending tracts from the brain. Monosynaptic reflexes are those reflexes in which a sensory neuron synapses directly onto a motor neuron. The most common monosynaptic reflex arc is the simple stretch reflex that helps provide automatic regulation of the length of skeletal muscles. In the stretch reflex, when a stimulus stretches a relaxed skeletal muscle, there is activation of a sensory neuron which triggers contraction of the muscle (Fig. 99-1).

A polysynaptic reflex involves more than interneuron synapses between the primary sensory neuron and the final motor neuron. A common example of a polysynaptic reflex is the patellar reflex (Fig. 99-2). The time it takes between stimulus and response is in direct proportion to the number of interneurons between the primary sensory neuron and the final motor neuron.

TABLE 99–1 The Spinal Reflex Arc

1. Arrival of stimulus and activation of receptor
2. Activation of a sensory neuron
3. Information processing in central nervous system
   a. Spinal reflexes are processed in spinal cord
   b. Cranial reflexes are processed in brain
4. Activation of motor neuron
5. Response by effector

SUGGESTED READINGS

Campbell W: DeJong's The Neurological Examination, ed 6. Philadelphia, Lippincott Williams and Wilkins, 2005.

Goetz CG: Textbook of Clinical Neurology, ed 2. Philadelphia, Saunders, 2003.

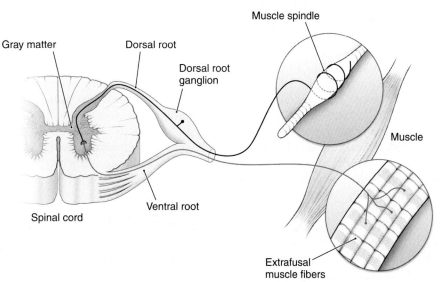

FIGURE 99–1 The monosynaptic spinal reflex.

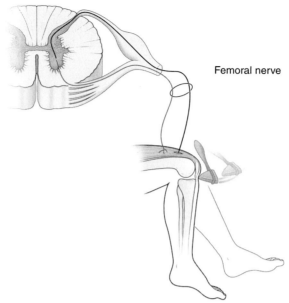

FIGURE 99–2 The polysynaptic spinal reflex.

CHAPTER 100

The Posterior Column Pathway

Delivering highly localized fine touch, pressure, vibratory, and proprioceptive information to the primary sensory cortex of the contralateral cerebral hemisphere, the posterior column pathway plays an important role in the maintenance of homeostasis (Fig. 100-1). First-order neurons carrying fine touch, pressure, vibratory, and proprioceptive information from the lower extremities enter the central nervous system via the dorsal roots and ascend via the fasciculus gracilis. First-order neurons carrying fine touch, pressure, vibratory, and proprioceptive information from the upper extremities enter the central nervous system via the dorsal roots and ascend via the fasciculus cuneatus. These fibers synapse at the nucleus gracilis or cuneatus, which are located in the medulla oblongata.

After synapsing at their respective nuclei in the medulla oblongata, second-order neurons leave the medulla oblongata and immediately cross to the opposite side of the brainstem to relay transmitted information via the ribbon-like medial lemniscus. The medial lemniscus continues to keep each type of information, such as fine touch, pressure, vibratory, and proprioception, segregated as it impinges on the ventral posterolateral thalamus. In the ventral posterolateral thalamus, incoming information is segregated according to the region of the body in which the data originated and is then projected via projection fibers to a specific region of the primary sensory cortex. The organization of the primary sensory cortex is oriented in what is known as the sensory homunculus with the toes projected on one end and the information from the head at the other (Fig. 100-2). It should be noted that a given area of the primary sensory cortex assigned to a specific region is proportional to the number of sensory receptors that the region contains rather than to the actual size of the area. Thus, the area of the primary sensory cortex devoted to the lips is much larger relative to the area of the primary sensory cortex devoted to the back despite the fact that the back is much larger in size compared with the lips.

SUGGESTED READINGS

Campbell W: DeJong's The Neurological Examination, ed 6. Philadelphia, Lippincott Williams and Wilkins, 2005.
Goetz CG: Textbook of Clinical Neurology, ed 2. Philadelphia, Saunders, 2003.

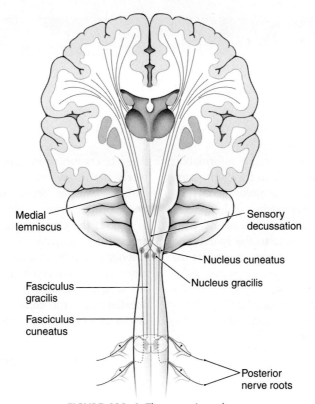

FIGURE 100–1 The posterior columns.

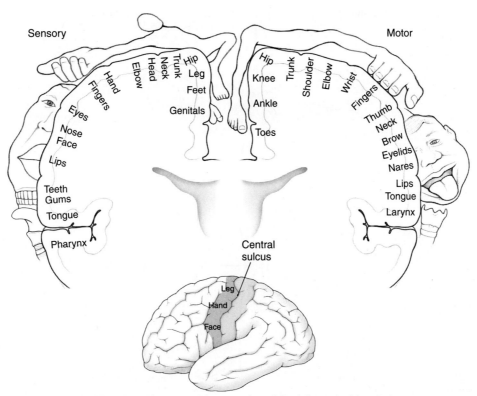

FIGURE 100–2 The sensory homunculus of the left cerebral hemisphere.

CHAPTER **101**

The Spinothalamic Pathway

The spinothalamic pathway carries affective information in that perception of information leads to the compulsion to act (e.g., withdraw from a painful stimulus, scratch an itch). The spinothalamic pathway begins as long first-order neurons that carry "crude" sensations of pain, touch, pressure, itch, and temperature to the spinal cord via the dorsal roots. These primary neurons synapse at the dorsal horns with secondary neurons known as tract cells. Unlike the posterior columns that decussate at the brainstem level, the tract cells of the spinothalamic pathway decussate to the opposite side of the spinal cord via the anterior white commissure to the contralateral anterolateral spinal cord where the tract neuron fibers form two tracts: (1) the anterior spinothalamic tract, which transmits touch, and (2) the lateral spinothalamic tract, which transmits pain and temperature (Fig. 101-1).

As these secondary tract neurons travel up the spinal cord in the anterior and lateral spinothalamic tracts, these tracts move dorsally within the spinal cord. These tracts ultimately impinge on the ventral posterolateral thalamic nuclei from which third-order projection fibers project information to the primary sensory cortex as well as the cingulate cortex and insular cortex. These areas are responsible for both the direct, or conscious, response to pain and the more subtle affective components of the pain response. Unilateral lesion affecting the lateral spinothalamic tracts of the spinal cord will cause anesthesia on the contralateral side of the body, which begins one to two segments below the lesion.

SUGGESTED READINGS

Campbell W: DeJong's The Neurological Examination, ed 6. Philadelphia, Lippincott Williams and Wilkins, 2005.
Goetz CG: Textbook of Clinical Neurology, ed 2. Philadelphia, Saunders, 2003.

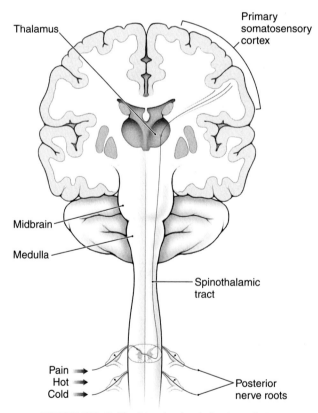

FIGURE 101-1 The lateral spinothalamic pathway.

The Spinocerebellar Pathway

Proprioceptive information from the Golgi tendon organs, muscle spindles, and joint capsules is carried by first-order sensory neurons to the dorsal roots to synapse with second-order neurons at the dorsal gray horns of the spinal cord (Fig. 102-1). Some of these second-order neurons decussate to the contralateral side of the spinal cord, while others do not decussate and remain on the ipsilateral side of the spinal cord. Those second-order neurons that decussate ascend the spinal cord via the anterior spinocerebellar tract to enter the cerebellum via the superior cerebellar peduncle. Those second-order neurons that do not decussate ascend the spinal cord via the posterior spinocerebellar tract to enter the cerebellum via the inferior cerebellar peduncle. The cerebellum then processes this position information to aid in coordination of fine motor movements throughout the body.

SUGGESTED READINGS

Campbell W: DeJong's The Neurological Examination, ed 6. Philadelphia, Lippincott Williams and Wilkins, 2005.

Goetz CG: Textbook of Clinical Neurology, ed 2. Philadelphia, Saunders, 2003.

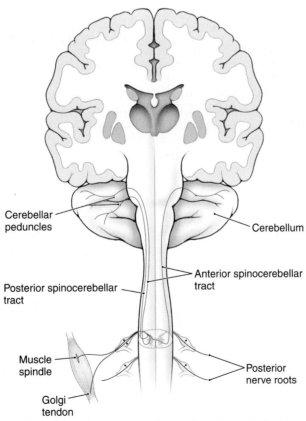

FIGURE 102–1 The anterior and posterior spinocerebellar tract.

Cerebellar peduncles

Cerebellum

Posterior spinocerebellar tract

Anterior spinocerebellar tract

Muscle spindle

Posterior nerve roots

Golgi tendon

CHAPTER 103

The Pyramidal System

Providing voluntary control of the skeletal muscles, the pyramidal system arises from the pyramidal cells of the primary motor cortex. These pyramid-shaped cells pass inferiorly either into the brainstem or directly into the spinal cord where they synapse directly on lower motor neurons. Because there are no interposed interneurons, the pyramidal system provides an extremely rapid communications pathway for the control of skeletal muscles.

The pyramidal system is made up of three pairs of descending motor tracts: (1) the corticobulbar tracts, (2) the lateral corticospinal tracts, and (3) the anterior corticospinal tracts (Fig. 103-1). The corticobulbar tracts find their origin in the primary motor cortex of the cerebrum and end at the brainstem motor nuclei of cranial nerves III, IV, VI, VII, IX, and XII, which are responsible for control of eye movements, the tongue, the muscles of facial expression, and the more superficial muscles of the neck and back. The corticospinal tracts, which are visible as a pair of thick elevated bands on the ventral surface of the medulla, pass inferiorly from the primary cerebral motor cortex directly into the spinal cord to synapse with motor neurons in the ventral gray horns of the spinal cord. Approximately 85% of these primary motor axons decussate at the level of the medulla to cross to the contralateral spinal cord to enter the lateral corticospinal tracts. The fibers of the lateral corticospinal tracts provide conscious control of

TABLE 103–1 Clinical Presentation of a Lower Motor Neuron Lesion

- Affected muscles are flaccid.
- Deep tendon reflexes are hyporeflexic or absent.
- Fasciculations of muscles are visible.
- Abnormal flail-like gait is present.
- Paresis is limited to specific muscle groups affected.
- With time, atrophy and contractures may develop.

the muscles of the limbs. The remaining 15% of these primary motor neurons remain on the ipsilateral side of the spinal cord and descend as the anterior corticospinal tracts. These uncrossed fibers then decussate within the spinal cord within the anterior gray commissure to synapse onto the ventral gray horns to provide conscious control over the muscles of the axial skeleton. Damage to the pyramidal system will present clinically as a lower motor neuron lesion (Table 103-1).

SUGGESTED READINGS

Campbell W: DeJong's The Neurological Examination, ed 6. Philadelphia, Lippincott Williams and Wilkins, 2005.

Goetz CG: Textbook of Clinical Neurology, ed 2. Philadelphia, Saunders, 2003.

Waldman SD: Pain Management. Philadelphia, Saunders, 2007.

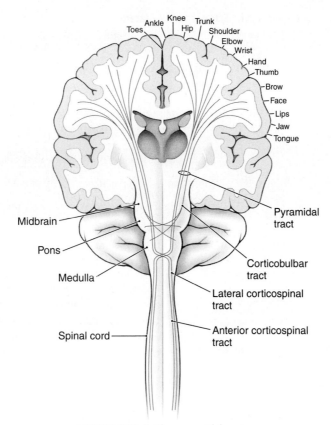

FIGURE 103–1 The pyramidal system.

The Extrapyramidal System

The extrapyramidal system is the name used to describe a number of centers and their associated tracts whose primary function is to coordinate and process motor commands performed at a subconscious level (Fig. 104-1). The anatomic centers and tracts are separate and apart from the pyramidal system, whose fibers reach their target muscles by traveling through the pyramids of the medulla and carrying their messages via the corticobulbar and corticospinal tracts. The processing centers of the extrapyramidal system are listed in Table 104-1. These processing centers produce output to a variety of targets, including (1) the primary motor cortex to modulate the activities of the pyramidal system; (2) the cranial nerve nuclei to

coordinate reflex activities in response to visual, auditory, and equilibrium input; and (3) descending pathways into the spinal cord including the vestibulospinal tracts, the tectospinal tracts, the rubrospinal tracts, and the reticulospinal tracts whose functions are outlined in Table 104-2.

The cerebral nuclei are the most important component of the extrapyramidal system. They are embedded just lateral to the thalamus in the cerebrum and serve as the processing center for voluntary motor activities. The cerebral nuclei carry out this function by fine-tuning the motor commands originating in other processing centers of the extrapyramidal system rather than by initiating specific motor commands via the lower motor neurons.

TABLE 104–1 The Primary Processing Centers of the Extrapyramidal System

Processing Center	Location	Primary Function
Vestibular nuclei	Pons and medulla oblongata	Processing of balance and control of associated reflexes of equilibrium
Superior colliculi	Mesencephalon	Processing of vision and control of associated reflexes
Inferior colliculi	Mesencephalon	Processing of hearing and control of associated reflexes
Red nucleus	Mesencephalon	Processing and control of skeletal muscle tone
Reticular formation	Mesencephalon	Processing of incoming sensory information and outgoing motor commands
Cerebral nuclei	Cerebrum	Organization and coordination of extremity and trunk movement
Cerebellar nuclei	Cerebellum	Coordination and integration of movement and integration of sensory feedback

TABLE 104–2 Extrapyramidal Tracts That Descend Directly into the Spinal Cord

Extrapyramidal Tracts	Function
Vestibulospinal tracts	Transmit balance information directly into the spinal cord from the vestibular nuclei
Tectospinal tracts	Transmit commands to change the position of the head, neck, eyes, and arms in response to sudden movements, loud noises, and/or bright lights
Rubrospinal tracts	Transmit motor commands to spinal motor neurons to maintain muscle tone
Reticulospinal tracts	Transmit motor commands from reticular formation

The cerebral nuclei also provide stereotypical motor commands necessary to initiate repetitive activities such as walking. Symptoms of extrapyramidal system dysfunction can take the form of Parkinson's disease or Parkinson's-like movement such as akinesia, which is the inability to initiate movement, or akathisia, which is the inability to remain motionless.

SUGGESTED READINGS

Campbell W: DeJong's The Neurological Examination, ed 6. Philadelphia, Lippincott Williams and Wilkins, 2005.

Goetz CG: Textbook of Clinical Neurology, ed 2. Philadelphia, Saunders, 2003.

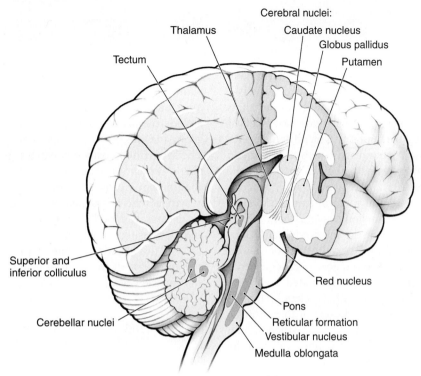

FIGURE 104–1 The extrapyramidal system.

CHAPTER 105

The Sympathetic Division of the Autonomic Nervous System

Often referred to as the "fight or flight" division of the autonomic nervous system, the sympathetic division helps maintain homeostasis by increasing alertness and cellular metabolism and making the body better able to deal with emergencies that threaten its integrity (Table 105-1). The sympathetic division is divided into three parts: (1) the preganglionic neurons, which have their cell bodies in the ventral gray horns of the spinal cord segments T1 though L2 with their axons occupying the corresponding ventral spinal roots; (2) the ganglionic neurons, which reside in ganglia which are located either within the sympathetic chain ganglia just lateral to the vertebral column or in the collateral ganglia just anterior to the vertebral column; and (3) the highly specialized neurons of the adrenal medulla (Fig. 105-1).

TABLE 105–1 Physiologic Effects of Sympathetic Activation

1. Decreased sensitivity to pain
2. Increased alertness via stimulation of the reticular activating system
3. Elevation of blood pressure
4. Increased heart rate
5. Increased respiratory rate
6. Increased depth of respiration
7. Mobilization of stored energy from increased breakdown of glycogen in the liver and muscle cells
8. Release of lipids by adipose cells
9. Increased muscle tone due to stimulation of the extrapyramidal system
10. A sense of increased energy and euphoria

The Sympathetic Chain Ganglion

The sympathetic chain ganglia are responsible for the sympathetic activity of the thoracic cavity, chest and abdominal wall, head, neck, and extremities. There is a sympathetic chain on each side of the vertebral columns with the average human having on each side 3 cervical, 11 or 12 thoracic, 3 to 5 lumbar, and 4 or 5 sacral ganglia with the coccygeal ganglion from each sympathetic chain fusing to form a single terminal ganglion known as the ganglion of Impar (Fig. 105-2).

Organizationally, the ventral roots of spinal segments T1 through L2 carry preganglionic sympathetic fibers that join the dorsal root to exit the intervertebral foramina as a spinal nerve root. As the spinal nerve root leaves the foramen, a white ramus communicans branches from its respective spinal nerve to carry myelinated preganglionic fibers into the adjacent sympathetic chain ganglion. These myelinated fibers will then do one of three things: (1) the fibers may synapse within the sympathetic chain ganglion at the same level at which the fibers entered the ganglion; (2) the fibers may ascend or descend within the sympathetic chain and then synapse with a sympathetic ganglion at a level different from the level of fiber entry; or (3) the fibers may simply pass through the sympathetic chain without synapsing with any sympathetic chain ganglion to ultimately synapse with a collateral ganglion or the adrenal medulla.

It should be noted that one of the hallmarks of the sympathetic division of the autonomic nervous system is that of divergence—that is, a single preganglionic sympathetic fiber may synapse on many sympathetic ganglionic neurons. Postganglionic fibers that innervate specific structures within the thoracic cavity (e.g., the heart or lungs) pass directly to these organs as sympathetic nerves to provide sympathetic innervation. Postganglionic fibers that innervate broader-ranging or more general somatic structures such as the smooth muscles of the blood vessels or sudoriferous glands of the skin enter the gray ramus communicans and reenter the spinal nerves for subsequent distribution to their target structures. To put in perspective the extent of postganglionic innervation to these diffuse structures, it has been estimated that between 8% and 9% of each spinal nerve is composed of these postganglionic sympathetic fibers.

The Sympathetic Collateral Ganglia

The sympathetic collateral ganglia are most often fused single ganglia rather than paired ganglia found in the sympathetic chain ganglia. The sympathetic collateral ganglia most often lie anterolateral to the descending aorta and include the celiac ganglion, the superior mesenteric ganglion, and the inferior sympathetic ganglion (Fig. 105-3). The sympathetic collateral ganglia give off postganglionic fibers, which provide sympathetic innervation to the abdominopelvic viscera. Activation of these postganglionic sympathetic fibers aids in maintenance of homeostasis by decreasing blood flow to the abdominopelvic viscera and decreasing activity of the nonvital digestive organs such as the intestines while at the same time increasing energy release in the form of glycogen stored in the liver and muscle cells.

The Adrenal Medulla

Preganglionic sympathetic fibers from the T3 through T8 spinal segments pass directly through the sympathetic chain ganglia without synapsing within the ganglia to end in the center of the adrenal medulla (Fig. 105-4). At this point, they synapse with a number of highly specialized modified neurons that function more like an endocrine gland than like a nerve. When these specialized neurons are stimulated, they release epinephrine and norepinephrine into the capillary bed of the adrenal medulla where they are transported to act on distant end organs in a manner analogous to a hormone. These circulating neurotransmitters allow tissues not innervated by postganglionic sympathetic fibers to receive stimulation by the sympathetic nervous system, provided they have receptors that are sensitive to epinephrine and norepinephrine.

SUGGESTED READINGS

Campbell W: DeJong's The Neurological Examination, ed 6. Philadelphia, Lippincott Williams and Wilkins, 2005.

Goetz CG: Textbook of Clinical Neurology, ed 2. Philadelphia, Saunders, 2003.

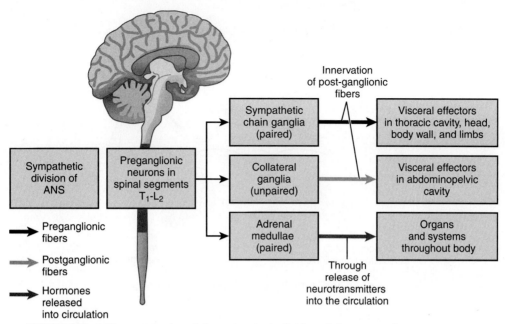

FIGURE 105–1 The organization of the sympathetic division of the autonomic nervous system.

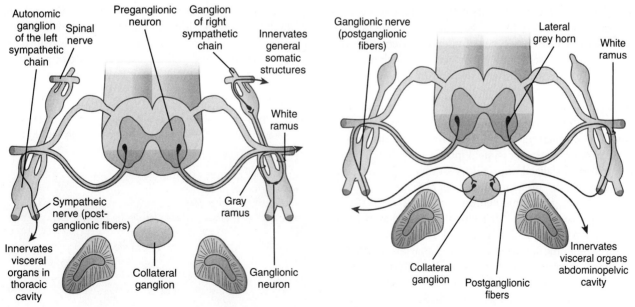

FIGURE 105–2 The anatomy of the sympathetic chain ganglia.

FIGURE 105–3 The anatomy of the collateral ganglia.

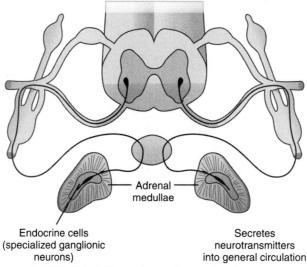

Adrenal
medullae

Endocrine cells
(specialized ganglionic
neurons)

Secretes
neurotransmitters
into general circulation

FIGURE 105–4 The anatomy of the adrenal medulla.

CHAPTER 106

The Parasympathetic Division of the Autonomic Nervous System

The parasympathetic division of the autonomic nervous system is often referred to as the "rest and repose" system as its primary function is that of energy conservation and the facilitation of sedentary bodily activities such as digestion. Unlike the sympathetic division of the autonomic nervous system, which is best characterized as a divergent system due to the far-reaching and diffuse impact that occurs when the sympathetic division neurons are stimulated, the stimulation of the parasympathetic division of the autonomic nervous system produces a much more targeted and localized impact. It is estimated that a typical parasympathetic preganglionic fiber synapses on only seven or eight ganglionic neurons.

The parasympathetic division of the autonomic nervous system has two basic units. (1) The first consists of the preganglionic neurons and nuclei that are located in the brain, mesencephalon, pons, and medulla oblongata as well as autonomic nuclei that reside in the lateral gray horns of spinal segments S2 through S4. These preganglionic fibers travel within cranial nerves III, VII, IX, and

X to synapse at the ciliary, sphenopalatine, otic, and submandibular ganglia. Short postganglionic fibers then carry parasympathetic commands to their respective target organs (Fig. 106-1). (2) The second consists of preganglionic neurons that do not enter the ventral rami of the

TABLE 106–1 Clinically Observed Responses to Stimulation of the Parasympathetic Division of the Autonomic Nervous System

- Reduction in heart rate
- Decrease in myocardial contractility
- Constriction of the airways
- Constriction of pupils
- Contraction of urinary bladder during micturition
- Sexual arousal and stimulation
- Stimulation and coordination of defecation
- Secretion of hormones that aid in the absorption of nutrients
- Increase in the secretion of digestive enzymes
- Increase in gastrointestinal mobility

spinal nerve but instead form discrete nerves that synapse with ganglia that are located in close proximity or within the walls of their target organs (e.g., the urinary bladder, uterus, etc.) (see Fig. 106-1). Stimulation of these parasympathetic nerves results in the release of acetylcholine by all preganglionic parasympathetic neurons, which causes stimulation of all nicotinic receptors and results in either stimulation or inhibition of muscarinic receptors depending on what enzymes are released when the acetylcholine binds to the muscarinic receptor. The specific clinically observed responses resulting from stimulation of the parasympathetic division of the autonomic nervous system are summarized in Table 106-1.

SUGGESTED READINGS

Campbell W: DeJong's The Neurological Examination, ed 6. Philadelphia, Lippincott Williams and Wilkins, 2005.
Goetz CG: Textbook of Clinical Neurology, ed 2. Philadelphia, Saunders, 2003.

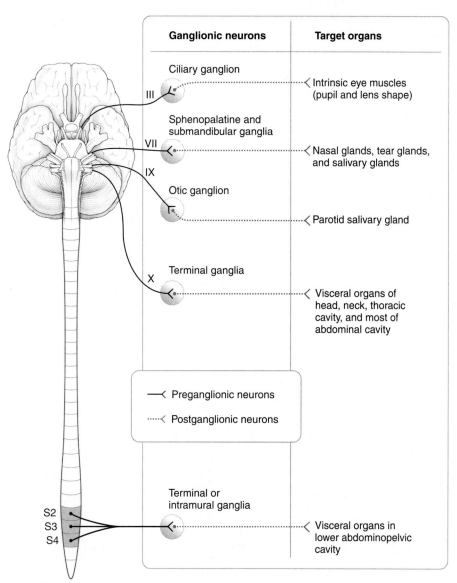

FIGURE 106–1 The organization of the parasympathetic division of the autonomic nervous system.

CHAPTER 107

The Relationship Between the Sympathetic and Parasympathetic Nervous Systems

Although some organs receive only sympathetic or parasympathetic innervation, the vast majority of organs receive innervation from both divisions of the autonomic nervous system. Conceptually, this dual innervation almost always works with each division having an antagonistic effect on one another. This antagonistic effect is most apparent in the cardiac, respiratory, and gastrointestinal systems. In situations in which the antagonistic effects of dual innervation are prominent, sympathetic postganglionic fibers and parasympathetic preganglionic fibers come together at the cardiac, pulmonary, esophageal, celiac, inferior mesenteric, and hypogastric plexuses with the nerves exiting the plexuses and traveling in tandem with blood vessels to innervate the thoracoabdominal organs (Fig. 107-1).

SUGGESTED READINGS

Campbell W: DeJong's The Neurological Examination, ed 6. Philadelphia, Lippincott Williams and Wilkins, 2005.
Goetz CG: Textbook of Clinical Neurology, ed 2. Philadelphia, Saunders, 2003.
Waldman SD: Pain Management. Philadelphia, Saunders, 2007.

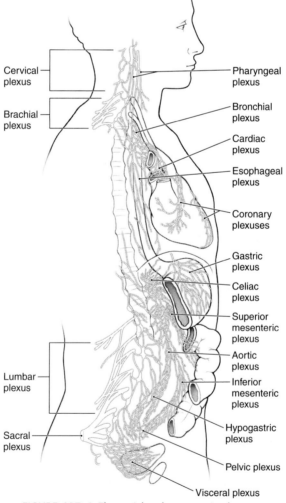

Cervical plexus
Brachial plexus
Lumbar plexus
Sacral plexus
Pharyngeal plexus
Bronchial plexus
Cardiac plexus
Esophageal plexus
Coronary plexuses
Gastric plexus
Celiac plexus
Superior mesenteric plexus
Aortic plexus
Inferior mesenteric plexus
Hypogastric plexus
Pelvic plexus
Visceral plexus

FIGURE 107–1 The peripheral autonomic plexuses.

Functional Anatomy of the Nociceptors

Nociceptors are pain receptors that are essential to the maintenance of homeostasis. Freely distributed in the outer layers of the skin, the walls of blood vessels, the periosteum of bone, and joint capsules, nociceptors are most often free nerve endings with large receptive fields. These large receptive fields make the exact localization of the origin of a painful stimulus somewhat difficult. There are significantly fewer nociceptors in the deep tissues and visceral organs when compared with the above mentioned structures.

There are three basic types of nociceptors: (1) receptors sensitive to temperature extremes; (2) receptors sensitive to mechanical damage; and (3) receptors sensitive to cytokines released from damaged cells, such as substance P (Fig. 108-1). Although each receptor is designed to identify a specific type of stimulus, it should be noted that each type of receptor will respond to extreme levels of any of these types of nociceptive stimuli.

When nociceptors are stimulated, the first response is the firing of the receptors to produce an immediate message to the central nervous system that there is a threat to homeostasis. This response is known as fast or sharp pain in recognition of the speed at which the message is received and processed by the central nervous system with the immediate triggering of somatic reflexes such as the withdrawal response being the first commands sent forth from the central nervous system. Fast pain information is carried by myelinated A-delta fibers into the dorsal horn and up the lateral spinothalamic tract to the thalamus, the reticular activating system, and the primary sensory cortex. Continued tissue damage will result in continued fast pain messages being transmitted to the central nervous system by the nociceptors with the central nervous system issuing commands to limit the amount of ongoing tissue damage or, if this is impossible, to begin attenuating the central perception of pain to allow the organism to continue with other tasks necessary to survive.

Following immediately after the first volley of fast pain impulses is sent to the central nervous system, a longer-lasting volley of impulses known as slow or dull pain is sent to the central nervous system. These slow pain impulses are carried by the only unmyelinated sensory fibers, which are known as C fibers. Slow pain impulses result in further activation of the reticular activating system and thalamus with a resultant awareness that a painful insult has occurred. This slow or dull pain tends to be perceived in a poorly localized fashion and is often described as more dull or aching in nature with the patient feeling the urge to rub or palpate the area of generalized pain.

As mentioned, there are significantly fewer nociceptors in the deep tissues and visceral organs than in the outer layers of the skin, the walls of blood vessels, the periosteum of bone, and joint capsules. When the deep tissues or visceral organs are injured, the pain tends to be poorly localized and often perceived in areas distant to the actual site of injury (Fig. 108-2). This phenomenon is known as referred pain and is thought to be at least in part due to the fact that these tissues are innervated by spinal nerves.

SUGGESTED READINGS

Campbell W: DeJong's The Neurological Examination, ed 6. Philadelphia, Lippincott Williams and Wilkins, 2005.

Goetz CG: Textbook of Clinical Neurology, ed 2. Philadelphia, Saunders, 2003.

Waldman SD: Pain Management. Philadelphia, Saunders, 2007.

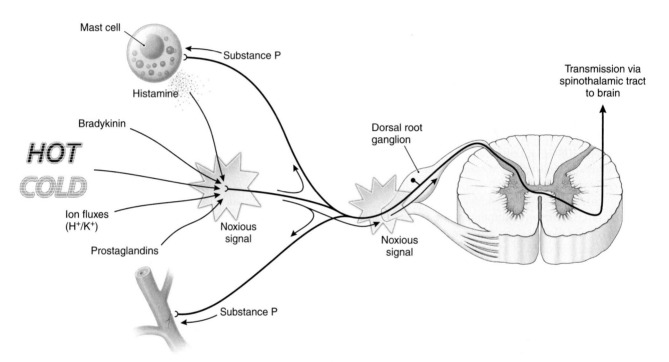

FIGURE 108–1 The nociceptive response to the release of cytokines.

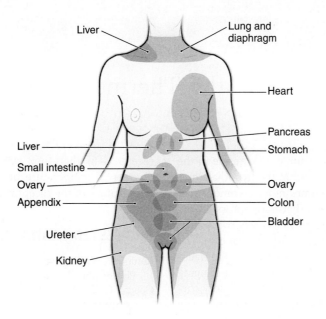

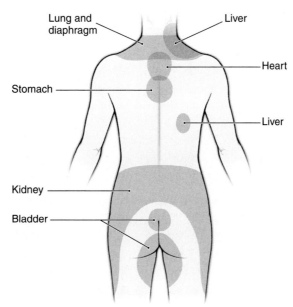

FIGURE 108–2 Patterns of referred pain.

CHAPTER 109

Functional Anatomy of the Thermoreceptors

Thermoreceptors are free nerve endings that reside in the skin, liver, and skeletal muscles, and in the hypothalamus, with cold thermoreceptors 3.5 times more common than heat receptors. Information from thermoreceptors is carried via the same A-delta and C fibers as carry pain information, and enters the dorsal horn of the spinal cord and then travels up the lateral spinothalamic tract to the thalamus with secondary thermoreceptor fibers also impinging on the reticular activating system and primary sensory cortex (Fig. 109-1). Thermoreceptors are called phasic-type receptors in that they respond very rapidly to minute changes in temperature but adapt and quit firing as the temperature of the receptor reaches steady state.

SUGGESTED READINGS

Campbell W: DeJong's The Neurological Examination, ed 6. Philadelphia, Lippincott Williams and Wilkins, 2005.
Goetz CG: Textbook of Clinical Neurology, ed 2. Philadelphia, Saunders, 2003.

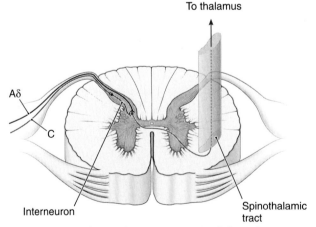

FIGURE 109–1 The pathway of temperature stimuli from thermoreceptors.

CHAPTER 110

Functional Anatomy of the Mechanoreceptors

Mechanoreceptors help maintain homeostasis by responding to stimuli that cause twisting, compression, distortion, or stretching of the mechanoreceptor's cell membrane. There are three basic types of mechanoreceptors: (1) tactile receptors, (2) baroreceptors, and (3) proprioceptors. Each type of mechanoreceptor has a specialized function that helps warn the organism that there is a threat of tissue injury.

Tactile Receptors

Tactile receptors can be divided into two subgroups: (1) encapsulated tactile receptors and (2) unencapsulated tactile receptors. Encapsulated tactile receptors include Meissner's corpuscles, Pacinian corpuscles, and Ruffinian corpuscles (Fig. 110-1). Unencapsulated receptors include Merkel's discs, free nerve endings, and the root hair plexuses (see Fig. 110-1).

Meissner's corpuscles are found in areas with the most highly developed tactile sensitivity—the nipples, lips, external genitalia, fingertips, and eyelids. Meissner's corpuscles are capable of detecting fine movement, light touch, and minute vibrations and are highly adaptable.

Pacinian corpuscles are the largest of the encapsulated tactile receptors and are located in the fingers, breast, and external genitalia as well as in the superficial and deep fascia, the joint capsules, the periostea of bone, urethra, urinary bladder, pancreas, and the mesentery. The Pacinian corpuscles respond primarily to deep pressure but will also respond to repetitive vibration or pulsing stimuli. Like the Meissner's corpuscles, the Pacinian corpuscles adapt very rapidly to repeat stimuli.

Ruffinian corpuscles are liberally distributed in the dermis and these encapsulated tactile receptors respond to distortion and stretching of the skin. Unlike the Meissner's and Pacinian corpuscles, the Ruffinian corpuscles are tonic receptors and adapt to repetitive stimuli very slowly if at all.

Located in the stratum germinativum of the epidermis, the unencapsulated Merkel's discs are tonic tactile receptors that are extremely sensitive to fine touch and pressure. They have very small receptive fields and aid in the precise localization of threats to tissue integrity.

The root hair plexuses monitor movement and distortion of large areas of the body's surface. Displacement of hair results in distortion of the sensory dendrites associated with the hair follicle producing immediate action potentials. The root hair plexuses are very adaptable, which explains why one only senses clothing when moving or changing position. Both the hair root plexuses and Merkel's disc closely interact with the ubiquitous free nerve endings that reside in the papillary layer of the dermis to further enhance the protective mechanism of these unencapsulated tactile receptors.

Baroreceptors

Located in the fibroelastic walls of blood vessels, hollow organs, and the respiratory, digestive, and urinary tracts, these baroreceptors are made of free nerve endings that monitor changes in pressure via the stretch and recoil of the tissue being monitored. Responding immediately to the most minute changes in pressure, the rate of action potential firing is in proportion to the rate at which the tissue being monitored is stretched. Large numbers of baroreceptors are located in the carotid and aortic sinuses and are crucial to the maintenance of homeostasis in health and disease (Fig. 110-2). It should be noted that baroreceptors trigger a number of complex cardiovascular and visceral reflexes when stimulated.

Proprioceptors

The primary function of proprioceptors is the preservation of joint integrity by the constant monitoring of joint position, tendon tension, ligament tension, and extent of muscle contraction. The muscle spindle apparatus and the Golgi tendon apparatus are examples of specialized proprioceptors (Fig. 110-3).

SUGGESTED READINGS

Campbell W: DeJong's The Neurological Examination, ed 6. Philadelphia, Lippincott Williams and Wilkins, 2005.
Goetz CG: Textbook of Clinical Neurology, ed 2. Philadelphia, Saunders, 2003.

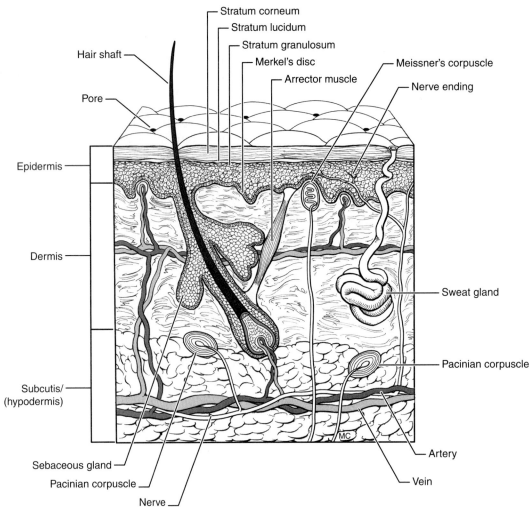

FIGURE 110–1 Tactile receptors.

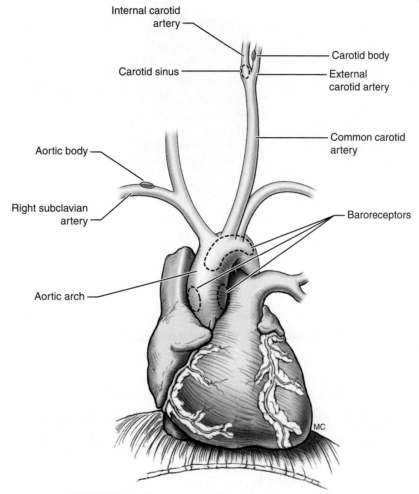

Internal carotid artery

Carotid sinus

Carotid body

External carotid artery

Common carotid artery

Aortic body

Right subclavian artery

Baroreceptors

Aortic arch

MC

FIGURE 110–2 Baroreceptors of the carotid artery and aorta.

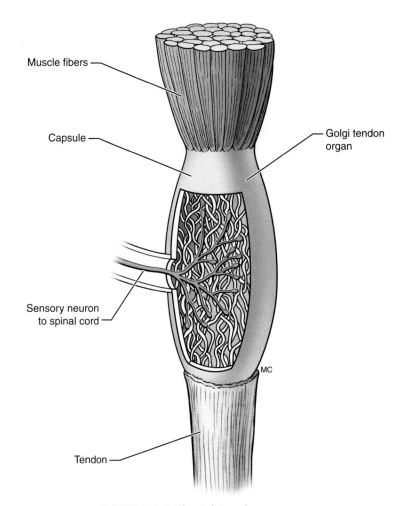

Muscle fibers

Capsule

Golgi tendon organ

Sensory neuron to spinal cord

MC

Tendon

FIGURE 110–3 The Golgi tendon apparatus.

CHAPTER 111

Functional Anatomy of the Chemoreceptors

Chemoreceptors are essential to the maintenance of homeostasis as they constantly monitor minute changes in the relative concentrations of both lipid and water-soluble compounds dissolved in the fluids that surround them. Chemoreceptors located the medulla oblongata respond to changes in the hydrogen ion and carbon dioxide concentrations in the cerebrospinal fluid by altering the rate and depth of respiration (Fig. 111-1). Additional chemoreceptors located in the carotid and aortic bodies monitor the concentration of carbon dioxide and oxygen in the arterial blood of the carotid arteries and aorta.

Changes in the concentration of the partial pressure of these gases trigger the firing of afferent fibers within cranial nerves IX and X to the respiratory centers to alter respiratory function.

SUGGESTED READINGS

Goetz CG: Textbook of Clinical Neurology, ed 2. Philadelphia, Saunders, 2003.
Waldman SD: Pain Management. Philadelphia, Saunders, 2007.

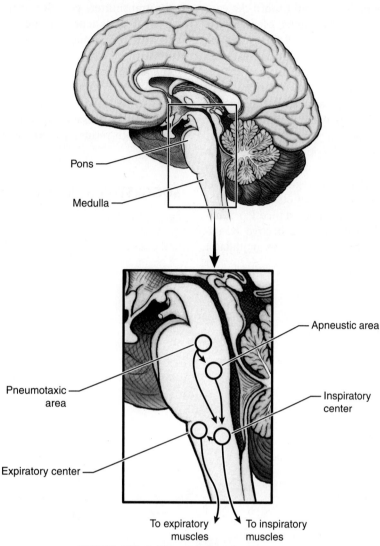

Pons

Medulla

Apneustic area

Pneumotaxic area

Inspiratory center

Expiratory center

To expiratory muscles

To inspiratory muscles

FIGURE 111–1 The central respiratory centers.

CHAPTER 112

Functional Anatomy of the Dorsal Root Ganglia and Dorsal Horn

Afferent sensory fibers coalesce to enter the spinal cord together via the dorsal root. The cell bodies of these afferent sensory fibers are grouped together just outside the bony spinal column forming the dorsal root ganglia. Entering the spinal cord at its dorsal surface at an area known as the dorsal root entry zone, small, medium-size, and large afferent fibers group together to perform their various functions with glutamate serving as the primary neurotransmitter (Fig. 112-1). Larger myelinated primary afferent sensory fibers transmit touch, vibratory, and pressure information and, after entering the dorsal root entry zone, cross to the contralateral side of the dorsal horn via

Lissauer's tract. These fibers then ascend toward the central nervous system via the dorsal columns. Medium-size and small myelinated and unmyelinated fibers, which carry important pain and temperature information, enter Lissauer's tract and diverge to impinge on gray matter neuronal cells at their level of entry into the spinal cord as well as traveling to spinal segments both craniad and caudad to level of entry. These primary afferent fibers are characterized by the presence of the neurotransmitter peptide calcitonin gene–related peptide (CGRP), which serves to modulate the transmission of the primary afferent fibers. In addition to CGRP, the region of the dorsal horn is richly endowed with a variety of other modulator neurotransmitter peptides, including substance P, adenosine triphosphate (ATP), somatostatin, vasoactive intestinal polypeptide (VIP), bombesin, etc. These modulator neurotransmitter peptides can enhance the activating effect of glutamate on the dorsal horn neurons and affect the processing of sensory information at the spinal cord level by either enhancing or inhibiting transmission to higher levels. The phenomenon of windup is an example of how modulatory neurotransmitter peptides can result in increased transmission of nociceptive information from the dorsal horn up the spinal cord to the higher centers with resultant increased perception of pain.

SUGGESTED READINGS

Goetz CG: Textbook of Clinical Neurology, ed 2. Philadelphia, Saunders, 2003.
Waldman SD: Pain Management. Philadelphia, Saunders, 2007.

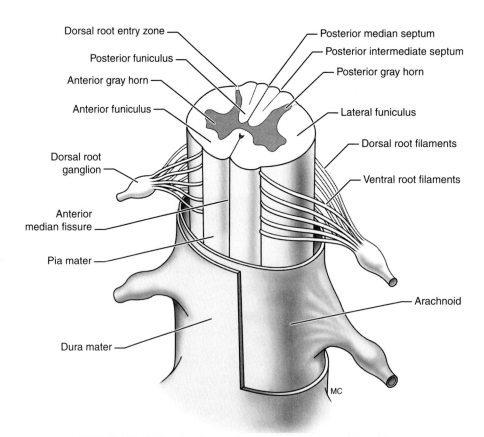

FIGURE 112–1 The dorsal root, dorsal root ganglion, and dorsal horn.

CHAPTER 113

The Gate Control Theory

The gate control theory of pain had a monumental impact on the field of pain as it provided basic scientists and clinicians with a unified theory to explain almost all clinically observed pain-related situations. Prior to the gate control theory, which was first promulgated by Ronald Melzack and Patrick Wall in 1965, the working model for painful conditions was based on the pain-pleasure theory put forth by René Descartes in the early 1600s. Under the Descartes model, the phenomenon of pain was viewed primarily as a linear stimulus-response curve, which did not explain a variety of commonly encountered clinical situations where there was either a lack of stimulus (e.g., phantom limb pain) or a lack of response (e.g., minimal pain complaints from a patient who has sustained massive trauma).

The afferent fibers that carry pain impulses are the faster, large myelinated A delta fibers and the slower, small unmyelinated C fibers (Fig. 113-1). Non-nociceptive A beta fibers enter the dorsal horn at the same place as the slow unmyelinated C fibers and can serve to "close the gate" to pain impulses by indirectly inhibiting the cephalad transmission of pain impulses to the brain. This indirect inhibition of the cephalad transmission of pain impulses by non-nociceptive A beta fibers occurs via inhibitory synapses with the projection neurons responsible to carry pain impulses to the brain. These non-nociceptive A beta fibers may also excite inhibitory interneurons within the dorsal horn, which will also inhibit transmission of pain impulses cephalad.

Inhibition of pain impulses may also occur centrally when descending inhibitory fibers that originate in the periaqueductal gray matter that surrounds the third ventricle and cerebral aqueduct are stimulated. Such stimulation results in activation of descending fibers that exert both direct and indirect inhibition of pain transmission at the spinal cord level. Stimulation of this anatomic area also causes activation of opioid receptors located in the spinal cord. The effects of the inhibition of pain at the spinal cord and central level allows the organism to protect itself by ignoring pain to pursue goals that the brain determines are of a higher priority.

SUGGESTED READINGS

Melzack R, Wall PD: Pain mechanisms: A new theory. Science 150:971-979, 1965.

McMahon S, Koltzenburg M (eds): Wall and Melzack's Textbook of Pain, ed 5. Philadelphia, Churchill Livingstone, 2006.

Waldman SD: Pain Management. Philadelphia, Saunders, 2007.

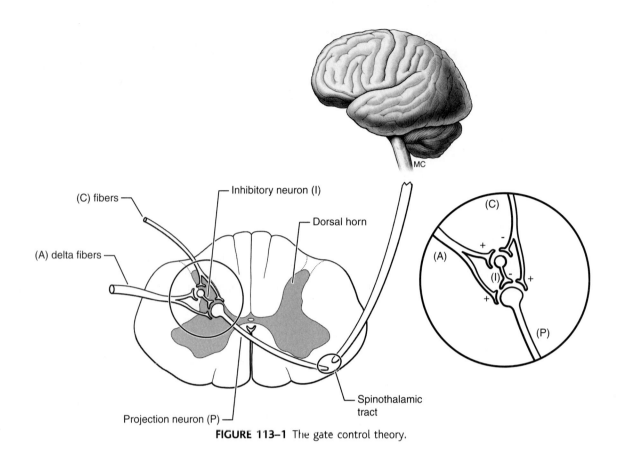

(C) fibers

(A) delta fibers

Inhibitory neuron (I)

Dorsal horn

MC

(C)

(A)

(I)

(P)

Spinothalamic
tract

Projection neuron (P)

FIGURE 113–1 The gate control theory.

CHAPTER **114**

The Cerebrum

Made up of two paired cerebral hemispheres, the cerebrum is the largest region of the brain. All conscious thought and the processing of somatosensory and somatomotor information are the cerebrum's primary functions. The paired cerebral hemispheres are covered with gray matter whose surface is covered with elevated ridges known as gyri and indented by depressions known as sulci, as well as deeper grooves known as fissures.

The gyri, sulci, and fissures increase the surface area of the cerebral hemispheres to accommodate the vast number of cerebral neurons necessary to perform the myriad complex functions required for humans to survive. Although each of the paired cerebral hemispheres appears grossly anatomically identical, some functional differences exist from individual to individual. It should

also be remembered that each cerebral hemisphere receives its afferent sensory information from the contralateral side of the body and sends efferent motor commands to the contralateral side of the body—for example, the right cerebral hemisphere controls the left side of the body.

The two cerebral hemispheres are divided by the deep medial longitudinal fissure (Fig. 114-1). Each individual hemisphere can be further subdivided into lobes which are named for the overlying bones of the cranium (Fig. 114-2). The central fissure or sulcus extends laterally from the medial longitudinal fissure and divides the frontal lobe anteriorly from the more posterior parietal lobe as well as separating the sensory and motor functional areas of the brain (see Fig. 114-2). The lateral sulcus marks the inferior border of the frontal lobe and separates it from the more inferior temporal lobe. Just deep to the lateral sulcus is a hidden island of cerebral cortex known as the insula, which is important in the affective component of pain (Fig. 114-3). The parieto-occipital sulcus extends posteriorly from the central fissure to separate the parietal lobe from the occipital lobe.

Important functional areas of the brain are illustrated in Figure 114-2, although it should be noted that many of the cerebrum's most important functions, such as consciousness, cannot be localized to a single region and are the result of complex interactions between multiple areas of the brain. The precentral gyrus of the frontal lobe at the anterior border of the central fissure is the area of the primary motor cortex with neurons controlling voluntary motor functions via the pyramidal cells of the pyramidal system (see Chapter 103). The postcentral gyrus of the parietal lobe lies at the posterior border of the central fissure and is the area of the primary sensory cortex that receives afferent sensory information. The visual cortex of the occipital lobe receives visual information, with the auditory and olfactory centers of the temporal lobe receiving auditory and olfactory information. The gustatory cortex located in the anterior portion of the insula and posterior frontal lobe receives gustatory information. Adjacent association centers help sort and interpret all of this incoming information and aid in formulating a coordinated response by forwarding this processed information to integrative centers, which further analyze this information, and formulate complex responses designed to maintain homeostasis and protect the organism from trauma.

Beneath the gray matter of the cerebral cortex are the myelinated fibers of the central white matter. There are three types of central white matter fibers, each serving a different major function: (1) commissural fibers including the corpus callosum and anterior commissure fibers, which facilitate communications between the two cerebral hemispheres; (2) association fibers, which provide interconnections between different portions of the same cerebral hemisphere; and (3) projection fibers, which link the cerebral cortex to the diencephalon, brainstem, cerebellum, and spinal cord.

The cerebral nuclei are paired aggregations of gray matter that are embedded into the central white matter just inferior to the lateral ventricles within each cerebral hemisphere (Fig. 114-4). Both commissural fibers and projection fibers interconnect these important components of the extrapyramidal system (see Chapter 104). The caudate nucleus and putamen serve the important functions of coordinating and perpetuating repetitive rhythmic movements such as walking. The claustrum

TABLE 114-1 The Anatomic Structures Supporting the Functions of the Limbic System

Cerebral Structures
• Cortical areas
• Cingulate gyrus
• Dentate gyrus
• Parahippocampal gyrus
• Nuclei
• Hippocampus
• Amygdaloid body
• Tracts
• Fornix
Diencephalon Components
• Thalamus
• Anterior nuclear group
• Hypothalamus
• Thirst center
• Hunger center
Other Components
• Reticular formation

performs the important function of processing huge amounts of visual information at the subconscious level by identifying previously seen patterns and features. The amygdaloid body performs important functions including regulation of basic drives like eating and sexual behavior. The globus pallidus performs the important function of adjusting body position and fine tuning the muscle tone prior to performing specific voluntary movements.

The limbic system is a functional grouping of gray matter nuclei and associated tracts that are located on the border between the cerebrum and diencephalon (Fig. 114-5). The functions of the limbic system are complex and include (1) the establishment of baseline emotional states, (2) behavior drives, (3) facilitation of storage and retrieval of memories, and (4) the coordination and linkage of the complex conscious functions of the cerebral cortex with the unconscious and autonomic functions necessary for the maintenance of homeostasis. Anatomic structures supporting the functions of the limbic system are listed in Table 114-1.

SUGGESTED READINGS

Campbell W: DeJong's The Neurological Examination, ed 6. Philadelphia, Lippincott Williams and Wilkins, 2005.

Goetz CG: Textbook of Clinical Neurology, ed 2. Philadelphia, Saunders, 2003.

Waldman SD: Pain Management. Philadelphia, Saunders, 2007.

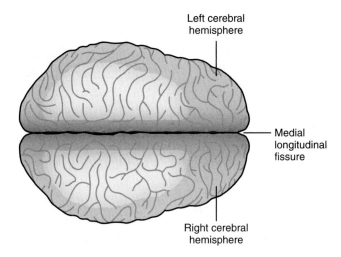

FIGURE 114–1 Superior view of the cerebral hemispheres.

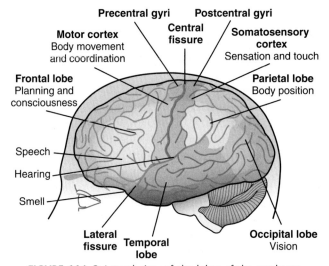

FIGURE 114–2 Lateral view of the lobes of the cerebrum.

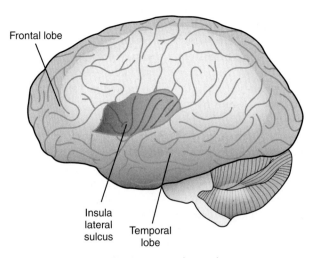

FIGURE 114–3 The insula.

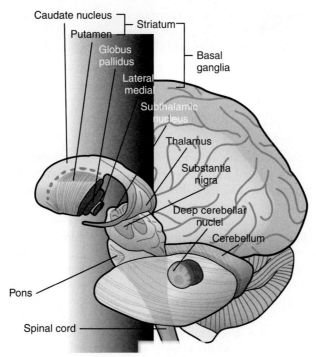

FIGURE 114–4 The cerebral nuclei.

THE LIMBIC SYSTEM

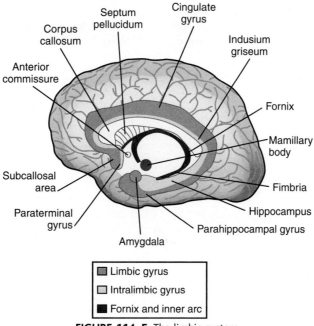

FIGURE 114–5 The limbic system.

CHAPTER 115

The Thalamus

The thalamus is located in the diencephalon and serves as the main relay and switching station as well as filter for both the sensory and motor pathways to and from the brain. With the exception of information from cranial nerve I (olfactory), all afferent sensory information from the other cranial nerves and spinal cord is processed by thalamic nuclei before it continues to the brainstem and cerebrum. The thalamus also serves the crucial function of coordinating and modulating the activities of the pyramidal and extrapyramidal systems. These functions occur primarily in the thalamic nuclei.

There are five thalamic nuclei: (1) the lateral nuclei, (2) the medial nuclei, (3) the anterior nuclei, (4) the ventral nuclei, and (5) the posterior nuclei (Fig. 115-1). The lateral nuclei provide feedback loops that allow modulation of the parietal lobe and cingulate gyrus, which helps control emotion and integrate sensory information. The medial nuclei provide integration of incoming sensory information arriving from other thalamic nuclei and then relays this information to the frontal lobes. The medial nuclei also provide the individual with a conscious awareness of his or her emotional states by sorting, relaying, and filtering information from the hypothalamus, cerebral prefrontal cortex, and the cerebral nuclei.

The anterior nuclei relay information from the hypothalamus and hippocampus to the cingulated gyrus and, as part of the limbic system, play an important role in the modulation of emotion as well as assisting in the learning and memory process. The ventral nuclei serve as the primary relay station of information to and from the cerebral nuclei and cerebral cortex. The ventral anterior and ventral lateral portions of the ventral nuclei are part of a feedback loop whose primary purpose is to fine tune anticipated movements by relaying, sorting, and filtering somatic motor information between the cerebral nuclei and cerebellum. The ventral posterior portion of the ventral nuclei is the primary relay station for the transmission of important sensory information including fine touch, pain, temperature, pressure, and proprioception from the spinal cord and brainstem to both the primary sensory cortex and the parietal lobe.

The posterior nuclei are made up of the pulvinar, lateral geniculate nuclei, and medial geniculate nuclei. The pulvinar integrates incoming sensory information and projects it to the primary association areas of the cerebral cortex. The lateral geniculate nuclei project incoming visual information onto the occipital lobe. The medial geniculate nuclei project incoming auditory information onto the temporal lobe.

SUGGESTED READINGS

Netter FH: The thalamus. In: Atlas of Human Anatomy, ed 4. Philadelphia, Saunders, 2006.
Waldman SD: Pain Management. Philadelphia, Saunders, 2007.

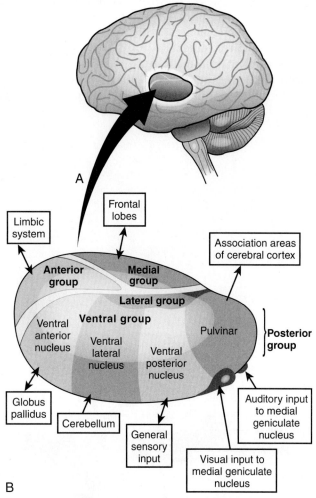

FIGURE 115–1 The thalamic nuclei.

CHAPTER 116

The Hypothalamus

The hypothalamus performs a variety of sorting, processing, modulating, and command functions crucial to the maintenance of homeostasis. Located at the floor of the third ventricle and extending from the region just above the optic chiasm to the posterior extent of the mamillary bodies, the hypothalamus is ideally situated to monitor the composition of the cerebrospinal fluid, the interstitial fluid of surrounding tissues, and the blood of the associated capillary bed (Fig. 116-1). Changes in the composition of these fluids can signal the hypothalamus to perform any and all of the following functions:

1. Raising or lowering of body temperature
2. Causing the release of antidiuretic hormone to signal the kidneys to restrict water loss

3. Causing the release of oxytocin to stimulate contractions of the uterus and prostate as well as the myoepithelial cells of the breasts
4. Coordination of circadian rhythms
5. Coordination and modulation of autonomic functions including blood pressure, heart rate, and respiration
6. Coordination and modulation of involuntary somatic motor activities associated with pain, pleasure, rage, and sexual arousal
7. Coordination of the complex interactions between the neuroendocrine system and the pituitary gland
8. Coordination and modulation of voluntary and involuntary behavioral patterns including thirst and hunger

SUGGESTED READING

Netter FH: Hypothalamus and hypophysis. In: Atlas of Human Anatomy, ed 4. Philadelphia, Saunders, 2006.

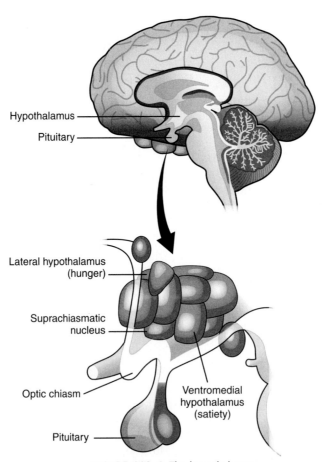

FIGURE 116–1 The hypothalamus.

The Mesencephalon

The mesencephalon contains the structures responsible for the processing of visual and auditory afferent impulses and for generating reflexive responses to help the organism avoid tissue damage. Just beneath the roof or tectum of the mesencephalon lies the corpora quadrigemina, which contain two pairs of sensory nuclei, the superior colliculi and the inferior colliculi (Fig. 117-1). Each superior colliculus receives afferent visual impulses from the geniculate nucleus on the ipsilateral side of the thalamus. Each inferior colliculus receives afferent auditory impulses from the medulla oblongata. The red nuclei on each side of the mesencephalon serve as the center that sorts and integrates volleys of information from the cerebellum and cerebrum and control and modulate muscle tone and posture. The substantia nigra on each side of the mesencephalon serves as the regulator of efferent motor output from the cerebral nuclei. Portions of the reticular activating system concerned with incoming sensory information, the maintenance of consciousness and involuntary motor responses, also reside on each side of the mesencephalon. The cerebral peduncles located on the ventrolateral surfaces of each side of the mesencephalon are composed of white matter and contain important ascending sensory fibers that connect to the thalamus and fibers that transmit voluntary motor commands from the primary motor cortex of each cerebral hemisphere to the brainstem and spinal cord.

SUGGESTED READING

Netter FH: Hypothalamus and hypophysis. In: Atlas of Human Anatomy, ed 4. Philadelphia, Saunders, 2006.

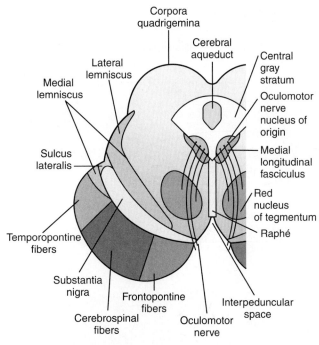

FIGURE 117–1 The mesencephalon: coronal section through mid-brain. 1. corpora quadrigemina; 2. cerebral aqueduct; 3. central gray stratum; 4. interpeduncular space; 5. sulcus lateralis; 6. substantia nigra; 7. red nucleus of tegmentum; 8. oculomotor nerve, with 8′ its nucleus of origin; a. lemniscus, with a′ the medial lemniscus and a″ the lateral lemniscus; b. medial longitudinal fasciculus; c. raphé; d. temporopontine fibers; e. portion of medial lemniscus, which runs to the lentiform nucleus and insula; f. cerebrospinal fibers; and g. frontopontine fibers.

CHAPTER 118

The Pons

The pons extends inferiorly from the mesencephalon to the medulla oblongata with the cerebral hemispheres lying astride the posterior surface of the pons (Fig. 118-1). The pons contains a number of important structures including:

1. The nuclei containing both the apneustic center and the pneumotaxic centers, which coordinate the involuntary control of respiration
2. The sensory and motor nuclei of cranial nerves V, VI, VII, and VIII
3. The nuclei that process and relay afferent information from the cerebellum that arrive in the pons via the middle cerebral peduncles

4. Tracts of ascending, descending, and transverse fibers that carry information from the spinal cord to the brain and from the brain to the spinal cord and information from opposite cerebral hemispheres

SUGGESTED READING

Netter FH: Cranial nerve nuclei in brainstem: Schema. In: Atlas of Human Anatomy, ed 4. Philadelphia, Saunders, 2006.

BRAINSTEM

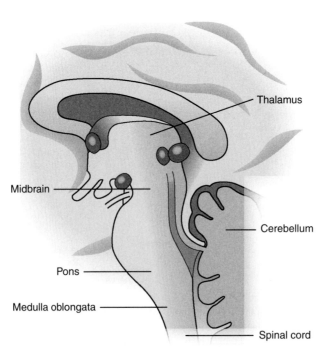

FIGURE 118–1 The pons.

CHAPTER 119

The Cerebellum

Without the cerebellum, coordinated voluntary and involuntary movement would be impossible and homeostasis would be difficult, if not impossible, to maintain (Fig. 119-1). The cerebellum is the primary site of the processing and integration of the functioning of the pyramidal and extrapyramidal systems. The cerebellum also modulates the muscle tone of the muscles of posture, whose coordinated function is necessary to almost all complex voluntary and involuntary movement. This information, as well as ever-changing proprioceptive information, is coordinated and processed in the cerebellum with constant motor commands being issued to increase and inhibit the number of motor units involved in a given motor action.

SUGGESTED READINGS

Campbell W: DeJong's The Neurological Examination, ed 6. Philadelphia, Lippincott Williams and Wilkins, 2005.

Goetz CG: Textbook of Clinical Neurology, ed 2. Philadelphia, Saunders, 2003.

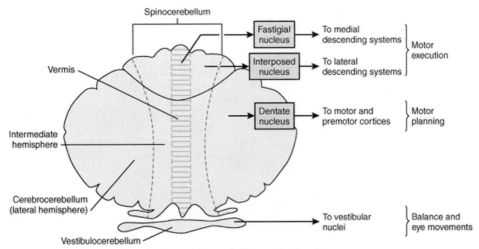

FIGURE 119–1 The cerebellum and related structures.

CHAPTER 120

The Medulla Oblongata

The medulla oblongata is home to all ascending and descending tracts that carry communications between the brain and the spinal cord (Fig. 120-1). Also housed within the medulla oblongata are a number of important nuclei and centers that sort, relay, and modulate a variety of activities necessary for the maintenance of homeostasis. These nuclei and centers include:

1. The cardiovascular center, which provides modulation and fine tuning of heart rate, the strength of myocardial contractility, and the dilatation and constriction of the peripheral vasculature
2. The respiratory rhythmicity center, which fine tunes and modulates afferent information received from the apneustic and pneumotaxic centers and provides baseline set points for the respiratory rate
3. The nucleus gracilis and nucleus cuneatus, which transmit afferent sensory information to the thalamus
4. The olivary nucleus, which relays information from the cerebral cortex, diencephalon, and brainstem to the cerebellum
5. The reticular formation of the medulla oblongata, which helps regulate vital autonomic functions via its interaction with the respiratory rhythmicity and cardiovascular centers
6. The sensory and motor nuclei of cranial nerves VIII, IX, X, XI, and XII

SUGGESTED READINGS

Jänig W: Organization of the sympathetic nervous system: Peripheral and central aspects. In del Rey A, Chrousos GP, Besedovsky HO (eds): Neuroimmune Biology, Volume 7: The Hypothalam–Pituitary–Adrenal Axis. Amsterdam, Elsevier, 2007, pp 55-85.

Romano S, Salvetti M, Ceccherini I, et al: Brainstem signs with progressing atrophy of medulla oblongata and upper cervical spinal cord. Lancet Neurol 6:562-570, 2007.

Sagen J, Proudfit HK: Evidence for pain modulation by pre- and postsynaptic noradrenergic receptors in the medulla oblongata. Brain Res 331:285-293, 1985.

Verberne AJM: Medulla oblongata. In Aminoff M (ed): Encyclopedia of the Neurological Sciences. San Diego, Academic Press, 2003, pp 54-63.

Zeng Z, McDonald TP, Wang R, et al: Neuropeptide FF receptor 2 (NPFF2) is localized to pain-processing regions in the primate spinal cord and the lower level of the medulla oblongata. J Chem Neuroanat 25:269-278, 2003.

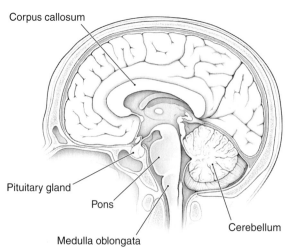

Corpus callosum

Pituitary gland

Pons

Medulla oblongata

Cerebellum

FIGURE 120–1 The medulla oblongata.

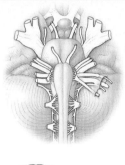

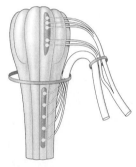

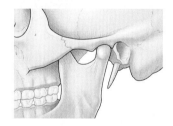

SECTION 3

Painful Conditions

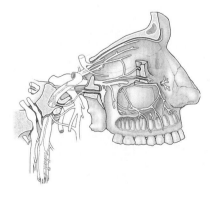

CHAPTER 121

Tension-Type Headache

Tension-type headache, formerly known as *muscle contraction headache*, is the most common type of headache that afflicts mankind. It can be episodic or chronic, and may or may not be related to muscle contraction. Significant sleep disturbance usually occurs, along with depression and, in some patients, somatization.

Signs and Symptoms

Tension-type headache is usually bilateral but it can be unilateral and often involves the frontal, temporal, and occipital regions (Fig. 121-1). It may mainfest as a bandlike nonpulsatile ache or tightness in the aforementioned anatomic areas. There is often associated neck symptomatology. Tension-type headache evolves over a period of hours or days and then tends to remain constant without progressive symptomatology. There is no aura associated with this headache. Significant sleep disturbance is usually present. This may manifest as difficulty in falling asleep, frequent awakening at night, or early awakening. These headaches most frequently occur between 4 and 8 AM and between 4 and 8 PM. Although both sexes are affected, females predominate. There is no hereditary pattern to tension-type headache, but it may occur in family clusters as children mimic and learn the pain behavior of their parents.

The triggering event for acute episodic tension-type headache is invariably either physical or psychological stress. Physical stress such as a long drive, working with the neck in a strained position, acute cervical spine injury due to whiplash, or prolonged exposure to the glare from a cathode ray tube may also precipitate a headache. A worsening of preexisting degenerative cervical spine conditions, such as cervical spondylosis, can also trigger a tension-type headache. The pathology responsible for the development of tension-type headache can also produce temporomandibular joint dysfunction.

Testing

There is no specific test for tension-type headache. Testing is aimed primarily at identifying occult pathology or other diseases that may mimic tension-type headaches. All patients with the recent onset of headache thought to be tension type should undergo magnetic resonance imaging of the brain and, if significant occipital or nuchal symptoms are present, of the cervical spine. Magnetic resonance imaging should also be performed in patients with previously stable tension-type headaches who have experienced a recent change in headache symptomatology. Screening laboratory testing consisting of complete blood count, erythrocyte sedimentation rate, and automated blood chemistry testing should be performed if the diagnosis of tension-type headache is in question.

Differential Diagnosis

Tension-type headache is usually diagnosed on clinical grounds by obtaining a careful targeted headache history. Despite their obvious differences, tension-type headache is often incorrectly diagnosed as migraine headache. Such misdiagnosis leads to illogical treatment plans and poor control of headache symptomatology. Table 122-1 helps distinguish tension-type headache from migraine headache and should aid the clinician in making the correct diagnosis.

Diseases of the cervical spine and surrounding soft tissues may also mimic tension-type headache. Arnold-Chiari malformations may also mainfest clinically as tension-type headache but will be easily identified on imaging of the cervical spine. Occasionally, frontal sinusitis can also be confused with tension-type headache, although individuals with acute frontal sinusitis appear systemically ill. Temporal arteritis, chronic subdural hematoma, and other intracranial pathology such as tumor may be incorrectly diagnosed as tension-type headache.

Treatment

ABORTIVE TREATMENT

In determining treatment, the physician must consider the frequency and severity of headaches, how the headaches affect the patient's lifestyle, the results of any previous therapy, and previous drug misuse and abuse. If the patient suffers from an attack of tension-type headache only once every 1 or 2 months, the condition can often be managed through teaching the patient to reduce or avoid stress. Analgesics or nonsteroidal anti-inflammatory drugs (NSAIDs) can provide symptomatic relief during acute attacks. Combination analgesic drugs used concomitantly with barbiturates and/or narcotic analgesics have no place in the management of headache patients. The risk of abuse and dependence more than outweighs any theoretical benefit. The physician should also avoid an abortive treatment approach in patients with a prior history of drug misuse or abuse. Many abortive drugs, including simple analgesics and NSAIDs, can produce serious consequences if abused.

PROPHYLACTIC TREATMENT

If the headaches occur more frequently than once every 1 or 2 months or are of such severity that the patient repeatedly misses work or social engagements, the following prophylactic therapy is indicated.

Antidepressants

These are generally the drugs of choice for prophylactic treatment of headaches. The antidepressants not only help decrease the frequency and intensity of tension-type headaches but also normalize sleep patterns and treat underlying depression. Patients should be educated about the potential side effects of sedation, dry mouth, blurred vision, constipation, and urinary retention that may be experienced when using this class of drugs. They should also be told that relief of headache pain generally takes 3 to 4 weeks. However, the normalization of sleep that occurs immediately may be sufficient to noticeably improve the headache symptomatology.

Amitriptyline, started at a single bedtime dose of 25 mg, is a reasonable initial choice. The dose may be increased in 25-mg increments as side effects allow. Other drugs that can be considered if the patient does not tolerate the sedation and anticholinergic effects of amitriptyline include trazodone (75 to 300 mg at bedtime) or fluoxetine (20 to 40 mg at lunchtime). Because of the sedating nature of these drugs (with the exception of fluoxetine), they must be used with caution in the elderly or in patients who are at risk for falling. Care should also be exercised when using these drugs in patients prone to cardiac arrhythmia because these drugs may be arrhythmogenic. Simple analgesics or the longer-acting NSAIDs may be used with the antidepressant compounds to treat exacerbations of headache pain.

Biofeedback

Monitored relaxation training combined with patient education about coping strategies and stress reduction techniques may be of value in the motivated tension-type headache sufferer. Appropriate patient selection is of paramount importance if good results are to be achieved. If the patient is significantly depressed at the time of initiation of therapy, it may be beneficial to treat the depression before trying biofeedback. The use of biofeedback may allow the patient to control the headache while at the same time avoiding the side effects of medications.

Cervical Steroid Epidural Nerve Blocks

Multiple studies have demonstrated the efficacy of cervical steroid epidural nerve blocks (CSENBs) in providing long-term relief of tension-type headache in a group of patients for whom all treatment modalities failed. CSENBs may be used early in the course of treatment while waiting for the antidepressant compounds to become effective. CSENBs may be performed on a daily to weekly basis as clinical symptoms dictate.

SUGGESTED READINGS

Goetz CG: Textbook of Clinical Neurology, ed 2. Philadelphia, Saunders, 2003.
Waldman SD: Tension-type headache. In: Atlas of Common Pain Syndromes, ed 2. Philadelphia, Saunders, 2008.

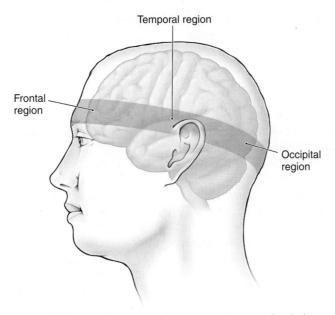

Temporal region

Frontal region

Occipital region

FIGURE 121–1 The location of pain in tension-type headache.

CHAPTER 122

Migraine Headache

Migraine headache is defined as a periodic unilateral headache that may begin in childhood but almost always develops before the age of 30. Attacks may occur with a variable frequency ranging from every few days to once every several months. More frequent migraine headaches are often associated with a phenomenon called *analgesic rebound*. Between 60% and 70% of patients suffering from migraine are female, and many report a family history of migraine headaches. Migraineurs have been described as having a unique personality type characterized by a meticulous, neat, compulsive, and often rigid nature. They tend to be obsessive in their daily routines and often find it hard to cope with the stresses of everyday life. Migraine headaches may be triggered by changes in sleep patterns or diet or by the ingestion of tyramine-containing foods, monosodium glutamate, nitrates, chocolate, or citrus fruits. Changes in endogenous and exogenous hormones such as occur with the use of birth control pills can also trigger migraine headache. Approximately 20% of patients suffering from migraine headache also experience a painless neurologic event before the onset of headache pain that is called *aura*.

Aura most often takes the form of visual disturbance but may also manifest as an alteration in smell or hearing; these are called olfactory and auditory aura, respectively.

Clinical Signs and Symptoms

Migraine headache is by definition a unilateral headache. Although with each episode the headache may change sides, the headache is never bilateral. The pain of migraine headache is usually periorbital or retro-orbital. It is pounding in nature, and its intensity is severe. The onset-to-peak of migraine headache is rapid, ranging from 20 minutes to 1 hour. In contradistinction to tension-type headache, migraine headache is often associated with systemic symptoms, including nausea and vomiting, photophobia, and sonophobia, as well as alterations in appetite, mood, and libido. Menstruation is also a common trigger of migraine headaches. Migraine that manifests without other neurologic symptoms is called *migraine without aura*.

As mentioned, approximately 20% of patients suffering from migraine headache also experience a painless neurologic event before the onset of headache pain called aura. Aura is thought to be the result of ischemia of specific regions of the cerebral cortex. Visual aura will often occur from 30 to 60 minutes before the onset of headache pain and may take the form of blind spots called *scotoma* or a zigzag disruption of the visual field called *fortification spectrum*. Occasionally, migraine patients may lose an entire visual field during aura. Auditory aura most often takes the form of hypersensitivity to sound, but other alterations of hearing, such as sounds perceived as farther away than they are, have also been reported. Olfactory aura may take the form of strong odors of substances that are not actually present or extreme hypersensitivity to otherwise normal odors of items such as coffee or copy machine toner. Migraine headache that is preceded by aura is called *migraine with aura*.

Rare patients who suffer from migraine will experience prolonged neurologic dysfunction associated with their headache pain. Such neurologic dysfunction may last for more than 24 hours and is termed *migraine with prolonged aura*. Although extremely rare, such patients are at risk for the development of permanent neurologic deficit, and risk factors such as hypertension, smoking, and oral contraceptives must be addressed. Even less common than migraine with prolonged aura is *migraine with complex aura*. Patients suffering from migraine with complex aura experience significant neurologic dysfunction associated with their headache pain. This dysfunction may include aphasia or hemiplegia. As with migraine with prolonged aura, patients suffering from migraine with complex aura may develop permanent neurologic deficits.

The patient suffering from all forms of migraine headache will appear systemically ill. Pallor, tremulousness, diaphoresis, and light sensitivity are common physical findings. Tenderness of the temporal artery and associated area may also be present. If aura is present, neurologic examination results will be abnormal; otherwise, the neurologic examination is within normal limits, before, during, and after migraine without aura.

Testing

There is no specific test for migraine headache. Testing is aimed primarily at identifying occult pathology or other diseases that may mimic migraine headache (see Differential Diagnosis). All patients with a recent onset of headache thought to be migraine should undergo magnetic resonance imaging (MRI) of the brain. If neurologic dysfunction accompanies the patient's headache symptomatology, the MRI should be performed with and without gadolinium contrast medium; magnetic resonance angiography should also be considered. MRI should also be performed in patients with previously stable migraine headache who are experiencing an inexplicable change in headache symptomatology. Screening laboratory testing that includes erythrocyte sedimentation rate, complete blood count, and automated blood chemistry should be performed if the diagnosis of migraine is in question. Ophthalmologic evaluation is indicated in those patients suffering from headache who experience significant ocular symptoms.

Differential Diagnosis

The diagnosis of migraine headache is usually made on clinical grounds by obtaining a careful targeted headache history. Tension-type headache is often confused with migraine headache, and such confusion leads to illogical treatment plans as the treatments for these two distinct headache syndromes are quite different. Table 122-1

TABLE 122–1 Comparison of Migraine Headache with Tension-Type Headache

	Migraine Headache	Tension-Type Headache
Onset-to-peak	Minutes to 1 hour	Hours to days
Frequency	Rarely more than 1 per week	Often daily or continuous
Location	Temporal	Nuchal or circumferential
Character	Pounding	Aching, pressure, bandlike
Laterality	Always unilateral	Usually bilateral
Aura	May be present	Never present
Nausea and vomiting	Common	Rare
Duration	Usually less than 24 hours	Often for days

distinguishes migraine headache from tension-type headache and should help clarify the correct diagnosis.

Diseases of the eye, ears, nose, and sinuses may also mimic migraine headache. The targeted history and physical examination combined with appropriate testing should help the astute clinician identify and properly treat underlying diseases of these organ systems. Glaucoma, temporal arteritis, sinusitis, intracranial pathology including chronic subdural hematoma, tumor, brain abscess, hydrocephalus, and pseudotumor cerebri, and inflammatory conditions including sarcoidosis may all mimic migraine and must be considered when treating the headache patient.

Treatment

When deciding how to best treat the patient suffering from migraine, the clinician should consider the frequency and severity of headache, the effect on the patient's lifestyle, the presence of focal or prolonged neurologic disturbances, the results of previous testing and treatment, the history of previous drug abuse or misuse, and the presence of other systemic disease, such as peripheral vascular or coronary artery disease, that might preclude the use of certain treatment modalities.

If the patient's migraine headaches occur infrequently, a trial of abortive therapy may be warranted. However, if headaches occur with greater frequency or cause the patient to miss work or be hospitalized, prophylactic therapy is warranted.

Abortive Therapy

For abortive therapy to be effective in the treatment of migraine headache, it must be initiated at the first sign of headache. This can often be difficult because of the short onset-to-peak of migraine headache coupled with the fact that migraine sufferers often experience nausea and vomiting that may limit the use of oral medications. By altering the route of administration to parenteral or transmucosal, this problem can be avoided.

Abortive medications that can be considered in migraine headache patients include compounds that contain isometheptene mucate (e.g., Midrin), the nonsteroidal anti-inflammatory drug naproxen, ergot alkaloids, the triptans including sumatriptan, and the intravenous administration of lidocaine combined with antiemetic compounds. The inhalation of 100% oxygen may also abort migraine headache, as well as the use of sphenopalatine ganglion block with local anesthetic. Caffeine-containing preparations, barbiturates, ergotamines, the triptans, and narcotics have a propensity to cause a phenomenon called *analgesic rebound headache*, which may ultimately be more difficult to treat than the patient's original migraine headaches. The ergotamines and triptans should not be used in patients with coexistent peripheral vascular disease, coronary artery disease, or hypertension.

Prophylactic Therapy

For most patients who suffer from migraine headaches, prophylactic therapy represents a better option. The mainstay of the prophylactic therapy of migraine is β-blocking agents. Propranolol and most of the other drugs of this class will help control or decrease the frequency and intensity of migraine headache and help prevent aura. Generally, an 80-mg daily dose of the long-acting formulation is a reasonable starting point for most patients with migraine. Propranolol should not be used in patients with asthma or other reactive airway diseases.

Valproic acid, the calcium channel blockers such as verapamil, clonidine, the tricyclic antidepressants, and the nonsteroidal anti-inflammatory drugs have also been used in the prophylaxis of migraine headache. Each of these drugs has its own profile of advantages and disadvantages, and the clinician should try to pharmacologically tailor a treatment plan that best meets the needs of the individual patient.

SUGGESTED READINGS

Goetz CG: Textbook of Clinical Neurology, ed 2. Philadelphia, Saunders, 2003.

Waldman SD: Migraine headache. In: Atlas of Common Pain Syndromes, ed 2. Philadelphia, Saunders, 2008.

CHAPTER 123

Cluster Headache

Cluster headache derives its name from the pattern by which cluster headaches occur—namely, the headaches occur in clusters followed by headache-free remission periods. Unlike other common headache disorders that affect primarily females, cluster headache happens much more commonly in males at a ratio of 5:1. Much less common than tension-type headache or migraine headache, cluster headache is thought to affect approximately 0.5% of the male population. Cluster headache is most often confused with migraine by clinicians unfamiliar with the headache syndrome.

The onset of cluster headache occurs in the late third or early fourth decade of life, in contradistinction to migraine, which almost always manifests itself by the early second decade. Unlike migraine, cluster headache does not appear to run in families and cluster sufferers do not experience aura. Attacks of cluster headache will generally occur approximately 90 minutes after the patient falls asleep. This association with sleep is reportedly maintained when a shift worker changes to and from nighttime to daytime hours of sleep. Cluster headache also appears to follow a distinct chronobiologic pattern that coincides with the seasonal change in the length of day. This results in an increased frequency of cluster headaches in the spring and fall.

During a cluster period, attacks occur two or three times a day and last for 45 minutes to 1 hour. Cluster periods usually last for 8 to 12 weeks, interrupted by remission periods of less than 2 years. In rare patients, the remission periods become shorter and shorter and the frequency may increase up to 10-fold. This situation is termed *chronic cluster headache* and differs from the more common episodic cluster headache described earlier.

Signs and Symptoms

Cluster headache is characterized as a unilateral headache that is retro-orbital and temporal in location. The pain has a deep burning or boring quality. Physical findings during an attack of cluster headache may include Horner's syndrome, consisting of ptosis, abnormal pupil constriction, facial flushing, and conjunctival injection. Additionally, profuse lacrimation and rhinorrhea are often present. The ocular changes may become permanent with repeated attacks. Peau d'orange skin over the malar region, deeply furrowed and glabellar folds, and telangiectasia may be observed.

Attacks of cluster headache may be provoked by small amounts of alcohol, nitrates, histamines, and other vasoactive substances and occasionally by high altitude. When the attack is in progress, the patient may not be able to lie still and may pace or rock back and forth in a chair. This behavior contrasts with that characterizing other headache syndromes, during which patients seeking relief will lie down in a dark, quiet room.

The pain of cluster headache is said to be among the worst pain from which mankind suffers. Because of the severity of pain associated with cluster headaches, the clinician must watch closely for medication overuse or misuse. Suicides have been associated with prolonged, unrelieved attacks of cluster headaches.

Testing

There is no specific test for cluster headache. Testing is aimed primarily at identifying occult pathology or other diseases that may mimic cluster headache (see Differential Diagnosis). All patients with a recent onset of headache thought to be cluster should undergo magnetic resonance imaging (MRI) of the brain. If neurologic dysfunction accompanies the patient's headache symptomatology, MRI should be performed with and without gadolinium contrast medium; magnetic resonance angiography should also be considered. MRI should also be performed in patients with previously stable cluster headache who are experiencing an inexplicable change in headache symptomatology. Screening laboratory testing including erythrocyte sedimentation rate, complete blood count, and automated blood chemistry should be performed if the diagnosis of cluster is in question. Ophthalmologic evaluation including measurement of intraocular pressures is indicated in those patients suffering with headache who experience significant ocular symptoms.

Differential Diagnosis

Cluster headache is usually made on clinical grounds by obtaining a careful, targeted headache history.

TABLE 123–1 Comparison of Cluster Headache with Migraine Headache

	Cluster Headache	Migraine Headache
Gender	Male 5:1	Female 2:1
Age of onset	Late 30s to early 40s	Menarche to early 20s
Family history	No	Yes
Aura	Never	Yes 20% of time
Chronobiologic pattern	Yes	No
Onset-to-peak	Seconds to minutes	Minutes to hours
Frequency	Two or three times per day	Once a week
Duration	45 minutes	Hours

Migraine headache is often confused with cluster headache, and such confusion leads to illogical treatment plans as the treatments of these two distinct headache syndromes are quite different. Table 123-1 distinguishes cluster headache from migraine headache and should help to clarify the correct diagnosis.

Diseases of the eyes, ears, nose, and sinuses may also mimic cluster headache. The targeted history and physical examination combined with appropriate testing should help the astute clinician identify and properly treat underlying diseases of these organ systems. Glaucoma, temporal arteritis, sinusitis, intracranial pathology including chronic subdural hematoma, tumor, brain abscess, hydrocephalus, and pseudotumor cerebri, and inflammatory conditions including sarcoidosis may all mimic cluster and must be considered when treating the headache patient.

Treatment

In contradistinction to migraine headache, in which most patients experience improvement with the implementation of therapy with β-blockers, patients suffering from cluster headache will usually require more individualized therapy. A reasonable starting place in the treatment of cluster headache is to begin treatment with prednisone combined with daily sphenopalatine ganglion blocks with local anesthetic. A reasonable starting dose of prednisone would be 80 mg given in divided doses tapered by 10 mg per dose per day. If headaches are not rapidly brought under control, inhalation of 100% oxygen via close-fitting mask is added.

If headaches persist and the diagnosis of cluster headache is not in question, a trial of lithium carbonate may be considered. It should be noted that the therapeutic window of lithium carbonate is small and this drug should be used with caution. A starting dose of 300 mg at bedtime may be increased after 48 hours to 300 mg twice a day. If no side effects are noted, after 48 hours the dose may again be increased to 300 mg three times a day. The patient should be continued at this dosage level for a total of 10 days, and the drug should then be tapered downward over a 1-week period. Other medications that can be considered if these treatments are ineffective include methysergide and sumatriptan and sumatriptan-like drugs.

In rare patients suffering from cluster headaches, the aforementioned treatments are ineffective. In this setting, given the severity of pain and the risk of suicide, more aggressive treatment is indicated. Destruction of the gasserian ganglion either by injection of glycerol or by radiofrequency lesioning may be a reasonable next step.

SUGGESTED READINGS

Goetz CG: Textbook of Clinical Neurology, ed 2. Philadelphia, Saunders, 2003.

Waldman SD: Cluster headache. In: Atlas of Common Pain Syndromes, ed 2. Philadelphia, Saunders, 2008.

CHAPTER 124

Pseudotumor Cerebri

Signs and Symptoms

An oft-missed diagnosis, pseudotumor cerebri is an uncommon cause of headache seen most frequently in overweight females between the ages of 20 and 45. More than 90% of patients suffering from pseudotumor cerebri present with the complaint of headache that increases with Valsalva maneuver. Associated nonspecific central nervous system signs and symptoms such as dizziness, visual disturbance including diplopia, tinnitus, nausea and vomiting, and ocular pain can often obfuscate what should otherwise be a reasonably straightforward diagnosis given that basically all patients suffering from pseudotumor cerebri exhibit papilledema on funduscopic examination. The extent of papilledema varies from patient to patient and may be associated with subtle visual field defects, including an enlarged blind spot and inferior nasal visual field defects.

The exact cause of pseudotumor cerebri has not be elucidated, but the common denominator appears to be a defect in the absorption of cerebrospinal fluid. Predisposing factors include ingestion of tetracycline, vitamin A, corticosteroids, and nalidixic acid. Other implicating factors include blood dyscrasias, anemias, endocrinopathies, and chronic respiratory insufficiency. However, in many patients, the exact cause of pseudotumor cerebri remains unknown.

Diagnosis

By convention, the diagnosis of pseudotumor cerebri is made when four criteria are identified: (1) signs and symptoms suggestive of increased intracranial pressure including papilledema; (2) normal magnetic resonance imaging (MRI) or computed tomography (CT) of the brain; (3) increased cerebrospinal fluid pressure documented by lumbar puncture; and (4) normal cerebrospinal fluid chemistry, cultures, and cytology (Table 124-1). Urgent MRI and CT scanning of the brain with contrast media should be obtained on all patients suspected of having

TABLE 124–1 The Diagnostic Criteria for Pseudotumor Cerebri

1. Signs and symptoms suggestive of increased intracranial pressure including papilledema
2. Normal MRI or CT of the brain performed with and without contrast media
3. Increased cerebrospinal fluid pressure documented by lumbar puncture
4. Normal cerebrospinal fluid chemistry, cultures, and cytology

increased intracranial pressure to rule out intracranial mass, infection, and other conditions. Patients suffering from pseudotumor cerebri will demonstrate small- to normal-sized ventricles on neuroimaging with an otherwise normal scan. Once the absence of space-occupying lesions of dilated ventricles are confirmed on neuroimaging, it is then safe to proceed with lumbar puncture to measure cerebrospinal fluid pressure and obtain fluid for chemistry, cultures, and cytology.

Treatment

A reasonable first step in the management of patients who exhibit all four criteria necessary for the diagnosis of pseudotumor cerebri is the initiation of oral acetazolamide. If poorly tolerated, the use of furosemide or chlorthalidone can be considered. A short course of systemic corticosteroids such as dexamethasone may also be used if the patient does not respond to diuretic therapy. For resistant cases, neurosurgical interventions including cerebrospinal fluid shunt procedures are a reasonable next step. If papilledema persists, decompression procedures on the optic nerve sheath have been advocated.

SUGGESTED READING

Goetz CG: Textbook of Clinical Neurology, ed 2. Philadelphia, Saunders, 2003.

Analgesic Rebound Headache

Analgesic rebound headache is a recently identified headache syndrome that occurs commonly in headache sufferers who overuse abortive medications to treat their headache symptomatology. The overuse of these abortive medications will result in increasingly frequent headaches that become unresponsive to both abortive and prophylactic medications. Over a period of weeks, the patient's episodic migraine or tension-type headache becomes more frequent and transforms into a chronic daily headache. This daily headache becomes increasingly unresponsive to analgesics and other headache medications, and patients will note an exacerbation of headache symptomatology if abortive or prophylactic analgesic medications are missed or delayed. Analgesic rebound headache is probably underdiagnosed by healthcare professionals, and its frequency is on the rise due to the heavy advertising by pharmaceutical companies of over-the-counter headache medications containing caffeine.

Signs and Symptoms

Clinically, analgesic rebound headache manifests as a transformed migraine or tension-type headache and may assume the characteristics of both of these common headache types, blurring their distinctive features and making correct diagnosis difficult. Common to all analgesic rebound headaches is the excessive use of the following medications (summarized in Table 125-1): simple analgesics, such as acetaminophen; sinus medications, including simple analgesics; combinations of aspirin, caffeine, and butalbital, such as Fiorinal; nonsteroidal anti-inflammatory drugs; opioid analgesics; ergotamines; and the triptans, such as sumatriptan. As with migraine and tension-type headache, the physical examination will most often be within normal limits.

Testing

There is no specific test for analgesic rebound headache. Testing is aimed primarily at identifying occult pathology or other diseases that may mimic tension-type or migraine headaches (see Differential Diagnosis). All patients with the recent onset of chronic daily headache thought to be analgesic rebound headache should undergo magnetic resonance imaging of the brain and, if significant occipital or nuchal symptoms are present, of the cervical spine. Magnetic resonance imaging should also be performed in patients with previously stable tension-type or migraine headaches who have experienced a recent change in headache symptomatology. Screening laboratory testing consisting of complete blood count, erythrocyte sedimentation rate, and automated blood chemistry testing should be performed if the diagnosis of analgesic rebound headache is in question.

Differential Diagnosis

Analgesic rebound headache is usually diagnosed on clinical grounds by obtaining a careful, targeted headache history. Because analgesic rebound headache assumes many of the characteristics of the underlying primary headache, diagnosis can be confusing at best if a careful medication history with specific questioning regarding the intake of over-the-counter headache medications and analgesics is not obtained. Any change in a previously stable headache pattern needs to be taken seriously and should not automatically be attributed to analgesic overuse without careful reevaluation of the patient.

Treatment

Treatment of analgesic rebound headache is the discontinuation of the overused or abused drugs and complete

TABLE 125–1 Drugs Implicated in Analgesic Rebound Headache

Simple analgesics
Nonsteroidal anti-inflammatory drugs
Opioid analgesics
Sinus medications
Ergotamines
Combination headache medications that include butalbital
The triptans (e.g., sumatriptan)

abstention from them for a period of at least 3 months. Many patients cannot tolerate outpatient discontinuation of these medications and will ultimately require hospitalization in a specialized inpatient headache unit. If outpatient discontinuation of the offending medications is considered, the following should be carefully explained to the patient:

- Their headaches and associated symptoms will get worse before they get better.
- Any use, no matter how small, of the offending medication will result in continued analgesic rebound headaches.
- The patient may not self-medicate with over-the-counter drugs.

- The significant overuse of opioids or combination medications containing butalbital or ergotamine will result in physical dependence, and their discontinuation must be done only under the supervision of a physician familiar with the treatment of physical dependencies.
- If the patient follows the physician's orders regarding discontinuation of the offending medications, he or she can expect the headaches to improve.

SUGGESTED READINGS

Waldman SD: Analgesic rebound headache. In: Atlas of Common Pain Syndromes, ed 2. Philadelphia, Saunders, 2007.

CHAPTER 126

Trigeminal Neuralgia

Trigeminal neuralgia occurs in many patients because of tortuous blood vessels that compress the trigeminal root as it exits the brainstem. Acoustic neuromas, cholesteatomas, aneurysms, angiomas, and bony abnormalities may also lead to the compression of nerve. The severity of pain produced by trigeminal neuralgia can only be rivaled by that of cluster headache. Uncontrolled pain has been associated with suicide and therefore should be treated as an emergency. Attacks can be triggered by daily activities involving contact with the face such as brushing the teeth, shaving, or washing. Pain can be controlled with medication in most patients (Table 126-1). About 2% to 3% of those patients experiencing trigeminal neuralgia also have multiple sclerosis. Trigeminal neuralgia is also called tic douloureux.

Signs and Symptoms

Trigeminal neuralgia is an episodic pain afflicting the areas of the face supplied by the trigeminal nerve. The pain is unilateral in 97% of cases reported. When it does occur bilaterally, it is in the same division of the nerve.

The second or third division of the nerve is affected in the majority of patients, with the first division affected less than 5% of the time. The pain develops on the right side of the face in unilateral disease 57% of the time. The pain is characterized by paroxysms of electric shock–like pain lasting from several seconds to less than 2 minutes. The progression from onset to peak is essentially instantaneous.

TABLE 126–1 Treatment Options for Trigeminal Neuralgia

Medications
• Carbamazepine
• Gabapentin
• Baclofen
Surgery
• Trigeminal nerve block
• Retrogasserian injection of glycerol
• Balloon compression of the gasserian ganglion
• Radiofrequency destruction of the gasserian ganglion
• Microvascular decompression of the trigeminal root

The patient with trigeminal neuralgia will go to great lengths to avoid any contact with trigger areas. Persons with other types of facial pain, such as temporomandibular joint dysfunction, tend to constantly rub the affected the area or apply heat or cold to it. Patients with uncontrolled trigeminal neuralgia frequently require hospitalization for rapid control of pain. Between attacks, the patient is relatively pain free. A dull ache remaining after the intense pain subsides may indicate a persistent compression of the nerve by a structural lesion. This disease is almost never seen in people under 30 unless it is associated with multiple sclerosis.

The patient with trigeminal neuralgia will often have severe and, at times, even suicidal depression with high levels of superimposed anxiety during acute attacks. Both of these problems may by exacerbated by the sleep deprivation that often occurs during episodes of pain. Patients with coexisting multiple sclerosis may exhibit the euphoric dementia characteristic of that disease. Physicians should reassure persons with trigeminal neuralgia that the pain can almost always be controlled.

Testing

All patients with a new diagnosis of trigeminal neuralgia should undergo magnetic resonance imaging of the brain and brainstem with and without gadolinium to rule out posterior fossa or brainstem lesions and demyelinating disease. Magnetic resonance angiography is also useful in confirming vascular compression of the trigeminal nerve by aberrant blood vessels. Additional imaging of the sinuses should also be considered if a question of occult or coexisting sinus disease is entertained. If the first division of the trigeminal nerve is affected, ophthalmic evaluation to measure intraocular pressure and to rule out intraocular pathology is indicated. Screening laboratory testing consisting of complete blood count, erythrocyte sedimentation rate, and automated blood chemistry testing should be performed if the diagnosis of trigeminal neuralgia is in question. A complete blood count will be required as a baseline before starting treatment with carbamazepine (see Treatment).

Differential Diagnosis

Trigeminal neuralgia is generally a straightforward clinical diagnosis that can be made on the basis of a targeted history and physical examination. Diseases of the eye, ears, nose, throat, and teeth may all mimic trigeminal neuralgia or may coexist and confuse the diagnosis. Atypical facial pain is sometimes confused with trigeminal neuralgia but can be distinguished by the character of pain, which is dull and aching, compared with the pain

of trigeminal neuralgia, which is sharp and neuritic in nature. Additionally, the pain of trigeminal neuralgia occurs in the distribution of the divisions of the trigeminal nerve, whereas the pain of atypical facial pain does not follow any specific nerve distribution. Multiple sclerosis should be considered in all patients who present with trigeminal neuralgia prior to the fifth decade of life.

Treatment

DRUG THERAPY

Carbamazepine

This drug is considered first-line treatment for trigeminal neuralgia. In fact, rapid response to this drug essentially confirms a clinical diagnosis of trigeminal neuralgia. Despite the safety and efficacy of carbamazepine compared with other treatments for trigeminal neuralgia, much confusion and unfounded anxiety surround its use. This medication, which may be the patient's best chance for pain control, is sometimes discontinued owing to laboratory abnormalities erroneously attributed to it. Therefore, baseline screening laboratory tests, consisting of a complete blood count, urinalysis, and automated chemistry profile, should be obtained before starting the drug.

Carbamazepine should be started slowly if the pain is not out of control. Start the dose at 100 to 200 mg at bedtime for 2 nights and caution the patient regarding side effects, including dizziness, sedation, confusion, and rash. The drug is increased in 100- to 200-mg increments, given in equally divided doses over 2 days, as side effects allow until pain relief is obtained or a total dose of 1200 mg daily is reached. Careful monitoring of laboratory parameters is mandatory to avoid the rare possibility of life-threatening blood dyscrasia. At the first sign of blood count abnormality or rash, this drug should be discontinued. Failure to monitor patients started on carbamazepine can be disastrous because aplastic anemia can occur. When pain relief is obtained, the patient should be kept at that dosage of carbamazepine for at least 6 months before considering tapering of this medication. The patient should be informed that under no circumstances should the dosage of drug be changed or the drug refilled or discontinued without the physician's knowledge.

Gabapentin

In the uncommon event that carbamazepine does not adequately control a patient's pain, gabapentin may be considered. As with carbamazepine, baseline blood tests should be obtained prior to starting therapy. Start with a 300-mg dose of gabapentin at bedtime for 2 nights and caution the patient about potential side effects, including dizziness, sedation, confusion, and rash. The drug is then increased in 300-mg increments, given in equally divided doses over 2 days, as side effects allow, until pain relief is obtained or a total dose of 2400 mg daily is reached. At this point, if the patient has experienced partial relief of pain, blood values are measured and the drug is carefully titrated upward using 100-mg tablets. Rarely will more than 3600 mg daily be required.

Baclofen

This drug has been reported to be of value in some patients who fail to obtain relief from the medications mentioned. Baseline laboratory tests should also be obtained prior to starting baclofen. Start with a 10-mg dose at bedtime for 2 nights and caution the patient about potential adverse effects, which are the same as those of carbamazepine and gabapentin. The drug is increased in 10-mg increments, given in equally divided doses over 7 days as side effects allow, until pain relief is obtained or a total dose of 80 mg daily is reached. This drug has significant hepatic and central nervous system side effects, including weakness and sedation. As with carbamazepine, careful monitoring of laboratory values is indicated during the initial use of this drug.

In treating individuals with any of the drugs mentioned, the physician should make the patient aware that premature tapering or discontinuation of the medication may lead to the recurrence of pain and that it will be more difficult to control pain thereafter.

INVASIVE THERAPY

Trigeminal Nerve Block

The use of trigeminal nerve block with local anesthetic and a steroid serves as an excellent adjunct to drug treatment of trigeminal neuralgia. This technique rapidly relieves pain while medications are being titrated to effective levels. The initial block is carried out with preservative-free bupivacaine combined with methylprednisolone. Subsequent daily nerve blocks are carried out in a similar manner substituting a lower-dose of methylprednisolone. This approach may also be used to obtain control of breakthrough pain.

Retrogasserian Injection of Glycerol and Balloon Compression

The injection of small quantities of glycerol into the area of the gasserian ganglion has been shown to provide long-term relief for patients suffering from trigeminal neuralgia who have not responded to optimal trials of the therapies mentioned. This procedure should be performed only by a physician well versed in the problems and pitfalls associated with neurodestructive procedures. Compression of the gasserian ganglion with a balloon has also been advocated for patients who are too sick to undergo microvascular decompression of the trigeminal root.

Radiofrequency Destruction of the Gasserian Ganglion

The destruction of the gasserian ganglion can be carried out by creating a radiofrequency lesion under biplanar fluoroscopic guidance. This procedure is reserved for patients who have failed to respond to all the above-mentioned treatments for intractable trigeminal neuralgia and are not candidates for microvascular decompression of the trigeminal root.

Microvascular Decompression of the Trigeminal Root

This technique, which is also called Jannetta's procedure, is the major neurosurgical procedure of choice for intractable trigeminal neuralgia. It is based on the theory that trigeminal neuralgia is in fact a compressive mononeuropathy. The operation consists of identifying the trigeminal root close to the brainstem and isolating the offending compressing blood vessel. A sponge is then interposed between the vessel and nerve, relieving the compression and thus the pain.

SUGGESTED READINGS

Campbell W: DeJong's The Neurological Examination, ed 6. Philadelphia, Lippincott Williams and Wilkins, 2005.

Goetz CG: Textbook of Clinical Neurology, ed 2. Philadelphia, Saunders, 2003.

Waldman SD: Trigeminal neuralgia. In: Atlas of Common Pain Syndromes, ed 2. Philadelphia, Saunders, 2008.

Temporal Arteritis

The Clinical Syndrome

As the name suggests, the headache associated with temporal arteritis is located primarily in the temples, with secondary pain often located in the frontal and occipital regions. A disease of the sixth decade and beyond, temporal arteritis affects whites almost exclusively, and there is a female gender predominance of 3:1. Temporal arteritis is also known as *giant cell arteritis* because of the finding of giant multinucleated cells that infiltrate arteries containing elastin, including the temporal, ophthalmic, and external carotid arteries. Approximately half of patients with temporal arteritis also suffer from polymyalgia rheumatica.

Signs and Symptoms

Headache is seen in the vast majority of patients suffering from temporal arteritis. The headache is located in the temples and is usually continuous. The character of the headache pain associated with temporal arteritis is aching in nature with a mild to moderate level of intensity. The patient suffering from temporal arteritis may also complain of soreness of the scalp, making the combing of hair or laying on a firm pillow extremely uncomfortable.

Although temporal headache is present in almost all patients suffering from temporal arteritis, it is the finding of intermittent jaw claudication that is pathognomonic for the disease. In the elderly patient, jaw pain while chewing should be considered to be secondary to temporal arteritis until proved otherwise. If there is a strong clinical suspicion that the patient has temporal arteritis, immediate treatment with corticosteroids is indicated (see Treatment). The reason for the need for immediate treatment is the potential for sudden painless deterioration of vision in one eye secondary to ischemia of the optic nerve.

In addition to the signs and symptoms mentioned, patients suffering from temporal arteritis experience myalgia and morning stiffness. Muscle weakness associated with inflammatory muscle disease and many of the other collagen vascular diseases is absent in temporal arteritis unless the patient has been treated with prolonged doses of corticosteroids for other systemic disease, such as polymyalgia rheumatica. The patient may also experience nonspecific systemic symptoms, including malaise, weight loss, night sweats, and depression.

On physical examination, a swollen, indurated, nodular temporal artery is present. Diminished pulses are often noted, as is tenderness to palpation. Scalp tenderness to palpation is often seen. Funduscopic examination may reveal a pale, edematous optic disc. The patient suffering from temporal arteritis often appears chronically ill, depressed, or both.

Testing

Erythrocyte sedimentation rate testing should be obtained on all patients suspected of having temporal arteritis. In temporal arteritis, the erythrocyte sedimentation rate is greater than 50 mm/hr in more than 90% of patients. Less than 2% of patients with biopsy-proved temporal arteritis have a normal erythrocyte sedimentation rate. Ideally, the blood for the erythrocyte sedimentation rate should be obtained before beginning corticosteroid therapy because the initial level of elevation of this test is useful not only to help diagnose the disease but also as a mechanism to establish the efficacy of therapy. It is important for the clinician to remember that the erythrocyte sedimentation rate is a nonspecific test and that other diseases that may present clinically in a manner similar to temporal arteritis, such as malignancy or infection, may also markedly elevate the erythrocyte sedimentation rate. Therefore, confirmation of the clinical diagnosis of temporal arteritis requires a temporal artery biopsy.

Given the simplicity and safety of temporal artery biopsy, this test should probably be performed in all patients suspected of suffering from temporal arteritis. The presence of an inflammatory infiltrate with giant cells in the biopsied artery is characteristic of the disease. Edema of the intima and disruption of the internal elastic lamina strengthen the diagnosis. A small percentage of patients with clinical signs and symptoms strongly suggestive of temporal arteritis who also exhibit a significantly elevated erythrocyte sedimentation rate will have a negative temporal artery biopsy. As mentioned, if there is a strong clinical impression that the patient in fact has temporal arteritis, an immediate blood sample for erythrocyte sedimentation rate testing should be obtained and the patient started on corticosteroids. Complete blood cell count and automated chemistries including thyroid testing are indicated in all patients with suspected temporal arteritis to help rule out other systemic disease that may mimic the clinical presentation of temporal arteritis.

If the diagnosis of temporal arteritis is in doubt, magnetic resonance imaging (MRI) of the brain provides the clinician with the best information regarding the cranial vault and its contents. MRI is highly accurate and helps to identify abnormalities that may put the patient at risk for neurologic disasters due to intracranial and brainstem pathology, including tumors and demyelinating disease. More important, MRI helps to identify bleeding associated with leaking intracranial aneurysms. Magnetic resonance angiography may be useful to help identify aneurysms responsible for the patient's neurologic symptomatology. In patients who cannot undergo MRI, such as a patient with a pacemaker, computed tomographic (CT) scanning is a reasonable second choice. Even if blood is not present on MRI or CT, if intracranial hemorrhage is suspected, lumbar puncture should be performed. Measurement of intraocular pressure should be performed if glaucoma is suspected.

Differential Diagnosis

Headache associated with temporal arteritis is a clinical diagnosis that is supported by a combination of clinical history, abnormal physical examination of the temporal artery, normal radiography, MRI, an elevated erythrocyte sedimentation rate, and positive results from a temporal artery biopsy. Pain syndromes that may mimic temporal arteritis include tension-type headache, brain tumor, other forms of arteritis, trigeminal neuralgia involving the first division of the trigeminal nerve, demyelinating disease, migraine headache, cluster headache, migraine, and chronic paroxysmal hemicrania. Trigeminal neuralgia involving the first division of the trigeminal nerve is uncommon and is characterized by trigger areas and ticlike movements. Demyelinating disease is generally associated with other neurologic findings, including optic neuritis and other motor and sensory abnormalities. The pain of chronic paroxysmal hemicrania and cluster is associated with redness and watering of the ipsilateral eye, nasal congestion, and rhinorrhea during the headache. These findings are absent in all types of sexual headache. Migraine headache may or may not be associated with nonpainful neurologic findings known as *aura*, but the patient almost always reports some systemic symptoms, such as nausea or photophobia, not typically associated with the headache of temporal arteritis.

Treatment

The mainstay of the treatment of temporal arteritis and its associated headaches and other systemic symptoms is the immediate use of corticosteroids. If visual symptoms are present, an initial dose of 80 mg prednisone is indicated. This dose should be continued until the symptoms of temporal arteritis have completely abated. At this point, the dose may be decreased by 5 mg/wk as long as the symptoms remain quiescent and the erythrocyte sedimentation rate does not rise. Consideration of cytoprotection of the stomach mucosa should be given because the possibility of ulceration and gastrointestinal bleeding remains a real problem. If the patient cannot tolerate the corticosteroids or the maintenance dose of steroids remains so high as to produce adverse effects, azathioprine is a reasonable next choice.

SUGGESTED READING

Waldman SD: Headache associated with temporal arteritis. In: Atlas of Uncommon Pain Syndromes, ed 2. Philadelphia, Saunders, 2008.

CHAPTER 128

Ocular Pain

The vast majority of patients presenting with ocular and periocular pain are relatively straightforward to diagnose and treat (Table 128-1). For those patients suffering from ocular and periocular pain that is unrelated to primary eye disease, it usually becomes the responsibility of the pain management specialist to identify and treat the painful condition. For those patients whose pain is related primarily to eye disease, ophthalmologic referral is generally the best course of action.

Common Causes of Ocular Pain

STYES (HORDEOLUM)

Styes, or hordeolums, are probably the most common cause of eye pain encountered in clinical practice. Styes are the result of bacterial infection of the small oil-producing meibomian glands and/or the eyelash follicles at the margin of the eyelid. More than 98% of styles are caused by *Staphylococcus aureus*. These pus-filled abscesses can appear quite suddenly and can run the gamut from small self-limited infections that produce little pain and resolve on their own to rapidly growing, extremely painful abscesses that require immediate surgical incision and drainage and systemic antibiotics for resolution. If identified early, the use of non–neomycin-containing antibiotic ointment such as gentamicin or polymyxin-B and bacitracin ophthalmic ointment combined with frequent applications of warm moist packs will usually resolve the problem. If fever is present or the stye does not drain with the conservative therapy mentioned, systemic antibiotics and immediate ophthalmologic referral for surgical incision and drainage are indicated. Untreated, what begins as a simple localized folliculitis or meibomianitis can evolve into a vision- and life-threatening periorbital cellulitis that has the potential to spread to the adjacent central nervous system.

TABLE 128–1 Common Causes of Eye Pain

- Styes/hordeolum
- Conjunctivitis
- Corneal abrasions
- Glaucoma
- Uveitis
- Optic neuritis

CORNEAL ABRASIONS

Corneal abrasions are another frequent cause of eye pain that prompts patients to seek urgent medical attention. The unique nature of the sensory innervation of the corneal results in the patient's perception of foreign body in the eye anytime the superficial corneal stroma is injured and the C-type polymodal nociceptors that richly innervate the cornea are stimulated. The foreign body sensation is usually felt by the patient as being located under the upper eyelid even when there is no foreign body present and damage is limited to the corneal stroma. The continued firing of the polymodal receptors and recruitment of the corneal mechanoreceptors are probably responsible for this foreign body sensation associated with corneal abrasion that occurs in almost all patients with corneal abrasion even in the absence of foreign body.

Patients presenting with corneal abrasion will usually relate a history of grit or a foreign body being blowing into the eye or a history of minor mechanical trauma to the cornea during the insertion of contact lens or while playing sports. Fluorescein staining will usually reveal the damage to the corneal stroma, and rarely will a foreign body will be seen. The patient will bitterly complain of severe pain that is out of proportion to the apparent injury and will insist that there is something trapped under the upper eyelid even after repeated attempts to convince the patient to the contrary. Photophobia and excessive lacrimation and scleral and conjunctival injection are often present, as is a significant substrate of anxiety.

In the presence of corneal abrasion, the clinician should evert the upper eyelid and rinse the eye with copious amounts of sterile saline solution to remove any residual foreign body that may not be readily apparent on initial investigation. If the corneal abrasion is the result of an accident that occurred during hammering or the use of power tools, a careful search for a metallic foreign body should be undertaken and a plain radiograph or computed tomographic scan of the orbit and orbital contents should be obtained to rule out occult intraocular metallic foreign body, which can present a significant risk to vision if undetected. Treatment with non–neomycin-containing antibiotic ointment such as gentamicin or polymyxin B and bacitracin ophthalmic ointment combined with patching of the eye and a large dose of reassurance will usually resolve the problem.

CONJUNCTIVITIS

Infection of the conjunctiva is a common cause of eye pain. Caused by bacteria, fungus, or virus, conjunctivitis can range from a mild self-limited disease requiring no treatment to a purulent eye infection that can be quite painful and upsetting to the patient. Bacterial and viral conjunctivitis, which is also known as pink eye, can be quite contagious, and all patients suffering from conjunctivitis should be instructed in good hand-washing techniques and informed of the need to sterilize fomites that they have in common with the family and coworkers, such as copy machines, faucets, telephones, computer keyboards, and so forth. In addition to infectious etiologies, conjunctivitis can also be caused by environmental irritants, including pollen, dust, smog, and fumes.

The patient with conjunctivitis will present with a red, irritated, and painful eye that is often associated with excessive lacrimation and some degree of photophobia. A purulent discharge is also often present. If the discharge is severe, the patient may awaken with the eyelids stuck together, resulting in extreme anxiety for the patient; this frequently results in trips to the nearest emergency department for treatment. Treatment of acute conjunctivitis begins with reassurance and the use of a warm moist pack applied to the affected eye to afford symptomatic relieve. Non–neomycin-containing antibiotic eye drops or ointment such as gentamicin or polymyxin B and bacitracin should be used, with care being taken to avoid touching the affected eye with the dropper or the tip of the tube of antibiotic ointment, to avoid reinfection. If the possibility of sexually transmitted conjunctivitis is present, a culture should be take and systemic antibiotics and ophthalmologic consultation on an urgent basis are indicated.

GLAUCOMA

Glaucoma is the most common eye disease that results in blindness in the United States. Glaucoma is not a single disease but a group of diseases that have in common dysfunction of the circulation and drainage of the aqueous humor inside the eyeball. Glaucoma is rarely seen in the absence of trauma or a congenital abnormality of the globe before the age of 40. It occurs more commonly in blacks and those with a family history of glaucoma. Any severe trauma to the globe increases the risk of glaucoma.

For purposes of this discussion, the pain management specialist must be aware that there are two types of glaucoma: (1) open angle glaucoma and (2) angle closure glaucoma. Open angle glaucoma has been called the "silent thief" in that the disease manifests with little or no symptoms and gradually causes permanent eye damage due to increased intraocular pressure, which causes ischemic damage to the optic nerve. Open angle glaucoma is caused by an inability of aqueous humor to drain from the anterior chamber of the eye even though the angle between the iris and cornea is opened. The causes of open angle glaucoma remain elusive. Initially, only the peripheral vision is affected, and as the disease progresses, the patient may present with painless vision loss and complaining of tunnel vision. Funduscopic examination will reveal disc cupping. Because of the lack of pain associated with open angle glaucoma, patients with this disease will rarely present to the pain management physician, although it should be remembered that all patients older than 60 years are at risk for glaucoma and an inquiry regarding visual loss should be part of every pain management assessment in this age group.

In contradistinction to open angle glaucoma, the pain management physician will in all likelihood encounter patients with eye pain and visual loss that may be the result of angle closure glaucoma. Angle closure glaucoma occurs when the angle between the iris and the cornea becomes blocked, impeding the drainage of aqueous humor. Angle closure glaucoma represents a true ophthalmologic emergency, and failure to rapidly identify the disease and help the patient receive immediate ophthalmologic care will invariably result in permanent visual loss. The patient with acute angle closure glaucoma will present with the acute onset of severe eye pain, blurred vision, the complaint of a halo effect around lights, nausea and vomiting, and a red eye. The cornea may appear steamy, like looking though a steamy window. The pupil may be poorly reactive or fixed in midposition, and the iris may have a whorled appearance. The patient will appear acutely ill, in contradistinction to the chronically ill–appearing patient with temporal arteritis, which can also manifest in this age group. The onset of angle closure glaucoma frequently occurs at night when the pupil dilates further, impeding the flow of aqueous humor by further narrowing or closing the angle between the iris and the cornea.

The first step is the diagnosis of glaucoma is for the clinician to think of it. The diagnosis of both of these types of glaucoma can be made by simple measurements of intraocular pressure. Although a rare low-pressure glaucoma exists, the vast majority of patients with glaucoma can be identified with simple ocular applanation or air-puff tonometry.

UVEITIS

Uveitis is a term used to describe inflammation of the uvea that is not due to infection. The uvea is divided into anterior and posterior parts. The anterior uvea consists of the ciliary body and iris, and the posterior uvea consists of the choroids layer. Uveitis is a common cause of eye pain, and the pain is frequently associated with a red eye. Uveitis is frequently associated with the autoimmune diseases, such as rheumatoid arthritis, Behçet's disease, among others, although the causes of uveitis may defy specific diagnosis. Patients with uveitis will present with eye pain, red eye, photophobia, blurred vision, and "floaters." The pain of uveitis can be exacerbated by shining a bright light into the eye, causing the inflamed iris to constrict. Uveitis is an ophthalmologic emergency, and immediate ophthalmologic evaluation and treatment with corticosteroids are mandatory if permanent visual loss is to be avoided.

OPTIC NEURITIS

Optic neuritis is another common cause of eye pain. Although pain is invariably present, it is the acute visual loss associated with the disease that usually prompts the patient to seek medical attention. The most common cause of optic neuritis is multiple sclerosis, with approximately 20% of patients suffering from multiple sclerosis having optic neuritis as their initial symptom. Approximately 70% of patients with multiple sclerosis will suffer from optic neuritis at some point in their disease.

Other causes of optic neuritis include temporal arteritis, tuberculosis, human immunodeficiency virus, hepatitis B, Lyme disease, and cytomegalovirus. Whether the optic neuritis is due to actual infection of the optic nerve or as part of a complex inflammatory response is the subject of debate. Optic neuritis is also seen as a sequelae to sinus infection and after radiation therapy.

The incidence of optic neuritis is approximately 7 cases per 100,000 patients, and it occurs most commonly in Caucasians of northern European ancestry. Blacks and Asians are rarely affected in the absence of an infectious etiology. Optic neuritis occurs more commonly in females and usually manifests between the ages of 20 and 50 years. In patients older than 50 years with acute vision loss in one eye, ischemic optic neuritis is a more likely diagnosis.

Patients with optic neuritis present with a triad of symptoms, including (1) acute vision loss, (2) eye pain, and (3) dyschromatopsia, which is impairment of accurate color vision. Some patients with optic neuritis also complain of sound- or sudden movement–induced flashing lights, which are known as phosgenes, as well as heat-induced visual loss. Approximately 70% of patients with optic neuritis have unilateral symptoms. On physical examination, the patient suffering from optic neuritis will exhibit a pale, swollen, optic disc. Magnetic resonance imaging and visual evoked responses will confirm the clinical diagnosis. Urgent ophthalmologic referral for treatment with intravenous corticosteroids and/or interferon therapy is indicated in all patients suspected of having optic neuritis.

SUGGESTED READING

Waldman SD: Pain of ocular origin. Waldman SD: Pain Management. Philadelphia, Saunders, 2007.

CHAPTER 129

Otalgia

Ear pain can result from local pathology (e.g., cellulitis, tumor) or can be referred from distant sites, most commonly from the nasopharynx (Table 129-1). Because of the complex functions of the ear, local disease may cause disturbances of hearing and balance, which can be quite distressing for the patient and may serve as a harbinger of serious diseases, such as acoustic neuroma.

Functional Anatomy of the Ear as It Relates to Pain

The ear and surrounding tissues are innervated both by the cranial nerves and from branches of nerves that have as their origin the spinal nerves. The auricle is innervated by the greater auricular nerve as well as the lesser occipital

TABLE 129–1 Common Causes of Otalgia

Auricular Pain
• Superficial infections
• Folliculitis
• Cellulitis
• Abscess
• Ramsay-Hunt syndrome
• Deep infections
• Chondritis
• Collagen vascular diseases
• Periarticular hematoma—"cauliflower ear"
• Malignancies, especially basal and squamous cell carcinomas
External Auditory Canal
• Otitis externa
• Foreign body
• Cholesteatoma
Tympanic Membrane and Middle Ear
• Myringitis
• Otitis media
• Mastoiditis
Referred Pain
• Nasopharynx
• Pyriformis sinuses
• Middle and posterior cranial fossa pathology

nerve, the auricular branch of the vagus nerve, and the auriculotemporal branch of the mandibular nerve. The external auditory canal receives innervation from branches of the glossopharyngeal and facial nerves. The inferoposterior portion of the tympanic membrane receives its innervation from the auriculotemporal branch of the mandibular nerve as well as the auricular branch of the vagus nerve and the tympanic branch of the glossopharyngeal nerve. The structures of the middle ear receive innervation from the tympanic branch of the glossopharyngeal nerve along with the caroticotympanic nerve, the superficial petrosal nerve. It is the overlap of these nerves as well as their diverse origin that can make localization of pathology responsible for the patient's pain quite challenging.

Painful Diseases of the Ear

AURICULAR PAIN

The skin of the auricle is richly innervated and is frequently the source of local ear pain. It should be noted that the auricular cartilage is poorly innervated and diseases that are limited to the cartilage may produce little or no pain until there is distention or inflammation of the overlying skin. Most painful conditions involving the auricle are due to infection, trauma, connective tissue disease, or tumor.

Superficial infections of the auricle include folliculitis, abscess, cellulitis, and infection from herpes simplex and zoster including the Ramsay-Hunt syndrome. Deep infections involving the cartilage, once uncommon, are now occurring with much greater frequency owing to the current increase in body piercing involving the auricular cartilage.

Both superficial and deep infections of the auricle are quite painful. Early incision and drainage, débridement of nonviable cartilage, and aggressive use of antibiotics are necessary to avoid spread of infection to the middle ear, bone, and intracranial structures, including the central nervous system.

Trauma to the auricle can be quite painful and, if not appropriately treated, can result in loss of cartilage and disfigurement. Blunt trauma to the auricle can cause superficial ecchymosis or, if severe enough, perichondral hematoma ("cauliflower ear"). Lacerations of the lobule, tragus, and cartilage from body piercings that have been torn from the ear are increasingly common occurrences at local emergency departments and urgent care centers. Prompt débridement and repair with careful observation for infection are crucial if disfiguring sequelae are to be avoided.

Thermal injuries from heat or cold are also common painful traumatic injuries to the ear that usually follow the use of heating pads or cold packs in patients who are also taking pain medications and/or self-medicating with alcohol. Frostbite injuries affecting the auricle are also common and are frequently related to alcohol and/or drug use. Thermal injuries can initially appear less severe that they really are. Initial treatment with topical antibiotics such as silver sulfadiazine and sterile dressings should be followed up with reevaluation and the redressing of the affected area on a daily basis until the thermal injury is well on the way to healing.

Connective tissue diseases can cause inflammation of the auricular cartilage. Usually manifesting as a bilateral acutely inflamed and painful swelling of the auricle, chondritis and perichondritis may initially be misdiagnosed as cellulitis. The bilateral nature of the disease as well as the involvement of other cartilage should alert the clinician to the possibility of a noninfectious cause of the pain, rubor, and swelling. Because many of the connective tissue diseases affect other organ systems, prompt diagnosis and treatment are essential.

Primary tumors of the auricle are usually basal cell or squamous cell carcinomas due to actinic damage of the skin. Rarely, primary tumors of the cartilage can occur. Metastatic lesions to the auricle are uncommon but not unheard of.

THE EXTERNAL AUDITORY CANAL

Far and away the most common painful condition of the external auditory meatus is otitis externa. Usually the result of swimming or digging in the ear with a fingernail, cotton swab, or hairpin, the initial symptom of otitis externa is usually pruritus. This is followed by pain that is made worse by yawning or chewing. On physical examination, there is a reddened, wet-appearing, edematous canal that may reveal abraded areas from previous digging or scratching from the patient's attempt to relieve the symptoms. Pulling on the auricle posteriorly will usually exacerbate the pain of otitis externa. The pain of this disease is often out of proportion to the findings on physical examination. Treatment of otitis externa consists of cleaning any debris out of the acoustic auditory canal and instilling topical antibiotic drops or solution. If significant edema is present, the use of topical antibiotic drops or solution containing corticosteroid will speed recovery.

Another cause of external auditory canal pain is cholesteatoma. Cholesteatoma most often occurs after trauma to the bone of the external auditory canal. Caused by invasion of the external auditory canal wall by exuberant tissue growth, cholesteatoma can become quite invasive if left untreated despite its benign tissue elements. The patient with cholesteatoma will present with a ball-like growth in the external auditory canal that has an onion skin–like appearance. Unless infected, the pain will most often be dull and aching in character. Secondary infection may cause foul-swelling purulent exudates to drain from the affected ear. Computed tomographic scanning will help the clinician determine the amount of bony destruction and help guide the microsurgical resection of this common cause of ear pain.

In the younger patient and the patient with impaired mentation, foreign bodies are a frequently overlooked cause of ear pain originating from the external auditory meatus. Most problematic are vegetable matter such as dried peas and beans, which swell once inside the acoustic auditory canal, making removal quite difficult. If the foreign body remains in the external auditory canal for any period of time, secondary infection invariably occurs. Insects may also fly or crawl into the external auditory meatus, causing the patient much distress. If the insect remains alive, instillation of lidocaine or mineral oil will stop the insect from moving around and make removal easier.

THE TYMPANIC MEMBRANE AND MIDDLE EAR

Myringitis is a painful condition that may be caused by viral infection of the tympanic membrane. Vesicles or blebs of the tympanic membrane may be present on physical examination or the tympanic membrane may appear normal. Antibiotic drops containing local anesthetic will usually provide symptomatic relief, although in the absence of physical findings, the diagnosis of idiopathic myringitis is one of exclusion. Other diseases of the middle ear or referred pain remains an ever-present possibility.

Acute otitis media is perhaps the second most common cause of otalgia after otitis externa. More common in children, otitis media can occur at any age. The pain of otitis media is caused primarily by distention and inflammation of the tympanic membrane. Young children with otitis media may pull on their ear, whereas older patients will complain bitterly of a deep, severe, unremitting pain. Fever is also usually present. Untreated, the pain will become increasingly severe as the tympanic membrane becomes more distended until the tympanic membrane ruptures. Although the pain may dramatically improve following spontaneous rupture, infection of the mastoid air cells can occur. Treatment of acute otitis media has its foundation in the administration of oral antibiotics and decongestants. Topical local anesthetic drops administered via the external auditory canal may provide symptomatic relief while waiting for the antibiotics and decongestants to work. For otitis media that does not promptly resolve, therapeutic tympanocentesis with placement of ear tubes should be considered.

As mentioned, acute mastoiditis is often the result of untreated or undertreated otitis media. Mastoiditis is characterized by pain, tenderness, and rubor in the posterior auricular region. The diagnosis is often misdiagnosed initially as recurrent otitis media as examination of the tympanic membrane will often reveal the findings of the unresolved otitis media. Fever is invariably present, and the patient will generally appear more ill than a patient with otitis media alone. Radiographic examination of the mastoid air cells will reveal opacification of the normally aerated structure and, as the disease progresses, bony destruction. Untreated, mastoiditis can become life threatening as the infection spreads to the central nervous system. The findings of headache, stiff neck, and visual disturbance are warning signs of central nervous system involvement and constitute a medical emergency. Surgical treatment combined with aggressive antibiotic therapy is required on an emergent basis for patients exhibiting signs of central nervous system infection.

A word of caution is in order whenever the clinician is unable to identify the cause of a patient's ear pain. Idiopathic otalgia, especially if unilateral, is a diagnosis of exclusion that should generally be resisted because it is invariably wrong. Repeat physical examination and a careful retaking of the history with special attention to areas where occult tumor might cause pain that is referred to the ear are essential if disaster is to be avoided. This is one clinical situation where serial magnetic resonance imaging of the brain and soft tissues of the neck as well as computed tomographic scanning of these areas will often yield results. All patients with unexplained ear pain should have a careful endoscopic examination of the aerodigestive tract with special attention to the region of the piriform sinuses to identify occult pathology responsible for the pain.

SUGGESTED READINGS

Goetz CG: Textbook of Clinical Neurology, ed 2. Philadelphia, Saunders, 2003.

Waldman SD: Pain of the ear, nose, and sinuses. In: Pain Management. Philadelphia, Saunders, 2007.

CHAPTER 130

Pain Involving the Nose, Sinuses, and Throat

Nose and Sinus Pain

Infection of the nose is the most common cause of nasal pain absent trauma. Superficial soft tissue infections can be quite painful and have the potential to spread to deep structures if left untreated. Folliculitis of the vestibule of the nose can also be quite painful and, when secondary to *Staphylococcus*, can be quite difficult to treat. Occurring more commonly as the use of intranasal steroid sprays to treat atrophic rhinitis increases, the early use of topical intranasal antibiotics such as mupirocin at the first sign of intranasal tenderness can help prevent more severe disease. Persistent foul-smelling discharge from the nose should alert the physician to the possibility of an intranasal foreign body, especially in children or mentally impaired individuals. Malignancy should always be considered in the differential diagnosis of nasal pain.

Acute sinusitis is another painful condition of the midface that can be caused by all infectious agents. Blockage of the ostia of the sinus is usually the cause of acute sinusitis, with the pressure within the sinuses increasing because mucus from the affected sinuses cannot flow into the nose. The maxillary sinuses are most commonly affected, and the pain associated with this disease can be quite severe. The pain of acute sinusitis is usually localized to the area over the sinus and may be worse with recumbency.

The diagnosis of acute sinusitis is usually made on clinical grounds and then confirmed with plain radiographs or computed tomography (CT). Treatment with decongestant nasal sprays and antibiotics will resolve most cases of acute sinusitis. Untreated, osteomyelitis may occur. Surgery may ultimately be required for recurrent disease or disease that remains unresponsive to conservative therapy or when radiographs reveal obstructive polyps or tumors.

Malignancies of the nose and sinuses can be notoriously difficult to diagnose. The most common tumors of the nose are basal cell and squamous cell carcinomas. Usually not painful unless infection intervenes or a painful structure is invaded, these tumors can become quite large before detected. Squamous cell carcinomas of the sinuses present in a manner identical to sinusitis, so diagnosis is often delayed. Nasopharyngeomas occur most commonly in patients of Asian decent. Thought to be caused by the Epstein-Barr virus, these tumors often cause referred pain to the face, neck, and retroauricular area. Other tumors known for their ability to cause referred nose and facial pain are tumors involving parapharyngeal space. Almost always causing unilateral symptoms such as facial paralysis and pain, parapharyngeal tumors are often of neural origin. As mentioned, delay in diagnosis of these tumors can complicate treatment and worsen prognosis.

Throat Pain

Pain emanating from this region is poorly localized owing to the mixed innervation of the anatomic structures by the trigeminal, glossopharyngeal, and vagus nerves as well as rich innervation by the sympathetic nervous system. For this reason, referred pain from this region is not the exception, but the rule. Because of the patient's difficulty in accurately localizing the source of the pain when pathology affects this anatomic region, extra vigilance on the part of the clinician is required.

Both superficial and deep infections are a common source of throat pain. Acute pharyngitis and laryngotracheobronchitis are among the most common reasons that patients seek medical attention. Dental infections are also common causes of pain in this anatomic region and often cause referred pain into the ear. Generally self-limited, these infections can become problematic if they spread to the deep structures of the neck and aerodigestive tract or if they occur in immunocompromised patients. In particular, parapharyngeal and retropharyngeal space abscesses following acute pharyngitis and tonsillitis can become life threatening if not promptly diagnosed and treated. Patients with these disorders will appear acutely ill and will talk with a characteristic muffled "hot potato voice." With the increased availability of magnetic resonance imaging (MRI) and CT scanning, early diagnosis of parapharyngeal and retropharyngeal abscess is much easier.

In addition to infections, tumors of this region can produce both local and referred pain. These tumors are often hard to diagnose, and by the time the pain is so severe as to cause the patient to seek medical attention, the tumors are already extremely problematic and in many cases already metastasized. Most primary tumors in this region are squamous cell tumors, although primary tumors of the neural structures and craniopharyngiomas occur with sufficient frequency to be part of the differential diagnosis. Metastatic lesions can also cause local and referred pain in this anatomic area. Given the silent nature of this area insofar as symptoms are concerned, the clinician should make early and frequent use of MRI and CT to identify occult tumors and other pathology. In particular, the clinician should never attribute pain in this region to idiopathic or psychogenic etiology without serial physical examinations, laboratory evaluations, and imaging. In particular, a unilateral otalgia in the absence of demonstrable ear pathology should be taking very seriously and considered to be referred pain from occult tumor until proved otherwise.

Other painful conditions unrelated to infection and tumor can occur in this anatomic region. These include Eagle's syndrome, carotidynia, and the hyoid syndrome.

Eagle's syndrome is caused by calcification of the stylohyoid ligament and is characterized by paroxysms of pain with movement of the mandible during chewing, yawning, and talking. Carotidynia consists of deep neck pain in the region of the carotid that radiates into the ear and jaw. It is made worse with palpation of the area overlying the carotid artery. Hyoid syndrome is characterized by sharp paroxysms of pain with swallowing or head turning. The pain radiates into the ear and the angle of the jaw. The pain can be reproduced with movement of the hyoid bone. For the most part, these unusual causes of ear, throat, and anterior neck pain are self-limited and will produce no long-lasting harm to the patient. However, before they are diagnosed, it is incumbent on the clinician to rule out other pathologic processes that may harm the patient as they are statistically much more common.

SUGGESTED READINGS

Goetz CG: Textbook of Clinical Neurology, ed 2. Philadelphia, Saunders, 2003.

Waldman SD: Pain of the ear, nose, and sinuses. In: Pain Management. Philadelphia, Saunders, 2007.

CHAPTER 131

Temporomandibular Joint Dysfunction

Temporomandibular joint (TMJ) dysfunction (TMD) (also known as myofascial pain dysfunction of the muscles of mastication) is characterized by pain in the joint itself that radiates into the mandible, ear, neck, and tonsillar pillars. Headache often accompanies the pain of TMD and is clinically indistinguishable from that of tension-type headache. Stress is often the precipitating or exacerbating factor in the development of TMD. Dental malocclusion may play a role in the evolution of TMD. Internal derangement and arthritis of the TMJ may manifest as clicking or grating when the joint is opened and closed. Untreated, the patient may experience increasing pain in the areas mentioned and limitation of jaw movement and opening.

Signs and Symptoms

The TMJ is a true joint that is divided into an upper and lower synovial cavity by a fibrous articular disc. Internal derangement of this disc may result in pain and TMD, but extracapsular causes of TMJ pain are much more common. The joint space between the mandibular condyle and the glenoid fossa of the zygoma may be injected with small amounts of local anesthetic and steroid. The TMJ is innervated by branches of the mandibular nerve. The muscles involved in TMD often include the temporalis, masseter, external pterygoid, and internal pterygoid and may include the trapezius and sternocleidomastoid. Trigger points may be identified when palpating these muscles. Crepitus on range of motion of the joint is suggestive of arthritis rather than dysfunction of myofascial origin. A history of bruxism and/or jaw clenching is often present.

Testing

Radiographs of the TMJ are usually within normal limits in patients suffering from TMD but may be useful to help identify inflammatory or degenerative arthritis of the joint. MRI of the joint will help the clinician to identify derangement of the disc as well as other abnormalities of the joint itself. Complete blood count, erythrocyte sedimentation rate, and antinuclear antibody testing are indicated if inflammatory arthritis or temporal arteritis is suspected. Injection of the joint with small amounts of local anesthetic will serve as a diagnostic maneuver to help determine if the TMJ is in fact the source of the patient's pain.

Differential Diagnosis

The clinical symptomatology of TMD may often be confused with pain of dental or sinus origin or may be characterized as atypical facial pain. Careful questioning and physical examination will usually allow the clinician to help separate these overlapping pain syndromes. Tumors of the zygoma and mandible as well as retropharyngeal tumors may produce ill-defined pain that may be attributed to TMD, and these potentially life-threatening diseases must be carefully searched for in any patient with facial pain. Reflex sympathetic dystrophy of the face should also be considered in any patient presenting with ill-defined facial pain following trauma, infection, or central nervous system injury. The pain of TMD is dull and aching in character, whereas the pain of reflex sympathetic dystrophy of the face is burning in nature with significant allodynia often present. Stellate ganglion block may help distinguish the two pain syndromes, because the pain of reflex sympathetic dystrophy of the face readily responds to this sympathetic nerve block and the pain of TMD does not. The pain of TMD must be distinguished from the pain of jaw claudication associated with temporal arteritis.

Treatment

The mainstay of TMD is the combination of pharmacologic treatment with tricyclic antidepressants, physical modalities such as oral orthotic devices and physical therapy, and intra-articular injection of the joint with small amounts of local anesthetic and steroid. Antidepressant compounds such as nortriptyline at a single bedtime dose of 25 mg will help normalize sleep disturbance and treat underlying myofascial pain syndrome. Orthotic devices help the patient avoid jaw clenching and bruxism, which may exacerbate the clinical syndrome. Intra-articular injection is useful both to provide palliation of acute pain to allow physical therapy and to treat joint arthritis that may contribute to the patient's pain symptomatology and joint dysfunction. Rarely, surgical treatment of the displaced intra-articular disc is required to restore the joint to normal function and reduce pain.

To perform intra-articular injection of the TMJ, the patient is placed in the supine position with the cervical spine in the neutral position. The TMJ is identified by asking the patient to open and close the mouth several times and palpating the area just anterior and slightly inferior to the acoustic auditory meatus. After the joint is identified, the patient is asked to hold his or her mouth in neutral position.

A total of 0.5 mL of local anesthetic is drawn up in a 3-mL sterile syringe. When treating TMD, internal derangement of the TMJ, arthritis pain of the TMJ, or other painful conditions involving the TMJ, a total of 20 mg of depot steroid is added to the local anesthetic with the first block and 10 mg of depot steroid is added to the local anesthetic with subsequent blocks. After the skin overlying the TMJ is prepared with antiseptic solution, a 25-gauge, 1-inch styletted needle is inserted just below the zygomatic arch directly in the middle of the joint space. The needle is advanced approximately ½ to ¾ inch in a plane perpendicular to the skull until a pop is felt, indicating the joint space has been entered. After careful aspiration, 1 mL of solution is slowly injected. Injection of the joint may be repeated in 5- to 7-day intervals if the symptoms persist.

SUGGESTED READING

Waldman SD: Temporomandibular joint dysfunction. In: Atlas of Common Pain Syndromes, ed 2. Philadelphia, Saunders, 2008.

Atypical Facial Pain

Atypical facial pain (also known as atypical facial neuralgia) is a term used to describe a heterogeneous group of pain syndromes that have in common the fact that the patient is suffering from facial pain that cannot be classified as trigeminal neuralgia. The pain is continuous but may vary in intensity. It is almost always unilateral and can be characterized as aching or cramping rather than shocklike neuritic pain typical of trigeminal neuralgia. The vast majority of patients suffering from atypical facial pain are female. The distribution of pain is in the distribution of the trigeminal nerve but invariably overlaps divisions of the nerve.

Headache often accompanies the pain of atypical facial pain and is clinically indistinguishable from that of tension-type headache. Stress is often the precipitating or exacerbating factor in the development of atypical facial pain. Depression and sleep disturbance are also manifest in a significant number of patients suffering from atypical facial pain. A history of facial trauma, infection, or tumor of the head and neck may be elicited in some patients with atypical facial pain, but in most cases, no precipitating event can be identified.

Signs and Symptoms

Table 132-1 compares atypical facial pain with trigeminal neuralgia. Unlike trigeminal neuralgia, which is characterized by sudden paroxysms of neuritic shocklike pain, the pain of atypical facial pain is constant and of a dull, aching quality, but it may vary in intensity. The pain of trigeminal neuralgia is always within the distribution of a division of the trigeminal nerve, whereas the pain of atypical facial pain will invariably overlap these divisional boundaries. The trigger areas that are characteristic of trigeminal neuralgia are absent in patients suffering from atypical facial pain.

Testing

Radiographs of the head are usually within normal limits in patients suffering from atypical facial pain but may be useful to help identify tumor or bony abnormality. Magnetic resonance imaging (MRI) of the brain and sinuses will help the clinician to identify intracranial pathology, including tumor, sinus disease, and infection. Complete blood count, erythrocyte sedimentation rate, and antinuclear antibody testing are indicated if inflammatory arthritis or temporal arteritis is suspected. Injection of the temporomandibular joint with small amounts of local anesthetic will serve as a diagnostic maneuver to help determine whether the temporomandibular joint is in fact the source of the patient's pain. MRI of the cervical spine is also indicated if the patient is experiencing significant occipital or nuchal pain symptomatology.

Differential Diagnosis

The clinical symptomatology of atypical facial pain may often be confused with pain of dental or sinus origin or may be erroneously characterized as trigeminal neuralgia.

TABLE 132–1 Comparison of Trigeminal Neuralgia and Atypical Facial Pain

	Trigeminal Neuralgia	Atypical Facial Pain
Temporal pattern of pain	Sudden and intermittent	Constant
Character of pain	Shocklike and neuritic	Dull, cramping, and aching
Pain-free Intervals	Usual	Rare
Distribution of pain	In division of trigeminal nerve	Overlaps division of trigeminal nerve
Trigger areas	Present	Absent
Underlying psychopathology	Rare	Common

Careful questioning and physical examination will usually allow the clinician to help separate these overlapping pain syndromes. Tumors of the zygoma and mandible, as well as posterior fossa tumors and retropharyngeal tumors, may produce ill-defined pain that may be attributed to atypical facial pain, and these potentially life-threatening diseases must be carefully searched for in any patient with facial pain. Reflex sympathetic dystrophy of the face should also be considered in any patient presenting with ill-defined facial pain following trauma, infection, or central nervous system injury. The pain of atypical facial pain is dull and aching in character, whereas the pain of reflex sympathetic dystrophy of the face is burning in nature, with significant allodynia often present. Stellate ganglion block may help distinguish the two pain syndromes, because the pain of reflex sympathetic dystrophy of the face readily responds to this sympathetic nerve block and atypical facial pain does not. The pain of atypical facial pain must be distinguished from the pain of jaw claudication associated with temporal arteritis.

Treatment

The mainstay of atypical facial pain is the combination of pharmacologic treatment with tricyclic antidepressants and physical modalities such as oral orthotic devices and physical therapy. Trigeminal nerve block and intra-articular injection of the temporomandibular joint with small amounts of local anesthetic and steroid may also be of value. Antidepressant compounds such as nortriptyline at a single bedtime dose of 25 mg will help normalize sleep disturbance and treat underlying myofascial pain syndrome. Orthotic devices help the patient avoid jaw clenching and bruxism, which may exacerbate the clinical syndrome. Treatment of underlying depression and anxiety is mandatory if the clinician hopes to help relieve the symptoms of atypical facial pain.

SUGGESTED READING

Waldman SD: Atypical facial pain. In: Atlas of Common Pain Syndromes, ed 2. Philadelphia, Saunders, 2008.

CHAPTER 133

Occipital Neuralgia

Occipital neuralgia is usually the result of blunt trauma to the greater and lesser occipital nerves. Repetitive microtrauma from working with the neck hyperextended (e.g., painting ceilings) or working for prolonged periods with computer monitors whose focal point is too high, causing extension of the cervical spine, may also cause occipital neuralgia. The pain of occipital neuralgia is characterized as persistent pain at the base of the skull with occasional sudden shocklike paresthesias in the distribution of the greater and lesser occipital nerves. Tension-type headache, which is much more common than occipital neuralgia, will occasionally mimic the pain of occipital neuralgia.

Signs and Symptoms

The greater occipital nerve arises from fibers of the dorsal primary ramus of the second cervical nerve and, to a lesser extent, from fibers from the third cervical nerve. The greater occipital nerve pierces the fascia just below the superior nuchal ridge along with the occipital artery. It supplies the medial portion of the posterior scalp as far anterior as the vertex (Fig. 133-1).

The lesser occipital nerve arises from the ventral primary rami of the second and third cervical nerves. The lesser occipital nerve passes superiorly along the posterior border of the sternocleidomastoid muscle, dividing into cutaneous branches that innervate the lateral portion of the posterior scalp and the cranial surface of the pinna of the ear (see Fig. 133-1).

The patient suffering from occipital neuralgia will experience neuritic pain in the distribution of the greater and lesser occipital nerves when the nerves are palpated at the level of the nuchal ridge. Some patients can elicit pain with rotation or lateral bending of the cervical spine.

Testing

There is no specific test for occipital neuralgia. Testing is aimed primarily at identifying occult pathology or other diseases that may mimic occipital neuralgia (see Differential Diagnosis). All patients with the recent onset of headache thought to be occipital neuralgia should undergo magnetic resonance imaging (MRI) of the brain and cervical spine. MRI should also be performed in patients with previously stable occipital neuralgia who have experienced a recent change in headache symptomatology. Screening laboratory testing consisting of complete blood count, erythrocyte sedimentation rate, and automated blood chemistry testing should be performed if the diagnosis of occipital neuralgia is in question.

Neural blockade of the greater and lesser occipital nerves can serve as a diagnostic maneuver to help confirm the diagnosis and to distinguish it from tension-type headache. The greater and lesser occipital nerves can easily be blocked at the nuchal ridge (see Fig. 133-1).

Differential Diagnosis

Occipital neuralgia is an infrequent cause of headaches and rarely occurs in the absence of trauma to the greater and lesser occipital nerves. More often, the patient with headaches involving the occipital region is in fact suffering from tension-type headaches. Tension-type headaches will not respond to occipital nerve blocks but are very amenable to treatment with antidepressant compounds such as amitriptyline in conjunction with cervical steroid epidural nerve blocks. Therefore, the clinician should reconsider the diagnosis of occipital neuralgia in those patients whose symptoms are consistent with occipital neuralgia but who fail to respond to greater and lesser occipital nerve blocks.

Treatment

The treatment of occipital neuralgia consists primarily of neural blockade with local anesthetic and steroid combined with the judicious use of nonsteroidal anti-inflammatory drugs, muscle relaxants, tricyclic antidepressants, and physical therapy. Neural blockade of the greater and lesser occipital nerves is a straightforward technique and is a reasonable early treatment of occipital neuralgia.

SUGGESTED READINGS

Campbell W: DeJong's The Neurological Examination, ed 6. Philadelphia, Lippincott Williams and Wilkins, 2005.

Goetz CG: Textbook of Clinical Neurology, ed 2. Philadelphia, Saunders, 2003.

Waldman SD: Occipital neuralgia. In: Atlas of Common Pain Syndromes, ed 2. Philadelphia, Saunders, 2008.

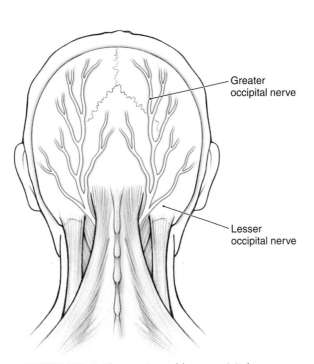

FIGURE 133–1 The greater and lesser occipital nerves.

CHAPTER 134

Cervical Radiculopathy

Cervical radiculopathy is a constellation of symptoms consisting of neurogenic neck and upper extremity pain emanating from the cervical nerve roots. In addition to the pain, the patient with cervical radiculopathy may experience associated numbness, weakness, and loss of reflexes. The causes of cervical radiculopathy include herniated disc, foraminal stenosis, tumor, osteophyte formation, and, rarely, infection.

Signs and Symptoms

The patient suffering from cervical radiculopathy will complain of pain, numbness, tingling, and paresthesias in the distribution of the affected nerve root or roots (Table 134-1). Patients may also note weakness and lack of coordination in the affected extremity. Muscle spasms and neck pain, as well as pain referred into the trapezius and intrascapular region, are common. Decreased sensation, weakness, and reflex changes are demonstrated on physical examination. Patients with C7 radiculopathy will commonly place the hand of the affected extremity on the top of their head in order to obtain relief. Occasionally, a patient suffering from cervical radiculopathy will experience compression of the cervical spinal cord resulting in myelopathy. Cervical myelopathy is most commonly due to midline herniated cervical disc, spinal stenosis, tumor, or, rarely, infection. Patients suffering from cervical myelopathy will experience lower extremity weakness and bowel and bladder symptomatology. This represents a neurosurgical emergency and should be treated as such.

Testing

Magnetic resonance imaging (MRI) of the cervical spine will provide the clinical with the best information regarding the cervical spine and its contents. MRI is highly accurate and will help identify abnormalities that may put the patient at risk for the development of cervical myelopathy. In patients who cannot undergo MRI (e.g., patients with a pacemaker), computed tomography or myelography is a reasonable second choice. Radionucleotide bone scanning and plain radiographs are indicated if fracture or bony abnormality such as metastatic disease is being considered.

Although the testing mentioned provides the clinician with useful neuroanatomic information, electromyography and nerve conduction velocity testing will provide the clinician with neurophysiologic information that can delineate that actual status of each individual nerve root and the brachial plexus. Screening laboratory testing consisting of complete blood count, erythrocyte sedimentation rate, and automated blood chemistry testing should be performed if the diagnosis of cervical radiculopathy is in question.

Differential Diagnosis

Cervical radiculopathy is a clinical diagnosis that is supported by a combination of clinical history, physical examination, radiography, and MRI. Pain syndromes that may mimic cervical radiculopathy include cervicalgia, cervical bursitis, cervical fibromyositis, inflammatory arthritis, and

TABLE 134–1 Clinical Features of Cervical Radiculopathy

Cervical Root	Pain	Sensory Changes	Weakness	Reflex Changes
C5 root	Neck, shoulder, anterolateral arm	Numbness In deltoid area	Deltoid and biceps	Biceps reflex
C6 root	Neck, shoulder, lateral aspect arm	Dorsolateral aspect of thumb and index finger	Biceps, wrist extensors, pollicis longus	Brachioradialis reflex
C7 root	Neck, shoulder, lateral aspect arm, dorsal forearm	Index and middle finger, dorsum of hand	Triceps	Triceps reflex

disorders of the cervical spinal cord, roots, plexus, and nerves. MRI of the cervical spine should be carried out in all patients suspected of suffering from cervical radiculopathy. Screening laboratory testing consisting of complete blood count, erythrocyte sedimentation rate, antinuclear antibody testing, HLA-B27 antigen screening, and automated blood chemistry testing should be performed if the diagnosis of cervical radiculopathy is in question, to help rule out other causes of the patient's pain.

Treatment

Cervical radiculopathy is best treated with a multimodality approach. Physical therapy including heat modalities and deep sedative massage, combined with nonsteroidal anti-inflammatory agents and skeletal muscle relaxants,

represents a reasonable starting point. The addition of cervical steroid epidural nerve blocks is a reasonable next step. Cervical epidural blocks with local anesthetic and steroid have been shown to be extremely effective in the treatment of cervical radiculopathy. Underlying sleep disturbance and depression are best treated with a tricyclic antidepressant compound such as nortriptyline, which can be started at a single bedtime dose of 25 mg.

SUGGESTED READINGS

Campbell W: DeJong's The Neurological Examination, ed 6. Philadelphia, Lippincott Williams and Wilkins, 2005.
Goetz CG: Textbook of Clinical Neurology, ed 2. Philadelphia, Saunders, 2003.
Waldman SD: Cervical radiculopathy. In: Atlas of Common Pain Syndromes, ed 2. Philadelphia, Saunders, 2008.

CHAPTER 135

Cervical Strain

Acute cervical strain is a constellation of symptoms consisting of nonradicular neck pain that radiates in a nondermatomal pattern into the shoulders and intrascapular region. Headaches often accompany the symptoms of cervical strain. The trapezius is often affected with resultant spasm and limitation in range of motion of the cervical spine. Cervical strain is usually the result of trauma to the cervical spine and associated soft tissues but may occur without an obvious inciting incident. The pathologic lesions responsible for this clinical syndrome may emanate from the soft tissues, facet joints, and/or intervertebral discs.

Signs and Symptoms

Neck pain is the hallmark of cervical strain. It may begin in the occipital region and radiate in a nondermatomal pattern into the shoulders and intrascapular region. The pain of cervical strain is often exacerbated by movement of the cervical spine and shoulders. Headaches often occur along with the symptoms mentioned and may worsen with emotional stress. Sleep disturbance is common, as is difficulty in concentrating on simple tasks. Depression may occur with prolonged symptomatology.

On physical examination, there is tenderness on palpation and spasm of the paraspinous musculature, and trapezius is often present. Decreased range if motion is invariably present, with pain increasing with this maneuver. The neurologic examination of the upper extremities is within normal limits despite the frequent complaint of upper extremity pain.

Testing

There is no specific test for cervical strain. Testing is aimed primarily at identifying occult pathology or other diseases that may mimic cervical strain (see Differential Diagnosis). Plain radiographs will help delineate bony abnormality of the cervical spine, including arthritis, fracture, congenital abnormalities such as Arnold-Chiari malformation, and tumor. Straightening of the lordotic curve will frequently be noted. All patients with the recent onset of cervical strain should undergo magnetic resonance imaging (MRI) of the cervical spine and, if significant occipital or headache symptoms are present, MRI of the brain. Screening laboratory testing consisting of complete blood count, erythrocyte sedimentation rate, antinuclear antibody testing, and automated blood chemistry testing should be performed to rule out occult inflammatory arthritis, infection, or tumor.

Differential Diagnosis

Cervical strain is a clinical diagnosis that is supported by a combination of clinical history, physical examination, radiography, and MRI. Pain syndromes that may mimic cervical strain include cervical bursitis, cervical fibromyositis, inflammatory arthritis, and disorders of the cervical spinal cord, roots, plexus, and nerves. MRI of the cervical spine should be carried out in all patients suspected of suffering from cervical strain. Screening laboratory testing consisting of complete blood count, erythrocyte sedimentation rate, antinuclear antibody testing, HLA-B27 antigen screening, and automated blood chemistry testing should be performed if the diagnosis of cervical strain is in question, to help rule out other causes of the patient's pain.

Treatment

Cervical strain is best treated with a multimodality approach. Physical therapy including heat modalities and deep sedative massage, combined with nonsteroidal anti-inflammatory agents and skeletal muscle relaxants, represents a reasonable starting point. The addition of cervical epidural nerve blocks and occasionally cervical facet blocks is a reasonable next step. For symptomatic relief, cervical epidural block and/or blockade of the medial branch of the dorsal ramus or intra-articular injection of the facet joint with local anesthetic and steroid has been shown to be extremely effective in the treatment of cervical strain. Underlying sleep disturbance and depression are best treated with a tricyclic antidepressant compound such as nortriptyline, which can be started at a single bedtime dose of 25 mg.

SUGGESTED READING

Waldman SD: Cervical strain. In: Atlas of Common Pain Syndromes, ed 2. Philadelphia, Saunders, 2008.

CHAPTER 136

Cervicothoracic Interspinous Bursitis

Cervicothoracic interspinous bursitis is an uncommon cause of pain in the lower cervical and upper thoracic spine. The interspinous ligaments of the lower cervical and upper thoracic spine and their associated muscles are susceptible to the development of acute and chronic pain symptomatology following overuse. It is thought that bursitis is responsible for this pain syndrome. Frequently, the patient presents with midline pain after prolonged activity requiring hyperextension of the neck such as painting a ceiling or following the prolonged use of a computer monitor with too high a focal point. The pain is localized to the interspinous region between C7 and T1 and does not radiate. It is constant, dull, and aching in character. The patient may attempt to relieve the constant ache by assuming a posture of dorsal kyphosis with a thrusting forward of the neck. The pain of cervicothoracic interspinous bursitis often improves with activity and is made worse with rest and relaxation.

Signs and Symptoms

The patient suffering from cervicothoracic bursitis will present with the complaint of dull, poorly localized pain in the lower cervical and upper thoracic region. The pain spreads from the midline to the adjacent paraspinous area but is nonradicular in nature. The patient often holds the cervical spine rigid with the head thrust forward to splint the affected ligament and bursae. Flexion and extension of the lower cervical spine and upper thoracic spine tend to cause more pain than does rotation of the head.

The neurologic examination of patients suffering from cervicothoracic bursitis should be normal. Focal or radicular neurologic findings suggest a central or spinal cord origin of the patient's pain symptomatology and should be followed up with magnetic resonance imaging (MRI) of the appropriate anatomic regions.

MRI of the lower cervical and upper thoracic spine should be carried out in all patients thought to be suffering from cervicothoracic bursitis. Electromyography of the brachial plexus and upper extremities is indicated if there are neurologic findings or pain that radiates into the arms. Clinical laboratory testing consisting of a complete blood cell count, automated chemistry profile, antinuclear antibody testing, and erythrocyte sedimentation rate are indicated to rule out infection, collagen vascular disease including ankylosing spondylitis, and malignancy that may mimic the clinical presentation of cervicothoracic bursitis. Injection of the affected interspinous bursae with local anesthetic and steroid may serve as both a diagnostic and therapeutic maneuver and may help strengthen the diagnosis of cervicothoracic bursitis. Plain radiography of the sacroiliac joints is indicated if ankylosing spondylitis is being considered in the differential diagnosis.

Differential Diagnosis

The diagnosis of cervicothoracic bursitis is usually made on clinical grounds as a diagnosis of exclusion. The clinician needs to rule intrinsic disease of the spinal cord, including syringomyelia and tumor, which may mimic the clinical presentation of cervicothoracic bursitis. Ankylosing spondylitis may also manifest in a manner similar to that of cervicothoracic bursitis. Fibromyalgia may coexist with cervicothoracic bursitis and should be identifiable by its characteristic trigger points and positive jump sign.

Treatment

Initial treatment of the pain and functional disability associated with cervicothoracic bursitis should include a combination of the nonsteroidal anti-inflammatory agents or cyclooxygenase-2 inhibitors and physical therapy. The local application of heat and cold may also be beneficial. For patients who do not respond to these treatment modalities, injection of the cervicothoracic bursae may be a reasonable next step. A series of two to five treatment sessions may be required to completely abolish the symptoms of cervicothoracic bursitis.

SUGGESTED READING

Waldman SD: Cervicothoracic bursitis. In: Atlas of Uncommon Pain Syndromes, ed 2. Philadelphia, Saunders, 2008.

CHAPTER 137

Fibromyalgia of the Cervical Musculature

Fibromyalgia of the cervical spine is one of the most common painful conditions encountered in clinical practice. Fibromyalgia is a chronic pain syndrome that affects a focal or regional portion of the body. The sine qua non of fibromyalgia of the cervical spine is the finding of myofascial trigger points on physical examination. Although these trigger points are generally localized to the cervical paraspinous musculature, trapezius, and other muscles of the neck, the pain of fibromyalgia of the cervical spine is often referred to other areas. This referred pain is often misdiagnosed or attributed to other organ systems, leading to extensive evaluations and ineffective treatment.

The trigger point is the pathognomonic lesion of fibromyalgia pain and is thought to be the result of microtrauma to the affected muscles. Stimulation of the myofascial trigger point will reproduce or exacerbate the patient's pain. Often, stiffness and fatigue will coexist with the pain of fibromyalgia of the cervical spine, increasing the functional disability associated with this disease and complicating its treatment. Fibromyalgia of the cervical spine may occur as a primary disease state or may occur in conjunction with other painful conditions, including radiculopathy and chronic regional pain syndromes. Psychological or behavioral abnormalities including depression frequently coexist with the muscle abnormalities associated with fibromyalgia of the cervical spine. Treatment of these psychological and behavioral abnormalities must be an integral part of any successful treatment plan for fibromyalgia of the cervical spine.

Although the exact cause of fibromyalgia of the cervical spine remains unknown, tissue trauma seems to be the common denominator. Acute trauma to muscle as a result of overstretching will commonly result in the development of fibromyalgia of the cervical spine. More subtle injury to muscle in the form of repetitive microtrauma can also result in the development of fibromyalgia of the cervical spine, as can damage to muscle fibers from exposure to extreme heat or cold. Extreme overuse or other coexistent disease processes such as radiculopathy may also result in the development of fibromyalgia of the cervical spine.

In addition to tissue trauma, a variety of other factors seem to predispose the patient to develop fibromyalgia of the cervical spine. The weekend athlete who subjects his or her body to unaccustomed physical activity may often develop fibromyalgia of the cervical spine. Poor posture while sitting at a computer keyboard or while watching television has also been implicated as a predisposing factor to the development of fibromyalgia of the cervical spine. Previous injuries may result in abnormal muscle function and predispose to the subsequent development of fibromyalgia of the cervical spine. All of these predisposing factors may be intensified if the patient also suffers from poor nutritional status or coexisting psychological or behavioral abnormalities, including depression.

Signs and Symptoms

The sine qua non of fibromyalgia of the cervical spine is the identification of myofascial trigger points. The trigger point is the pathologic lesion of fibromyalgia of the cervical spine and is characterized by a local point of exquisite tenderness in affected muscle. Mechanical stimulation of the trigger point by palpation or stretching will produce not only intense local pain but referred pain as well. In addition to this local and referred pain, there will often be an involuntary withdrawal of the stimulated muscle that is called a *jump sign*. This jump sign is also characteristic of fibromyalgia of the cervical spine, as is stiffness of the neck, pain of range of motion of the cervical spine, and pain referred into the upper extremities in a nondermatomal pattern.

Although the patterns of referred pain have been well studied and occur in a characteristic pattern, this referred pain is often misdiagnosed and attributed to diseases of organ systems in the distribution of the referred pain. This often leads to extensive evaluation and ineffective treatments. Taut bands of muscle fibers are often identified when myofascial trigger points are palpated. Despite this consistent physical finding in patients suffering from fibromyalgia of the cervical spine, the pathophysiology of the myofascial trigger point remains elusive, although many theories have been advanced. Common to all of these theories is the belief that trigger points are the result of microtrauma to the affected muscle.

This microtrauma may occur as a single injury to the affected muscle or may occur as the result of repetitive microtrauma or as the result of chronic deconditioning of the agonist and antagonist muscle unit.

Testing

The exact pathophysiologic processes responsible for the development of fibromyalgia of the cervical spine remain elusive. Biopsy specimens of clinically identified trigger points have not revealed consistently abnormal histology. The muscle hosting the trigger points has been alternatively described as "moth eaten" or as containing "waxy degeneration." Increased plasma myoglobin has been reported in some patients with fibromyalgia of the cervical spine, but this finding has not been reproduced by other investigators. Electrodiagnostic testing of patients suffering from fibromyalgia of the cervical spine has revealed an increase in muscle tension in some patients. Again, this finding has not been reproducible. However, regardless of the pathophysiology of fibromyalgia of the cervical spine, there is little doubt that the clinical findings of trigger points in the cervical paraspinous muscles and associated jump sign exist in combination with a clinically recognizable constellation of symptoms that are consistently diagnosed as fibromyalgia of the cervical spine by clinicians.

The diagnosis of fibromyalgia of the cervical spine is made on the basis of clinical findings rather than specific diagnostic laboratory, electrodiagnostic, or radiographic testing. For this reason, a targeted history and physical examination with a systematic search for trigger points and identification of a positive jump sign must be carried out on every patient suspected of suffering from fibromyalgia of the cervical spine. Because of the lack of objective diagnostic testing, the clinician must also rule out other coexisting disease processes that may mimic fibromyalgia of the cervical spine, including primary inflammatory muscle disease and collagen vascular disease. The judicious use of electrodiagnostic and radiographic testing will also help identify coexisting pathology such as herniated nucleus pulposus and rotator cuff tears. The clinician must also identify coexisting psychological and behavioral abnormalities that may mask or exacerbate the symptoms associated with fibromyalgia of the cervical spine and other coexisting pathologic processes.

Differential Diagnosis

The diagnosis of fibromyalgia of the cervical spine is made on the basis of clinical findings rather than specific diagnostic laboratory, electrodiagnostic, or radiographic testing. For this reason, a targeted history and physical examination with a systematic search for trigger points and identification of a positive jump sign must be carried out on every patient suspected of suffering from fibromyalgia of the cervical spine. Because of the lack of objective diagnostic testing, the clinician must also rule out other coexisting disease processes that may mimic fibromyalgia of the cervical spine, including primary inflammatory muscle disease, multiple sclerosis, and collagen vascular disease. The judicious use of electrodiagnostic and radiographic testing will also help identify coexisting pathology such as herniated nucleus pulposus and rotator cuff tears. The clinician must also identify coexisting psychological and behavioral abnormalities that may mask or exacerbate the symptoms associated with fibromyalgia of the cervical spine and other coexisting pathologic processes.

Treatment

The treatment of fibromyalgia of the cervical spine involves the use of techniques that will help eliminate the trigger point that may serve as the source of the perpetuation of this painful condition. It is hoped that the interruption of the pain cycle by the elimination of trigger points will allow the patient to experience prolonged relief. The mechanism of action of each of the modalities mentioned is poorly understood, and thus an element of trial and error in developing a treatment plan is the expected norm.

Because underlying depression and a substrate of anxiety are present in many patients suffering from fibromyalgia of the cervical spine, the inclusion of antidepressant compounds as an integral part of most treatment plans represents a reasonable choice.

In addition to the treatment modalities mentioned, a variety of additional treatments are available for the treatment of fibromyalgia of the cervical spine. The therapeutic use of heat and cold is often combined with trigger point injections and antidepressant compounds to effect pain relief. Some patients will experience decreased pain with the use of transcutaneous nerve stimulation or the use of electrical stimulation to fatigue-affected muscles. Although not currently approved by the Food and Drug Administration, the injection of minute quantities of botulinum toxin A directly into trigger points has recently gained favor in the treatment of persistent fibromyalgia of the cervical spine that has not responded to traditional treatment modalities.

SUGGESTED READING

Waldman SD: Fibromyalgia of the cervical musculature. In: Atlas of Common Pain Syndromes, ed 2. Philadelphia, Saunders, 2008.

CHAPTER 138

Cervical Facet Syndrome

Cervical facet syndrome is a constellation of symptoms consisting of neck, head, shoulder, and proximal upper extremity pain that radiates in a nondermatomal pattern. The pain is dull and ill defined in character. It may be unilateral or bilateral and is thought to be the result of pathology of the facet joint. The pain of cervical facet syndrome is exacerbated by flexion, extension, and lateral bending of the cervical spine. It is often worse in the morning after physical activity. Each facet joint receives innervation from two spinal levels. Each joint receives fibers from the dorsal ramus at the same level as the vertebra as well as fibers from the dorsal ramus of the vertebra above (Fig. 138-1). This fact has clinical import in that it provides an explanation for the ill-defined nature of facet-mediated pain and also explains why the dorsal nerve from the vertebra above the offending level often must also be blocked to provide complete pain relief.

Signs and Symptoms

Most patients with cervical facet syndrome have tenderness to deep palpation of the cervical paraspinous musculature. Spasm of these muscles may also be present. The patient will exhibit decreased range of motion of the cervical spine and will usually complain of pain on flexion, extension, rotation, and lateral bending of the cervical spine. There will be no motor or sensory deficit unless there is coexisting radiculopathy, plexopathy, or entrapment neuropathy.

If the C1-2 facet joints are involved, the pain will be referred to the posterior auricular and occipital region. If the C2-3 facet joints are involved, the pain may radiate to the nuchal ridge as well as the forehead and eyes (Fig. 138-2). Pain emanating from the C3-4 facet joints will be referred superiorly to the suboccipital region and inferiorly to the posterolateral neck, with pain from the C4-5 facet joints radiating to the base of the neck. Pain from the C5-6 joints produces pain that is referred to the shoulders and intrascapular region, with pain from the C6-7 facet joints radiating to the supraspinous and infraspinous fossa.

Testing

As patients enter the fifth decade, almost all of them will exhibit some degree of abnormality of the facet joints of the cervical spine on plain radiographs (see Fig. 138-2). The clinical import of the findings has long been debated by pain specialists but it was not until the advent of computed tomography (CT) scanning and magnetic resonance imaging (MRI) that the relationship of these abnormal facet joints to the cervical nerve roots and other surrounding anatomic structures was clearly understood. However, any data gleaned from these sophisticated imaging techniques can provide only a presumptive diagnosis to guide the clinician. To prove that in fact a specific facet joint is contributing to the patient's pain, a diagnostic intra-articular injection of that joint with local anesthetic is required.

Differential Diagnosis

Cervical facet syndrome is a diagnosis of exclusion that is supported by a combination of clinical history, physical examination, radiography, and MRI and by intra-articular injection of the suspect facet joints. Pain syndromes that may mimic cervical facet syndrome include cervicalgia, cervical bursitis, cervical fibromyositis, inflammatory arthritis, and disorders of the cervical spinal cord, roots, plexus, and nerves. MRI of the cervical spine should be carried out on all patients suspected of suffering from cervical facet syndrome. Screening laboratory testing consisting of complete blood count, erythrocyte sedimentation rate, antinuclear antibody testing, HLA-B27 antigen screening, and automated blood chemistry testing should be performed if the diagnosis of cervical facet syndrome is in question, to help rule out other causes of the patient's pain.

Treatment

Cervical facet syndrome is best treated with a multimodality approach. Physical therapy including heat modalities and deep sedative massage, combined with nonsteroidal anti-inflammatory agents and skeletal muscle relaxants, represents a reasonable starting point. The addition of cervical facet blocks is a reasonable next step. For symptomatic relief, blockade of the medial branch of the dorsal ramus or intra-articular injection of the facet joint with local anesthetic and steroid has been shown to be extremely effective in the treatment of cervical facet syndrome. Underlying sleep disturbance and depression are best treated with a tricyclic antidepressant compound such as nortriptyline, which can be started at a single bedtime dose of 25 mg.

SUGGESTED READING

Waldman SD: Cervical facet syndrome. In: Atlas of Common Pain Syndromes, ed 2. Philadelphia, Saunders, 2008.

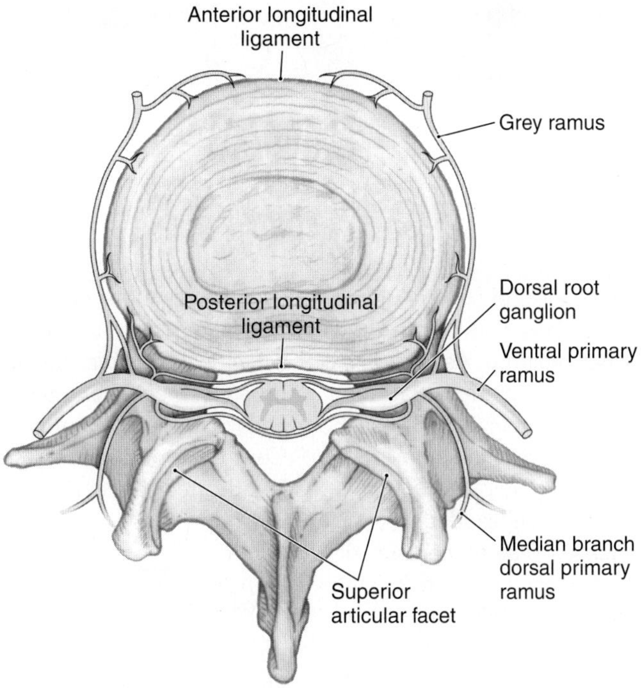

Anterior longitudinal
ligament

Grey ramus

Posterior longitudinal
ligament

Dorsal root
ganglion

Ventral primary
ramus

Median branch
dorsal primary
ramus

Superior
articular facet

FIGURE 138–1 Innervation of the facet joint.

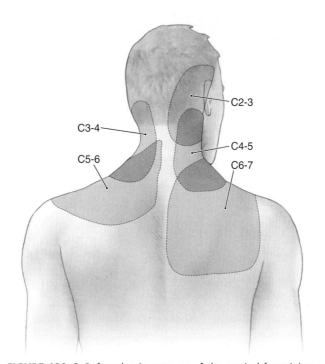

C2-3

C3-4

C4-5

C5-6

C6-7

FIGURE 138–2 Referred pain patterns of the cervical facet joints.

CHAPTER 139

Intercostal Neuralgia

In contradistinction to most other causes of pain involving the chest wall, which are musculoskeletal in nature, the pain of intercostal neuralgia is neuropathic. As with costosternal joint pain, and rib fractures, a significant number of patients who suffer from intercostal neuralgia first seek medical attention because they believe they are suffering a heart attack. If the subcostal nerve is involved, patients may believe they are suffering from gallbladder disease. The pain of intercostal neuralgia is due to damage or inflammation of the intercostal nerves. The pain is constant and burning in nature and may involve any of the intercostal nerves as well as the subcostal nerve of the twelfth rib. The pain usually begins at the posterior axillary line and radiates anteriorly into the distribution of the affected intercostal and/or subcostal nerves.

Deep inspiration or movement of the chest wall may slightly increase the pain of intercostal neuralgia, but to a much lesser extent compared with the pain associated with the musculoskeletal causes of chest wall pain such as costosternal joint pain, Tietze's syndrome, or broken ribs.

Signs and Symptoms

Physical examination of the patient suffering from intercostal neuralgia will generally reveal minimal physical findings unless there was a history of previous thoracic or subcostal surgery or cutaneous findings of herpes zoster involving the thoracic dermatomes. In contradistinction to the above-mentioned musculoskeletal causes of chest wall and subcostal pain, the patient suffering from intercostal neuralgia does not attempt to splint or protect the affected area. Careful sensory examination of the affected dermatomes may reveal decreased sensation or allodynia. With significant motor involvement of the subcostal nerve, the patient may complain that his or her abdomen bulges out.

Testing

Plain radiographs are indicated in all patients who present with pain thought to be emanating from the intercostal nerve to rule out occult bony pathology, including tumor. If trauma is present, radionuclide bone scanning may be useful to rule out occult fractures of the ribs and/or sternum. Based on the patient's clinical presentation, additional testing including complete blood count, prostate-specific antigen, erythrocyte sedimentation rate, and antinuclear antibody testing may be indicated. Computed tomographic scanning of the thoracic contents is indicated if occult mass is suspected.

Differential Diagnosis

As mentioned, the pain of intercostal neuralgia is often mistaken for pain of cardiac or gallbladder origin and can lead to visits to the emergency department and unnecessary cardiac and gastrointestinal workups. If trauma has occurred, intercostal neuralgia may coexist with fractured ribs or fractures of the sternum itself, which can be missed on plain radiographs and may require radionuclide bone scanning for proper identification. Tietze's syndrome, which is painful enlargement of the upper costochondral cartilage associated with viral infections, can be confused with intercostal neuralgia.

Neuropathic pain involving the chest wall may also be confused or coexist with costosternal syndrome. Examples of such neuropathic pain include diabetic polyneuropathies and acute herpes zoster involving the thoracic nerves. The possibility of diseases of the structures of the mediastinum remains ever present and at times can be difficult to diagnose. Pathologic processes such as pulmonary embolism, infection, and Bornholm disease can be responsible for the inflammation of the pleura.

Treatment

Initial treatment of intercostal neuralgia should include a combination of simple analgesics and the nonsteroidal anti-inflammatory agents or the cyclooxygenase-2 inhibitors. If these medications do not adequately control the patient's symptomatology, a tricyclic antidepressant or gabapentin should be added.

Traditionally, the tricyclic antidepressants have been a mainstay in the palliation of pain secondary to intercostal neuralgia. Controlled studies have demonstrated the efficacy of amitriptyline for this indication. Other tricyclic antidepressants including nortriptyline and desipramine have also been shown to be clinically useful. Unfortunately, this class of drugs is associated with significant anticholinergic side effects, including dry mouth, constipation, sedation, and urinary retention. These drugs should be used with caution in those suffering from glaucoma, cardiac arrhythmia, and prostatism. In order to minimize side effects and encourage compliance, the primary care physician should start amitriptyline or nortriptyline at a 10-mg dose at bedtime. The dose can be then titrated upward to 25 mg at bedtime as side effects allow. Upward titration of dosage in 25-mg increments can be carried out each week as side effects allow. Even at lower doses, patients will generally report a rapid improvement in sleep disturbance and will begin to experience some pain relief in 10 to 14 days. If the patient does not experience any improvement in pain as the dose is being titrated upward, the addition of gabapentin alone or in combination with nerve blocks with local anesthetics and/or steroid is recommended (see later). The selective serotonin reuptake inhibitors such as fluoxetine have also been used to treat the pain of intercostal neuralgia and, although better tolerated than the tricyclic antidepressants, they appear to be less efficacious.

If the antidepressant compounds are ineffective or contraindicated, gabapentin represents a reasonable alternative.

Gabapentin should be started with a 300-mg dose redundant at bedtime for 2 nights. The patient should be cautioned about potential side effects, including dizziness, sedation, confusion, and rash. The drug is then increased in 300-mg increments, given in equally divided doses over 2 days as side effects allow, until pain relief is obtained or a total dose of 2400 mg daily is reached. At this point, if the patient has experienced partial relief of pain, blood values are measured and the drug is carefully titrated upward using 100-mg tablets. Rarely will more than 3600 mg daily be required.

The local application of heat and cold may also be beneficial to provide symptomatic relief of the pain of intercostal neuralgia. The use of an elastic rib belt may also help provide symptomatic relief. For patients who do not respond to these treatment modalities, intercostal nerve block using local anesthetic and steroid may be a reasonable next step.

SUGGESTED READING

Waldman SD: Intercostal neuralgia. In: Atlas of Common Pain Syndromes, ed 2. Philadelphia, Saunders, 2008.

CHAPTER 140

Thoracic Radiculopathy

Thoracic radiculopathy is a common source of chest wall and upper abdominal pain that emanates from the thoracic nerve roots. In addition to the dorsal spine pain, which radiates in a thoracic dermatomal distribution, the patient with thoracic radiculopathy may experience associated paresthesias, numbness, weakness, and, rarely, loss of superficial abdominal reflexes. The causes of thoracic radiculopathy include herniated disc, foraminal stenosis, tumor, osteophyte formation, vertebral compression fractures, and, rarely, infection.

Signs and Symptoms

The patient suffering from thoracic radiculopathy will complain of pain, numbness, tingling, and paresthesias in the distribution of the affected nerve root or roots.

Muscle spasms of the paraspinous musculature are also common. Decreased sensation, weakness, and, rarely, superficial abdominal reflex changes are demonstrated on physical examination. Patients with thoracic radiculopathy will commonly experience a reflex shifting of the trunk to one side. This reflex shifting is called *list*. Occasionally, a patient suffering from thoracic radiculopathy will also experience compression of the thoracic spinal nerve roots resulting in myelopathy. Thoracic myelopathy is most commonly due to midline herniated thoracic disc, spinal stenosis, demyelinating disease, tumor, or, rarely, infection. Patients suffering from thoracic myelopathy will experience varying degrees of neurologic disturbance based on the level and extent of cord compression. Significant compression of the thoracic spinal cord will result in a Brown-Séquard syndrome, with spastic paralysis of the ipsilateral muscles below the lesion and loss of sensation on the contralateral side. Thoracic myelopathy represents a neurosurgical emergency and should be treated as such.

Testing

Magnetic resonance imaging (MRI) of the thoracic spine will provide the clinician with the best information regarding the thoracic spine and its contents. MRI is highly accurate and will help identify abnormalities that may put the patient at risk for the development of thoracic myelopathy. In patients who cannot undergo MRI (e.g., patients with a pacemaker), computed tomography (CT) or myelography followed by CT of the affected area is a reasonable second choice. Radionuclide bone scanning and plain radiographs are indicated if fracture or bony abnormality such as metastatic disease is being considered.

Although this testing provides the clinician with useful neuroanatomic information, electromyography and nerve conduction velocity testing will provide the clinician with neurophysiologic information that can delineate the actual status of each individual nerve root and the thoracic plexus. Screening laboratory testing consisting of complete blood count, erythrocyte sedimentation rate, and automated blood chemistry testing should be performed if the diagnosis of thoracic radiculopathy is in question.

Differential Diagnosis

Thoracic radiculopathy is a clinical diagnosis that is supported by a combination of clinical history, physical examination, radiography, and MRI. Pain syndromes that may mimic thoracic radiculopathy include dorsal spine strain, thoracic bursitis, thoracic fibromyositis, inflammatory arthritis, mononeuritis multiplex, infectious lesions such as epidural abscess, and disorders of the thoracic spinal cord, roots, plexus, and nerves. MRI of the thoracic spine should be carried out on all patients suspected of suffering from thoracic radiculopathy. Screening laboratory testing consisting of complete blood count, erythrocyte sedimentation rate, antinuclear antibody testing, HLA-B27 antigen screening, and automated blood chemistry testing should be performed if the diagnosis of thoracic radiculopathy is in question to help rule out other causes of the patient's pain.

Treatment

Thoracic radiculopathy is best treated with a multimodality approach. Physical therapy including heat modalities and deep sedative massage, combined with nonsteroidal anti-inflammatory agents and skeletal muscle relaxants, represents a reasonable starting point. The addition of thoracic steroid epidural nerve blocks is a reasonable next step. Thoracic epidural blocks with local anesthetic and steroid have been shown to be extremely effective in the treatment of thoracic radiculopathy. Underlying sleep disturbance and depression are best treated with a tricyclic antidepressant compound such as nortriptyline, which can be started at a single bedtime dose of 25 mg.

SUGGESTED READING

Waldman SD: Thoracic radiculopathy. In: Pain Management. Philadelphia, Saunders, 2007.

CHAPTER 141

Costosternal Syndrome

A significant number of patients who suffer from noncardiogenic chest pain suffer from costosternal joint pain. Most commonly, the costosternal joints become a source of pain due to inflammation as a result of overuse or misuse or due to trauma secondary to acceleration/deceleration injuries or blunt trauma to the chest wall. With severe trauma, the joints may sublux or dislocate.

The costosternal joints are also susceptible to the development of arthritis, including osteoarthritis, rheumatoid arthritis, ankylosing spondylitis, Reiter's syndrome, and psoriatic arthritis. In addition, the joints are subject to invasion by tumor either from primary malignancies, including thymoma, or from metastatic disease.

Signs and Symptoms

Physical examination of the patient suffering from costosternal syndrome will reveal that the patient will vigorously attempt to splint the joints by keeping the shoulders stiffly in neutral position. Pain is reproduced with active protraction or retraction of the shoulder, deep inspiration, and full elevation of the arm. Shrugging of the shoulder may also reproduce the pain. Coughing may be difficult, and this may lead to inadequate pulmonary toilet in patients who have sustained trauma to the anterior chest wall. The costosternal joints and adjacent intercostal muscles may also be tender to palpation. The patient may also complain of a clicking sensation with movement of the joint.

Testing

Plain radiographs are indicated in all patients who present with pain thought to be emanating from the costosternal joints to rule out occult bony pathology, including tumor. If trauma is present, radionuclide bone scanning may be useful to rule out occult fractures of the ribs and/or sternum. Based on the patient's clinical presentation, additional testing including complete blood count, prostate-specific antigen, erythrocyte sedimentation rate, and antinuclear antibody testing may be indicated. Magnetic resonance imaging of the joints is indicated if joint instability or occult mass is suspected.

Differential Diagnosis

As mentioned, the pain of costosternal syndrome is often mistaken for pain of cardiac origin and can lead to visits to the emergency department and unnecessary cardiac workups. If trauma has occurred, costosternal syndrome may coexist with fractured ribs or fractures of the sternum itself, which can be missed on plain radiographs and may require radionuclide bone scanning for proper identification. Tietze's syndrome, which is painful enlargement of the upper costochondral cartilage associated with viral infections, can be confused with costosternal syndrome.

Neuropathic pain involving the chest wall may also be confused or coexist with costosternal syndrome. Examples of such neuropathic pain include diabetic polyneuropathies and acute herpes zoster involving the thoracic nerves. The possibility of diseases of the structures of the mediastinum remains ever present and at times can be difficult to diagnose. Pathologic processes such as pulmonary embolus, infection, and Bornholm disease can inflame the pleura.

Treatment

Initial treatment of the pain and functional disability associated with costosternal syndrome should include a combination of the nonsteroidal anti-inflammatory agents or the cyclooxygenase-2 inhibitors. The local application of heat and cold may also be beneficial. The use of an elastic rib belt may also help provide symptomatic relief and help protect the costosternal joints from additional trauma. For patients who do not respond to these treatment modalities, injection of the costosternal joints may be a reasonable next step.

SUGGESTED READING

Waldman SD: Costosternal syndrome. In: Atlas of Common Pain Syndromes, ed 2. Philadelphia, Saunders, 2008.

CHAPTER 142

Manubriosternal Joint Syndrome

The manubriosternal joint can serve as a source of pain that often mimics the pain of cardiac origin. The manubrium articulates with the body of the sternum via the manubriosternal joint. The joint articulates at an angle called the angle of Louis, which allows for easy identification. The joint is a fibrocartilaginous joint, or synchondrosis, that lacks a true joint cavity. The manubriosternal joint allows protraction and retraction of the thorax. Above, the manubrium articulates with the sternal end of the clavicle and the cartilage of the first rib. Below, the body of the sternum articulates with the xiphoid process. Posterior to the manubriosternal joint are the structures of the mediastinum.

The manubriosternal joint is susceptible to the development of arthritis, including osteoarthritis, rheumatoid arthritis, ankylosing spondylitis, Reiter's syndrome, and psoriatic arthritis. The joint is often traumatized during acceleration/deceleration injuries and blunt trauma to the chest. With severe trauma, the joint may sublux or dislocate. Overuse or misuse can also result in acute inflammation of the manubriosternal joint, which can be quite debilitating for the patient. The joint is also subject to invasion by tumor from primary malignancies, including thymoma, or metastatic disease.

Signs and Symptoms

Physical examination will reveal that the patient will vigorously attempt to splint the joint by keeping the shoulders stiffly in neutral position. Pain is reproduced by active protraction or retraction of the shoulder, deep inspiration, and full elevation of the arm. Shrugging of the shoulder may also reproduce the pain. The manubriosternal joint may be tender to palpation and feel hot and swollen if acutely inflamed. The patient may also complain of a clicking sensation with movement of the joint.

Testing

Plain radiographs are indicated in all patients who present with pain thought to be emanating from the manubriosternal joint to rule out occult bony pathology, including tumor. Based on the patient's clinical presentation, additional testing including complete blood count, prostate-specific antigen, erythrocyte sedimentation rate, and antinuclear antibody testing may be indicated. Magnetic resonance imaging of the joint is indicated if joint instability is suspected. Injection of the manubriosternal joint with local anesthetic will serve as both a diagnostic and therapeutic maneuver.

Differential Diagnosis

As mentioned, the pain of manubriosternal joint syndrome is often mistaken for pain of cardiac origin and can lead to visits to the emergency department and unnecessary cardiac workups. If trauma has occurred, costosternal syndrome may coexist with fractured ribs or fractures of the sternum itself, which can be missed on plain radiographs and may require radionuclide bone scanning for proper identification. Tietze's syndrome, which is painful enlargement of the upper costochondral cartilage associated with viral infections, can be confused with costosternal syndrome.

Neuropathic pain involving the chest wall may also be confused or coexist with manubriosternal joint syndrome. Examples of such neuropathic pain include diabetic polyneuropathies and acute herpes zoster involving the thoracic nerves. The possibility of diseases of the structures of the mediastinum remains ever present and at times can be difficult to diagnose. Pathologic processes such as pulmonary embolus, infection, and Bornholm disease can inflame the pleura.

Treatment

Initial treatment of the pain and functional disability associated with manubriosternal joint syndrome should include a combination of the nonsteroidal anti-inflammatory agents or the cyclooxygenase-2 inhibitors. The local application of heat and cold may also be beneficial. The use of an elastic rib belt may also help provide symptomatic relief and help protect the manubriosternal joints from additional trauma. For patients who do not respond to these treatment modalities, injection of manubriosternal joints may be a reasonable next step.

Patients suffering from pain emanating from the manubriosternal joint will often attribute their pain symptomatology to a heart attack. Reassurance is required, although it should be remembered that this musculoskeletal pain syndrome and coronary artery disease can coexist. Care must be taken to use sterile technique to avoid infection as well as the use of universal precautions to avoid risk to the operator. The incidence of ecchymosis and hematoma formation can be decreased if pressure is placed on the injection site immediately following injection. The use of physical modalities including local heat and gentle range of motion exercises should be introduced several days after the patient undergoes this injection technique for manubriosternal joint pain. Vigorous exercises should be avoided as they will exacerbate the patient's symptomatology. Simple analgesics and nonsteroidal anti-inflammatory agents may be used concurrently with this injection technique. Laboratory evaluation for collagen vascular disease is indicated in patients suffering from manubriosternal joint pain in whom other joints are involved.

SUGGESTED READING

Waldman SD: Manubriosternal joint syndrome. In: Atlas of Common Pain Syndromes, ed 2. Philadelphia, Saunders, 2008.

Thoracic Vertebral Compression Fracture

Thoracic vertebral compression fracture is one of the most common causes of dorsal spine pain. Vertebral compression fracture is most commonly the result of osteoporosis of the dorsal spine. It is also associated with trauma to the dorsal spine due to acceleration/deceleration injuries. In osteoporotic patients or in patients with primary tumors or metastatic disease involving the thoracic vertebra, the fracture may occur with coughing (tussive fractures) or spontaneously.

The pain and functional disability associated with fractures of the vertebra are determined in large part by the severity of injury (e.g., the number of vertebra involved) and the nature of the injury (e.g., whether the fracture allows impingement on the spinal nerves or the spinal cord itself). The severity of pain associated with thoracic vertebral compression fracture may range from a dull, deep ache with minimal compression of the vertebra without nerve impingement to severe sharp, stabbing pain that limits the patient's ability to ambulate and cough.

Signs and Symptoms

Compression fractures of the thoracic vertebrae are aggravated by deep inspiration, coughing, and any movement of the dorsal spine. Palpation of the affected vertebra may elicit pain and reflex spasm of the paraspinous musculature of the dorsal spine. If trauma has occurred, hematoma and ecchymosis overlying the fracture site may be present. If trauma has occurred, the clinician should be aware of the possibility of damage to the bony thorax and the intra-abdominal and intrathoracic contents. Damage to the spinal nerves may produce abdominal ileus and severe pain with resulting splinting of the paraspinous muscles of the dorsal spine, further compromising the patient's ability to walk and his or her pulmonary status. Failure to aggressively treat this pain and splinting may result in a negative cycle of hypoventilation, atelectasis, and ultimately pneumonia.

Testing

Plain radiographs of the vertebra are indicated in all patients who present with pain from thoracic vertebral compression fracture to rule out other occult fractures and other bony pathology, including tumor. If trauma is present, radionuclide bone scanning may be useful to rule out occult fractures of the vertebra and/or sternum. If no trauma is present, bone density testing to rule out osteoporosis is appropriate, as are serum protein electrophoresis and testing for hyperparathyroidism. Based on the patient's clinical presentation, additional testing including complete blood count, prostate-specific antigen, erythrocyte sedimentation rate, and antinuclear antibody testing may be indicated. Computed tomography scan of the thoracic contents is indicated if occult mass or significant trauma to the thoracic contents is suspected. Electrocardiogram to rule out cardiac contusion is indicated in all patients with traumatic sternal fractures or significant anterior dorsal spine trauma.

Differential Diagnosis

In the setting of trauma, the diagnosis of thoracic vertebral compression fracture is usually easily made. It is in the setting of spontaneous vertebral fracture secondary to osteoporosis or metastatic disease that the diagnosis may be confusing. In this setting, the pain of occult rib fracture is often mistaken for pain of cardiac or gallbladder origin and can lead to visits to the emergency department and unnecessary cardiac and gastrointestinal workups. Acute sprain of the thoracic paraspinous muscles can be confused with thoracic vertebral compression fracture, especially if the patient has been coughing. Because the pain of acute herpes zoster may precede the rash by 24 to 72 hours, the pain may be erroneously attributed to vertebral compression fracture.

Treatment

Initial treatment of pain secondary to compression fracture of the thoracic spine should include a combination of simple analgesics and the nonsteroidal anti-inflammatory agents or the cyclooxygenase-2 inhibitors. If these medications do not adequately control the patient's symptomatology, short-acting potent opioid analgesics such as hydrocodone represent a reasonable next step. As the opioid analgesics have the potential to suppress the cough reflex and respiration, the clinician must be careful to monitor the patient closely and to instruct the patient in adequate pulmonary toilet techniques.

The local application of heat and cold may also be beneficial to provide symptomatic relief of the pain of vertebral fracture. The use of an orthotic (e.g., the Cash brace) may also help provide symptomatic relief. For patients who do not respond to these treatment modalities, thoracic epidural block with local anesthetic and steroid is a reasonable next step.

SUGGESTED READING

Waldman SD: Thoracic vertebral compression fracture. In: Atlas of Common Pain Syndromes, ed 2. Philadelphia, Saunders, 2008.

CHAPTER 144

Lumbar Radiculopathy

Lumbar radiculopathy is a constellation of symptoms consisting of neurogenic back and lower extremity pain emanating from the lumbar nerve roots. In addition to the pain, the patient with lumbar radiculopathy may experience associated numbness, weakness, and loss of reflexes. The causes of lumbar radiculopathy include herniated disc, foraminal stenosis, tumor, osteophyte formation, and, rarely, infection. Many patients and their physicians will use the term *sciatica* to refer to the constellation of symptoms known as lumbar radiculopathy.

experience a reflex shifting of the trunk to one side. This reflex shifting is called a *list*. Occasionally, a patient suffering from lumbar radiculopathy will experience compression of the lumbar spinal nerve roots and cauda equina, resulting in myelopathy or cauda equina syndrome. Lumbar myelopathy is most commonly due to midline herniated lumbar disc, spinal stenosis, tumor, or, rarely, infection. Patients suffering from lumbar myelopathy or cauda equina syndrome will experience varying degrees of lower extremity weakness and bowel and bladder symptomatology. This represents a neurosurgical emergency and should be treated as such.

Signs and Symptoms

The patient suffering from lumbar radiculopathy will complain of pain, numbness, tingling, and paresthesias in the distribution of the affected nerve root or roots (Table 144-1). Patients may also note weakness and lack of coordination in the affected extremity. Muscle spasms and back pain, as well as pain referred into the buttocks, are common. Decreased sensation, weakness, and reflex changes are demonstrated on physical examination. Patients with lumbar radiculopathy will commonly

Testing

Magnetic resonance imaging (MRI) of the lumbar spine will provide the clinician with the best information regarding the lumbar spine and its contents. MRI is highly accurate and will help identify abnormalities that may put the patient at risk for the development of lumbar myelopathy. In patients who cannot undergo MRI (e.g., patients with a pacemaker), computed tomography or myelography is a reasonable second choice.

TABLE 144–1 Clinical Features of Lumbar Radiculopathy

Lumbar Root	Pain	Sensory Changes	Weakness	Reflex Changes
L4 root	Back, shin, thigh, leg	Shin numbness	Ankle dorsiflexors	Knee jerk
L5 root	Back, posterior thigh, leg	Numbness top of foot and first web space	Extensor hallucis longus	None
S1 root	Back, posterior calf, leg	Numbness lateral foot	Gastrocnemius and soleus	Ankle jerk

Radionuclide bone scanning and plain radiographs are indicated if fracture or bony abnormality such as metastatic disease is being considered.

Although this testing provides the clinician with useful neuroanatomic information, electromyography and nerve conduction velocity testing will provide the clinician with neurophysiologic information that can delineate the actual status of each individual nerve root and the lumbar plexus. Screening laboratory testing consisting of complete blood count, erythrocyte sedimentation rate, and automated blood chemistry testing should be performed if the diagnosis of lumbar radiculopathy is in question.

Differential Diagnosis

Lumbar radiculopathy is a clinical diagnosis that is supported by a combination of clinical history, physical examination, radiography, and MRI. Pain syndromes that may mimic lumbar radiculopathy include low back strain, lumbar bursitis, lumbar fibromyositis, inflammatory arthritis, and disorders of the lumbar spinal cord, roots, plexus, and nerves. MRI of the lumbar spine should be carried out on all patients suspected of suffering from lumbar radiculopathy. Screening laboratory testing consisting of complete blood count, erythrocyte sedimentation rate, antinuclear antibody testing, HLA-B27 antigen screening, and automated blood chemistry testing should be performed if the diagnosis of lumbar radiculopathy is in question, to help rule out other causes of the patient's pain.

Treatment

Lumbar radiculopathy is best treated with a multimodality approach. Physical therapy including heat modalities and deep sedative massage, combined with nonsteroidal anti-inflammatory agents and skeletal muscle relaxants, represents a reasonable starting point. The addition of lumbar steroid epidural nerve blocks is a reasonable next step. Caudal or lumbar epidural blocks with local anesthetic and steroid have been shown to be extremely effective in the treatment of lumbar radiculopathy. Underlying sleep disturbance and depression are best treated with a tricyclic antidepressant compound such as nortriptyline, which can be started at a single bedtime dose of 25 mg.

SUGGESTED READING

Waldman SD: Lumbar radiculopathy. In: Atlas of Common Pain Syndromes, ed 2. Philadelphia, Saunders, 2008.

CHAPTER 145

Sacroiliac Joint Pain

Pain emanating from the sacroiliac joint commonly occurs after the patient lifts in an awkward position, putting strain on the joint and supporting ligaments and soft tissues. The sacroiliac joint is also susceptible to the development of arthritis from a variety of conditions that have in common the ability to damage the joint cartilage. Osteoarthritis of the joint is the most common form of arthritis that results in sacroiliac joint pain. However, rheumatoid arthritis and post-traumatic arthritis are also common causes of sacroiliac pain secondary to arthritis. Less common causes of arthritis-induced sacroiliac pain include the collagen vascular diseases such as ankylosing spondylitis, infection, and Lyme disease. The collagen vascular diseases will generally present as a polyarthropathy rather than a monoarthropathy limited to the sacroiliac joint, although sacroiliac pain secondary to the collagen vascular disease ankylosing spondylitis responds exceedingly well to the intra-articular injection technique. Occasionally, the clinician will encounter patients with iatrogenically induced sacroiliac joint dysfunction due to overaggressive bone graft harvesting for spinal fusions.

Signs and Symptoms

The majority of patients presenting with sacroiliac pain secondary to strain or arthritis will present with the complaint of pain that is localized around the sacroiliac joint and upper leg. The pain of sacroiliac joint strain or arthritis radiates into the posterior buttocks and the back of the legs. The pain does not radiate below the knees. Activity makes the pain worse, with rest and heat providing some relief. The pain is constant and characterized as aching in nature. The pain may interfere with sleep. On physical examination, there will be tenderness to palpation of the affected sacroiliac joint. The patient will often favor the affected leg and exhibit a list to the unaffected side. Spasm of the lumbar paraspinal musculature is often present, as is limitation of range of motion of the lumbar spine in the erect position that improves in the sitting position due to relaxation of the hamstring muscles. Patients with pain emanating from the sacroiliac joint will exhibit a positive pelvic rock test. The pelvic rock test is performed by placing the hands on the iliac crests and the thumbs on the anterior superior iliac spines and then forcibly compressing the pelvis toward the midline. A positive test is indicated by the production of pain around the sacroiliac joint.

Testing

Plain radiographs are indicated in all patients who present with sacroiliac pain. Based on the patient's clinical presentation, additional testing including complete blood count, erythrocyte sedimentation rate, HLA-B27 antigen, and antinuclear antibody testing may be indicated.

Differential Diagnosis

Pain emanating from the sacroiliac joint can often be confused with include low back strain, lumbar bursitis, lumbar fibromyositis, inflammatory arthritis, and disorders of the lumbar spinal cord, roots, plexus, and nerves. Plain radiographs of the lumbar spine and sacroiliac joints should be obtained on all patients thought to be suffering from sacroiliac joint pain. Magnetic resonance imaging of the lumbar spine and sacroiliac joint should be carried out on those patients suspected of suffering from sacroiliac joint pain whose cause is not clearly defined. Radionuclide bone scanning should also be considered in such patients to rule out tumor and unsuspected insufficiency fractures that may be missed on conventional radiographs. Screening laboratory testing consisting of complete blood count, erythrocyte sedimentation rate, antinuclear antibody testing, HLA-B27 antigen screening, and automated blood chemistry testing should be performed if the diagnosis is in question to help rule out other causes of the patient's pain.

Treatment

Initial treatment of the pain and functional disability associated with sacroiliac joint pain should include a combination of the nonsteroidal anti-inflammatory agents or cyclooxygenase-2 inhibitors and physical therapy. The local application of heat and cold may also be beneficial. For patients who do not respond to these treatment modalities, injection of the sacroiliac joint with local anesthetic and steroid may be a reasonable next step.

SUGGESTED READING

Waldman SD: Sacroiliac joint pain. In: Atlas of Common Pain Syndromes, ed 2. Philadelphia, Saunders, 2008.

CHAPTER 146

Coccydynia

Coccydynia is a common pain syndrome characterized by pain localized to the tailbone that radiates into the lower sacrum and perineum. Coccydynia affects females more frequently than males. Coccydynia occurs most commonly following direct trauma to the coccyx from a kick or a fall directly onto the coccyx. Coccydynia can also occur following difficult vaginal delivery. The pain of coccydynia is thought to be the result of strain of the sacrococcygeal ligament or occasionally due to fracture of the coccyx. Less commonly, arthritis of the sacrococcygeal joint can result in coccydynia.

Signs and Symptoms

On physical examination, the patient will exhibit point tenderness over the coccyx with the pain being increased with movement of the coccyx. Movement of the coccyx may also cause sharp paresthesias into the rectum, which can be quite distressing to the patient. On rectal examination, the levator ani, piriformis, and coccygeus muscles may feel indurated, and palpation of these muscles may induce severe spasm. Sitting may exacerbate the pain of coccydynia, and the patient may attempt to sit on one buttock to avoid pressure on the coccyx.

Testing

Plain radiographs are indicated in all patients who present with pain thought to be emanating from the coccyx, to rule out occult bony pathology and tumor. Based on the patient's clinical presentation, additional testing including complete blood count, prostate-specific antigen, erythrocyte sedimentation rate, and antinuclear antibody testing may be indicated. Magnetic resonance imaging of the pelvis is indicated if occult mass or tumor is suspected. Radionuclide bone scanning may be useful to rule out stress fractures not seen on plain radiographs.

Differential Diagnosis

Primary pathology of the rectum and anus may occasionally be confused with the pain of coccydynia. Primary tumors or metastatic lesions of the sacrum and/or coccyx may also present as coccydynia. Proctalgia fugax may also mimic the pain of coccydynia but can be distinguished as movement of the coccyx will not reproduce the pain. Insufficiency fractures of the pelvis and sacrum may on occasion also mimic coccydynia, as can pathology of the sacroiliac joints.

Treatment

A short course of conservative therapy consisting of simple analgesics, nonsteroidal anti-inflammatory agents or cyclooxygenase-2 inhibitors, and a foam donut to prevent further irritation to the sacrococcygeal ligament is a reasonable first step in the treatment of patients suffering from coccydynia. If the patient does not experience rapid improvement, injection of the sacrococcygeal joint is a reasonable next step.

SUGGESTED READING

Waldman SD: Coccydynia. In: Atlas of Common Pain Syndromes, ed 2. Philadelphia, Saunders, 2008.

CHAPTER 147

Reflex Sympathetic Dystrophy of the Face

Reflex sympathetic dystrophy (RSD) is an infrequent cause of face and neck pain. Although the symptom complex in this disorder is relatively constant from patient to patient, the diagnosis is often missed. This diagnosis is overlooked despite the fact that RSD of the face and neck presents in a manner that closely parallels its presentation in the upper or lower extremity. This difficulty in diagnosis often results in extensive diagnostic and therapeutic endeavors in an effort to palliate the patient's pain. The common denominator in all patients suffering from RSD of the face is trauma to tissue. This trauma may take the form of actual injury to the soft tissues, dentition, or bones of the face; infection; cancer; arthritis; or insults to the central nervous system or cranial nerves.

Signs and Symptoms

The hallmark of RSD of the face is pain that is burning in nature. The pain is frequently associated with cutaneous or mucosal allodynia and does not follow the path of either cranial or peripheral nerves. Trigger areas, especially in the oral mucosa, are common, as are trophic skin and mucosal changes in the area affected by the RSD. Sudomotor and vasomotor changes may also be identified but are often less obvious than in patients suffering from RSD of the extremities. Often, patients suffering from RSD of the face will have evidence of previous dental extractions that were performed in an effort to provide the patient with pain relief. Patients suffering from RSD of the face frequently experience significant sleep disturbance and depression.

Testing

Although there is not a specific test for RSD, a presumptive diagnosis of RSD of the face can be made if the patient experiences significant pain relief following stellate ganglion block with local anesthetic. It should be noted that given the diverse nature of tissue injury that can cause RSD of the face, the clinician must assiduously search for occult pathology that may mimic or coexist with the RSD. Testing is aimed primarily at identifying occult pathology or other diseases that may mimic RSD of the face (see Differential Diagnosis). All patients with a presumptive diagnosis of RSD of the face should undergo magnetic resonance imaging (MRI) of the brain and, if significant occipital or nuchal symptoms are present, MRI of the cervical spine. Screening laboratory testing consisting of complete blood count, erythrocyte sedimentation rate, and automated blood chemistry testing should be performed to rule out infection or other inflammatory causes of tissue injury that may serve as the nidus for the RSD.

Differential Diagnosis

The clinical symptomatology of RSD of the face may often be confused with pain of dental or sinus origin or may be erroneously characterized as atypical facial pain or trigeminal neuralgia (Table 147-1). Careful questioning and physical examination will usually allow the clinician to help separate these overlapping pain syndromes. Tumors of the zygoma and mandible, as well as posterior fossa tumors and retropharyngeal tumors, may produce ill-defined pain that may be attributed to RSD of the face, and these potentially life-threatening diseases must be carefully searched for in any patient with facial pain.

The pain of atypical facial pain is constant and dull and aching in character, whereas the pain of trigeminal neuralgia is intermittent and shocklike in nature. Stellate ganglion block may help distinguish it from these two pain syndromes, as the pain of RSD of the face readily responds to this sympathetic nerve block, whereas atypical facial pain does not. The pain of RSD of the face must be distinguished from the pain of jaw claudication associated with temporal arteritis.

Treatment

The successful treatment of RSD of the face requires two things. First, any nidus of tissue trauma that is contributing to the ongoing sympathetic dysfunction responsible for the symptoms of RSD of the face must be identified and removed; second, interruption of the sympathetic innervation of the face via stellate ganglion block with local anesthetics must be implemented. This may require daily stellate ganglion block for a significant period of time. Occupational therapy consisting of tactile desensitization of the affected skin may also be of value. Underlying depression and sleep disturbance are best treated with a tricyclic antidepressant such as nortriptyline given as a single bedtime dose of 25 mg. Gabapentin may help palliate any component of neuritic pain. Opioid analgesics and benzodiazepines should be avoided to prevent iatrogenic chemical dependence.

SUGGESTED READING

Waldman SD: Reflex sympathetic dystrophy. In: Atlas of Common Pain Syndromes, ed 2. Philadelphia, Saunders, 2008.

TABLE 147-1 The Differential Diagnosis of Reflex Dystrophy of the Face

	Trigeminal Neuralgia	Atypical Facial Pain	RSD of the Face
Temporal pattern of pain	Sudden and intermittent	Constant	Constant
Character of pain	Shocklike and neuritic	Dull, cramping, and aching	Burning with allodynia
Pain-free intervals	Usual	Rare	Rare
Distribution of pain	In division of trigeminal nerve	Overlaps division of trigeminal nerve	Overlaps division of trigeminal nerve
Trigger areas	Present	Absent	Present
Underlying psychopathology	Rare	Common	Common
Trophic skin changes	Absent	Absent	Present
Sudomotor and vasomotor changes	Absent	Absent	Often present

Post-Dural Puncture Headache

Whenever the dura is intentionally or accidentally punctured, the potential for headache exists. The clinical presentation of post-dural puncture headache is classic and makes the diagnosis straightforward if one simply thinks about this diagnostic category of headache. The diagnosis may be obscured if the clinician is unaware that the possibility of dural puncture has occurred or in the rare instance when this type of headache occurs spontaneously after a bout of sneezing or coughing. The etiology of the symptoms and rare physical findings associated with post-dural puncture headache are due to low cerebrospinal fluid pressure resulting from continued leakage of spinal fluid out of the subarachnoid space. The symptoms of post-dural puncture headache begin almost immediately after the patient moves from a horizontal to an upright position. The intensity peaks within 1 or 2 minutes and abates within several minutes of the patient again assuming the horizontal position. The headache is pounding in character and its intensity is severe, with the intensity increasing the longer the patient remains upright. The headache is almost always bilateral and located in the frontal, temporal, and occipital region. Nausea and vomiting as well as dizziness frequently accompany the headache pain, especially if the patient remains upright for long periods. If cranial nerve palsy occurs, visual disturbance may occur.

Signs and Symptoms

The diagnosis of post-dural puncture headache is most often made on the basis of clinical history rather than on physical findings on examination. The neurologic examination in the vast majority of patients suffering from post-dural puncture headache will be normal. If the spinal fluid leak is allowed to persist or if the patient remains in the upright position for long periods of time despite the headache, cranial nerve palsies may occur, with the sixth cranial nerve affected most commonly. This complication may be transient but may become permanent, especially in patients with vulnerable nerves such as diabetics.

If the neurologic examination is abnormal, other causes of headache should be considered, including subarachnoid hemorrhage.

The onset of headache pain and other associated symptoms such as nausea and vomiting that appear when the patient moves from the horizontal to the upright position and then abates when the patient resumes a horizontal position is the sine qua non of post-dural puncture headache. A history of intentional dural puncture, such as lumbar puncture, spinal anesthesia, or myelography, or accidental dural puncture, such as failed epidural block or dural injury during spinal surgery, points strongly to the diagnosis of post-dural puncture headache. As mentioned, a spontaneous postural headache that presents identically to headache after dural puncture can occur after bouts of heavy sneezing or coughing and is thought to be due to traumatic rents in the dura. In this setting, a diagnosis of post-dural puncture headache is one of exclusion.

Testing

Magnetic resonance imaging (MRI) with and without gadolinium is highly accurate in helping confirm the diagnosis of post-dural puncture headache. Enhancement of the dura with low lying cerebellar tonsils will invariably be present. Poor visualization of the cisterns and subdural and epidural fluid collections may also be identified.

No additional testing is indicated for the patient who has undergone dural puncture and then develops a classic postural headache unless infection or subarachnoid hemorrhage is suspected. In this setting, lumbar puncture, complete blood cell count, and erythrocyte sedimentation rate are indicated on an emergent basis.

Differential Diagnosis

If the clinician is aware that the patient has undergone dural puncture, then the diagnosis of post-dural puncture headache is usually made. It is in those settings in which dural puncture is not suspected that delayed diagnosis most often occurs. Occasionally, post-dural puncture is misdiagnosed as migraine headache due to the associated nausea and vomiting coupled with visual disturbance. In any patient with dural puncture, infection remains an ever-present possibility. If fever is present, immediate lumbar puncture and blood cultures should be obtained and the patient started on antibiotics that cover resistant strains of *Staphylococcus*. MRI to rule out epidural abscess should also be considered if fever is present. Subarachnoid hemorrhage may also mimic post-dural puncture headache but should be identified on MRI of the brain.

Treatment

The mainstay of the treatment of post-dural puncture headache is the administration of autologous blood into the epidural space. This technique is known as *epidural blood patch* and is highly successful in the treatment of post-dural puncture headache. A volume of 12 to 18 mL of autologous blood is injected slowly into the epidural space at the level of dural puncture under strict aseptic precautions. The patient should remain in the horizontal position for the next 12 to 24 hours. Relief will occur within 2 to 3 hours in more than 90% of patients. Approximately 10% of patients will experience temporary relief but will experience a recurrence of symptoms when assuming the upright position. These patients should undergo a second epidural blood patch within 24 hours.

If the patient has experienced significant nausea and vomiting, antiemetics combined with intravenous fluids will help speed recovery. Some clinicians have advocated the use of alcoholic beverages to suppress the secretion of antidiuretic hormone and to increase cerebrospinal fluid production. Caffeine has also been reported to be of value in helping to treat the headache pain.

Failure to promptly recognize, diagnose, and treat post-dural puncture headache may result in considerable pain and suffering for the patient. If the low spinal fluid pressure is allowed to persist, cranial nerve deficits may occur. In most instances, the cranial nerve deficits are temporary, but in rare instances, these deficits may become permanent, especially in those patients with vulnerable nerves, such as diabetics. MRI of the brain is indicated in all patients thought to be suffering from headaches associated with dural puncture. Failure to correctly diagnose central nervous system infection can result in significant mortality and morbidity.

SUGGESTED READINGS

Goetz CG: Textbook of Clinical Neurology, ed 2. Philadelphia, Saunders, 2003.
Waldman SD: Post-dural puncture headache. In: Atlas of Uncommon Pain Syndromes, ed 2. Philadelphia, Saunders, 2008.

CHAPTER 149

Glossopharyngeal Neuralgia

Glossopharyngeal neuralgia is a rare condition characterized by paroxysms of pain in the sensory division of the ninth cranial nerve. Although the pain of glossopharyngeal neuralgia is similar to that of trigeminal neuralgia, it occurs 100 times less frequently. Glossopharyngeal neuralgia occurs more commonly in patients older than 50 years. The pain is located in the tonsil, laryngeal region, and posterior tongue. The pain is unilateral in the majority of patients but can occur bilaterally 2% of the time. In rare patients, the pain of glossopharyngeal neuralgia is associated with bradyarrhythmias and, in some patients, syncope. These cardiac symptoms are thought to be due to overflow of neural impulses from the glossopharyngeal nerve to the vagus nerve. Although rare, this unusual combination of pain and cardiac arrhythmia can be lethal.

Signs and Symptoms

The pain of glossopharyngeal neuralgia is in the distribution of the ninth cranial nerve. In some patients, there may be overflow pain into areas innervated by the trigeminal nerve and/or upper cervical segments. The pain is unilateral in 98% of patients and is neuritic in nature. It is often described as shooting or stabbing with a severe intensity level. The pain of glossopharyngeal neuralgia is often triggered by swallowing, chewing, coughing, or talking. With the exception of trigger areas in the distribution of the ninth cranial nerve, the patient's neurologic examination should be normal. Because tumors at the cerebellopontine angle may produce symptoms identical to glossopharyngeal neuralgia, an abnormal neurologic examination is cause for serious concern. Dull, aching pain that persists between the paroxysms of pain normally associated with glossopharyngeal neuralgia is highly suggestive of a space-occupying lesion and requires a thorough evaluation.

Testing

Magnetic resonance imaging (MRI) of the brain and brainstem should be performed on all patients suspected of suffering from glossopharyngeal neuralgia. MRI of the brain provides the clinician with the best information regarding the cranial vault and its contents. MRI is highly accurate and helps to identify abnormalities that may put the patient at risk for neurologic disasters due to intracranial and brainstem pathology, including tumors and demyelinating disease. Magnetic resonance angiography may be useful to help identify aneurysms responsible for the patient's neurologic symptomatology. In patients who cannot undergo MRI, such as a patient with a pacemaker, computed tomography (CT) scanning is a reasonable second choice.

Clinical laboratory testing consisting of a complete blood cell count, automated chemistry profile, and erythrocyte sedimentation rate are indicated to rule out infection, temporal arteritis, and malignancy that may mimic glossopharyngeal neuralgia. Endoscopy of the hypopharynx with special attention to the piriform sinuses is also indicated to rule out occult malignancy. Differential neural blockade of the glossopharyngeal nerve may help strengthen the diagnosis of glossopharyngeal neuralgia.

Differential Diagnosis

Glossopharyngeal neuralgia is generally a straightforward clinical diagnosis that can be made on the basis of a targeted history and physical examination. Diseases of the eye, ears, nose, throat, and teeth may all mimic glossopharyngeal neuralgia or may coexist and confuse the diagnosis. Tumors of the hypopharynx, including the tonsillar fossa and piriform sinus, may mimic the pain of glossopharyngeal neuralgia, as will tumors at the cerebellopontine angle. Occasionally, demyelinating disease may produce a clinical syndrome identical to glossopharyngeal neuralgia. The jaw claudication associated with temporal arteritis also sometimes confuses the clinical picture, as may trigeminal neuralgia.

Treatment

DRUG THERAPY

Carbamazepine

This drug is considered first-line treatment for glossopharyngeal neuralgia. In fact, rapid response to this drug essentially confirms a clinical diagnosis of glossopharyngeal neuralgia. Despite the safety and efficacy of carbamazepine compared with other treatments for glossopharyngeal neuralgia, much confusion and unfounded anxiety surround its use. This medication, which may be the patient's best chance for pain control, is sometimes discontinued due to laboratory abnormalities erroneously attributed to it. Therefore, baseline screening laboratory tests, consisting of a complete blood cell count, urinalysis, and automated chemistry profile, should be obtained before starting the drug.

Carbamazepine should be started slowly if the pain is not out of control, at a starting dose of 100 to 200 mg at bedtime for 2 nights, and the patient should be cautioned regarding side effects, including dizziness, sedation, confusion, and rash. The drug is increased in 100- to 200-mg increments, given in equally divided doses over 2 days as side effects allow, until pain relief is obtained or a total dose of 1200 mg daily is reached. Careful monitoring of laboratory parameters is mandatory to avoid the rare possibility of life-threatening blood dyscrasia. At the first sign of blood count abnormality or rash, this drug should be discontinued. Failure to monitor patients started on carbamazepine can be disastrous because aplastic anemia can occur. When pain relief is obtained, the patient should be kept at that dosage of carbamazepine for at least 6 months before considering tapering of this medication. The patient should be informed that under no circumstances should the dosage of drug be changed or the drug refilled or discontinued without the physician's knowledge.

Gabapentin

In the uncommon event that carbamazepine does not adequately control a patient's pain, gabapentin may be considered. As with carbamazepine, baseline blood tests should be obtained before starting therapy. Start with a 300-mg dose of gabapentin at bedtime for 2 nights, and caution the patient about potential side effects, including dizziness, sedation, confusion, and rash. The drug is then increased in 300-mg increments, given in equally divided doses over 2 days as side effects allow, until pain relief is obtained or a total dose of 2400 mg daily is reached. At this point, if the patient has experienced partial relief of pain, blood values are measured and the drug is carefully titrated upward using 100-mg tablets. Rarely will more than 3600 mg daily be required.

Baclofen

This drug has been reported to be of value in some patients who fail to obtain relief from the above-mentioned medications. Baseline laboratory tests should also be obtained before starting baclofen. Start with a 10-mg dose at bedtime for 2 nights, and caution the patient about potential adverse effects, which are the same as those of carbamazepine and gabapentin. The drug is increased in 10-mg increments, given in equally divided doses over 7 days as side effects allow, until pain relief is obtained or a total dose of 80 mg daily is reached. This drug has significant hepatic and central nervous system side effects, including weakness and sedation. As with carbamazepine, careful monitoring of laboratory values is indicated during the initial use of this drug.

In treating individuals with any of the drugs mentioned, the clinician should make the patient aware that premature tapering or discontinuation of the medication may lead to the recurrence of pain and that it will be more difficult to control pain thereafter.

INVASIVE THERAPY

Glossopharyngeal Nerve Block

The use of glossopharyngeal nerve block with local anesthetic and a steroid serves as an excellent adjunct to drug treatment of glossopharyngeal neuralgia.

This technique rapidly relieves pain while medications are being titrated to effective levels. The initial block is carried out with preservative-free bupivacaine combined with methylprednisolone. Subsequent daily nerve blocks are carried out in a similar manner substituting a lower dose of methylprednisolone. This approach may also be used to obtain control of breakthrough pain.

Radiofrequency Destruction of the Glossopharyngeal Nerve

The destruction of the glossopharyngeal nerve can be carried out by creating a radiofrequency lesion under biplanar fluoroscopic guidance. This procedure is reserved for patients who have failed to respond to all the treatments mentioned for intractable glossopharyngeal neuralgia and are not candidates for microvascular decompression of the glossopharyngeal root.

Microvascular Decompression of the Glossopharyngeal Root

This technique, which is also called *Jannetta's procedure*, is the major neurosurgical procedure of choice for intractable glossopharyngeal neuralgia. It is based on the theory that glossopharyngeal neuralgia is in fact a compressive mononeuropathy. The operation consists of identifying the glossopharyngeal root close to the brainstem and isolating the offending compressing blood vessel. A sponge is then interposed between the vessel and nerve, relieving the compression and thus the pain.

SUGGESTED READINGS

Goetz CG: Textbook of Clinical Neurology, ed 2. Philadelphia, Saunders, 2003.

Waldman SD: Glossopharyngeal neuralgia. In: Atlas of Uncommon Pain Syndromes, ed 2. Philadelphia, Saunders, 2008.

CHAPTER 150

Spasmodic Torticollis

Spasmodic torticollis is a rare condition characterized by involuntary movement of the head. It is classified as a focal or segmental dystonia and occurs in approximately 3 in 10,000 people. It begins in early adult life. There are three varieties of spasmodic torticollis:

- Tonic, which involves involuntary turning of the head to one side
- Clonic, which involves involuntary shaking of the head
- Tonic/clonic, which involves both types of involuntary movement

Spasmodic torticollis can also be subclassified as to the specific movement of the head: (1) rotation, which involves the turning of the head to the side;

(2) laterocollis, which involves the leaning of the head against the shoulder; (3) retrocollis, which involves the leaning of the head toward the back; and (4) anterocollis, which involves the leaning of the head toward the chest. The disease occurs more commonly in women and is often initially diagnosed as a hysterical reaction or tic.

Thought to be due to dysfunction centrally, rather than a disease of the affected muscles, spasmodic torticollis often begins a subtle involuntary movement of the head. Early in the disease, the dystonia is often intermittent. As the disease progresses, the symptoms become more severe and harder for the patient to hide. The dystonic movements may become more sustained and associated with constant, aching pain in the affected muscles. The pain often becomes the primary reason for the patient to seek medical attention, with the patient almost indifferent to the dystonic movements. The dystonia often disappears with sleep and becomes less pronounced on first awakening, with the dystonic movements and pain worsening as the day progresses. Spontaneous recovery has been reported, but overall, treatment is difficult and of limited success.

Signs and Symptoms

The patient suffering from spasmodic torticollis exhibits involuntary, dystonic movements of the head. In extreme cases, the dystonia will be continuous and the laterocollis so marked that the patient's ear will rest on the ipsilateral shoulder. Pain may be a predominant feature of the syndrome, and spasms of the cervical paraspinous musculature, the strap muscles of the neck, and the sternocleidomastoid are often present. Hypertrophy of the affected muscles may occasionally occur. Other than the dystonic movements, the neurologic examination is normal. As mentioned, the patient may exhibit a seeming indifference to his or her abnormal head movements or position. Often, touching the opposite side of the face or chin will cause the dystonia to momentarily cease.

Testing

Magnetic resonance imaging (MRI) of the brain and brainstem should be performed on all patients suspected of suffering from spasmodic torticollis. MRI of the brain provides the clinician with the best information regarding the cranial vault and its contents. MRI is highly accurate and helps to identify abnormalities that may put the patient at risk for neurologic disasters due to intracranial and brainstem pathology, including tumors and demyelinating disease. Magnetic resonance angiography may be useful to help identify aneurysms responsible for the patient's neurologic symptomatology. In patients who cannot undergo MRI, such as a patient with a pacemaker, computed tomography scanning is a reasonable second choice.

Clinical laboratory testing consisting of a complete blood cell count, automated chemistry profile, and erythrocyte sedimentation rate is indicated to rule out infection and malignancy.

Differential Diagnosis

Spasmodic torticollis is generally a straightforward clinical diagnosis that can be made on the basis of a targeted history and physical examination. The involuntary nature of this movement disorder is the hallmark of the disease and helps distinguish it from tics and habit spasms that are voluntary and worsen when the patient is tense. Both tics and habit spasms resemble volitional movement. Behavioral abnormalities such as hysterical conversion reactions must also be considered. Acute spasm and pain of the muscles of the neck or wry neck can mimic spasmodic torticollis, but its onset is acute and the symptoms usually resolve within days to a week. Occasionally, patients with clonic spasmodic torticollis are initially diagnosed as having Parkinson's disease.

Treatment

In general, the treatment of spasmodic torticollis is disappointing. Pharmacologic treatment with the skeletal muscle relaxants, drugs that act at the spinal cord level such as baclofen, and centrally acting drugs, including the anticonvulsants and L-dopa, may provide some symptomatic relief in mild cases. Trihexyphenidyl and diazepam have also been advocated.

For those patients for whom pharmacologic treatment fails, injection of the affected muscles with botulinum toxin is a reasonable next step. Frequent injections may result in the development of antibodies against the toxin, which makes the toxin less effective. By changing to different subtypes of toxin, efficacy may be restored. For intractable cases, bilateral thalamotomy has been advocated. The results of this radical treatment are variable at best.

SUGGESTED READINGS

Goetz CG: Textbook of Clinical Neurology, ed 2. Philadelphia, Saunders, 2003.

Waldman SD: Spasmodic torticollis. In: Atlas of Uncommon Pain Syndromes, ed 2. Philadelphia, Saunders, 2008.

CHAPTER 151

Brachial Plexopathy

There are numerous causes of the clinical syndrome called brachial plexopathy. In common to all of them is the constellation of symptoms consisting of neurogenic pain and associated weakness that radiates into the supraclavicular region and upper extremity. More common causes of brachial plexopathy include compression of the plexus by cervical ribs or abnormal muscles (e.g., thoracic outlet syndrome), invasion of the plexus by tumor (e.g., Pancoast's tumor), direct trauma to the plexus (e.g., stretch injuries and avulsions), inflammatory causes (e.g., Parsonage-Turner syndrome), and post-radiation plexopathy.

Signs and Symptoms

Patients suffering from brachial plexopathy will complain of pain radiating to the supraclavicular region and upper extremity. The pain is neuritic in character and may take on a deep, boring quality with invasion of the plexus by tumor. Movement of the neck and shoulder will exacerbate the pain, and patients suffering from brachial plexopathy will often avoid such movements in an effort to palliate the pain. Frozen shoulder often results and may confuse the diagnosis. If thoracic outlet syndrome is suspected, Adson's test may be performed. A positive test is indicated if the radial pulse disappears with neck extended and the head turned toward the affected side. It must be noted that this test is nonspecific and treatment decisions should not be based on this finding alone (see Testing). If the patient presents with severe pain that is shortly followed by profound weakness, brachial plexitis should be considered and can be confirmed with electromyography.

Testing

All patients presenting with brachial plexopathy, especially without a clear history of antecedent trauma, must undergo MRI of the cervical spine and the brachial plexus. Computed tomography testing is a reasonable second choice if MRI is contraindicated. Electromyography and nerve conduction velocity testing are extremely sensitive, and the skilled electromyographer can help delineate the specific portion of the plexus that is abnormal. If an inflammatory basis for the plexopathy is suspected, serial electromyography is indicated. If Pancoast's tumor or other tumors of the brachial plexus are suspected, chest radiographs with apical lordotic views may be helpful. Screening laboratory testing consisting of complete blood count, erythrocyte sedimentation rate, antinuclear antibody testing, and automated blood chemistry testing should be performed if the diagnosis of brachial plexopathy is in question, to help rule out other causes of the patient's pain.

Differential Diagnosis

Diseases of the cervical spinal cord, the bony cervical spine, and disc can mimic brachial plexopathy. Appropriate testing including MRI and electromyography will help sort out the myriad possibilities, but the clinician should also be aware that more than one pathologic process may coexist and contribute to the patient's symptomatology. Syringomyelia, tumors of the cervical spinal cord, and tumors of the cervical nerve roots as they exit the spinal cord (e.g., schwannomas) can be of insidious onset and quite difficult to diagnosis. Pancoast's tumor should be high on the list of diagnostic possibilities in all patients presenting with brachial plexopathy in the absence of clear antecedent trauma, especially if there is a past history of tobacco abuse. Lateral herniated cervical disc, metastatic tumor, or cervical spondylosis that results in significant nerve root compression may also present as a brachial plexopathy. Rarely, infection involving the apex of the lung may compress and irritate the plexus.

Treatment

DRUG THERAPY

Gabapentin

Gabapentin is the first-line treatment for the neuritic pain of brachial plexopathy. Start with a 300-mg dose of gabapentin at bedtime for 2 nights and caution the patient about potential side effects, including dizziness, sedation, confusion, and rash. The drug is then increased in 300-mg increments, given in equally divided doses over 2 days, as side effects allow until pain relief is obtained or a total dose of 2400 mg daily is reached. At this point, if the patient has experienced partial relief of pain, blood values are measured and the drug is carefully titrated upward using 100-mg tablets. Rarely will more than 3600 mg daily be required.

Carbamazepine

This drug is useful in those patients suffering from brachial plexopathy who do not experience pain relief with gabapentin. Despite carbamazepine's safety and efficacy compared with other treatments for brachial plexopathy, much confusion and unfounded anxiety surround its use. This medication, which may be the patient's best chance for pain control, is sometimes discontinued due to laboratory abnormalities erroneously attributed to it. Therefore, baseline screening laboratory tests, consisting of a complete blood count, urinalysis, and automated chemistry profile, should be obtained before starting the drug.

Carbamazepine should be started slowly if the pain is not out of control. Start with a dose of 100 to 200 mg at bedtime for 2 nights and caution the patient regarding side effects, including dizziness, sedation, confusion, and rash. The drug is increased in 100- to 200-mg increments, given in equally divided doses over 2 days, as side effects allow until pain relief is obtained or a total dose of 1200 mg daily is reached. Careful monitoring of laboratory parameters is mandatory to avoid the rare possibility of life-threatening blood dyscrasia. At the *first* sign of blood count abnormality or rash, this drug should be discontinued. Failure to monitor patients started on carbamazepine can be disastrous as aplastic anemia can occur. When pain relief is obtained, the patient should be kept at that dosage of carbamazepine for at least 6 months before considering tapering of this medication. The patient should be informed that under no circumstances should the dosage of drug be changed or the drug refilled or discontinued without the physician's knowledge.

Baclofen

This drug has been reported to be of value in some patients who fail to obtain relief from the above-mentioned medications. Baseline laboratory tests should also be obtained prior to starting baclofen. Start with a 10-mg dose at bedtime for 2 nights and caution the patient about potential adverse effects, which are the same as those of carbamazepine and gabapentin. The drug is increased in 10-mg increments, given in equally divided doses over 7 days as side effects allow, until pain relief is obtained or a total dose of 80 mg daily is reached. This drug has significant hepatic and central nervous system side effects, including weakness and sedation. As with carbamazepine, careful monitoring of laboratory values is indicated during the initial use of this drug.

In treating individuals with any of the above-mentioned drugs, the physician should make the patient aware that premature tapering or discontinuation of the medication may lead to the recurrence of pain and that it will be more difficult to control pain thereafter.

INVASIVE THERAPY

Brachial Plexus Block

The use of brachial plexus block with local anesthetic and a steroid serves as an excellent adjunct to drug treatment of brachial plexopathy. This technique rapidly relieves pain while medications are being titrated to effective levels. The initial block is carried out with preservative-free bupivacaine combined with methylprednisolone. Subsequent daily nerve blocks are carried out in a similar manner, substituting a lower dose of methylprednisolone. This approach may also be used to obtain control of breakthrough pain.

Radiofrequency Destruction of the Brachial Plexus

The destruction of the brachial plexus can be carried out by creating a radiofrequency lesion under biplanar fluoroscopic guidance. This procedure is reserved for patients for whom all the above-mentioned treatments for brachial plexopathy have failed and whose pain is secondary to tumor or avulsion of the brachial plexus.

Dorsal Root Entry Zone (DREZ) Lesioning

This technique, which is called DREZ lesioning, is the neurosurgical procedure of choice for intractable brachial plexopathy in those patients for whom all the above-mentioned treatments for brachial plexopathy have failed and whose pain is secondary to tumor or avulsion of the brachial plexus. This is a major neurosurgical procedure and carries significant risks.

PHYSICAL MODALITIES

The use of physical and occupational therapy to maintain function and help palliate pain is a crucial part of the treatment plan for patients suffering from brachial plexopathy. Shoulder abnormalities, including subluxation and adhesive capsulitis, must be aggressively searched for and treated. Occupational therapy to assist in activities of daily living is also important to avoid further deterioration of function.

SUGGESTED READINGS

Goetz CG: Textbook of Clinical Neurology, ed 2. Philadelphia, Saunders, 2003.

Waldman SD: Brachial plexopathy. In: Atlas of Common Pain Syndromes, ed 2. Philadelphia, Saunders, 2008.

CHAPTER 152

Thoracic Outlet Syndrome

Thoracic outlet syndrome is the name given to a constellation of signs and symptoms, including paresthesias and aching pain of the neck, shoulder, and arm, that are thought to be due to compression of the brachial plexus and subclavian artery and vein as they exit the space between the shoulder girdle and the first rib or congenitally abnormal structures such as cervical ribs. Either one or all of the structures may be compressed giving the syndrome a varied clinical expression. Thoracic outlet syndrome is seen most commonly in women between 25 and 50 years of age. The subject of significant debate, the diagnosis and treatment of thoracic outlet syndrome remain controversial.

Signs and Symptoms

Although the symptoms of thoracic outlet syndrome vary, compression of neural structures account for most clinical symptomatology. Paresthesias of the upper extremity radiating into the distribution of the ulnar nerve may be misdiagnosed as tardy ulnar palsy. Aching and incoordination of the affected extremity are also common findings. If vascular compression exists, edema or discoloration of the arm may be noted and, in rare instances, venous or arterial thrombosis may occur.

Rarely, the symptoms of thoracic outlet syndrome can be caused by arterial aneurysm, and auscultation of the supraclavicular region will reveal a bruit.

Provocation of the symptoms of thoracic outlet syndrome may be elicited by a variety of maneuvers, including Adson's test and the elevated arm stress test. Adson's test is carried out by palpating the radial pulse on the affected side with the patient's neck extended and the head turned toward the affected side. A diminished pulse is suggestive of thoracic outlet syndrome. The elevated arm stress test is performed by having the patient hold their arms over head and open and close their hands. A patient without thoracic outlet syndrome can perform this maneuver for approximately 3 minutes, whereas patients suffering from thoracic outlet syndrome will experience the onset of symptoms within 30 seconds.

Testing

Plain radiographs of the cervical spine should be performed on all patients suspected of suffering from thoracic outlet syndrome. Careful review for congenital abnormalities such as cervical ribs or overly elongated transverse processes should be carried out. Patients should also undergo chest radiography with apical lordotic views to rule out Pancoast's tumor. Magnetic resonance imaging (MRI) of the cervical spine is indicated to rule out lesions of the cervical spinal cord and exiting nerve roots. If a diagnosis is still in doubt, MRI of the brachial plexus is also indicated to rule out occult pathology, including primary tumors of the plexus. Screening laboratory testing consisting of complete blood count, erythrocyte sedimentation rate, antinuclear antibody testing, and automated blood chemistry testing should be performed if the diagnosis of brachial plexopathy is in question, to help rule out other causes of the patient's pain.

Differential Diagnosis

Diseases of the cervical spinal cord, the bony cervical spine, and disc can mimic brachial plexopathy. Appropriate testing including MRI and electromyography will help sort out the myriad possibilities, but the clinician should also be aware that more than one pathologic process may coexist and contribute to the patient's symptomatology. Syringomyelia, tumors of the cervical spinal cord, and tumors of the cervical nerve roots as they exit the spinal cord (e.g., schwannomas) can be of insidious onset and quite difficult to diagnosis. Pancoast's tumor should be high on the list of diagnostic possibilities in all patients presenting with brachial plexopathy in the absence of clear antecedent trauma, especially if there is a past history of tobacco abuse. Lateral herniated cervical disc, metastatic tumor, or cervical spondylosis that results in significant nerve root compression may also present as a brachial plexopathy. Rarely, infection involving the apex of the lung may compress and irritate the plexus.

Treatment

PHYSICAL MODALITIES

The primary treatment for patients suffering from thoracic outlet syndrome is the rational use of physical therapy to maintain function and help palliate pain. Shoulder abnormalities, including subluxation and adhesive capsulitis, must be aggressively searched for and treated. Occupation therapy to assist in activities of daily living is also important to avoid further deterioration of function.

DRUG THERAPY

Gabapentin

Gabapentin is the first-line pharmacologic treatment for the neuritic pain of thoracic outlet syndrome. Start with a 300-mg dose of gabapentin at bedtime for 2 nights and caution the patient about potential side effects, including dizziness, sedation, confusion, and rash. The drug is then increased in 300-mg increments, given in equally divided doses over 2 days as side effects allow, until pain relief is obtained or a total dose of 2400 mg daily is reached. At this point, if the patient has experienced partial relief of pain, blood values are measured and the drug is carefully titrated upward using 100-mg tablets. Rarely will more than 3600 mg daily be required.

Carbamazepine

This drug is useful in those patients suffering from thoracic outlet syndrome who do not experience pain relief with gabapentin. Despite the safety and efficacy of carbamazepine compared with other treatments for thoracic outlet syndrome, much confusion and unfounded anxiety surround its use. This medication, which may be the patient's best chance for pain control, is sometimes discontinued due to laboratory abnormalities erroneously attributed to it. Therefore, baseline screening laboratory tests, consisting of a complete blood count, urinalysis, and automated chemistry profile, should be obtained before starting the drug.

Carbamazepine should be started slowly if the pain is not out of control. Start with a dose of 100 to 200 mg at bedtime for 2 nights and caution the patient regarding side effects, including dizziness, sedation, confusion, and rash. The drug is increased in 100- to 200-mg increments, given in equally divided doses over 2 days as side effects allow, until pain relief is obtained or a total dose of 1200 mg daily is reached. Careful monitoring of laboratory parameters is mandatory to avoid the rare possibility of life-threatening blood dyscrasia. At the *first* sign of blood count abnormality or rash, this drug should be discontinued. Failure to monitor patients started on carbamazepine can be disastrous as aplastic anemia can occur. When pain relief is obtained, the patient should be kept at that dosage of carbamazepine for at least 6 months before considering tapering of this medication. The patient should be informed that under no circumstances should the dosage of drug be changed or the drug refilled or discontinued without the physician's knowledge.

Baclofen

This drug has been reported to be of value in some patients who fail to obtain relief from the above-mentioned medications. Baseline laboratory tests should also be obtained prior to starting baclofen. Start with a 10-mg dose at bedtime for 2 nights and caution the patient about potential adverse effects, which are the same as those of carbamazepine and gabapentin. The drug is increased in 10-mg increments, given in equally divided doses over 7 days as side effects allow, until pain relief is obtained or a total dose of 80 mg daily is reached. This drug has significant hepatic and central nervous system side effects, including weakness and sedation. As with carbamazepine, careful monitoring of laboratory values is indicated during the initial use of this drug.

In treating individuals with any of the drugs mentioned, the physician should make the patient aware that premature tapering or discontinuation of the medication may lead to the recurrence of pain and that it will be more difficult to control pain thereafter.

INVASIVE THERAPY

Brachial Plexus Block

The use of brachial plexus block with local anesthetic and a steroid serves as an excellent adjunct to drug treatment of thoracic outlet syndrome. This technique rapidly relieves pain while medications are being titrated to effective levels. The initial block is carried out with preservative-free bupivacaine combined with methylprednisolone. Subsequent daily nerve blocks are carried out in a similar manner, substituting a lower dose of methylprednisolone. This approach may also be used to obtain control of breakthrough pain.

SURGICAL TREATMENTS

In the absence of demonstrable pathology (e.g., a cervical rib), the outcome of the surgical treatment for thoracic outlet syndrome is dismal regardless of the surgical technique chosen. In patients with a clear etiology for their symptoms for whom all attempts at conservative therapy have failed, the judicious use of surgical treatment may be a reasonable last step.

SUGGESTED READINGS

Campbell W: DeJong's The Neurological Examination, ed 6. Philadelphia, Lippincott Williams and Wilkins, 2005.

Goetz CG: Textbook of Clinical Neurology, ed 2. Philadelphia, Saunders, 2003.

Waldman SD: Adson's test. In: Physical Diagnosis of Pain: An Atlas of Signs and Symptoms. Philadelphia, Saunders, 2006.

Waldman SD: Thoracic outlet syndrome. In: Atlas of Common Pain Syndromes, ed 2. Philadelphia, Saunders, 2008.

CHAPTER 153

Pancoast's Tumor Syndrome

Pancoast's tumor syndrome is the result of local growth of tumor from the apex of the lung directly into the brachial plexus. Such tumors usually involve the first and second thoracic nerves as well as the eighth cervical nerve, producing a classic clinical syndrome consisting of severe arm pain and, in some patients, a Horner syndrome. Destruction of the first and second ribs is also common. Diagnosis is usually delayed, and patients are often erroneously treated for cervical radiculopathy or primary shoulder pathology until the diagnosis becomes clear.

Signs and Symptoms

Patients suffering from Pancoast's tumor syndrome will complain of pain radiating to the supraclavicular region and upper extremity. Initially, the lower portion of the brachial plexus is involved as the tumor growth is from below, causing pain in the upper thoracic and lower cervical dermatomes. The pain is neuritic in character and may take on a deep, boring quality, with invasion of the brachial plexus by tumor. Movement of the neck and shoulder will exacerbate the pain, and patients suffering from brachial plexopathy will often avoid such movements in an effort to palliate the pain. Frozen shoulder often results and may confuse the diagnosis. As the disease progresses, Horner's syndrome may occur.

Testing

All patients presenting with brachial plexopathy, especially without a clear history of antecedent trauma, must undergo magnetic resonance imaging (MRI) of the cervical spine and the brachial plexus. Computed tomography (CT) testing is a reasonable second choice if MRI is contraindicated. Electromyography and nerve conduction velocity testing are extremely sensitive, and the skilled electromyographer can help delineate the specific portion of the plexus that is abnormal. All patients with a significant smoking history in whom Pancoast's tumor or other tumors of the brachial plexus are suspected should undergo chest radiography with apical lordotic views or CT scanning through the apex of the lung. Screening laboratory testing consisting of complete blood count,

erythrocyte sedimentation rate, antinuclear antibody testing, and automated blood chemistry testing should be performed if the diagnosis of brachial plexopathy is in question, to help rule out other causes of the patient's pain.

Differential Diagnosis

Diseases of the cervical spinal cord, the bony cervical spine, and disc can mimic the brachial plexopathy associated with Pancoast's tumor syndrome. Appropriate testing including MRI and electromyography will help sort out the myriad possibilities, but the clinician should also be aware that more than one pathologic process may coexist and contribute to the patient's symptomatology. Syringomyelia, tumors of the cervical spinal cord, and tumors of the cervical nerve roots as they exit the spinal cord (e.g., schwannomas) can be of insidious onset and quite difficult to diagnosis. Pancoast's tumor should be high on the list of diagnostic possibilities in all patients presenting with brachial plexopathy in the absence of clear antecedent trauma, especially if there is a past history of tobacco abuse. Lateral herniated cervical disc, metastatic tumor, or cervical spondylosis, which result in significant nerve root compression, may also present as a brachial plexopathy. Rarely, infection involving the apex of the lung may compress and irritate the plexus.

Treatment

The primary treatment of Pancoast's tumor syndrome should be aimed at the tumor itself. Based on the cell type and extent of involvement, chemotherapy and radiation therapy may be indicated. Primary surgical treatment of tumors involving the brachial plexus is difficult and the results are disappointing.

DRUG THERAPY

Opioid Analgesics

The mainstay of the treatment of pain associated with Pancoast's tumor syndrome is the opioid analgesics. Although as a general rule, neuropathic pain responds poorly to opioid analgesics, given the severity of pain and lack of options available to treat the pain of Pancoast's tumor syndrome, a trial of opioid analgesics is warranted. The use of a short-acting potent opioid such as oxycodone is a reasonable starting point. Immediate-release morphine or methadone can also be considered. These drugs can be used in combination with nonsteroidal anti-inflammatory agents and the adjuvant analgesics described next.

Gabapentin

Gabapentin is the first-line treatment for the neuritic pain of Pancoast's tumor syndrome. Start with a 300-mg dose of gabapentin at bedtime for 2 nights and caution the patient about potential side effects, including dizziness, sedation, confusion, and rash. The drug is then increased in 300 mg increments, given in equally divided doses over 2 days as side effects allow, until pain relief is obtained or a total dose of 2400 mg daily is reached. At this point, if the patient has experienced partial relief of pain, blood values are measured and the drug is carefully titrated upward using 100-mg tablets. Rarely will more than 3600 mg daily be required.

Carbamazepine

This drug is useful in those patients suffering from Pancoast's tumor syndrome who do not experience pain relief with gabapentin. Despite the safety and efficacy of carbamazepine compared with other treatments for brachial plexopathy, much confusion and unfounded anxiety surround its use. This medication, which may be the patient's best chance for pain control, is sometimes discontinued due to laboratory abnormalities erroneously attributed to it. Therefore, baseline screening laboratory tests, consisting of a complete blood count, urinalysis, and automated chemistry profile, should be obtained before starting the drug.

Carbamazepine should be started slowly if the pain is not out of control. Start with a dose of 100 to 200 mg at bedtime for 2 nights and caution the patient regarding side effects, including dizziness, sedation, confusion, and rash. The drug is increased in 100- to 200-mg increments, given in equally divided doses over 2 days as side effects allow, until pain relief is obtained or a total dose of 1200 mg daily is reached. Careful monitoring of laboratory parameters is mandatory to avoid the rare possibility of life-threatening blood dyscrasia. At the *first* sign of blood count abnormality or rash, this drug should be discontinued. Failure to monitor patients started on carbamazepine can be disastrous as aplastic anemia can occur. When pain relief is obtained, the patient should be kept at that dosage of carbamazepine for at least 6 months before considering tapering of this medication. The patient should be informed that under no circumstances should the dosage of drug be changed or the drug refilled or discontinued without the physician's knowledge.

Baclofen

This drug has been reported to be of value in some patients who fail to obtain relief from the above-mentioned medications. Baseline laboratory tests should also be obtained prior to starting baclofen. Start with a 10-mg dose at bedtime for 2 nights and caution the patient about potential adverse effects, which are the same as those of carbamazepine and gabapentin. The drug is increased in 10-mg increments, given in equally divided doses over 7 days as side effects allow, until pain relief is obtained or a total dose of 80 mg daily is reached. This drug has significant hepatic and central nervous system side effects, including weakness and sedation. As with carbamazepine, careful monitoring of laboratory values is indicated during the initial use of this drug.

INVASIVE THERAPY

Brachial Plexus Block

The use of brachial plexus block with local anesthetic and a steroid serves as an excellent adjunct to drug treatment of Pancoast's tumor syndrome. This technique rapidly relieves pain while medications are being titrated to effective levels. The initial block is carried out with preservative-free bupivacaine combined with methylprednisolone. Subsequent daily nerve blocks are carried out in a similar manner, substituting a lower dose of methylprednisolone. This approach may also be used to obtain control of breakthrough pain.

Radiofrequency Destruction of the Brachial Plexus

The destruction of the brachial plexus can be carried out by creating a radiofrequency lesion under biplanar fluoroscopic guidance. This procedure is reserved for patients for whom all the above-mentioned treatments for Pancoast's tumor syndrome have failed.

Dorsal Root Entry Zone (DREZ) Lesioning

This technique, which is called DREZ lesioning, is the neurosurgical procedure of choice for intractable brachial plexopathy associated with Pancoast's tumor in those patients for whom all the above-mentioned treatments for brachial plexopathy have failed. This is a major neurosurgical procedure and carries significant risks.

Other Neurosurgical Options

The pain of Pancoast's tumor syndrome is notoriously difficult to treat. Cordotomy, deep brain stimulation, and thalamotomy have all been tried in such patients with varying degrees of success.

PHYSICAL MODALITIES

The use of physical and occupational therapy to maintain function and help palliate pain is a crucial part of the treatment plan for patients suffering from Pancoast's tumor syndrome. Shoulder abnormalities including subluxation and adhesive capsulitis must be aggressively searched for and treated. Occupational therapy to assist in activities of daily living is also important to avoid further deterioration of function.

SUGGESTED READINGS

Campbell W: DeJong's The Neurological Examination, ed 6. Philadelphia, Lippincott Williams and Wilkins, 2005.
Goetz CG: Textbook of Clinical Neurology, ed 2. Philadelphia, Saunders, 2003.
Waldman SD: Pancoast's tumor syndrome. In: Atlas of Common Pain Syndromes, ed 2. Philadelphia, Saunders, 2008.

CHAPTER 154

Tennis Elbow

Tennis elbow (also known as lateral epicondylitis) is caused by repetitive microtrauma to the extensor tendons of the forearm. The pathophysiology of tennis elbow is initially caused by microtearing at the origin of extensor carpi radialis and extensor carpi ulnaris. Secondary inflammation may occur, which can become chronic as the result of continued overuse or misuse of the extensors of the forearm. Coexistent bursitis, arthritis, and gout may also perpetuate the pain and disability of tennis elbow.

Tennis elbow occurs in patients engaged in repetitive activities that include hand grasping, such as politicians shaking hands, or high-torque wrist turning, such as scooping ice cream at an ice cream parlor. Tennis players develop tennis elbow via two separate mechanisms: first, increased pressure grip strain as a result of playing with too heavy a racquet, and, second, making backhand shots with a leading shoulder and elbow rather than keeping the shoulder and elbow parallel to the net. Other racquet sport players are also susceptible to the development of tennis elbow.

Signs and Symptoms

The pain of tennis elbow is localized to the region of the lateral epicondyle. It is constant and is made worse with active contraction of the wrist. Patients will note the inability to hold a coffee cup or hammer. Sleep disturbance is common. On physical examination, there will be tenderness along the extensor tendons at or just below the lateral epicondyle. Many patients with tennis elbow will exhibit a bandlike thickening within the affected extensor tendons. Elbow range of motion will be normal. Grip strength on the affected side will be diminished. Patients with tennis elbow will demonstrate a positive tennis elbow test. The test is performed by stabilizing the patient's forearm and then having the patient clench his or her fist and actively extend the wrist. The examiner then attempts to force the wrist into flexion. Sudden severe pain is highly suggestive of tennis elbow.

Testing

Electromyography will help distinguish cervical radiculopathy and radial tunnel syndrome from tennis elbow. Plain radiographs are indicated in all patients who present with tennis elbow to rule out joint or occult bony pathology. Based on the patient's clinical presentation, additional testing including complete blood count, uric acid, erythrocyte sedimentation rate, and antinuclear antibody testing may be indicated. Magnetic resonance imaging of the elbow is indicated if joint instability is suspected.

Differential Diagnosis

Radial tunnel syndrome and occasionally C6-7 radiculopathy can mimic tennis elbow. Radial tunnel syndrome is an entrapment neuropathy that is the result of entrapment of the radial nerve below the elbow. Radial tunnel syndrome can be distinguished from tennis elbow in that with radial tunnel syndrome, the maximal tenderness to palpation is distal to the lateral epicondyle over the radial nerve, whereas with tennis elbow, the maximal tenderness to palpation is over the lateral epicondyle.

The most common nidus of pain from tennis elbow is the bony origin of the extensor tendon of extensor carpi radialis brevis at the anterior facet of the lateral epicondyle. Less commonly, tennis elbow pain can originate from the origin of the extensor carpi radialis longus at the supracondylar crest or, rarely, more distally at the point where the extensor carpi radialis brevis overlies the radial head. As mentioned, bursitis may accompany tennis elbow. The olecranon bursa lies in the posterior aspect of the elbow joint and may also become inflamed as a result of direct trauma or overuse of the joint. Other bursae susceptible to the development of bursitis exist between the insertion of the biceps and the head of the radius as well as in the antecubital and cubital area.

Treatment

Initial treatment of the pain and functional disability associated with tennis elbow should include a combination of the nonsteroidal anti-inflammatory agents or cyclooxygenase-2 inhibitors and physical therapy. The local application of heat and cold may also be beneficial. Any repetitive activity that may exacerbate the patient's symptomatology should be avoided. For patients who do not respond to these treatment modalities, injection of the lateral epicondyle may be a reasonable next step.

SUGGESTED READINGS

Waldman SD: Tennis elbow. In: Atlas of Common Pain Syndromes, ed 2. Philadelphia, Saunders, 2008.

Waldman SD: The tennis elbow test. In: Physical Diagnosis of Pain: An Atlas of Signs and Symptoms. Philadelphia, Saunders, 2006.

CHAPTER 155

Golfer's Elbow

Golfer's elbow (also known as medial epicondylitis) is caused by repetitive microtrauma to the flexor tendons of the forearm in a manner analogous to tennis elbow. The pathophysiology of golfer's elbow is initially caused by microtearing at the origin of pronator teres, flexor carpi radialis, and flexor carpi ulnaris and the palmaris longus. Secondary inflammation may occur, which can become chronic as the result of continued overuse or misuse of the flexors of the forearm. The most common nidus of pain from golfer's elbow is the bony origin of the flexor tendon of flexor carpi radialis and the humeral heads of the flexor carpi ulnaris and pronator teres at the medial epicondyle of the humerus. Less commonly, golfer's elbow pain can originate from the ulnar head of the flexor carpi ulnaris at the medial aspect of the olecranon process. Coexistent bursitis, arthritis, and gout may also perpetuate the pain and disability of golfer's elbow.

Golfer's elbow occurs in patients engaged in repetitive flexion activities, which includes throwing baseballs, carrying heavy suitcases, and driving golf balls. These activities have in common repetitive flexion of the wrist and strain on the flexor tendons due to excessive weight or sudden arrested motion. Interestingly, many of the activities that can cause tennis elbow can also cause golfer's elbow.

Signs and Symptoms

The pain of golfer's elbow is localized to the region of the medial epicondyle. It is constant and is made worse with active contraction of the wrist. Patients will note the inability to hold a coffee cup or hammer. Sleep disturbance is common. On physical examination, there will be tenderness along the flexor tendons at or just below the medial epicondyle. Many patients with golfer's elbow will exhibit a bandlike thickening within the affected flexor tendons. Elbow range of motion will be normal. Grip strength on the affected side will be diminished. Patients with golfer's elbow will demonstrate a positive golfer's elbow test. The test is performed by stabilizing the patient's forearm and then having the patient actively flex the wrist. The examiner then attempts to force the wrist into extension. Sudden severe pain is highly suggestive of golfer's elbow.

Testing

Plain radiographs are indicated in all patients who present with golfer's elbow to rule out joint mice and other occult bony pathology. Based on the patient's clinical presentation, additional testing including complete blood count, uric acid, erythrocyte sedimentation rate, and antinuclear antibody testing may be indicated. Magnetic resonance imaging (MRI) of the elbow is indicated if joint instability is suspected. Electromyography is indicated to diagnose entrapment neuropathy at the elbow and to help distinguish golfer's elbow from cervical radiculopathy. The injection technique described below will serve as both a diagnostic and therapeutic maneuver.

Differential Diagnosis

Occasionally, C6-7 radiculopathy can mimic golfer's elbow. The patient suffering from cervical radiculopathy will usually have neck pain and proximal upper extremity pain in addition to symptoms below the elbow. Electromyography will help distinguish radiculopathy from golfer's elbow. Bursitis, arthritis, and gout may also mimic golfer's elbow and may confuse the diagnosis. The olecranon bursa lies in the posterior aspect of the elbow joint and may also become inflamed as a result of direct trauma or overuse of the joint. Other bursae susceptible to the development of bursitis exist between the insertion of the biceps and the head of the radius, as well as in the antecubital and cubital area.

Treatment

Initial treatment of the pain and functional disability associated with golfer's elbow should include a combination of the nonsteroidal anti-inflammatory agents or cyclooxygenase-2 inhibitors and physical therapy. The local application of heat and cold may also be beneficial. Any repetitive activity that may exacerbate the patient's symptomatology should be avoided. For patients who do not respond to these treatment modalities, the following injection technique may be a reasonable next step.

SUGGESTED READINGS

Waldman SD: Golfer's elbow. In: Atlas of Common Pain Syndromes, ed 2. Philadelphia, Saunders, 2008.
Waldman SD: The golfer's elbow test. In: Physical Diagnosis of Pain: An Atlas of Signs and Symptoms. Philadelphia, Saunders, 2006.

CHAPTER 156

Radial Tunnel Syndrome

Radial tunnel syndrome is an uncommon cause of lateral elbow pain that has the unique distinction among the entrapment neuropathies of almost always being initially misdiagnosed. The incidence of misdiagnosis of radial tunnel syndrome is in fact so common that it is often incorrectly referred to under the name of *resistant tennis elbow*. As will be seen from the following discussion, the only major similarity that radial tunnel syndrome and tennis elbow share is the fact that both clinical syndromes produce lateral elbow pain.

The lateral elbow pain of radial tunnel syndrome is aching in nature and is localized to the deep extensor muscle mass. The pain may radiate proximally and distally into the upper arm and forearm. The intensity of the pain of radial tunnel syndrome is mild to moderate but may produce significant functional disability.

In radial tunnel syndrome, the posterior interosseous branch of the radial nerve is entrapped by a variety of mechanisms that have in common a similar clinical presentation. These mechanisms include aberrant fibrous bands in front of the radial head, anomalous blood vessels that compress the nerve, and/or a sharp tendinous margin of the extensor carpi radialis brevis. These entrapments may exist alone or in combination.

Signs and Symptoms

Regardless of the mechanism of entrapment of the radial nerve, the common clinical feature of radial tunnel syndrome is pain just below the lateral epicondyle of the humerus. The pain of radial tunnel syndrome may develop after an acute twisting injury or direct trauma to the soft tissues overlying the posterior interosseous branch of the radial nerve, or the onset may be more insidious without an obvious inciting factor. The pain is constant and is made worse with active supination of the wrist. Patients will often note the inability to hold a coffee cup or hammer. Sleep disturbance is common. On physical examination, elbow range of motion will be normal. Grip strength on the affected side may be diminished.

In the classic text on entrapment neuropathies, Dawson et al. (Entrapment Neuropathies, ed 2. Boston, Little, Brown, 1990) note three important signs that will allow the clinician to distinguish radial tunnel syndrome from tennis elbow: (1) tenderness to palpation distal to the radial head in the muscle mass of the extensors rather than over the more proximal lateral epicondyle, as in tennis elbow; (2) increasing pain on active resisted supination of the forearm due to compression of the radial nerve by the arcade of Frohse as a result of contraction of the muscle mass; and (3) a positive result on the middle finger test. The middle finger test is performed by having the patient extend his or her forearm, wrist, and middle finger and sustain this action against resistance. Patients suffering from radial tunnel syndrome will exhibit increased lateral elbow pain due to fixation and compression of the radial nerve by the extensor carpi radialis brevis muscle.

Testing

Because of the ambiguity and confusion surrounding this clinical syndrome, testing is important to help confirm the diagnosis of radial tunnel syndrome. Electromyography helps to distinguish cervical radiculopathy and radial tunnel syndrome from tennis elbow. Plain radiographs are indicated in all patients who present with radial tunnel syndrome to rule out occult bony pathology. Based on the patient's clinical presentation, additional testing including complete blood cell count, uric acid, sedimentation rate, and antinuclear antibody testing may be indicated.

Magnetic resonance imaging of the elbow is indicated if internal derangement of the joint is suspected and may also help identify the factors responsible for the nerve entrapment, such as ganglion cysts, lipomas, etc.

The injection technique of the radial nerve at the elbow with a local anesthetic and steroid may help confirm the diagnosis as well as treat the syndrome.

Differential Diagnosis

Cervical radiculopathy and tennis elbow can mimic radial tunnel syndrome. Radial tunnel syndrome can be distinguished from tennis elbow in that with radial tunnel syndrome, the maximal tenderness to palpation is distal to the lateral epicondyle over the posterior interosseous branch of the radial nerve, whereas with tennis elbow, the maximal tenderness to palpation is over the lateral epicondyle. Increased pain with active supination as well as a positive middle finger test (see earlier) will help strengthen the diagnosis of radial tunnel syndrome. Acute gout affecting the elbow will present as a diffuse acute inflammatory condition that may be difficult to distinguish from infection of the joint, rather than a localized nerve entrapment.

Treatment

Initial treatment of the pain and functional disability associated with radial tunnel syndrome should include a combination of the nonsteroidal anti-inflammatory agents or cyclooxygenase-2 inhibitors and physical therapy. The local application of heat and cold may also be beneficial. The repetitive movements that incite the syndrome should be avoided. For patients who do not respond to these treatment modalities, injection of the radial nerve at the elbow with a local anesthetic and steroid may be a reasonable next step. If the symptoms of radial tunnel syndrome persist, surgical exploration and decompression of the radial nerve are indicated.

SUGGESTED READINGS

Waldman SD: Radial tunnel syndrome. In: Atlas of Uncommon Pain Syndromes, ed 2. Philadelphia, Saunders, 2008.
Waldman SD: The compression test for radial tunnel syndrome. In: Physical Diagnosis of Pain: An Atlas of Signs and Symptoms. Philadelphia, Saunders, 2006.

CHAPTER 157

Ulnar Nerve Entrapment at the Elbow

Ulnar nerve entrapment at the elbow is one of the most common entrapment neuropathies encountered in clinical practice. The causes include compression of the ulnar nerve by an aponeurotic band that runs from the medial epicondyle of the humerus to the medial border of the olecranon, direct trauma to the ulnar nerve at the elbow, and repetitive elbow motion. Ulnar nerve entrapment at the elbow is also called tardy ulnar palsy, cubital tunnel syndrome, and ulnar nerve neuritis. This entrapment neuropathy presents as pain and associated paresthesias in the lateral forearm that radiates to the wrist and ring and little finger. Some patients suffering from ulnar nerve entrapment at the elbow may also notice pain referred to the medial aspect of the scapula on the affected side. Untreated, ulnar nerve entrapment at the elbow can result in a progressive motor deficit and ultimately flexion contracture of the affected fingers can result. The onset of symptoms is usually after repetitive elbow motions or from repeated pressure on the elbow such as using the elbows to arise from bed. Direct trauma to the ulnar nerve as it enters the cubital tunnel may also result in a similar clinical presentation. Patients with vulnerable nerve syndrome, e.g., diabetics and alcoholics, are at greater risk for the development of ulnar nerve entrapment at the elbow.

Signs and Symptoms

Physical findings include tenderness over the ulnar nerve at the elbow. A positive Tinel sign over the ulnar nerve as it passes beneath the aponeurosis is usually present. Weakness of the intrinsic muscles of the forearm and hand that are innervated by the ulnar nerve may be identified with careful manual muscle testing, although early in the course of the evolution of cubital tunnel syndrome, the only physical finding other than tenderness over the nerve may be the loss of sensation on the ulnar side of the little finger. Muscle wasting of the intrinsic muscles of the hand can best be identified by viewing the hand with the palm down. Tinel's sign at the elbow is often present when the ulnar nerve is stimulated.

Testing

Electromyography and nerve conduction velocity testing are extremely sensitive tests; the skilled electromyographer can diagnose ulnar nerve entrapment at the elbow with a high degree of accuracy as well as help sort out other neuropathic causes of pain that may mimic ulnar nerve entrapment at the elbow, including radiculopathy and plexopathy (see later). Plain radiographs are indicated in all patients who present with ulnar nerve entrapment at the elbow to rule out occult bony pathology. If surgery is contemplated, a magnetic resonance imaging (MRI) scan of the affected elbow may help further delineate the pathologic process responsible for the nerve entrapment, e.g., bone spur or aponeurotic band thickening. If Pancoast's tumor or other tumors of the brachial plexus are suspected, chest x-rays with apical lordotic views may be helpful. Screening laboratory testing consisting of complete blood count, erythrocyte sedimentation rate, antinuclear antibody testing, and automated blood chemistry testing should be performed if the diagnosis of ulnar nerve entrapment at the elbow is in question to help rule out other causes of the patient's pain. The injection technique described below will serve as both a diagnostic and therapeutic maneuver.

Differential Diagnosis

Ulnar nerve entrapment at the elbow is often misdiagnosed as golfer's elbow and this fact accounts for the many patients whose "golfer's elbow" fails to respond to conservative measures. Cubital tunnel syndrome can be distinguished from golfer's elbow in that in cubital tunnel syndrome, the maximal tenderness to palpation is over the ulnar nerve, one inch below the medial epicondyle, whereas with golfer's elbow, the maximal tenderness to palpation is directly over the medial epicondyle. Cubital tunnel syndrome should also be differentiated from cervical radiculopathy involving the C7 or C8 roots and golfer's elbow. Furthermore, it should be remembered that cervical radiculopathy and ulnar nerve entrapment may coexist as the so-called "double crush" syndrome. The double crush syndrome is seen most commonly with median nerve entrapment at the wrist or carpal tunnel syndrome.

Treatment

A short course of conservative therapy consisting of simple analgesics, nonsteroidal anti-inflammatory agents or cyclooxygenase-2 inhibitors, and splinting to avoid elbow flexion is indicated in patients who present with ulnar nerve entrapment at the elbow. If the patient does not experience a marked improvement in symptoms within 1 week, careful injection of the ulnar nerve at the elbow is a reasonable next step.

If the patient does not respond to the above-mentioned treatments or if the patient is experiencing progressive neurologic deficit, strong consideration of surgical decompression of the ulnar nerve is indicated. As mentioned, MRI scanning of the affected elbow

should help clarify the pathology responsible for compression of the ulnar nerve.

SUGGESTED READINGS

Campbell W: DeJong's The Neurological Examination, ed 6. Philadelphia, Lippincott Williams and Wilkins, 2005.

Goetz CG: Textbook of Clinical Neurology, ed 2. Philadelphia, Saunders, 2003.

Waldman SD: Ulnar nerve entrapment at the elbow. In: Atlas of Common Pain Syndromes, ed 2. Philadelphia, Saunders, 2008.

CHAPTER 158

Anterior Interosseous Syndrome

Anterior interosseous syndrome is an uncommon cause of forearm and wrist pain. The onset of symptoms in patients suffering from anterior interosseous syndrome is usually after acute trauma to the forearm or after repetitive forearm and elbow motions such as using an ice pick. It is thought that in this setting, the pain and muscle weakness of anterior interosseous syndrome are secondary to median nerve compression just below the elbow by the tendinous origins of the pronator teres muscle and flexor digitorum superficialis muscle of the long finger or by aberrant blood vessels. In some patients, no antecedent trauma is identified and an inflammatory etiology analogous to Parsonage-Turner syndrome has been suggested as the etiology of anterior interosseous syndrome in the absence of trauma.

Clinically, anterior interosseous syndrome presents as an acute pain in the proximal forearm and deep in the wrist. As the syndrome progresses, patients with anterior interosseous syndrome may complain about a tired or heavy sensation in the forearm with minimal activity as well as the inability to pinch items between the thumb and index finger due to paralysis of the flexor pollicis longus and the flexor digitorum profundus.

Signs and Symptoms

Physical findings include the inability to flex the interphalangeal joint of the thumb and the distal interphalangeal joint of the index finger due to paralysis of the flexor pollicis longus and the flexor digitorum profundus.

Tenderness over the forearm in the region of the pronator teres muscle is seen in some patients suffering from anterior interosseous syndrome. A positive Tinels sign over the anterior interosseous branch of the median nerve approximately 6 to 8 cm below the elbow may also be present.

Testing

Electromyography helps to distinguish cervical radiculopathy, thoracic outlet syndrome, and carpal tunnel syndrome from anterior interosseous syndrome. Plain radiographs are indicated in all patients who present with anterior interosseous syndrome to rule out occult bony pathology. Based on the patient's clinical presentation, additional testing including complete blood cell count, uric acid, sedimentation rate, and antinuclear antibody testing may be indicated. Magnetic resonance imaging of the forearm is indicated if primary elbow pathology or a space-occupying lesion is suspected. The injection of the median nerve at the elbow will serve as both a diagnostic and therapeutic maneuver.

Differential Diagnosis

The anterior interosseous syndrome should also be differentiated from cervical radiculopathy involving the C6 or C7 roots that may at times mimic median nerve compression. Furthermore, it should be remembered that cervical radiculopathy and median nerve entrapment may coexist as the "double crush" syndrome. The double crush syndrome is seen most commonly with median nerve entrapment at the wrist or carpal tunnel syndrome. Anterior interosseous syndrome can be distinguished from pronator syndrome and median nerve compression by the ligament of Struthers in that the pain of anterior interosseous syndrome occurs more distally and is accompanied by the characteristic loss of ability to pinch items between the thumb and index finger.

Treatment

The nonsteroidal anti-inflammatory agents or cyclooxygenase-2 inhibitors represent a reasonable first step in the treatment of anterior interosseous syndrome.

The use of the tricyclic antidepressants such as nortriptyline at a single bedtime dose of 25 mg titrating upward as side effects allow will also be useful, especially if sleep disturbance is also present. Avoidance of repetitive trauma thought to be contributing to this entrapment neuropathy is also important. If these maneuvers fail to produce rapid symptomatic relief, injection of the median nerve at the elbow with a local anesthetic and steroid is a reasonable next step. If symptoms continue to persist, surgical exploration and release of the anterior interosseous branch of the median nerve are indicated.

SUGGESTED READING

Waldman SD: Anterior interosseous syndrome. In: Atlas of Uncommon Pain Syndromes, ed 2. Philadelphia, Saunders, 2008.

CHAPTER 159

Olecranon Bursitis

Olecranon bursitis may develop gradually, owing to repetitive irritation of the olecranon bursa, or acutely because of trauma or infection. The olecranon bursa lies in the posterior aspect of the elbow between the olecranon process of the ulna and the overlying skin. It may exist as a single bursal sac or, in some patients, as a multisegmented series of sacs that may be loculated in nature. With overuse or misuse, these bursae may become inflamed, enlarged, and, on rare occasions, infected. The swelling associated with olecranon bursitis may at times be quite impressive, and the patient may complain about difficulty in wearing a long-sleeved shirt.

The olecranon bursa is vulnerable to injury from both acute trauma and repeated microtrauma. Acute injuries frequently take the form of direct trauma to the elbow when playing sports such as hockey or falling directly onto the olecranon process. Repeated pressure from leaning on the elbow to arise or from working long hours at a drafting table may result in inflammation and swelling of the olecranon bursa. Gout or bacterial infection may rarely precipitate acute olecranon bursitis. If the inflammation of the olecranon bursa becomes chronic, calcification of the bursa may occur with residual nodules called *gravel* resulting.

Signs and Symptoms

The patient suffering from olecranon bursitis will frequently complain of pain and swelling with any movement of the elbow but especially with extension. The pain is localized to the olecranon area with referred pain often noted above the elbow joint. Often, the patient will be more concerned about the swelling around the bursa than the pain. Physical examination will reveal point tenderness over the olecranon and swelling of the bursa, which at times can be quite extensive. Passive extension and resisted shoulder flexion will reproduce the pain, as will any pressure over the bursa. Fever and chills will usually accompany infection of the bursa. If infection is suspected, aspiration, Gram stain, and culture of the bursa followed by treatment with appropriate antibiotics are indicated on an emergent basis.

Testing

The diagnosis of olecranon bursitis is usually made on clinical grounds alone. Plain radiographs of the posterior elbow are indicated if there is a history of elbow trauma or arthritis of the elbow is suspected. Plain radiographs may also reveal calcification of the bursa and associated structures consistent with chronic inflammation. Magnetic resonance imaging is indicated if joint instability is suspected. Complete blood count, automated chemistry profile including uric acid, sedimentation rate, and antinuclear antibody testing are indicated if collagen vascular disease is suspected. If infection is considered, aspiration, Gram stain, and culture of bursal fluid are indicated on an emergent basis.

Differential Diagnosis

Olecranon bursitis is usually a straightforward clinical diagnosis. Occasionally, rheumatoid nodules or gouty arthritis of the elbow may confuse the clinician. Synovial cysts of the elbow may also mimic olecranon bursitis. It should be remembered that coexistent tendinitis (e.g., tennis elbow and golfer's elbow) may require additional treatment.

Treatment

A short course of conservative therapy consisting of simple analgesics, nonsteroidal anti-inflammatory agents or cyclooxygenase-2 inhibitors, and an elbow protector to prevent further trauma is a reasonable first step in the treatment of patients suffering from olecranon bursitis. If the patient does not experience rapid improvement, injection of the inflamed bursa with local anesthetic and methylprednisolone is a reasonable next step.

SUGGESTED READING

Waldman SD: Olecranon bursitis. In: Atlas of Common Pain Syndromes, ed 2. Philadelphia, Saunders, 2008.

CHAPTER 160

Carpal Tunnel Syndrome

Carpal tunnel syndrome is the most common entrapment neuropathy encountered in clinical practice. It is caused by compression of the median nerve as it passes through the carpal canal at the wrist. The most common causes of compression of the median nerve at this anatomic location include flexor tenosynovitis, rheumatoid arthritis, pregnancy, amyloidosis, and other space-occupying lesions that compromise the median nerve as it passes though this closed space. This entrapment neuropathy presents as pain, numbness, paresthesias, and associated weakness in the hand and wrist that radiate to the thumb, index, middle, and radial half of the ring fingers (Fig. 160-1). These symptoms may also radiate proximal to the entrapment into the forearm. Untreated, progressive motor deficit and, ultimately, flexion contracture of the affected fingers can result. The onset of symptoms is usually after repetitive wrist motions or from repeated pressure on the wrist such as resting the wrists on the edge of a computer keyboard. Direct trauma to the median nerve as it enters the carpal tunnel may result in a similar clinical presentation.

Signs and Symptoms

Physical findings include tenderness over the median nerve at the wrist. A positive Tinel sign over the median nerve as it passes beneath the flexor retinaculum is usually present. A positive Phalen test is highly suggestive of carpal tunnel syndrome. Phalen's test is performed by having patients place their wrists in complete unforced flexion for at least 30 seconds. If the median nerve is entrapped at the wrist, this maneuver will reproduce the symptoms of carpal tunnel syndrome. Weakness of thumb opposition and wasting of the thenar eminence are often seen in advanced carpal tunnel syndrome, although because of the complex motion of the thumb, subtle motor deficits may easily be missed. Early in the course of the evolution of carpal tunnel syndrome, the only physical finding other than tenderness over the nerve may be the loss of sensation on the above-mentioned fingers.

Testing

Electromyography will help distinguish cervical radiculopathy and diabetic polyneuropathy from carpal tunnel syndrome. Plain radiographs are indicated in all patients who present with carpal tunnel syndrome to rule out occult bony pathology. Based on the patient's clinical presentation, additional testing including complete blood count, uric acid, erythrocyte sedimentation rate, and antinuclear antibody testing may be indicated. Magnetic resonance imaging of the wrist is indicated if joint instability or a space-occupying lesion is suspected.

Differential Diagnosis

Carpal tunnel syndrome is often misdiagnosed as arthritis of the carpometacarpal joint of the thumb, cervical radiculopathy, or diabetic polyneuropathy. Patients with arthritis of the carpometacarpal joint of the thumb will have a positive Watson's test and radiographic evidence of arthritis. Most patients suffering from a cervical radiculopathy will have reflex, motor, and sensory changes associated with neck pain, whereas patients with carpal tunnel syndrome will have no reflex changes and motor and sensory changes will be limited to the distal median nerve. Diabetic polyneuropathy will generally present as symmetrical sensory deficit involving the entire hand rather than limited just in the distribution of the median nerve. It should be remembered that cervical radiculopathy and median nerve entrapment may coexist as the so-called "double crush" syndrome. Furthermore, because carpal tunnel syndrome is commonly seen in patients with diabetes, it is not surprising that diabetic polyneuropathy is usually present in diabetic patients with carpal tunnel syndrome.

Treatment

Mild cases of carpal tunnel syndrome will usually respond to conservative therapy, and surgery should be reserved for more severe cases. Initial treatment of carpal tunnel syndrome should consist of simple analgesics, nonsteroidal anti-inflammatory agents or cyclooxygenase-2 inhibitors, and splinting of the wrist. At a minimum, the splint should be worn at night, but ideally it should be worn for 24 hours a day. Avoidance of repetitive activities thought to be responsible for the evolution of carpal tunnel syndrome (e.g., keyboard use, hammering, etc.) will also help ameliorate the patient's symptoms. If the patient fails to respond to these conservative measures, a next reasonable step is injection of the carpal tunnel with local anesthetic and steroid.

SUGGESTED READINGS

Campbell W: DeJong's The Neurological Examination, ed 6. Philadelphia, Lippincott Williams and Wilkins, 2005.

Goetz CG: Textbook of Clinical Neurology, ed 2. Philadelphia, Saunders, 2003.

Waldman SD: Carpal tunnel syndrome. In: Atlas of Common Pain Syndromes, ed 2. Philadelphia, Saunders, 2008.

Waldman SD: The Tinel sign for carpal tunnel syndrome. In: Physical Diagnosis of Pain: An Atlas of Signs and Symptoms. Philadelphia, Saunders, 2006.

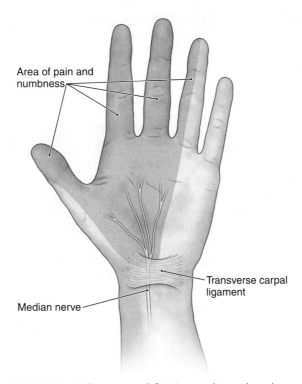

FIGURE 160–1 The sensory deficit in carpal tunnel syndrome.

Area of pain and numbness

Transverse carpal ligament

Median nerve

CHAPTER 161

Cheiralgia Paresthetica

Cheiralgia paresthetica is an uncommon cause of wrist and hand pain and numbness. It is also known as *handcuff neuropathy*. The onset of symptoms of cheiralgia paresthetica is usually after compression of the sensory branch of the radial nerve. Radial nerve dysfunction secondary to compression by tight handcuffs, wristwatch bands, or casts is a common cause of cheiralgia paresthetica.

Direct trauma to the nerve may also result in a similar clinical presentation. Fractures or lacerations frequently completely disrupt the nerve, resulting in sensory deficit in the distribution of the radial nerve. The sensory branch of the radial nerve may also be damaged during surgical treatment of de Quervain's tenosynovitis.

Cheiralgia paresthetica presents as pain and associated paresthesias and numbness of the radial aspect of the dorsum of the hand to the base of the thumb. Because there is significant interpatient variability in the distribution of the sensory branch of the radial nerve due to overlap of the lateral antebrachial cutaneous nerve, the signs and symptoms of cheiralgia paresthetica may vary from patient to patient.

Signs and Symptoms

Physical findings include tenderness over the radial nerve at the wrist. A positive Tinel's sign over the radial nerve at the distal forearm is usually present. Decreased sensation in the distribution of the sensory branch of the radial nerve is often present, although as mentioned, the overlap of the lateral antebrachial cutaneous nerve may result in a confusing clinical presentation. A positive wristwatch sign may also be present. Flexion and pronation of the wrist, as well as ulnar deviation, often cause paresthesias in the distribution of the sensory branch of the radial nerve in patients suffering from cheiralgia paresthetica.

Testing

Electromyography can help to identify the exact source of neurologic dysfunction and to clarify the differential diagnosis and thus should be the starting point of the evaluation of all patients suspected of having cheiralgia paresthetica. Plain radiographs are indicated in all patients who present with cheiralgia paresthetica to rule out occult bony pathology. Based on the patient's clinical presentation, additional testing including complete blood cell count, uric acid, erythrocyte sedimentation rate, and antinuclear antibody testing may be indicated. Magnetic resonance imaging of the elbow is indicated if joint instability is suspected. Injection of the sensory branch of the radial nerve at the wrist will serve as both a diagnostic and therapeutic maneuver and may be used as an anatomic differential neural blockade to distinguish lesions of the sensory branch of the radial nerve from lesions involving the lateral antebrachial cutaneous nerve.

Differential Diagnosis

Cheiralgia paresthetica is often misdiagnosed as lateral antebrachial cutaneous nerve syndrome. Cheiralgia paresthetica should also be differentiated from cervical radiculopathy involving the C6 or C7 roots, although patients with cervical radiculopathy will generally present not only with pain and numbness but also with reflex and motor changes. Furthermore, it should be remembered that cervical radiculopathy and radial nerve entrapment may coexist as the "double crush" syndrome. The double crush syndrome is seen most commonly with median nerve entrapment at the wrist or carpal tunnel syndrome.

Treatment

The first step in the treatment of cheiralgia paresthetica is the removal of the cause of pressure on the radial nerve. A trial of the nonsteroidal anti-inflammatory agents or the cyclooxygenase-2 inhibitors represents a reasonable next step. For patients for whom these treatment modalities fail, injection of the sensory branch of the radial nerve at the wrist with a local anesthetic and steroid should be considered. For persistent symptoms, surgical exploration and decompression of the radial nerve are indicated.

SUGGESTED READINGS

Campbell W: DeJong's The Neurological Examination, ed 6. Philadelphia, Lippincott Williams and Wilkins, 2005.
Goetz CG: Textbook of Clinical Neurology, ed 2. Philadelphia, Saunders, 2003.
Waldman SD: Cheiralgia paraesthetica. In: Atlas of Uncommon Pain Syndromes, ed 2. Philadelphia, Saunders, 2008.
Waldman SD: The wristwatch test for cheiralgia paresthetica. In: Physical Diagnosis of Pain: An Atlas of Signs and Symptoms. Philadelphia, Saunders, 2006.

CHAPTER 162

de Quervain's Tenosynovitis

de Quervain's tenosynovitis is caused by an inflammation and swelling of the tendons of the abductor pollicis longus and extensor pollicis brevis at the level of the radial styloid process. This inflammation and swelling are usually the result of trauma to the tendon from repetitive twisting motions. If the inflammation and swelling become chronic, a thickening of the tendon sheath occurs with a resulting constriction of the sheath. A triggering phenomenon may result with the tendon catching within the sheath, causing the thumb to lock or "trigger." Arthritis and gout of the first metacarpal joint may also coexist with de Quervain's tenosynovitis and exacerbate the pain and disability of de Quervain's tenosynovitis.

de Quervain's tenosynovitis occurs in patients engaged in repetitive activities that include hand grasping, such as politicians shaking hands, or high-torque wrist turning, such as scooping ice cream at an ice cream parlor. de Quervain's tenosynovitis may also develop without obvious antecedent trauma in the parturient.

The pain of de Quervain's tenosynovitis is localized to the region of the radial styloid. It is constant and is made worse with active pinching activities of the thumb or ulnar deviation of the wrist. Patients will note the inability to hold a coffee cup or turn a screwdriver. Sleep disturbance is common.

Signs and Symptoms

On physical examination, there will be tenderness and swelling over the tendons and tendon sheaths along the distal radius with point tenderness over the radial styloid. Many patients with de Quervain's tenosynovitis will exhibit a creaking sensation with flexion and extension of the thumb. Range of motion of the thumb may be decreased due to the pain, and a trigger thumb phenomenon may be noted. Patients with de Quervain's tenosynovitis will demonstrate a positive Finkelstein test. The Finkelstein test is performed by stabilizing the patient's forearm and then having the patient fully flex his or her thumb into the palm and then actively forcing the wrist toward the ulna. Sudden severe pain is highly suggestive of de Quervain's tenosynovitis.

Testing

There is no specific test to diagnose de Quervain's tenosynovitis. The diagnosis is generally made on clinical grounds. Electromyography will help distinguish de Quervain's tenosynovitis from neuropathic processes such as cervical radiculopathy and cheiralgia paresthetica. Plain radiographs are indicated in all patients who present with de Quervain's tenosynovitis to rule out occult bony pathology. Based on the patient's clinical presentation, additional testing including complete blood count, uric acid, erythrocyte sedimentation rate, and antinuclear antibody testing may be indicated. Magnetic resonance imaging of the wrist is indicated if joint instability is suspected.

Differential Diagnosis

Entrapment of the lateral antebrachial cutaneous nerve, arthritis of the first metacarpal joint, gout, cheiralgia paresthetica, and occasionally C6-7 radiculopathy can mimic de Quervain's tenosynovitis. Cheiralgia paresthetica is an entrapment neuropathy that is the result of entrapment of the superficial branch of the radial nerve at the wrist. All of these painful conditions can coexist with de Quervain's tenosynovitis.

Treatment

Initial treatment of the pain and functional disability associated with de Quervain's tenosynovitis should include a combination of the nonsteroidal anti-inflammatory agents or cyclooxygenase-2 inhibitors and physical therapy. The local application of heat and cold may also be beneficial. Any repetitive activity that may exacerbate the patient's symptomatology should be avoided. Night-time splinting of the affected thumb may also help avoid the "trigger finger" phenomenon that can occur upon awakening in many patients suffering from this condition. For patients who do not respond to these treatment modalities, injection of the tenosynovitis is a reasonable next step.

SUGGESTED READING

Waldman SD: de Quervain's tenosynovitis. In: Atlas of Common Pain Syndromes, ed 2. Philadelphia, Saunders, 2008.

CHAPTER 163

Dupuytren's Contracture

Dupuytren's contracture is a common complaint encountered in clinical practice. Although initially painful, patients suffering from Dupuytren's contracture generally seek medical help due to the functional disability rather than the pain. Dupuytren's contracture is caused by a progressive fibrosis of the palmar fascia. Initially, the patient may notice fibrotic nodules along the course of the flexor tendons of the hand that are tender to palpation. These nodules arise from the palmar fascia and initially do not involve the flexor tendons. As the disease advances, these fibrous nodules coalesce and form fibrous bands that gradually thicken and contract around the flexor tendons, which has the effect of drawing the affected fingers into flexion. Although all fingers can develop Dupuytren's contracture, the ring and little finger are most commonly affected. If untreated, the fingers will develop permanent flexion contractures. The pain of Dupuytren's contracture seems to burn itself out as the disease progresses.

Dupuytren's contracture is thought to have a genetic basis and occurs most frequently in males of northern

Scandinavian descent. The disease may also be associated with trauma to the palm, diabetes, alcoholism, and chronic barbiturate use. The disease rarely occurs before the fourth decade. The plantar fascia may also be concurrently affected.

Signs and Symptoms

In the early stages of the disease, hard fibrotic nodules along the path of the flexor tendons may be palpated. These nodules are often misdiagnosed as calluses or warts. At this early stage, pain is invariably present. As the disease progresses, the clinician will note taut fibrous bands that may cross the metacarpophalangeal joint and ultimately the proximal interphalangeal joint. These bands are not painful to palpation, and although they limit finger extension, finger flexion remains relatively normal. It is at this point that patients will often seek medical advice as they began having difficulty putting on gloves and reaching into their pocket to retrieve keys. In the final stages of the disease, the flexion contracture develops with its attendant negative impact on function. Coexistent arthritis, gout of the metacarpal and interphalangeal joints, and trigger finger may also coexist with Dupuytren's contracture and exacerbate the pain and disability of Dupuytren's contracture.

Testing

Plain radiographs are indicated in all patients who present with Dupuytren's contracture to rule out underlying occult bony pathology. Based on the patient's clinical presentation, additional testing including complete blood count, uric acid, erythrocyte sedimentation rate, and antinuclear antibody testing also may be indicated. Magnetic resonance imaging of the hand is indicated if joint instability or tumor is suspected. Electromyography is indicated if coexistent ulnar or carpal tunnel is suspected. Injection treatment may provide transient improvement of the pain and disability of this disease, but surgical treatment may ultimately be required to restore function.

Differential Diagnosis

Dupuytren's contracture is the result of the thickening of the palmar fascia and its effect on the flexor tendons, and it represents a clinically distinct entity that is rarely misdiagnosed once the syndrome is well established. Coexistent flexor tendinitis or occasionally trigger finger may be confused with Dupuytren's contracture early in the course of the disease.

Treatment

Initial treatment of the pain and functional disability associated with Dupuytren's contracture should include a combination of the nonsteroidal anti-inflammatory agents or cyclooxygenase-2 inhibitors and physical therapy. The use of physical modalities, including local heat, as well as gentle range of motion exercises, may also be helpful. A nighttime splint to protect the fingers may also help relieve the symptoms of trigger thumb. Vigorous exercises should be avoided as they will exacerbate the patient's symptomatology. Injection of Dupuytren's contracture with local anesthetic and steroid may also be effective in the management of the symptoms associated with this disease.

SUGGESTED READING

Waldman SD: Dupuytren's contracture. In: Atlas of Common Pain Syndromes, ed 2. Philadelphia, Saunders, 2008.

Diabetic Truncal Neuropathy

Diabetic neuropathy is the name used by clinicians to describe a heterogeneous group of diseases that affect the autonomic and peripheral nervous systems of patients suffering from diabetes mellitus. Diabetic neuropathy is now thought to be the most common form of peripheral neuropathy that afflicts humankind, with an estimated 220 million people suffering from this malady worldwide.

One of the most commonly encountered forms of diabetes neuropathy is diabetic truncal neuropathy. The pain and motor dysfunction of diabetic truncal neuropathy is often attributed to intrathoracic or intra-abdominal pathology leading to extensive workups for appendicitis, cholecystitis, renal calculi, etc. The onset of symptoms will frequently coincide with periods of extreme hypoglycemia or hyperglycemia or with weight loss or weight gain. The patient presenting with diabetic truncal neuropathy will complain of severe dysesthetic pain with patchy sensory deficits in the distribution of the lower thoracic and/or upper thoracic dermatomes. The pain will often be worse at night, and significant sleep disturbance may result, further worsening the patient's pain symptomatology. The symptoms of diabetic truncal neuropathy will often spontaneously resolve over a period of 6 to 12 months. However, due to the severity of symptoms associated with this condition, aggressive symptomatic relief with pharmacotherapy and neural blockade with local anesthetics and steroids is indicated.

Signs and Symptoms

Physical examination of the patient suffering from diabetic truncal neuropathy will generally reveal minimal physical findings unless there was a history of previous thoracic or subcostal surgery or cutaneous findings of herpes zoster involving the thoracic dermatomes. In contradistinction to the above-mentioned musculoskeletal causes of chest wall and subcostal pain, the patient suffering from diabetic truncal neuropathy does not attempt to splint or protect the affected area. Careful sensory examination of the affected dermatomes may reveal decreased sensation or allodynia. With significant motor involvement of the subcostal nerve, the patient may complain that the abdomen bulges out.

Testing

The presence of diabetes should raise a high index of suspicion that diabetic truncal neuropathy is present given the high incidence of this condition in patients suffering from diabetes mellitus. The targeted history and physical examination should allow the primary care physician to make the diagnosis of peripheral neuropathies in a large percentage of their patients suffering from diabetes.

If a diagnosis of diabetic truncal neuropathy is entertained on the basis of the targeted history and physical, screening laboratory testing including a complete blood count, chemistry profile, erythrocyte sedimentation rate, thyroid function studies, antinuclear antibody testing, and urinalysis should help rule out most peripheral neuropathies that may mimic diabetic truncal neuropathy and that are easily treatable. Electromyography and nerve conduction velocity testing are indicated in all patients suffering from peripheral neuropathy to help identify treatable entrapment neuropathies and further delineate the type of peripheral neuropathy that is present. Electromyography and nerve conduction velocity testing may also help quantify the severity of peripheral and/or entrapment neuropathy. Additional laboratory testing is indicated as the clinical situation dictates (e.g., Lyme disease titers, heavy metal screens, etc.). Magnetic resonance imaging of the spinal canal and cord should be performed if myelopathy is suspected. Nerve and/or skin biopsy is occasionally indicated if no etiology for the peripheral neuropathy can be ascertained. Lack of response to the therapies presented later should cause the primary care physician to reconsider the working diagnosis and repeat testing as clinically indicated.

Differential Diagnosis

It should be remembered that diseases other than diabetic neuropathy may cause peripheral neuropathies in diabetic patients. These diseases may exist alone and may be clinically misdiagnosed as diabetic truncal neuropathy or may coexist with diabetic truncal neuropathy, making their identification and subsequent treatment more difficult.

Although uncommon in the United States, globally, Hansen's disease is a common cause of peripheral neuropathy that may mimic or coexist with diabetic truncal neuropathy. Other infectious etiologies of peripheral neuropathies include Lyme disease and human immunodeficiency virus infection. Substances that are toxic to nerves may also cause peripheral neuropathies that are indistinguishable from diabetic neuropathy on clinical grounds. Such substances include alcohol, heavy metals, chemotherapeutic agents, and hydrocarbons. Heritable disorders such as Charcot-Marie-Tooth disease and other familial diseases of the peripheral nervous system must also be considered. although treatment options are somewhat limited. Metabolic and endocrine causes of peripheral neuropathy that must be ruled out include vitamin deficiencies, pernicious anemia, hypothyroidism, uremia, and acute intermittent porphyria. Other causes of peripheral neuropathy that may confuse the clinical picture include Guillain-Barré syndrome, amyloidosis, entrapment neuropathies, carcinoid, paraneoplastic syndromes, and sarcoidosis. Because many of these causes of peripheral neuropathy are treatable (e.g., pernicious anemia), it is imperative that the clinician rule out these treatable diagnosis prior to attributing a patient's symptomatology solely to his or her diabetes.

Intercostal neuralgia and the musculoskeletal causes of chest wall and subcostal pain may also be confused with diabetic truncal neuropathy. As with these conditions, the patient's pain may be erroneously attributed to cardiac or upper abdominal pathology, leading to unnecessary testing and treatment.

Treatment

CONTROL OF BLOOD SUGAR

Current thinking suggests that the better the glycemic control, the less severe is the symptomatology of diabetic truncal neuropathy. Significant swings in blood sugars seem to predispose diabetic patients to the development of clinically significant diabetic truncal neuropathy. Some investigators believe that oral hypoglycemic agents, although controlling blood sugars, do not protect the patient from the development of diabetic truncal neuropathy as well as does insulin. In fact, some patients with diabetic truncal neuropathy who are on hypoglycemic agents will experience improvement in symptomatology when switched to insulin.

PHARMACOLOGIC TREATMENT

Antidepressant Compounds

Traditionally, the tricyclic antidepressants have been a mainstay in the palliation of pain secondary to diabetic truncal neuropathy. Controlled studies have demonstrated the efficacy of amitriptyline for this indication. Other tricyclic antidepressants, including nortriptyline and desipramine, have also been shown to be clinically useful. Unfortunately, this class of drugs is associated with significant anticholinergic side effects, including dry mouth, constipation, sedation, and urinary retention. These drugs should be used with caution in those suffering from glaucoma, cardiac arrhythmia, and prostatism. In order to minimize side effects and encourage compliance, the primary care physician should start amitriptyline or nortriptyline at a 10-mg dose at bedtime. The dose can be then titrated upward to 25 mg at bedtime as side effects allow. Upward titration of dosage in 25-mg increments can be carried out each week as side effects allow. Even at lower doses, patients will generally report a rapid improvement in sleep disturbance and will begin to experience some pain relief in 10 to 14 days. If the patient does not experience any improvement in pain as the dose is being titrated upward, the addition of gabapentin alone or in combination with nerve blocks with local anesthetics and/or steroid is recommended (see later). The selective serotonin reuptake inhibitors such as fluoxetine have also be used to treat the pain of diabetic truncal neuropathy, and although they are better tolerated than the tricyclic antidepressants, they appear to be less efficacious.

Anticonvulsants

The anticonvulsants have long been used to treat neuropathic pain, including diabetic truncal neuropathy. Both phenytoin and carbamazepine have been used with varying degrees of success either alone or in combination with the antidepressant compounds. Unfortunately, the side effect profiles of these drugs have limited their clinical utility. Recently, the anticonvulsant gabapentin has been shown to be highly efficacious in the treatment of a variety of neuropathic painful conditions, including postherpetic neuralgia and diabetic truncal neuropathy. Used properly, gabapentin is extremely well tolerated compared with other drugs, including the antidepressant compounds and anticonvulsants mentioned earlier that previously had routinely been used to treat diabetic truncal neuropathy. In fact, in most pain centers, gabapentin has become the adjuvant analgesic of choice when treating diabetic truncal neuropathy. Gabapentin has a large therapeutic window, but the primary care physician is cautioned to start this medication at the lower end of the dosage spectrum and titrate upward slowly to avoid central nervous system side effects, including sedation and fatigue. The following recommended dosage schedule will minimize side effects and encourage compliance. A single bedtime dose of 300 mg for two nights can be followed with a 300-mg twice-daily dose for an additional 2 days. If the patient is tolerating this twice-daily dosage, the dosage may be increased to 300 mg three times daily. Most patients will begin to experience pain relief at this dosage level. Additional titration upward can be carried out in 300-mg increments as side effects allow. Daily doses above 3600 mg in divided doses are not currently recommended. Recently, 600-mg and 800-mg tables have been made available to simplify maintenance dosing after titration has been completed. Clinical trials are currently under way with a gabapentin analogue, which may provide additional therapeutic options for patients suffering from diabetic truncal neuropathy.

Antiarrhythmics

Mexiletine is an antiarrhythmic compound that has been shown to be possibly effective in the management of diabetic truncal neuropathy. Some pain specialists believe that mexiletine is especially useful in those patients with diabetic truncal neuropathy whose pain manifests primarily as sharp lancinating or burning pain. Unfortunately, this drug is poorly tolerated by most patients and should be reserved for those patients who have failed to respond to first-line pharmacologic treatments such as gabapentin or nortriptyline alone or in combination with neural blockade.

Topical Agents

Some clinicians have reported success in the treatment of diabetic truncal neuropathy with topical application of capsaicin. An extract of chili peppers, capsaicin is thought to relieve neuropathic pain by depleting substance P. The side effects of capsaicin include significant burning and erythema and limit the use of this substance by many patients.

Topical lidocaine administered via transdermal patch or in a gel has also been shown to provide short-term relief of the pain of diabetic truncal neuropathy. This drug should be used with caution in patients that are on mexiletine as there is the potential for cumulative local anesthetic toxicity. Whether topical lidocaine will have a role in the long-term treatment of diabetic truncal neuropathy remains to be seen.

Analgesics

In general, neuropathic pain such as diabetic truncal neuropathy responds poorly to analgesic compounds. The simple analgesics, including acetaminophen and aspirin, can be used in combination with the antidepressant and anticonvulsant compounds, but care must be taken not to exceed the recommended daily dose or renal or hepatic side effects may occur. The nonsteroidal anti-inflammatory agents may also provide a modicum of pain relief when used with the antidepressants and anticonvulsant compounds, but given the nephrotoxicity of this class of drugs, they should be used with extreme caution in diabetic patients due to the high incidence of diabetic nephropathy, even early in the course of the disease. The role of the cyclooxygenase-2 inhibitors in the palliation of the pain has not been adequately studied.

Narcotic analgesics treat neuropathic pain such as diabetic truncal neuropathy poorly. Given the significant central nervous system and gastrointestinal side effects coupled with the problems of tolerance, dependence, and addiction, the narcotic analgesics should rarely, if ever, be used as a primary treatment for the pain of diabetic truncal neuropathy. If a narcotic analgesic is being considered in the setting, consideration should be given to the analgesic tramadol, which binds weakly to the opioid receptors and may provide some symptomatic relief. Tramadol should be used with care in combination with the antidepressant compounds to avoid the increased risk of seizures.

Neural Blockade

The use of neural blockade with local anesthetics either alone or in combination with steroids has been shown to been useful in the management of both the acute and chronic pain associated with diabetic truncal neuropathy. For truncal neuropathic pain, thoracic epidural or intercostal nerve block with local anesthetic and/or steroid may be beneficial. Occasionally, neuroaugmentation via spinal cord stimulation may provide significant relief of the pain of diabetic truncal neuropathy in those patients who have failed to respond to more conservative measures. Neurodestructive procedures are rarely, if ever, indicated to treat the pain of diabetic truncal neuropathy as they will often worsen the patient's pain and cause functional disability.

SUGGESTED READINGS

Campbell W: DeJong's The Neurological Examination, ed 6. Philadelphia, Lippincott Williams and Wilkins, 2005.

Goetz CG: Textbook of Clinical Neurology, ed 2. Philadelphia, Saunders, 2003.

Waldman SD: Diabetic truncal neuropathy. In: Atlas of Common Pain Syndromes, ed 2. Philadelphia, Saunders, 2008.

CHAPTER 165

Tietze's Syndrome

Tietze's syndrome is a common cause of chest wall pain encountered in clinical practice. Distinct from costosternal syndrome, Tietze's syndrome was first described in 1921, and it is characterized by acute painful swelling of the costal cartilages. The second and third costal cartilages are most commonly involved, and in contradistinction to costosternal syndrome, which usually occurs no earlier than the fourth decade, Tietze's syndrome is a disease of the second and third decades. The onset is acute and is often associated with a concurrent viral respiratory tract infection. It has been postulated that microtrauma to the costosternal joints from severe coughing or heavy labor may be the cause of Tietze's syndrome. Painful swelling of the second and third costochondral joints is the sine qua non of Tietze's syndrome. Such swelling is absent in costosternal syndrome, which occurs much more frequently than Tietze's syndrome.

Signs and Symptoms

Physical examination will reveal that the patient suffering from Tietze's syndrome will vigorously attempt to splint the joints by keeping the shoulders stiffly in neutral position. Pain is reproduced with active protraction or retraction of the shoulder, deep inspiration, and full elevation of the arm. Shrugging of the shoulder may also reproduce the pain. Coughing may be difficult, and this may lead to inadequate pulmonary toilet in patients suffering from Tietze's syndrome. The costosternal joints, especially the second and third, will be swollen and exquisitely tender to palpation. The adjacent intercostal muscles may also be tender to palpation. The patient may also complain of a clicking sensation with movement of the joint.

Testing

Plain radiographs are indicated in all patients who present with pain thought to be emanating from the costosternal joints to rule out occult bony pathology, including tumor. If trauma is present, radionuclide bone scanning should be considered to rule out occult fractures or the ribs and/or sternum. Based on the patient's clinical presentation, additional testing including complete blood count, prostate-specific antigen, erythrocyte sedimentation rate, and antinuclear antibody testing may be indicated. Magnetic resonance imaging of the joints is indicated if joint instability or occult mass is suspected.

Differential Diagnosis

It should be remembered that there are a variety of other painful conditions that affect the costosternal joints and occur with a much greater frequency than Tietze's syndrome. The costosternal joints are susceptible to the development of arthritis, including osteoarthritis, rheumatoid arthritis, ankylosing spondylitis, Reiter's syndrome, and psoriatic arthritis. The joints are often traumatized during acceleration/deceleration injuries and blunt trauma to the chest. With severe trauma, the joints may sublux or dislocate. Overuse or misuse can also result in acute inflammation of the costosternal joint, which can be quite debilitating for the patient. The joints are also subject to invasion by tumor either from primary malignancies including thymoma or from metastatic disease.

Treatment

Initial treatment of the pain and functional disability associated with Tietze's syndrome should include a combination of the nonsteroidal anti-inflammatory agents or the cyclooxygenase-2 inhibitors. The local application of heat and cold may also be beneficial. The use of an elastic rib belt may also help provide symptomatic relief and help protect the costovertebral joints from additional trauma. For patients who do not respond to these treatment modalities, injection of the costosternal joints using local anesthetic and steroid may be a reasonable next step.

SUGGESTED READING

Waldman SD: Tietze's syndrome. In: Atlas of Common Pain Syndromes, ed 2. Philadelphia, Saunders, 2008.

Post-Thoracotomy Pain Syndrome

Essentially all patients who undergo thoracotomy will suffer from acute postoperative pain. This acute pain syndrome will invariably respond to the rational use of systemic and spinal opioids as well as intercostal nerve block. Unfortunately, a small percentage of patients who undergo thoracotomy will suffer persistent pain beyond the usual course of postoperative pain. This pain syndrome is called post-thoracotomy pain syndrome and can be difficult to treat. The causes of post-thoracotomy pain are listed in Table 166-1 and include direct surgical trauma to the intercostal nerves, fractured ribs due to use of the rib spreader, compressive neuropathy of the intercostal nerves due to direct compression to the intercostal nerves, cutaneous neuroma formation, and stretch injuries to the intercostal nerves at the costovertebral junction. With the exception of fractured ribs, which produce characteristic local pain that is worse with deep inspiration, coughing, or movement of the affected ribs, the other causes of post-thoracotomy pain result in moderate to severe pain that is constant in nature and follows the distribution of the affected intercostal nerves. The pain may be characterized as neuritic and may occasionally have a dysesthetic quality.

Signs and Symptoms

Physical examination of the patient suffering from post-thoracotomy syndrome will generally reveal tenderness along the healed thoracotomy incision. Occasionally, palpation of the scar will elicit paresthesias suggestive of neuroma formation. The patient suffering from post-thoracotomy syndrome may attempt to splint or protect the affected area. Careful sensory examination of the affected dermatomes may reveal decreased sensation or allodynia. With significant motor involvement of the subcostal nerve, the patient may complain that the abdomen bulges out. Occasionally, patients suffering from post-thoracotomy syndrome will develop a reflex sympathetic dystrophy of the ipsilateral upper extremity. If the reflex sympathetic dystrophy is left untreated, a frozen shoulder may develop.

Testing

Plain radiographs are indicated in all patients who present with pain thought to be emanating from the intercostal

TABLE 166–1 Causes of Post-Thoracotomy Pain Syndrome

- Direct surgical trauma to the intercostal nerves
- Fractured ribs due to the rib spreader
- Compressive neuropathy of the intercostal nerves due to direct compression to the intercostal nerves by retractors
- Cutaneous neuroma formation
- Stretch injuries to the intercostal nerves at the costovertebral junction

nerve to rule out occult bony pathology, including tumor. Radionuclide bone scanning may be useful to rule out occult fractures of the ribs and/or sternum. Based on the patient's clinical presentation, additional testing including complete blood count, prostate-specific antigen, erythrocyte sedimentation rate, and antinuclear antibody testing may be indicated. Computed tomography scan of the thoracic contents is indicated if occult mass or pleural disease is suspected. Electromyography is useful in distinguishing injury of the distal intercostal nerve from stretch injuries of the intercostal nerve at the costovertebral junction.

Differential Diagnosis

The pain of post-thoracotomy syndrome may be mistaken for pain of cardiac or gallbladder origin and can lead to visits to the emergency department and unnecessary cardiac and gastrointestinal workups. If trauma has occurred, post-thoracotomy syndrome may coexist with fractured ribs or fractures of the sternum itself, which can be missed on plain radiographs and may require radionuclide bone scanning for proper identification. Tietze's syndrome, which is painful enlargement of the upper costochondral cartilage associated with viral infections, can be confused with post-thoracotomy syndrome.

Neuropathic pain involving the chest wall may also be confused or coexist with post-thoracotomy syndrome. Examples of such neuropathic pain include diabetic polyneuropathies and acute herpes zoster involving the thoracic nerves. The possibility of diseases of the structures of the mediastinum remains ever present and at times can be difficult to diagnose. Pathologic processes that inflame the pleura (e.g., pulmonary embolus, infection,

Bornholm disease) may also confuse the diagnosis and complicate treatment.

Treatment

Initial treatment of post-thoracotomy syndrome should include a combination of simple analgesics and the non-steroidal anti-inflammatory agents or the cyclooxygenase-2 inhibitors. If these medications do not adequately control the patient's symptomatology, a tricyclic antidepressant or gabapentin should be added.

Traditionally, the tricyclic antidepressants have been a mainstay in the palliation of pain secondary to post-thoracotomy syndrome. Controlled studies have demonstrated the efficacy of amitriptyline for this indication. Other tricyclic antidepressants including nortriptyline and desipramine have also been shown to be clinically useful. Unfortunately, this class of drugs is associated with significant anticholinergic side effects, including dry mouth, constipation, sedation, and urinary retention. These drugs should be used with caution in those suffering from glaucoma, cardiac arrhythmia, and prostatism. In order to minimize side effects and encourage compliance, the primary care physician should start amitriptyline or nortriptyline at a 10-mg dose at bedtime. The dose can be then titrated upward to 25 mg at bedtime as side effects allow. Upward titration of dosage in 25-mg increments can be carried out each week as side effects allow. Even at lower doses, patients will generally report a rapid improvement in sleep disturbance and will begin to experience some pain relief in 10 to 14 days. If the patient does not experience any improvement in pain as the dose is being titrated upward, the addition of gabapentin alone or in combination with nerve blocks with local

anesthetics and/or steroid is recommended (see later). The selective serotonin reuptake inhibitors such as fluoxetine have also been used to treat the pain of post-thoracotomy pain syndrome, and although better tolerated than the tricyclic antidepressants, they appear to be less efficacious.

If the antidepressant compounds are ineffective or contraindicated, gabapentin represents a reasonable alternative. Gabapentin should be started with a 300-mg dose of gabapentin at bedtime for 2 nights. The patient should be cautioned about potential side effects, including dizziness, sedation, confusion, and rash. The drug is then increased in 300-mg increments, given in equally divided doses over 2 days as side effects allow, until pain relief is obtained or a total dose of 2400 mg daily is reached. At this point, if the patient has experienced partial relief of pain, blood values are measured and the drug is carefully titrated upward using 100-mg tablets. Rarely will more than 3600 mg daily be required.

The local application of heat and cold may also be beneficial to provide symptomatic relief of the pain of post-thoracotomy syndrome. The use of an elastic rib belt may also help provide symptomatic relief. For patients who do not respond to these treatment modalities, injection of local anesthetic and steroid into the structures that are thought to be responsible for the patient's pain may be a reasonable next step.

SUGGESTED READINGS

Goetz CG: Textbook of Clinical Neurology, ed 2. Philadelphia, Saunders, 2003.
Waldman SD: Post-thoracotomy pain syndrome. In: Atlas of Common Pain Syndromes, ed 2. Philadelphia, Saunders, 2008.

CHAPTER 167

Postmastectomy Pain

Postmastectomy pain syndrome is a constellation of symptoms that include pain in the anterior chest, breast, axilla, and medial upper extremity after surgical procedures on the breast. *Postmastectomy pain* is somewhat of a misnomer in that the clinical syndrome includes the pain mentioned here even if the patient has had only a lumpectomy or if another less-extensive surgical

procedure is performed on the breast. The pain is often described as constricting with a continuing dull ache. In addition to these symptoms, many patients with postmastectomy pain syndrome will also complain of sudden paresthesia radiating into the breast and/or axilla. In some patients, a burning, allodynic pain reminiscent of reflex sympathetic dystrophy may be the principal complaint.

The intensity of postmastectomy pain is moderate to severe. It is important to note that the onset of postmastectomy pain may occur immediately after surgery and initially be confused with the expected postsurgical pain, or the onset may be more insidious, occurring gradually 2 to 6 weeks after the inciting surgical procedure. If complete mastectomy is performed, phantom breast pain may further confound the diagnosis, as may associated lymphedema. Sleep disturbance is a common finding in patients suffering from postmastectomy pain.

Signs and Symptoms

Evaluation of the patient suffering from postmastectomy syndrome requires that the clinician take a careful history designed to delineate the various components that make up the patient's pain to help guide the physical examination. The clinician should question the patient specifically about the presence of phantom breast pain, which may be quite distressing to the patient when superimposed on the pain of postmastectomy syndrome.

Typical physical findings in patients suffering from postmastectomy syndrome include areas of decreased sensation, hyperpathia, and dysesthesia in the distribution of the intercostal brachial nerve, which is a branch of the second intercostal nerve.

This nerve is frequently damaged during breast surgery. Allodynia outside the distribution of the intercostal brachial nerve is also often present. Movement of the arm and axilla will often exacerbate the pain, which leads to splinting and disuse of the affected shoulder and upper extremity. This disuse will often worsen any lymphedema that is present. If the disuse of the upper extremity continues, frozen shoulder may develop, further complicating the clinical picture.

The clinician should always be alert to the possibility of metastatic disease or direct extension of tumor into the chest wall, which may mimic the pain of postmastectomy syndrome.

The findings of the targeted history and physical examination will assist the clinician to make an assessment of the sympathetic, neuropathic, and musculoskeletal components of the pain and design a rational treatment plan.

Testing

Plain radiographs are indicated in all patients who present with pain thought to be due to postmastectomy syndrome to rule out occult bony pathology, including tumor. Electromyography will help rule out damage to the nerve or plexopathy that may be contributing to the patient's pain. Radionuclide bone scanning may be useful to rule out occult pathologic fractures of the ribs and/or sternum. Based on the patient's clinical presentation, additional testing including complete blood cell count, prostate-specific antigen, erythrocyte sedimentation rate, and antinuclear antibody testing may be indicated. Computed tomography scan of the thoracic contents is indicated if occult mass is suspected. Magnetic resonance imaging of the brachial plexus should also be considered if plexopathy secondary to tumor involvement is a consideration.

Differential Diagnosis

As mentioned, the pain of postmastectomy syndrome is often mistaken for postoperative pain. If the breast surgery was performed for malignancy, a careful search for metastatic disease or tumor invasion of the chest wall is mandatory. Postmastectomy syndrome may coexist with pathologic fractured ribs or pathologic fractures of the sternum itself, which can be missed on plain radiographs and may require radionuclide bone scanning for proper identification.

Neuropathic pain involving the chest wall may also be confused or coexist with postmastectomy syndrome. Examples of such neuropathic pain include diabetic polyneuropathies and acute herpes zoster involving the thoracic nerves. The possibility of diseases of the structures of the mediastinum remains ever present and at times can be difficult to diagnose. Pathologic processes that inflame the pleura, such as pulmonary embolus, infection, and Bornholm disease, may also mimic the pain of postmastectomy syndrome.

Treatment

Initial treatment of postmastectomy syndrome should include a combination of simple analgesics and the nonsteroidal anti-inflammatory agents or the cyclooxygenase-2 inhibitors. If these medications do not adequately control the patient's symptomatology, a tricyclic antidepressant or gabapentin should be added.

Traditionally, the tricyclic antidepressants have been a mainstay in the palliation of pain secondary to postmastectomy syndrome. Controlled studies have demonstrated the efficacy of amitriptyline for this indication. Other tricyclic antidepressants including nortriptyline and desipramine have also been shown to be clinically useful. Unfortunately, this class of drugs is associated with significant anticholinergic side effects, including dry mouth, constipation, sedation, and urinary retention. These drugs should be used with caution in those suffering from glaucoma, cardiac arrhythmia, and prostatism. To minimize side effects and encourage compliance, the primary care physician should start amitriptyline or nortriptyline at a 10-mg dose at bedtime. The dose can be then titrated upward to 25 mg at bedtime as side effects allow. Upward titration of dosage in 25-mg increments can be carried out each week as side effects allow. Even at lower doses, patients will generally report a rapid improvement in sleep disturbance and will begin to experience some pain relief in 10 to 14 days. If the patient does not experience any improvement in pain as the dose is being titrated upward, the addition of gabapentin alone or in combination with nerve blocks of the intercostal nerves with local anesthetics and/or steroid is recommended. The selective serotonin reuptake inhibitors such as fluoxetine have also been used to treat postmastectomy pain, and although better tolerated than the tricyclic antidepressants, they appear to be less efficacious.

If the antidepressant compounds are ineffective or contraindicated, gabapentin represents a reasonable alternative. Gabapentin should be started with a 300-mg dose of gabapentin at bedtime for 2 nights. The patient should be cautioned about potential side effects, including dizziness, sedation, confusion, and

rash. The drug is then increased in 300-mg increments, given in equally divided doses over 2 days as side effects allow, until pain relief is obtained or a total dose of 2400 mg daily is reached. At this point, if the patient has experienced partial relief of pain, blood values are measured and the drug is carefully titrated upward using 100-mg tablets. Rarely will more than 3600 mg daily be required.

The local application of heat and cold may also be beneficial to provide symptomatic relief of the pain of postmastectomy syndrome. The use of an elastic rib belt may also help provide symptomatic relief.

For patients who do not respond to these treatment modalities, injection of the affected intercostal nerves or thoracic epidural nerve block using local anesthetic and steroid may be a reasonable next step.

SUGGESTED READING

Waldman SD: Post-mastectomy pain. In: Atlas of Uncommon Pain Syndromes, ed 2. Philadelphia, Saunders, 2008.

CHAPTER 168

Acute Herpes Zoster of the Thoracic Dermatomes

Herpes zoster is an infectious disease that is caused by the varicella-zoster virus (VZV), which also is the causative agent of chickenpox (varicella). The thoracic nerve roots are the most common site for the development of acute herpes zoster. Primary infection in the nonimmune host manifests itself clinically as the childhood disease chickenpox. It is postulated that during the course of primary infection with VZV, the virus migrates to the dorsal root of the thoracic nerves. The virus then remains dormant in the ganglia, producing no clinically evident disease. In some individuals, the virus may reactivate and travel along the sensory pathways of the first division of the trigeminal nerve, producing the pain and skin lesions characteristic of shingles. The reason that reactivation occurs in only some individuals is not fully understood, but it is theorized that a decrease in cell-mediated immunity may play an important role in the evolution of this disease entity by allowing the virus to multiply in the ganglia and spread to the corresponding sensory nerves, producing clinical disease. Patients who are suffering from malignancies

(particularly lymphoma), receiving immunosuppressive therapy (chemotherapy, steroids, radiation), or suffering from chronic diseases are generally debilitated and much more likely than the healthy population to develop acute herpes zoster. These patients all have in common a decreased cell-mediated immune response, which may be the reason for their propensity to develop shingles. This may also explain why the incidence of shingles increases dramatically in patients older than 60 years and is relatively uncommon in persons younger than 20 years.

Signs and Symptoms

As viral reactivation occurs, ganglionitis and peripheral neuritis cause pain, which is generally localized to the segmental distribution of the thoracic nerve roots. This pain may be accompanied by flulike symptoms and generally progresses from a dull, aching sensation to dysesthetic to neuritic pain in the distribution of the thoracic nerve roots.

In most patients, the pain of acute herpes zoster precedes the eruption of rash by 3 to 7 days, often leading to erroneous diagnosis (see Differential Diagnosis). However, in most patients, the clinical diagnosis of shingles is readily made when the characteristic rash appears. Like chickenpox, the rash of herpes zoster appears in crops of macular lesions, which rapidly progress to papules and then to vesicles. As the disease progresses, the vesicles coalesce and crusting occurs. The area affected by the disease can be extremely painful, and the pain tends to be exacerbated by any movement or contact (e.g., with clothing or sheets). As healing takes place, the crusts fall away, leaving pink scars in the distribution of the rash that gradually become hypopigmented and atrophic.

In most patients, the hyperesthesia and pain generally resolve as the skin lesions heal. In some, however, pain may persist beyond lesion healing. This most common and feared complication of acute herpes zoster is called postherpetic neuralgia, and the elderly are affected at a higher rate than the general population suffering from acute herpes zoster. The symptoms of postherpetic neuralgia can vary from a mild self-limited problem to a debilitating, constantly burning pain that is exacerbated by light touch, movement, anxiety, or temperature change or a combination. This unremitting pain may be so severe that it completely devastates the patient's life, and ultimately it can lead to suicide. It is the desire to avoid this disastrous sequel to a usually benign self-limited disease that dictates the clinician use all possible therapeutic efforts for the patient suffering from acute herpes zoster in the thoracic nerve roots.

Testing

Although in most instances the diagnosis of acute herpes zoster involving the thoracic nerve roots is easily made on clinical grounds, occasionally confirmatory testing is required. Such testing may be desirable in patients with other skin lesions that confuse the clinical picture, such as patients with human immunodeficiency virus infection who are suffering from Kaposi's sarcoma. In such patients, the diagnosis of acute herpes zoster may be confirmed by obtaining a Tzanck smear from the base of a fresh vesicle, which will reveal multinucleated giant cells and eosinophilic inclusions. To differentiate acute herpes zoster from localized herpes simplex infection, the clinician can obtain fluid from a fresh vesicle and submit it for immunofluorescent testing.

Differential Diagnosis

Careful initial evaluation, including a thorough history and physical examination, is indicated in all patients suffering from acute herpes zoster involving the thoracic nerve roots to rule out occult malignancy or systemic disease that may be responsible for the patient's immunocompromised state and to allow early recognition of changes in clinical status that may presage the development of complications, including myelitis or dissemination of the disease. Other causes of pain in the distribution of the thoracic nerve roots include thoracic radiculopathy and peripheral neuropathy. Intrathoracic and intra-abdominal pathology may also mimic the pain of acute herpes zoster involving the thoracic dermatomes.

Treatment

The therapeutic challenge of the patient presenting with acute herpes zoster involving the thoracic nerve roots is twofold: (1) the immediate relief of acute pain and symptoms and (2) the prevention of complications, including postherpetic neuralgia. It is the consensus of most pain specialists that the earlier in the natural course of the disease that treatment is initiated, the less likely it is that the patient will develop postherpetic neuralgia. Furthermore, because the older patient is at highest risk for developing postherpetic neuralgia, early and aggressive treatment of this group of patients is mandatory.

NERVE BLOCKS

Sympathetic neural blockade with local anesthetic and steroid via thoracic epidural nerve block appears to be the treatment of choice to relieve the symptoms of acute herpes zoster involving the thoracic nerve roots as well as to prevent the occurrence of postherpetic neuralgia. Sympathetic nerve block is thought to achieve these goals by blocking the profound sympathetic stimulation that is a result of the viral inflammation of the nerve and dorsal root ganglion. If untreated, this sympathetic hyperactivity can cause ischemia secondary to decreased blood flow of the intraneural capillary bed. If this ischemia is allowed to persist, endoneural edema forms, increasing endoneural pressure and causing a further reduction in endoneural blood flow with irreversible nerve damage.

As vesicular crusting occurs, the addition of steroids to the local anesthetic may decrease neural scarring and further decrease the incidence of postherpetic neuralgia. These sympathetic blocks should be continued aggressively until the patient is pain free and should be reimplemented at the return of pain. Failure to use sympathetic neural blockade immediately and aggressively, especially in the elderly, may sentence the patient to a lifetime of suffering from postherpetic neuralgia. Occasionally, some patients suffering from acute herpes zoster involving the thoracic nerve roots may not experience pain relief from thoracic epidural nerve block but will respond to blockade of the thoracic sympathetic nerves.

OPIOID ANALGESICS

Opioid analgesics may be useful in relieving the aching pain that is often present during the acute stages of herpes zoster as sympathetic nerve blocks are being implemented. They are less effective in the relief of the neuritic pain that is often present. Careful administration of potent, long-acting narcotic analgesics (e.g., oral morphine elixir or methadone) on a time-contingent rather than an as-needed basis may represent a beneficial adjunct to the pain relief provided by sympathetic neural blockade. Because many patients suffering from acute herpes zoster are elderly or may have severe multisystem disease, close monitoring for the potential side effects of potent narcotic analgesics (e.g., confusion or dizziness, which may cause a patient to fall) is warranted. Daily dietary fiber supplementation and milk of magnesia should be started along with opioid analgesics to prevent the side effect of constipation.

ADJUVANT ANALGESICS

The anticonvulsant gabapentin represents a first-line treatment in the palliation of neuritic pain of acute herpes zoster involving the thoracic nerve roots. Studies also suggest that gabapentin may help prevent the development of postherpetic neuralgia. Treatment with gabapentin should begin early in the course of the disease, and this drug may be used concurrently with neural blockade, opioid analgesics, and other adjuvant analgesics, including the antidepressant compounds if care is taken to avoid central nervous system side effects. Gabapentin is started at a dose of 300 mg at bedtime and is titrated upward in 300-mg increments to a maximum dosage of 3600 mg daily given in divided doses as side effects allow. Carbamazepine should be considered in patients suffering from severe neuritic pain who have failed to respond to nerve blocks and gabapentin. If this drug is used, rigid monitoring for hematologic parameters, especially in patients receiving chemotherapy or radiation therapy, is indicated. Phenytoin may also be beneficial to treat neuritic pain but should not be used in patients with lymphoma because the drug may induce a pseudo-lymphoma–like state that is difficult to distinguish from the actual lymphoma itself.

ANTIDEPRESSANT COMPOUNDS

Antidepressants may also be useful adjuncts in the initial treatment of the patient suffering from acute herpes zoster. On an acute basis, these drugs will help alleviate the significant sleep disturbance that is commonly seen in this setting. In addition, the antidepressants may be valuable in helping ameliorate the neuritic component of the pain, which is treated less effectively with narcotic analgesics. After several weeks of treatment, the antidepressants may exert a mood-elevating effect that may be desirable in some patients. Care must be taken to observe closely for central nervous system side effects in this patient population. These drugs may cause urinary retention and constipation that may be mistakenly attributed to herpes zoster myelitis.

ANTIVIRAL AGENTS

A limited number of antiviral agents, including famciclovir and acyclovir, have been shown to shorten the course of acute herpes zoster and may help prevent the development of postherpetic neuralgia. They are probably useful in attenuating the disease in immunosuppressed patients. These antiviral agents can be used in conjunction with the aforementioned treatment modalities. Careful monitoring for side effects is mandatory with the use of these drugs.

ADJUNCTIVE TREATMENTS

The application of ice packs to the lesions of acute herpes zoster may provide relief in some patients. The application of heat will increase pain in most patients, presumably because of increased conduction of small fibers, but is beneficial in an occasional patient and may be worth trying if the application of cold is ineffective. Transcutaneous electrical nerve stimulation and vibration may also be effective in a limited number of patients. The favorable risk-to-benefit ratio of all these modalities makes them reasonable alternatives for patients who cannot or will not undergo sympathetic neural blockade or tolerate pharmacologic interventions.

Topical application of aluminum sulfate as a tepid soak provides excellent drying of the crusting and weeping lesions of acute herpes zoster, and most patients find these soaks to be soothing. Zinc oxide ointment may also be used as a protective agent, especially during the healing phase, when temperature sensitivity is a problem. Disposable diapers can be used as an absorbent padding to protect healing lesions from contact with clothing and sheets.

SUGGESTED READINGS

Campbell W: DeJong's The Neurological Examination, ed 6. Philadelphia, Lippincott Williams and Wilkins, 2005.

Goetz CG: Textbook of Clinical Neurology, ed 2. Philadelphia, Saunders, 2003.

Waldman SD: Acute herpes zoster of the thoracic dermatomes. In: Atlas of Common Pain Syndromes, ed 2. Philadelphia, Saunders, 2008.

Postherpetic Neuralgia

One of the most difficult pain syndromes to treat, postherpetic neuralgia will occur in 10% of patients following a bout of acute herpes zoster. The reason that this painful condition occurs in some patients but not in others is unknown, but the condition occurs more frequently in older patients and appears to occur more frequently following acute herpes zoster of the trigeminal nerve as opposed to acute herpes zoster involving the thoracic dermatomes. Conditions that cause vulnerable nerve syndrome (e.g., diabetes) may also predispose the patient to develop postherpetic neuralgia. It is the current consensus among pain specialists that aggressive treatment of acute herpes zoster will help the patient avoid postherpetic neuralgia.

The pain of postherpetic neuralgia is characterized as a constant, dysesthetic pain that may be exacerbated by movement or stimulation of the affected cutaneous regions. There may be sharp, shooting neuritic pain superimposed on the constant dysesthetic symptoms. Some patients suffering from postherpetic neuralgia will also note a burning component reminiscent of reflex sympathetic dystrophy.

Signs and Symptoms

As the lesions of acute herpes zoster heal, the crusts fall away, leaving pink scars in the distribution of the rash that gradually become hypopigmented and atrophic. These affected cutaneous areas are often allodynic, although hypesthesia and, rarely, anesthesia of the affected areas may occur. In most patients, these sensory abnormalities and pain generally resolve as the skin lesions heal. In some, however, pain may persist beyond lesion healing.

Testing

In most instances, the diagnosis of postherpetic neuralgia roots is easily made of clinical grounds. Testing is generally used to identify other treatable coexisting diseases such as vertebral compression fractures or to rule out the underlying disease responsible for the patient's immunocompromised state. Such testing should include basic screening laboratory testing, rectal examination, mammography, and testing for collagen vascular diseases and human immunodeficiency virus infection. Skin biopsy may help confirm the presence of previous infection with herpes zoster if the history is in question.

Differential Diagnosis

Careful initial evaluation, including a thorough history and physical examination, is indicated in all patients suffering from postherpetic neuralgia to rule out occult malignancy or systemic disease that may be responsible for the patient's immunocompromised state and to allow early recognition of changes in clinical status that may presage the development of complications, including myelitis or dissemination of the disease. Other causes of pain in the distribution of the thoracic nerve roots include thoracic radiculopathy and peripheral neuropathy. Intrathoracic and intra-abdominal pathology may also mimic the pain of acute herpes zoster involving the thoracic dermatomes. For pain in the distribution of the first division of the trigeminal nerve, the clinician must rule out diseases of the eye, ear, nose, and throat, as well as intracranial pathology.

Treatment

The primary goal of all clinicians caring for patients with acute herpes zoster is the rapid and aggressive treatment of symptoms to help decrease the incidence of postherpetic neuralgia. It is the consensus of most pain specialists that the earlier in the natural course of the disease that treatment is initiated, the less likely it is that the patient will develop postherpetic neuralgia. Furthermore, because the older patient is at highest risk for developing postherpetic neuralgia, early and aggressive treatment of this group of patients is mandatory. If despite everyone's best efforts postherpetic neuralgia occurs, the following treatments are appropriate.

ADJUVANT ANALGESICS

The anticonvulsant gabapentin represents a first-line treatment in the palliation of pain of postherpetic neuralgia. Treatment with gabapentin should begin early in the course of the disease, and this drug may be used concurrently with neural blockade, opioid analgesics, and other adjuvant analgesics, including the antidepressant compounds if care is taken to avoid central nervous system side effects. Gabapentin is started at a bedtime dose of 300 mg and is titrated upward in 300-mg increments to a maximum dose of 3600 mg given in divided doses as side effects allow.

Carbamazepine should be considered in patients suffering from severe neuritic pain who have failed to respond to nerve blocks and gabapentin. If this drug is used, rigid monitoring for hematologic parameters, especially in patients receiving chemotherapy or radiation therapy, is indicated. Phenytoin may also be beneficial to treat neuritic pain but should not be used in patients with lymphoma because the drug may induce a pseudo-lymphoma–like state that is difficult to distinguish from the actual lymphoma itself.

Antidepressants may also be useful adjuncts in the initial treatment of the patient suffering from postherpetic neuralgia. On an acute basis, these drugs will help alleviate the significant sleep disturbance that is commonly seen in this setting. In addition, the antidepressants may be valuable in helping ameliorate the neuritic component of the pain, which is treated less effectively with narcotic analgesics. After several weeks of treatment, the antidepressants may exert a mood-elevating effect that may be desirable in some patients. Care must be taken to observe closely for central nervous system side effects in this patient population. These drugs may cause urinary retention and constipation that may be mistakenly attributed to herpes zoster myelitis.

NERVE BLOCKS

Sympathetic neural blockade with local anesthetics and steroids via either epidural nerve block or blockade of the sympathetic nerves subserving the painful area appears to be a reasonable next step if the pharmacologic modalities mentioned fail to control the pain of postherpetic neuralgia. The exact mechanism of pain relief from neural blockade when treating postherpetic neuralgia is unknown, but it may be related to modulation of pain transmission at the spinal cord level. In general, neurodestructive procedures have a very low success rate and should be used only after all other treatments have been optimized if at all.

OPIOID ANALGESICS

Opioid analgesics have a limited role in the management of postherpetic neuralgia and in the experience of this author frequently do more harm than good. Careful administration of potent, long-acting narcotic analgesics (e.g., oral morphine elixir or methadone) on a time-contingent basis rather than on an as-needed (prn) basis may represent a beneficial adjunct to the pain relief provided by sympathetic neural blockade. Because many patients suffering from postherpetic neuralgia are elderly or may have severe multisystem disease, close monitoring for the potential side effects of potent narcotic analgesics (e.g., confusion or dizziness, which may cause a patient to fall) is warranted. Daily dietary fiber supplementation and milk of magnesia should be started along with opioid analgesics to prevent the side effect of constipation.

ADJUNCTIVE TREATMENTS

The application of ice packs to the areas affected with postherpetic neuralgia may provide relief in some patients. Application of heat will increase pain in most patients, presumably because of increased conduction of small fibers, but is beneficial in an occasional patient and may be worth trying if the application of cold is ineffective. Transcutaneous electrical nerve stimulation and vibration may also be effective in a limited number of patients. The favorable risk-to-benefit ratio of all these modalities makes them reasonable alternatives for patients who cannot or will not undergo sympathetic neural blockade or tolerate pharmacologic interventions. The topical application of capsaicin may be beneficial in some patients suffering from postherpetic neuralgia. However, the burning associated with this drug when applied to the painful area will often limit the utility of this intervention.

SUGGESTED READINGS

Campbell W: DeJong's The Neurological Examination, ed 6. Philadelphia, Lippincott Williams and Wilkins, 2005.

Goetz CG: Textbook of Clinical Neurology, ed 2. Philadelphia, Saunders, 2003.

Waldman SD: Postherpetic neuralgia. In: Atlas of Common Pain Syndromes, ed 2. Philadelphia, Saunders, 2008.

CHAPTER **170**

Epidural Abscess

Epidural abscess is an uncommon cause of spine pain that, if undiagnosed, can result in paralysis and/or life-threatening complications. Epidural abscess can occur anywhere in the spine as well as intracranially. It can occur spontaneously via hematogenous seeding, most frequently as a result of urinary tract infections that spread to the spinal epidural space via Batson's plexus. More commonly, epidural abscess occurs after instrumentation of the spine, including surgery and epidural nerve blocks. The literature has suggested that the administration of steroids into the epidural space results in immunosuppression with a resultant increase in the incidence of epidural abscess. Although theoretically plausible, the statistical evidence given the thousands of epidural steroid injections performed around the country on a daily basis calls this belief into question.

The patient with epidural abscess initially presents with ill-defined pain in the segment of the spine affected (e.g., cervical, thoracic, or lumbar). This pain will become more intense and localized as the abscess increases in size and compresses neural structures. Low-grade fever and vague constitutional symptoms, including malaise and anorexia, will progress to frank sepsis with a high-grade fever, rigors, and chills. At this point, the patient will begin to experience sensory and motor deficits as well as bowel and bladder symptomatology as the result of neural compromise. As the abscess continues to expand, compromise of the vascular supply to the affected spinal cord and nerve will occur with resultant ischemia and, if untreated, infarction and permanent neurologic deficits.

TABLE 170–1 Algorithm for Spinal Cord Compression Due to Epidural Abscess

- Obtain stat blood and urine cultures.
- Immediately start high-dose antibiotics that cover *Staphylococcus aureus*.
- Immediately obtain the most readily available spinal imaging technique that can confirm the presence of spinal cord compression, such as abscess, tumor, and others.
- Computed tomography
- Magnetic resonance imaging
- Myelography
- Simultaneously obtain emergency consultation from a spinal surgeon.
- Continuously and carefully monitor the patient's neurologic status.
- If any of the above are unavailable, arrange emergency transfer of the patient to a tertiary care center via the most rapidly available transportation.
- Repeat imaging and obtain a repeat surgical consultation if there is any deterioration in the patient's neurologic status.

The clinician may be able to identify neurologic findings suggestive of spinal nerve root and/or spinal cord compression. Subtle findings that point toward the development of myelopathy (e.g., Babinski's sign, clonus, and decreased perineal sensation) may be overlooked if not carefully sought. As compression of the involved neural structures continues, the patient's neurologic status may deteriorate quite rapidly. If diagnosis is not made, irreversible motor and sensory deficit will result.

Signs and Symptoms

The patient with epidural abscess initially presents with ill-defined pain in the general area of the infection. Table 170-1 provides an algorithm for the evaluation and treatment of epidural abscess. At this point, there may be mild pain on range of motion of the affected segments. The neurologic examination will be within normal limits. A low-grade fever and/or night sweats may be present. Theoretically, if the patient has received steroids, these constitutional symptoms may be attenuated or their onset delayed. As the abscess increases in size, the patient will appear acutely ill with fever, rigors, and chills.

Testing

Myelography is still considered the best test to ascertain compromise of the spinal cord and exiting nerve roots by an extrinsic mass such as an epidural abscess. However, in this era of readily available magnetic resonance imaging (MRI) and high-speed computed tomographic (CT) scanning, it may be more prudent to obtain this noninvasive testing first rather than wait for a radiologist or spine surgeon to perform a myelogram. Both MRI and CT are highly accurate in the diagnosis of epidural abscess and are probably more accurate than myelography in the diagnosis of intrinsic disease of the spinal cord, spinal tumor, and so forth. All patients suspected of suffering from epidural abscess should undergo laboratory testing consisting of complete blood cell count, erythrocyte sedimentation rate, and automated blood chemistries. Blood and urine cultures should be immediately obtained in all patients thought to be suffering from epidural abscess to allow immediate implementation of antibiotic therapy while the workup is in progress. Gram stains and cultures of the abscess material should also be obtained, but antibiotic treatment should not be delayed while waiting for this information.

Differential Diagnosis

The diagnosis of epidural abscess should be strongly considered in any patient with spine pain and fever, especially if the patient has undergone spinal instrumentation or epidural nerve blocks for either surgical anesthesia or pain control. Other pathologic processes that must be considered in the differential diagnosis include intrinsic disease of the spinal cord, such as demyelinating disease and syringomyelia, as well as other processes that can result in compression of the spinal cord and exiting nerve roots, such as metastatic tumor, Paget's disease, and neurofibromatosis. As a general rule, unless the patient has concomitant infection, none of these diseases will routinely be associated with fever, just with back pain.

Treatment

The rapid initiation of treatment of epidural abscess is mandatory if the patient is to avoid the sequelae of permanent neurologic deficit or death. The treatment of epidural abscess is aimed at two goals: (1) treatment of the infection with antibiotics and (2) drainage of the abscess to relieve compression on neural structures. Because the vast majority of epidural abscesses are caused by *Staphylococcus aureus*, antibiotics such as vancomycin that will treat staphylococcal infection should be started immediately after blood and urine culture samples are taken. Antibiotic therapy can be tailored to the culture and sensitivity reports as they become available. As mentioned, antibiotic therapy should not be delayed while waiting for definitive diagnosis if epidural abscess is being considered as part of the differential diagnosis.

Antibiotics alone will rarely successfully treat an epidural abscess unless the diagnosis is made very early in the course of the disease; thus, drainage of the abscess will be required to effect full recovery. Drainage of the epidural abscess is usually accomplished via decompression laminectomy and evacuation of the abscess. More recently, interventional radiologists have been successful in draining epidural abscesses percutaneously using drainage catheters placed with the use of CT or MRI guidance. Serial CT or MRI scans are useful in following the resolution of epidural abscess and should be repeated immediately at the first sign of negative change in the patient's neurologic status.

SUGGESTED READINGS

Campbell W: DeJong's The Neurological Examination, ed 6. Philadelphia, Lippincott Williams and Wilkins, 2005.
Waldman SD: Epidural abscess. In: Atlas of Uncommon Pain Syndromes, ed 2. Philadelphia, Saunders, 2008.

CHAPTER 171

Spondylolisthesis

Spondylolisthesis is a degenerative disease of the lumbar spine that results in pain and functional disability. It occurs more commonly in women and is most often seen after the age of 40. This disease is caused by the slippage of one vertebral body onto another due to degeneration of the facet joints and intervertebral disc. Usually, the upper vertebral body moves anteriorly relative to the vertebral body below it, which causes narrowing of the spinal canal. This results in a relative spinal stenosis and back pain. Occasionally, the upper vertebral body slides posteriorly relative to the vertebral body below it, which compromises the neural foramina.

Clinically, the patient with spondylolisthesis will complain of back pain with lifting, twisting, or bending of the lumbar spine. Patients may complain that it feels like they have "a catch in their back." The patient with spondylolisthesis will often complain of radicular pain of the lower extremity and will often experience pseudoclaudication with walking. Rarely, the slippage of the vertebra is so extreme that myelopathy or cauda equina syndrome develops.

Signs and Symptoms

The patient suffering from spondylolisthesis will complain of back pain with motion of the lumbar spine. Rising from a sitting to a standing position will often reproduce the pain. Many patients with spondylolisthesis will experience radicular symptoms that will manifest on physical examination as weakness and sensory abnormality in the affected dermatomes. Often more than one dermatome will be affected. Occasionally, a patient suffering from spondylolisthesis experiences compression of the lumbar spinal nerve roots and cauda equina, resulting in myelopathy or cauda equina syndrome. Lumbar myelopathy is most commonly due to midline herniated lumbar disc, spinal stenosis, tumor, or, rarely, infection. Patients suffering from lumbar myelopathy or cauda equina syndrome will experience varying degrees of lower extremity weakness and bowel and bladder symptomatology. This represents a neurosurgical emergency and should be treated as such.

Testing

Plain radiographs of the lumbar spine usually allow the clinician to diagnose spondylolisthesis. The lateral view will demonstrate the slippage of one vertebra onto another.

Magnetic resonance imaging (MRI) of the lumbar spine provides the clinician with the best information regarding the contents of the lumbar spine. MRI is highly accurate and will help identify abnormalities that may put the patient at risk of lumbar myelopathy. In patients who cannot undergo MRI, such as a patient with a pacemaker, computed tomography and myelography are reasonable second choices. Radionuclide bone scanning and plain radiographs are indicated if fracture or bony abnormality such as metastatic disease is being considered.

Although this testing provides the clinician with useful neuroanatomic information, electromyography and nerve conduction velocity testing will provide the clinician with neurophysiologic information that can delineate the actual status of each individual nerve root and the lumbar plexus. Screening laboratory testing consisting of complete blood cell count, erythrocyte sedimentation rate, and automated blood chemistry testing should be performed if the diagnosis of spondylolisthesis is in question.

Differential Diagnosis

Spondylolisthesis is a radiographic diagnosis that is supported by a combination of clinical history, physical examination, radiography, and MRI. Pain syndromes that may mimic spondylolisthesis include lumbar radiculopathy, low back strain, lumbar bursitis, lumbar fibromyositis, inflammatory arthritis, and disorders of the lumbar spinal cord, roots, plexus, and nerves. MRI of the lumbar spine should be carried out in all patients suspected of suffering from spondylolisthesis. Screening laboratory testing consisting of complete blood cell count, erythrocyte sedimentation rate, antinuclear antibody testing, HLA-B27 antigen screening, and automated blood chemistry testing should be performed if the diagnosis of spondylolisthesis is in question, to help rule out other causes of the patient's pain.

Treatment

Spondylolisthesis is best treated with a multimodality approach. Physical therapy including flexion exercises, heat modalities, and deep sedative massage, combined with nonsteroidal anti-inflammatory agents and skeletal muscle relaxants, represents a reasonable starting point. The addition of steroid epidural nerve blocks is a reasonable next step. Caudal or lumbar epidural blocks with a local anesthetic and steroid have been shown to be extremely effective in the treatment of pain secondary to spondylolisthesis. Underlying sleep disturbance and depression are best treated with a tricyclic antidepressant compound such as nortriptyline, which can be started at a single bedtime dose of 25 mg.

SUGGESTED READING

Waldman SD: Spondylolisthesis. In: Atlas of Uncommon Pain Syndromes, ed 2. Philadelphia, Saunders, 2008.

CHAPTER 172

Ankylosing Spondylitis

Ankylosing spondylitis is an inflammatory disease of the spine, sacroiliac joints, and occasionally the extra-articular structures including the eye. It is also known as *Marie-Strümpell disease*. The etiology of ankylosing spondylitis is unknown, but autoimmune-mediated mechanisms have been implicated. Approximately 90% of patients suffering from ankylosing spondylitis have the histocompatibility antigen HLA-B27, compared with 7% of the general population. The significance of this fact is unknown but provides the basis for a diagnostic test to aid in the diagnosis of the disease. Ankylosing spondylitis occurs three times more frequently in men, and symptoms usually appear by the third decade of life. Onset of the disease after the age of 40 is rare.

Sacroiliitis is often one of the earliest manifestations of ankylosing spondylitis. This finding usually presents as morning stiffness and a deep aching pain of insidious onset in the low back and over the sacroiliac joints. This stiffness improves with activity and then reappears with periods of inactivity. The pain will worsen as the disease progresses, and nocturnal exacerbations with significant sleep disturbance are common. Tenderness over the spine, sacroiliac joints, costosternal junction, and greater trochanters are common. Pain and stiffness of the peripheral joints including the hips and shoulders are present in 30% to 40% of patients suffering from ankylosing spondylitis. The character of the pain of ankylosing spondylitis is dull and aching, and its intensity is mild to moderate. Occasionally, acute uveitis can occur, as can aortic valvular disease.

Signs and Symptoms

Clinically, the patient with ankylosing spondylitis will complain of back and sacroiliac pain and stiffness that is worse in the morning and after periods of prolonged activity. The patient may complain of a limitation of range of motion of the lateral spine and, on occasion, chest expansion. This limitation of range of motion is due to a combination of bony ankylosis and muscle spasm that the clinician may be able to identify on physical examination. Tenderness to palpation of the iliac crests, greater trochanter, and axial skeleton is a common finding in ankylosing spondylitis. As the disease progresses, the lumbar lordosis disappears and atrophy of the gluteal muscles may occur. A thoracic kyphosis develops, and the neck is forward flexed. Hip ankylosis may occur with hip involvement, and the patient will often compensate with flexion at the knee. Spinal fracture with resultant spinal cord injury may occur due to the rigid and inflexible nature of the spine. Anterior uveitis will manifest with photophobia, decreased visual acuity, and excessive lacrimation and represents an ophthalmologic emergency.

Testing

Plain radiographs of the sacroiliac joints will usually allow the clinician to diagnose ankylosing spondylitis. Erosion of the sacroiliac joints produces a characteristic symmetrical "pseudo-widening" that is diagnostic of the disease. Magnetic resonance imaging (MRI) of the spine provides the clinician with the best information regarding the contents of the lumbar spine and sacroiliac joints. MRI is highly accurate and helps to identify abnormalities that may put the patient at risk for the development of myelopathy.

In patients who cannot undergo MRI, such as a patient with a pacemaker, computed tomography or myelography is a reasonable second choice. Radionuclide bone scanning and plain radiography are indicated if fracture or bony abnormality such as metastatic disease is being considered in the differential diagnosis.

Although there is no test that is diagnostic for ankylosing spondylitis, the finding of the HLA-B27 antigen is highly suggestive of the disease in patients with the clinical findings mentioned. This antigen is present in 90% of patients suffering from ankylosing spondylitis. Complete blood cell count may reveal normocytic normochromic anemia. The erythrocyte sedimentation rate is usually elevated, as are the serum IgA levels.

Differential Diagnosis

Ankylosing spondylitis is a radiographic diagnosis that is supported by a combination of clinical history, physical examination, and laboratory testing. Pain syndromes that may mimic ankylosing spondylitis include low back strain, lumbar bursitis, lumbar fibromyositis, inflammatory arthritis, Reiter's syndrome, the collagen vascular diseases, and disorders of the lumbar spinal cord, roots, plexus, and nerves. Screening laboratory testing consisting of complete blood cell count, erythrocyte sedimentation rate, antinuclear antibody testing, HLA-B27 antigen screening, and automated blood chemistry testing should be performed if the diagnosis of ankylosing spondylitis is in question, to help rule out other causes of the patient's pain.

Treatment

Ankylosing spondylitis is best treated with a multimodality approach. Physical therapy, including exercises to maintain function, heat modalities, and deep sedative massage, combined with nonsteroidal anti-inflammatory agents and skeletal muscle relaxants represents a reasonable starting point. Sulfasalazine may also be useful in managing the arthritis associated with the disease. The addition of steroid epidural nerve blocks is a reasonable next step. Caudal or lumbar epidural blocks with a local anesthetic and steroid have been shown to be extremely effective in the treatment of pain secondary to ankylosing spondylitis. Underlying sleep disturbance and depression are best treated with a tricyclic antidepressant compound such as nortriptyline, which can be started at a single bedtime dose of 25 mg. Acute uveitis should be managed with corticosteroids and mydriatic agents.

SUGGESTED READING

Waldman SD: Ankylosing spondylitis. In: Atlas of Uncommon Pain Syndromes, ed 2. Philadelphia, Saunders, 2008.

CHAPTER **173**

Acute Pancreatitis

Acute pancreatitis is one of the most common causes of abdominal pain. The incidence of acute pancreatitis is approximately 0.5% of the general population, with a mortality rate between 1% and 1.5%. In the United States, acute pancreatitis is most commonly caused by alcohol, with gallstones being the most common cause in most European countries. There are many causes of acute pancreatitis, which are summarized in Table 173-1. In addition to alcohol and gallstones, other common causes of acute pancreatitis are viral infections, tumor, and medications.

Abdominal pain is a common feature in acute pancreatitis. It may range from mild to severe and is characterized by steady, boring epigastric pain that radiates to the flanks and chest. The pain is worse with the supine position, and the patient with acute pancreatitis will often prefer sitting with the dorsal spine flexed and the knees drawn up to the abdomen. Nausea, vomiting, and anorexia are also common features of acute pancreatitis.

Signs and Symptoms

The patient with acute pancreatitis will appear ill and anxious. Tachycardia and hypotension due to

TABLE 173–1 Common Causes of Acute Pancreatitis

- Alcohol
- Gallstones
- Viral infections
- Medications
- Metabolic causes
- Connective tissue diseases
- Tumor obstruction of ampulla of Vater
- Hereditary

hypovolemia are common, as is low-grade fever. Saponification of subcutaneous fat is seen in approximately 15% of patients suffering from acute pancreatitis, as are pulmonary complications including pleural effusions and pleuritic pain that may compromise respiration. Diffuse abdominal tenderness with peritoneal signs is invariably present. A pancreatic mass or pseudocyst due to pancreatic edema may be palpable. If hemorrhage occurs, periumbilical ecchymosis (Cullen's sign) and flank ecchymosis (Turner's sign) may be present. Both of these findings suggest severe necrotizing pancreatitis and indicate a poor prognosis. If hypocalcemia is present, Chvostek's or Trousseau's signs may be present.

Testing

Elevation of the serum amylase is the sine qua non of acute pancreatitis. Levels tend to peak at 48 to 72 hours and then begin to drift toward normal. Serum lipase will remain elevated and may actually correlate better with the actual severity of the disease. Since elevated serum amylase may be caused by other diseases, such as parotitis, amylase isoenzymes may be necessary to confirm a pancreatic basis for this laboratory finding. Plain radiographs of the chest are indicated in all patients who present with pain from acute pancreatitis to identify pulmonary complications, including pleural effusion, that are the result of the acute pancreatitis. Given the extrapancreatic manifestations of acute pancreatitis (e.g., acute renal or hepatic failure), serial complete blood count, serum calcium, serum glucose, liver function tests, and electrolytes are indicated in all patients suffering from acute pancreatitis. Computed tomographic (CT) scan of the abdomen will help identify pancreatic pseudocyst and may help the clinician gauge the severity and progress of the disease. Gallbladder evaluation with radionuclides is indicated if gallstones are being considered as a cause of acute pancreatitis. Arterial blood gases will help identify respiratory failure and metabolic acidosis.

Differential Diagnosis

The differential diagnosis should consider perforated peptic ulcer, acute cholecystitis, bowel obstruction, renal calculi, myocardial infarction, mesenteric infarction, diabetic ketoacidosis, and pneumonia. Rarely, the collagen vascular diseases including systemic lupus erythematosus and polyarteritis nodosa may mimic pancreatitis. Because the pain of acute herpes zoster may precede the rash by 24 to 72 hours, the pain may erroneously be attributed to acute pancreatitis.

Treatment

Most cases of acute pancreatitis are self-limited and will resolve within 5 to 7 days. Initial treatment of acute pancreatitis is aimed primarily at putting the pancreas at rest. This is accomplished by holding the patient NPO (nothing by mouth) to decrease serum gastrin secretion and, if ileus is present, instituting nasogastric suction. Short-acting potent opioid analgesics such as hydrocodone represent a reasonable next step if conservative measures do not control the patient's pain. If ileus is present, parenteral narcotics such as meperidine are a good alternative. As the opioid analgesics have the potential to suppress the cough reflex and respiration, the clinician must be careful to monitor the patient closely and to instruct the patient in adequate pulmonary toilet techniques. If the symptoms persist, CT-guided celiac plexus block with local anesthetic and steroid is indicated and may help decrease the mortality and morbidity associated with the disease. As an alternative, continuous thoracic epidural block with local anesthetic and/or opioid may provide adequate pain control and allow the patient to avoid the respiratory depression associated with systemic opioid analgesics.

Hypovolemia should be treated aggressively with crystalloid and colloid infusions. For prolonged cases of acute pancreatitis, parenteral nutrition is indicated to avoid malnutrition. Surgical drainage and removal of necrotic tissue may be required in severe necrotizing pancreatitis that fails to respond to the treatment modalities mentioned.

SUGGESTED READING

Waldman SD: Acute pancreatitis. In: Atlas of Common Pain Syndromes, 2nd ed. Philadelphia, WB Saunders, 2007.

CHAPTER 174

Chronic Pancreatitis

Chronic pancreatitis is one result of acute pancreatitis. Chronic pancreatitis may manifest as recurrent episodes of acute inflammation of the pancreas superimposed on chronic pancreatic dysfunction or as a more constant problem. As the exocrine function of the pancreas deteriorates, malabsorption with steatorrhea and isorrhea develops. Abdominal pain is usually present, but it may be characterized by exacerbations and remissions. In the United States, chronic pancreatitis is most commonly caused by alcohol, followed by cystic fibrosis and pancreatic malignancies. Hereditary causes such as alpha-1 antitrypsin deficiency are also common causes of chronic pancreatitis. In the developing countries, the most common cause of chronic pancreatitis is severe protein-calorie malnutrition.

Abdominal pain is a common feature in chronic pancreatitis. It mimics the pain of acute pancreatitis, may range from mild to severe, and is characterized by steady, boring epigastric pain that radiates to the flanks and chest. The pain is worse with alcohol and fatty meals. Nausea, vomiting, and anorexia are also common features of chronic pancreatitis, but as mentioned, the clinical symptoms frequently encountered in chronic pancreatitis are characterized by exacerbations and remissions.

Signs and Symptoms

The patient with chronic pancreatitis will present as does the patient with acute pancreatitis but may appear more chronically ill than acutely ill. Tachycardia and hypotension due to hypovolemia are much less common in chronic pancreatitis and if present represent an extremely ominous prognostic indicator or suggest that another pathologic process, such as perforated peptic ulcer, is present. Diffuse abdominal tenderness with peritoneal signs may be present if acute inflammation occurs. A pancreatic mass or pseudocyst due to pancreatic edema may be palpable.

Testing

Although elevation of serum amylase levels is the sine qua non of acute pancreatitis, amylase levels in chronic pancreatitis may be only mildly elevated or even within normal limits. Amylase levels tend to peak at 48 to 72 hours and then begin to drift toward normal. Serum lipase levels will also be attenuated in chronic pancreatitis compared with the findings seen in acute pancreatitis. Serum lipase may remain elevated longer than serum amylase in this setting and may correlate better with the actual severity of the disease. Because elevated serum amylase may be caused by other diseases, such as parotitis, amylase isozymes may be necessary to confirm a pancreatic basis for this laboratory finding. Plain radiographs of the chest are indicated for all patients who present with pain from chronic pancreatitis to identify pulmonary complications, including pleural effusion, that are the result of the chronic pancreatitis. Given the extrapancreatic manifestations of chronic pancreatitis (e.g., acute renal or hepatic failure), serial complete blood count, serum calcium, serum glucose, liver function tests, and electrolytes are indicated in all patients suffering from chronic pancreatitis. Computed tomographic (CT) scanning of the abdomen will help identify a pancreatic pseudocyst or pancreatic tumor that may have been previously overlooked and may help the clinician gauge the severity and progress of the disease. Gallbladder evaluation with radionuclides is indicated if gallstones are being considered as a cause of chronic pancreatitis. Arterial blood gases will help identify respiratory failure and metabolic acidosis.

Differential Diagnosis

The differential diagnosis should consider perforated peptic ulcer, acute cholecystitis, bowel obstruction, renal calculi, myocardial infarction, mesenteric infarction, diabetic ketoacidosis, and pneumonia. Rarely, the collagen vascular diseases, including systemic lupus erythematosus and polyarteritis nodosa, may mimic chronic pancreatitis. Because the pain of acute herpes zoster may precede the rash by 24 to 72 hours, the pain may be erroneously attributed to chronic pancreatitis in patients who have had previous bouts of the disease. The clinician should always consider the possibility of pancreatic malignancy in patients who are thought to be suffering from chronic pancreatitis.

Treatment

The initial treatment of patients suffering from chronic pancreatitis should be focused on the treatment of the pain and malabsorption. As with acute pancreatitis, the treatment of chronic pancreatitis is aimed primarily at putting the pancreas at rest. This is accomplished by holding the patient NPO (nothing by mouth) to decrease serum gastrin secretion and, if ileus is present, instituting nasogastric suction. Short-acting potent opioid analgesics such as hydrocodone represent a reasonable next step if conservative measures do not control the patient's pain. If ileus is present, parenteral narcotics such as meperidine are a good alternative. Because the opioid analgesics have the potential to suppress the cough reflex and respiration, the clinician must be careful to monitor the patient closely and to instruct the patient in adequate pulmonary toilet techniques. As with all chronic diseases, the use of opioid analgesics must be monitored carefully as the potential for misuse and dependence is high.

If the symptoms persist, CT-guided celiac plexus block with local anesthetic and steroid is indicated and may help decrease the mortality and morbidity rates associated with the disease. If the relief from this technique is short lived, neurolytic CT-guided celiac plexus block with alcohol or phenol represents a reasonable next step. As an alternative, continuous thoracic epidural block with local anesthetic, opioid, or both may provide adequate pain control and allow the patient to avoid the respiratory depression associated with systemic opioid analgesics.

Hypovolemia should be treated aggressively with crystalloid and colloid infusions. For prolonged cases of chronic pancreatitis, parenteral nutrition is indicated to avoid malnutrition. Surgical drainage and removal of necrotic tissue may be required in patients with severe necrotizing pancreatitis that fails to respond to the treatment modalities mentioned.

SUGGESTED READING

Waldman SD: Chronic pancreatitis. In: Atlas of Common Pain Syndromes, ed 2. Philadelphia, Saunders, 2008.

CHAPTER 175

Ilioinguinal Neuralgia

Ilioinguinal neuralgia is one of the most common causes of lower abdominal and pelvic pain encountered in clinical practice. Ilioinguinal neuralgia is caused by compression of the ilioinguinal nerve as it passes through the transverse abdominal muscle at the level of the anterior superior iliac spine. The most common causes of compression of the ilioinguinal nerve at this anatomic location involve injury to the nerve induced by trauma including direct blunt trauma to the nerve as well as damage during inguinal herniorrhaphy and pelvic surgery. Rarely, ilioinguinal neuralgia will occur spontaneously.

Signs and Symptoms

Ilioinguinal neuralgia presents as paresthesias, burning pain, and, occasionally, numbness over the lower abdomen that radiates into the scrotum or labia and occasionally into the inner upper thigh. The pain does not radiate below the knee. The pain of ilioinguinal neuralgia is made worse by extension of the lumbar spine, which puts traction on the nerve. Patients suffering from ilioinguinal neuralgia will often assume a bent-forward "novice skier's" position. Untreated, progressive motor deficit consisting of bulging of the anterior abdominal wall muscles may occur. This bulging may be confused with inguinal hernia.

Physical findings include sensory deficit in the inner thigh, scrotum, or labia in the distribution of the ilioinguinal nerve. Weakness of the anterior abdominal wall musculature may be present. Tinel's sign may be elicited by tapping over the ilioinguinal nerve at the point at which it pierces the transverse abdominal muscle. As mentioned, the patient may assume a bent-forward novice skier's position.

Testing

Electromyography will help distinguish ilioinguinal nerve entrapment from lumbar plexopathy, lumbar radiculopathy, and diabetic polyneuropathy. Plain radiographs of the hip and pelvis are indicated in all patients who present with ilioinguinal neuralgia, to rule out occult bony pathology. Based on the patient's clinical presentation, additional testing including complete blood count, uric acid, erythrocyte sedimentation rate, and antinuclear antibody testing may be indicated. Magnetic resonance imaging scan of the lumbar plexus is indicated if tumor or hematoma is suspected.

Differential Diagnosis

It should be remembered that lesions of the lumbar plexus from trauma, hematoma, tumor, diabetic neuropathy, or inflammation can mimic the pain, numbness, and weakness of ilioinguinal neuralgia and must be included in the differential diagnosis. Furthermore, there is significant intrapatient variability in the anatomy of the ilioinguinal nerve, which can result in significant variation in the patient's clinical presentation. The ilioinguinal nerve is a branch of the L1 nerve root with contribution from T12 in some patients. The nerve follows a curvilinear course that takes it from its origin of the L1 and occasionally T12 somatic nerves to inside the concavity of the ilium. The ilioinguinal nerve continues anteriorly to perforate the transverse abdominal muscle at the level of the anterior superior iliac spine. The nerve may interconnect with the iliohypogastric nerve as it continues to pass along its course medially and inferiorly where it accompanies the spermatic cord through the inguinal ring and into the inguinal canal. The distribution of the sensory innervation of the ilioinguinal nerves varies from patient to patient as there may be considerable overlap with the iliohypogastric nerve. In general, the ilioinguinal nerve provides sensory innervation to the upper portion of the skin of the inner thigh and the root of the penis and upper scrotum in men or the mons pubis and lateral labia in women.

Treatment

Pharmacologic management of ilioinguinal neuralgia is generally disappointing, and general nerve block will be required to provide pain relief. Initial treatment of ilioinguinal neuralgia should consist of treatment with simple analgesics, nonsteroidal anti-inflammatory agents or cyclooxygenase-2 inhibitors. Avoidance of repetitive activities thought to exacerbate the symptoms of ilioinguinal neuralgia (e.g., squatting or sitting for prolonged periods) will also help ameliorate the patient's symptoms. If the patient fails to respond to these conservative measures, a next reasonable step is ilioinguinal nerve block with local anesthetic and steroid. Because of overlapping innervation of the ilioinguinal and iliohypogastric nerve, it is not unusual to block branches of each nerve when performing ilioinguinal nerve block.

SUGGESTED READING

Waldman SD: Ilioinguinal neuralgia. In: Atlas of Common Pain Syndromes, ed 2. Philadelphia, Saunders, 2008.

CHAPTER 176

Genitofemoral Neuralgia

Genitofemoral neuralgia is one of the most common causes of lower abdominal and pelvic pain encountered in clinical practice. Genitofemoral neuralgia may be caused by compression or damage to the genitofemoral nerve anywhere along its path. The genitofemoral nerve arises from fibers of the L1 and L2 nerve roots. The genitofemoral nerve passes through the substance of the psoas muscle where it divides into a genital and a femoral branch. The femoral branch passes beneath the inguinal ligament along with the femoral artery and provides sensory innervation to a small area of skin on the inside of the thigh. The genital branch passes through the inguinal canal to provide innervation to the round ligament of the uterus and labia majora in women. In men, the genital branch of the genitofemoral nerve passes with the spermatic cord to innervate the cremasteric muscles and provide sensory innervation to the bottom of the scrotum.

The most common causes of genitofemoral neuralgia involve injury to the nerve induced by trauma including direct blunt trauma to the nerve as well as damage during inguinal herniorrhaphy and pelvic surgery. Rarely, genitofemoral neuralgia will occur spontaneously.

Signs and Symptoms

Genitofemoral neuralgia presents as paresthesias, burning pain, and occasionally numbness over the lower abdomen that radiates into the inner thigh in both men and women and into the labia majora in women and the bottom of the scrotum and cremasteric muscles in men. The pain does not radiate below the knee. The pain of genitofemoral neuralgia is made worse by extension of the lumbar spine, which puts traction on the nerve. Patients suffering from genitofemoral neuralgia will often assume a bent-forward "novice skier's" position.

Physical findings include sensory deficit in the inner thigh, base of the scrotum, or labia majora in the distribution of the genitofemoral nerve. Weakness of the anterior abdominal wall musculature may occasionally be present. Tinel's sign may be elicited by tapping over the genitofemoral nerve at the point where it passes beneath the inguinal ligament. As mentioned, the patient may assume a bent-forward novice skier's position.

Testing

Electromyography will help distinguish genitofemoral nerve entrapment from lumbar plexopathy, lumbar radiculopathy, and diabetic polyneuropathy. Plain radiographs of the hip and pelvis are indicated in all patients who present with genitofemoral neuralgia, to rule out occult bony pathology. Based on the patient's clinical presentation, additional testing including complete blood count, uric acid, erythrocyte sedimentation rate, and antinuclear antibody testing may be indicated. Magnetic resonance imaging (MRI) of the lumbar plexus is indicated if tumor or hematoma is suspected.

Differential Diagnosis

It should be remembered that lesions of the lumbar plexus from trauma, hematoma, tumor, diabetic neuropathy, or inflammation can mimic the pain, numbness, and weakness of genitofemoral neuralgia and must be included in the differential diagnosis. Furthermore, there is significant intrapatient variability in the anatomy of the genitofemoral nerve, which can result in significant variation in the patient's clinical presentation.

Treatment

Pharmacologic management of genitofemoral neuralgia is generally disappointing, and general nerve block will be required to provide pain relief. Initial treatment of genitofemoral neuralgia should consist of treatment with simple analgesics, nonsteroidal anti-inflammatory agents, or cyclooxygenase-2 inhibitors. Avoidance of repetitive activities thought to exacerbate the symptoms of genitofemoral neuralgia, such as squatting or sitting for prolonged periods, will also help ameliorate the patient's symptoms. If the patient fails to respond to these conservative measures, a next reasonable step is genitofemoral nerve block with local anesthetic and steroid. Because of overlapping innervation of the ilioinguinal and iliohypogastric nerve, it is not unusual to block branches of each nerve when performing genitofemoral nerve block.

If a patient presents with pain suggestive of genitofemoral neuralgia and does not respond to genitofemoral nerve blocks, a diagnosis of lesions more proximal in the lumbar plexus or an L1 radiculopathy should be considered. Such patients will often respond to epidural steroid blocks. Electromyography and MRI of the lumbar plexus are indicated in this patient population to help rule out other causes of genitofemoral pain including malignancy invading the lumbar plexus or epidural or vertebral metastatic disease at T12-L1.

SUGGESTED READING

Waldman SD: Genitofemoral neuralgia. In: Atlas of Common Pain Syndromes, ed 2. Philadelphia, Saunders, 2008.

CHAPTER 177

Meralgia Paresthetica

Meralgia paresthetica is caused by compression of the lateral femoral cutaneous nerve by the inguinal ligament as it passes through or under the inguinal ligament. This entrapment neuropathy presents as pain, numbness, and dysesthesias in the distribution of the lateral femoral cutaneous nerve. These symptoms often begin as a burning pain in the lateral thigh with associated cutaneous sensitivity. Patients suffering from meralgia paresthetica note that sitting, squatting, or wearing wide belts that compress the lateral femoral cutaneous nerve will cause the symptoms of meralgia paresthetica to worsen. Although traumatic lesions to the lateral femoral cutaneous nerve have been implicated in the onset of meralgia paresthetica, in most patients, no obvious antecedent trauma can be identified.

Signs and Symptoms

Physical findings include tenderness over the lateral femoral cutaneous nerve at the origin of the inguinal ligament at the anterior superior iliac spine. A positive Tinel's sign over the lateral femoral cutaneous nerve as it passes beneath the inguinal ligament may be present. Careful sensory examination of the lateral thigh will reveal a sensory deficit in the distribution of the lateral femoral cutaneous nerve. No motor deficit should be present. Sitting or the wearing of tight waistbands or wide belts that compress the lateral femoral cutaneous nerve may exacerbate the symptoms of meralgia paresthetica.

Testing

Electromyography will help distinguish lumbar radiculopathy and diabetic femoral neuropathy from meralgia paresthetica. Plain radiographs of the back, hip, and pelvis are indicated in all patients who present with meralgia paresthetica to rule out occult bony pathology. Based on the patient's clinical presentation, additional testing including complete blood count, uric acid, erythrocyte sedimentation rate, and antinuclear antibody testing may be indicated. Magnetic resonance imaging of the back is indicated if herniated disc, spinal stenosis, or a space-occupying lesion is suspected.

Differential Diagnosis

Meralgia paresthetica is often misdiagnosed as lumbar radiculopathy or trochanteric bursitis, or attributed to primary hip pathology. Radiographs of the hip and electromyography will help distinguish meralgia paresthetica from radiculopathy or pain emanating from the hip. Most patients suffering from a lumbar radiculopathy will have back pain associated with reflex, motor, and sensory changes, whereas patients with meralgia paresthetica will have no back pain and no motor or reflex changes. The sensory changes of meralgia paresthetica will be limited to the distribution of the lateral femoral cutaneous nerve and should not extend below the knee. It should be remembered that lumbar radiculopathy and lateral femoral cutaneous nerve entrapment may coexist as the so-called "double crush" syndrome. Occasionally, diabetic femoral neuropathy may produce anterior thigh pain, which may confuse the diagnosis.

Treatment

The patient suffering from meralgia paresthetica should be instructed in avoidance techniques to help reduce the unpleasant symptoms and pain associated with this entrapment neuropathy. A short course of conservative therapy consisting of simple analgesics, nonsteroidal anti-inflammatory agents, or cyclooxygenase-2 inhibitors is a reasonable first step in the treatment of patients suffering from meralgia paresthetica. If the patient does not experience rapid improvement, the injection of the lateral femoral cutaneous nerve is a reasonable next step.

SUGGESTED READING

Waldman SD: Meralgia paresthetic. In: Atlas of Common Pain Syndromes, ed 2. Philadelphia, Saunders, 2008.

CHAPTER 178

Spinal Stenosis

Spinal stenosis is the result of a congenital or acquired narrowing of the spinal canal. Clinically, the pain of spinal stenosis usually manifests in a characteristic manner as pain and weakness in the legs and calves when walking. This neurogenic pain is called pseudo-claudication or neurogenic claudication. These symptoms are usually accompanied with lower extremity pain emanating from the lumbar nerve roots. In addition to the pain, the patient with spinal stenosis may experience associated numbness, weakness, and loss of reflexes. The causes of spinal stenosis include bulging or herniated disc, facet arthropathy, and thickening and bucking of the interlaminar ligaments. All of these inciting factors tend to worsen with age.

Signs and Symptoms

The patient suffering from spinal stenosis will complain of calf and leg pain and fatigue with walking, standing, or lying supine. This fatigue and pain will disappear if the patient flexes the lumbar spine or assumes the sitting position. Extension of the spine may also cause an increase in symptoms. Patients will also complain of pain, numbness, tingling, and paresthesias in the distribution of the affected nerve root or roots. Patients may also note weakness and lack of coordination in the affected extremity. Muscle spasms and back pain, as well as pain referred into the trapezius and intrascapular region, are common. Decreased sensation, weakness, and reflex changes are demonstrated on physical examination.

Occasionally, a patient suffering from spinal stenosis will experience compression of the lumbar spinal nerve roots and cauda equina resulting in myelopathy or cauda equina syndrome. Patients suffering from lumbar myelopathy or cauda equina syndrome will experience varying degrees of lower extremity weakness and bowel and bladder symptomatology. This represents a neurosurgical emergency and should be treated as such, although often the onset of symptoms is insidious.

Testing

Magnetic resonance imaging (MRI) of the lumbar spine will provide the clinician with the best information regarding the lumbar spine and its contents. MRI is highly accurate and will help identify abnormalities that may put the patient at risk for the development of lumbar myelopathy. In patients who cannot undergo MRI (e.g., patients with a pacemaker), computed tomography or myelography is a reasonable second choice. Radionuclide bone scanning and plain radiographs are indicated if coexistent fracture or bony abnormality such as metastatic disease is being considered.

Although the testing mentioned provides the clinician with useful neuroanatomic information, electromyography and nerve conduction velocity testing will provide the clinician with neurophysiologic information that can delineate the actual status of each individual nerve root and the lumbar plexus. Screening laboratory testing consisting of complete blood count, erythrocyte sedimentation rate, and automated blood chemistry testing should be performed if the diagnosis of spinal stenosis is in question.

Differential Diagnosis

Spinal stenosis is a clinical diagnosis that is supported by a combination of clinical history, physical examination, radiography, and MRI. Pain syndromes that may mimic spinal stenosis include low back strain, lumbar bursitis, lumbar fibromyositis, inflammatory arthritis, and disorders of the lumbar spinal cord, roots, plexus, and nerves including diabetic femoral neuropathy. MRI of the lumbar spine should be carried out on all patients suspected of suffering from spinal stenosis. Screening laboratory testing consisting of complete blood count, erythrocyte sedimentation rate, antinuclear antibody testing, HLA-B27 antigen screening, and automated blood chemistry testing should be performed if the diagnosis of spinal stenosis is in question, to help rule out other causes of the patient's pain.

Treatment

Spinal stenosis is best treated with a multimodality approach. Physical therapy including heat modalities and deep sedative massage, combined with nonsteroidal anti-inflammatory agents and skeletal muscle relaxants, represents a reasonable starting point. The addition of lumbar steroid epidural nerve blocks is a reasonable next step. Caudal epidural blocks with local anesthetic and steroid have been shown to be extremely effective in the treatment of spinal stenosis. Underlying sleep disturbance and depression are best treated with a tricyclic antidepressant compound such as nortriptyline, which can be started at a single bedtime dose of 25 mg.

SUGGESTED READING

Waldman SD: Spinal stenosis. In: Atlas of Common Pain Syndromes, ed 2. Philadelphia, Saunders, 2008.

CHAPTER 179

Arachnoiditis

Arachnoiditis is a term used to describe thickening, scarring, and inflammation of the arachnoid membrane. These abnormalities may be self-limited or may lead to compression of the nerve roots and spinal cord. In addition to pain, the patient with arachnoiditis may experience associated numbness, weakness, loss of reflexes, and bowel and bladder symptomatology. The cause of arachnoiditis is unknown but may occur following a herniated disc, infection, tumor, myelography, spine surgery, or intrathecal administration of drugs. Anecdotal reports of arachnoiditis following epidural and subarachnoid administration of depot-steroid preparations have been reported.

Signs and Symptoms

The patient suffering from arachnoiditis will complain of pain, numbness, tingling, and paresthesias in the distribution of the affected nerve root or roots (Table 179-1). Patients may also note weakness and lack of coordination in the affected extremity. Muscle spasms and back pain, as well as pain referred into the buttocks, are common. Decreased sensation, weakness, and reflex changes are demonstrated on physical examination. Occasionally, a patient suffering from arachnoiditis will experience compression of the lumbar spinal cord, nerve roots, and cauda equina resulting in myelopathy or cauda equina syndrome.

Patients suffering from lumbar myelopathy or cauda equina syndrome due to arachnoiditis will experience varying degrees of lower extremity weakness and bowel and bladder symptomatology.

Testing

Magnetic resonance imaging (MRI) of the lumbar spine will provide the clinician with the best information regarding the lumbar spine and its contents. MRI is highly accurate and will help identify abnormalities that may put the patient at risk for the development of lumbar myelopathy or cauda equina syndrome. In patients who cannot undergo MRI (e.g., patients with a pacemaker), computed tomography or myelography is a reasonable second choice. Radionuclide bone scanning and plain radiographs are indicated if fracture or bony abnormality such as metastatic disease is being considered.

Although the testing mentioned provides the clinician with useful neuroanatomic information, electromyography and nerve conduction velocity testing will provide the clinician with neurophysiologic information that can delineate the actual status of each individual nerve root and the lumbar plexus. Screening laboratory testing consisting of complete blood count, erythrocyte sedimentation rate, and automated blood chemistry testing should

TABLE 179–1 Anatomic Localization of Lumbar Nerve Roots Affected by Arachnoiditis

Lumbar Root	Pain	Sensory Changes	Weakness	Reflex Changes
L4	Back, shin, thigh, and leg	Shin numbness	Ankle dorsiflexors	Knee jerk
L5	Back, posterior thigh, and leg	Numbness of top of foot and first web space	Extensor hallucis longus	None
S1	Back, posterior calf, and leg	Numbness of lateral foot	Gastrocnemius and soleus	Ankle jerk

be performed if the diagnosis of arachnoiditis is in question.

Differential Diagnosis

Arachnoiditis is a clinical diagnosis that is supported by a combination of clinical history, physical examination, radiography, and MRI. Pain syndromes that may mimic arachnoiditis include tumor, infection, and disorders of the lumbar spinal cord, roots, plexus, and nerves. MRI of the lumbar spine should be carried out on all patients suspected of suffering from arachnoiditis. Screening laboratory testing consisting of complete blood count, erythrocyte sedimentation rate, antinuclear antibody testing, HLA-B27 antigen screening, and automated blood chemistry testing should be performed if the diagnosis of arachnoiditis is in question, to help rule out other causes of the patient's pain.

Treatment

There is little consensus as to how best to treat the patient suffering from arachnoiditis, and most efforts are aimed at decompressing nerve roots and spinal cord and/or treating the inflammatory component of the disease. Epidural neurolysis and/or caudal administration of steroids may help decompress nerve roots if the pathology is localized. More generalized cases of arachnoiditis will often require surgical decompressive laminectomy. The results of all modalities are disappointing at best. Underlying sleep disturbance and depression are best treated with a tricyclic antidepressant compound such as nortriptyline, which can be started at a single bedtime dose of 25 mg. Neuropathic pain associated with arachnoiditis may respond to gabapentin. Spinal cord stimulation may also help provide symptomatic relief. Opioid analgesics should be used with caution if at all.

SUGGESTED READING

Waldman SD: Arachnoiditis. In: Atlas of Common Pain Syndromes, ed 2. Philadelphia, Saunders, 2008.

CHAPTER 180

Orchialgia

Orchialgia, or testicular pain, can be a difficult clinical situation for the patient and clinician alike owing to the unique significance the testicle has as part of the male psyche. This fact is crucial if the clinician is to successfully evaluate and treat patients who present with orchialgia.

Acute orchialgia represents a medical emergency and may be the result of trauma, infection, or inflammation of the testes or torsion of the testes and spermatic cord.

Chronic orchialgia is defined as testicular pain that is of more than 3 months' duration and significantly interferes with the patient's activities of daily living. Chronic orchialgia can be the result of pathologic processes that are extrascrotal (e.g., ureteral calculi, inguinal hernia, ilioinguinal or genitofemoral nerve entrapment) or of diseases of the lumbar spine and roots, or it can be intrascrotal in origin (e.g., tumor, chronic epididymitides, hydrocele, varicocele). The history of all patients suffering from chronic orchialgia should include specific questioning regarding a past history of sexual abuse.

Signs and Symptoms

Physical examination of patients suffering from acute orchialgia is directed at identifying acute torsion of the testes and spermatic cord, which is a surgical emergency. Patients with acute orchitis secondary to infections including sexually transmitted diseases present with testes that are exquisitely tender to palpation. For patients with chronic orchialgia, the physical findings are often nonspecific with the testicle mildly tender to palpation unless specific pathologic processes are present. For example, patients with chronic testicular pain secondary to varicocele will present with a scrotum that feels like a "bag of worms." Patients with chronic epididymitis will present with tenderness that is localized to the epididymis. Testicular malignancy should always be considered in any patient presenting with orchialgia. Physical findings in this setting vary, but testicular enlargement is often an early finding.

As mentioned, extrascrotal pathologic processes can also manifest with the primary symptom of orchialgia. One of the most common causes of orchialgia of extrascrotal origin is ilioinguinal and/or genitofemoral neuralgia. Ilioinguinal neuralgia manifests as a sensory deficit in the inner thigh and scrotum in the distribution of the ilioinguinal nerve. Weakness of the anterior abdominal wall musculature may be present. Tinel's sign may be elicited by tapping over the ilioinguinal nerve at the point it pierces the transverse abdominal muscle. The patient suffering from ilioinguinal and/or genitofemoral neuralgia may assume a bent-forward "novice skier's" position to remove pressure on the affected nerve.

Testing

Ultrasound examination of the scrotal contents is indicated in all patients suffering from orchialgia. Radionuclide and Doppler studies are indicated if vascular compromise is suspected. Transillumination of the scrotal contents can also help identify varicocele.

Electromyography will help distinguish ilioinguinal nerve entrapment from lumbar plexopathy, lumbar radiculopathy, and diabetic polyneuropathy. Based on the patient's clinical presentation, additional testing including complete blood cell count, uric acid, erythrocyte sedimentation rate, and antinuclear antibody testing may be indicated. Magnetic resonance imaging of the lumbar plexus and pelvis is indicated if tumor or hematoma is suspected.

Differential Diagnosis

It should be remembered that extrascrotal pathology, including inguinal hernia, ilioinguinal neuralgia, and lesions of the lumbar plexus, nerve roots, and spinal cord, can mimic the pain of orchialgia and must be included in the differential diagnosis. Furthermore, there is significant intrapatient variability in the anatomy of the ilioinguinal and genitofemoral nerves, which can result in significant variation in the patient's clinical presentation. The ilioinguinal nerve is a branch of the L1 nerve root with contribution from T12 in some patients. The nerve follows a curvilinear course that takes it from its origin of the L1 and occasionally T12 somatic nerves to inside the concavity of the ilium. The ilioinguinal nerve continues anteriorly to perforate the transverse abdominal muscle at the level of the anterior superior iliac spine. The nerve may interconnect with the iliohypogastric nerve as it continues to pass along its course medially and inferiorly, where it accompanies the spermatic cord through the inguinal ring and into the inguinal canal. The distribution of the sensory innervation of the ilioinguinal nerves varies from patient to patient as there may be considerable overlap with the iliohypogastric nerve. In general, the ilioinguinal nerve provides sensory innervation to the upper portion of the skin of the inner thigh and the root of the penis and upper scrotum in men.

Treatment

Initial treatment of the pain associated with orchialgia should include a combination of the nonsteroidal anti-inflammatory agents or cyclooxygenase-2 inhibitors and physical therapy. The local application of heat and cold may also be beneficial. The use of supportive undergarments or an athletic supporter may also provide symptomatic relief.

For patients who do not respond to these treatment modalities, injection of the spermatic cord and/or ilioinguinal and genitofemoral nerves with a local anesthetic and steroid may be a reasonable next step. If the symptoms of orchialgia persist, surgical exploration of the scrotal contents should be considered. Psychological evaluation and interventions should take place concurrently with the treatment modalities mentioned.

SUGGESTED READING

Waldman SD: Orchialgia. In: Atlas of Uncommon Pain Syndromes, ed 2. Philadelphia, Saunders, 2008.

CHAPTER 181

Vulvodynia

The Clinical Syndrome

Vulvodynia is an uncommon cause of pelvic pain encountered in clinical practice. Vulvodynia probably is not a single clinical entity but rather the conglomeration of a variety of disorders that can cause pain in this anatomic region. Included in these disorders are chronic infections of the female urogenital tract; chronic inflammation of the skin and mucosa of the vulva without demonstrable bacterial, viral, or fungal infection; and bladder abnormalities including interstitial cystitis, pelvic floor muscle disorders, reflex sympathetic dystrophy, and psychogenic causes. All have in common the ability to cause chronic, ill-defined pain of the vulva that is the hallmark of vulvodynia.

The pain of vulvodynia is characterized by dull, stinging, aching, or burning pain of the vulva. The intensity of pain is mild to moderate and may worsen with bathing, urination, or sexual activity. The pain may be referred to the perineum, rectum, or inner thigh. Irritative urinary outflow symptoms and sexual dysfunction often coexist with the pain of vulvodynia, with vulvodynia being one of the leading causes of dyspareunia. The history of all patients suffering from chronic vulvodynia should include specific questioning regarding a past history of sexual abuse, sexually transmitted diseases, and psychological abnormalities related to sexuality.

Signs and Symptoms

Physical examination of patients suffering from acute vulvodynia is directed at identifying acute infections of the vulva and/or urinary tract that may be readily treatable. Patients with acute infections, including yeast infections and sexually transmitted diseases, will present with a vulva that is irritated, inflamed, raw to the touch, and tender to palpation. For patients with chronic vulvodynia, the physical findings are often nonspecific, with the vulva mildly tender to palpation and an otherwise normal pelvic examination. Changes of the skin and mucous membranes of the vulva due to herpes, chronic itching, irritation, or douching may also be present. In a small number of patients suffering from vulvodynia, spasm of the muscles of the pelvic floor may be demonstrated on pelvic examination. Allodynia of the vulva and perineum may be present, especially if there is a history of prior trauma, such as surgery, radiation therapy, straddle injuries, etc. Vulvar malignancy should always be considered in any patient presenting with vulvodynia.

Extravulva pathologic processes can also present with the primary symptom of vulvodynia. One of the most common causes of vulvodynia of extravulvar origin is malignancy involving the pelvic contents other than the vulva. Tumor involving the lumbar plexus, cauda equina, and/or hypogastric plexus can rarely present as pain localized to the vulva and perineum. Postradiation neuropathy can occur after radiation therapy for the treatment of malignancy of the vulva and rectum and can mimic the pain of vulvodynia. Ilioinguinal or genitofemoral entrapment neuropathy can also present clinically as vulvodynia.

Testing

Pelvic examination is the cornerstone of the diagnosis of patients suffering from vulvodynia. Careful examination for infection, cutaneous or mucosal abnormalities, tenderness, muscle spasm, and/or tumor is crucial to avoid overlooking vulvar malignancy. Ultrasound examination of the pelvis is indicated in all patients suffering from vulvodynia.

If there is any question of occult malignancy of the vulva or pelvic contents, magnetic resonance imaging (MRI) or computed tomography scanning of the pelvis is mandatory to rule out malignancy or disease of the pelvic organs, such as endometriosis, that may be responsible for the patient's pain symptomatology. Urinalysis to rule out urinary tract infection is also indicated in all patients suffering from vulvodynia. Culture for sexually transmitted diseases including herpes is also indicated in the evaluation of all patients thought to be suffering from vulvodynia.

Electromyography will help distinguish entrapment neuropathy of the genitofemoral or ilioinguinal nerves from lumbar plexopathy or lumbar radiculopathy. Based on the patient's clinical presentation, additional testing including complete blood cell count, erythrocyte sedimentation rate, and antinuclear antibody testing may be indicated. MRI of the lumbar plexus is indicated if tumor or hematoma is suspected.

Differential Diagnosis

It should be remembered that extravulvar pathology, including reflex sympathetic dystrophy and lesions of the lumbar plexus, nerve roots, and spinal cord, can mimic the pain of vulvodynia and must be included in the differential diagnosis. As mentioned, because of the disastrous results of missing a diagnosis of pelvic or vulvar malignancy when evaluating and treating patients thought to be suffering from vulvodynia, it is mandatory that malignancy be high on the list of differential diagnostic possibilities.

Treatment

Initial treatment of the pain associated with vulvodynia should include a combination of the nonsteroidal anti-inflammatory agents or cyclooxygenase-2 inhibitors. The local application of heat and cold via sitz baths may also be beneficial. An empirical treatment course of antibiotics such as doxycycline 100 mg twice a day for 2 weeks may also be worth a try even though urine cultures are negative. A course of treatment for vaginal yeast infection concurrently with the antibiotics should also be considered. Anecdotal reports of decreased pain after treatment with adjuvant analgesics including the tricyclic antidepressants, such as nortriptyline, 25 mg at bedtime and titrating upward as side effects allow, or gabapentin make these drugs a consideration for patients who continue to have pain in the absence of demonstrable treatable disease.

For patients who do not respond to these treatment modalities, caudal epidural or hypogastric nerve block with a local anesthetic and steroid may be a reasonable next step.

If the symptoms of vulvodynia persist, laparoscopy should be considered. Psychologic evaluation and interventions should take place concurrently with the treatment modalities mentioned, given the high incidence of coexistent psychological issues associated with all pelvic pain syndromes.

SUGGESTED READING

Waldman SD: Vulvodynia. In: Atlas of Uncommon Pain Syndromes, ed 2. Philadelphia, Saunders, 2008.

CHAPTER 182

Proctalgia Fugax

Proctalgia fugax is a disease of unknown etiology that is characterized by paroxysms of rectal pain with pain-free periods between attacks. The pain-free periods between attacks can last seconds to minutes. Like cluster headache, spontaneous remissions of the disease occur and may last from weeks to years. Proctalgia fugax is more common in females and occurs with greater frequency in those patients suffering from irritable bowel syndrome.

The pain of proctalgia fugax is sharp or gripping in nature and is severe in intensity. Like other urogenital focal pain syndromes such as vulvodynia and proctodynia, the causes remain obscure. Increased stress will often increase the frequency and intensity of attacks of proctalgia fugax, as will sitting for prolonged periods. Patients will often feel an urge to defecate with the onset of the paroxysms of pain.

Depression often accompanies the pain of proctalgia fugax but is not thought to be the primary cause. The symptoms of proctalgia fugax can be so severe as to limit the patient's ability to carry out activities of daily living.

Signs and Symptoms

The physical examination of the patient suffering from proctalgia fugax is usually normal. The patient may be depressed or appear anxious. Rectal examination is normal, although deep palpation of the surrounding musculature may trigger paroxysms of pain. Interestingly, the patient suffering from proctalgia fugax will often report that he or she can abort the attack of pain by placing a finger in the rectum. Rectal suppositories may also interrupt the attacks.

Testing

As with the physical examination, testing in patients suffering from proctalgia fugax is usually within normal limits. Because of the risk of overlooking rectal malignancy that may be responsible for pain that may be attributed to a benign etiology, by necessity proctalgia fugax must be a diagnosis of exclusion. Rectal examination is mandatory in all patients thought to be suffering from proctalgia fugax. Sigmoidoscopy or colonoscopy is also strongly recommended in such patients. Testing of the stool for occult blood is also indicated. Screening laboratory studies consisting of a complete blood cell count, automated chemistries, and erythrocyte sedimentation rate should also be performed. Magnetic resonance imaging (MRI) or computed tomographic (CT) scanning of the pelvis should also be considered in all patients suffering from proctalgia fugax to rule out occult pathology. If psychological problems are suspected or if there is a history of sexual abuse, psychiatric evaluation is indicated concurrently with laboratory and radiographic testing.

Differential Diagnosis

As mentioned, because of the risk of overlooking serious pathology of the anus and rectum, proctalgia fugax must be a diagnosis of exclusion. First and foremost, the clinician must rule out rectal malignancy to avoid disaster. Proctitis can mimic the pain of proctalgia fugax and can be diagnosed on sigmoidoscopy or colonoscopy. Hemorrhoids will usually present with bleeding associated with pain and can be distinguished from proctalgia fugax on physical examination. Proctodynia may sometimes be confused with proctalgia fugax, but the pain is more constant and duller and aching in character.

Treatment

Initial treatment of proctalgia fugax should include a combination of simple analgesics and the nonsteroidal anti-inflammatory agents or the cyclooxygenase-2 inhibitors. If these medications do not adequately control the patient's symptomatology, a tricyclic antidepressant or gabapentin should be added.

Traditionally, the tricyclic antidepressants have been a mainstay in the palliation of pain secondary to proctalgia fugax. Controlled studies have demonstrated the efficacy of amitriptyline for this indication. Other tricyclic antidepressants including nortriptyline and desipramine have also been shown to be clinically useful. Unfortunately, this class of drugs is associated with significant anticholinergic side effects, including dry mouth, constipation, sedation, and urinary retention. These drugs should be used with caution in those suffering from glaucoma, cardiac arrhythmia, and prostatism. To minimize side effects and encourage compliance, the primary care physician should start amitriptyline or nortriptyline at a 10-mg dose at bedtime. The dose can then be titrated upward to 25 mg at bedtime as side effects allow. Upward titration of dosage in 25-mg increments can be carried out each week as side effects allow. Even at lower doses, patients will generally report a rapid improvement in sleep disturbance and will begin to experience some pain relief in 10 to 14 days. If the patient does not experience any improvement in pain as the dose is being titrated upward, the addition of gabapentin alone or in combination with nerve blocks of the intercostal nerves with local anesthetics and/or steroid is recommended. The selective serotonin reuptake inhibitors such as fluoxetine have also been used to treat the pain of proctalgia fugax and, although better tolerated than the tricyclic antidepressants, they appear to be less efficacious.

If the antidepressant compounds are ineffective or contraindicated, gabapentin represents a reasonable alternative. Gabapentin should be started with a 300-mg dose at bedtime for 2 nights. The patient should be cautioned about potential side effects, including dizziness, sedation, confusion, and rash. The drug is then increased in 300-mg increments, given in equally divided doses over 2 days as side effects allow, until pain relief is obtained or a total dose of 2400 mg daily is reached. At this point, if the patient has experienced partial relief of pain, blood values are measured and the drug is carefully titrated upward using 100-mg tablets. Rarely will more than 3600 mg daily be required.

The local application of heat and cold may also be beneficial to provide symptomatic relief of the pain of proctalgia fugax. The use of bland rectal suppositories may also help provide symptomatic relief. For patients who do not respond to these treatment modalities, injection of the peroneal nerves or caudal epidural nerve block using a local anesthetic and steroid may be a reasonable next step. The clinician should be aware that there are anecdotal reports that the calcium channel blockers, topical nitroglycerin, and inhalation of albuterol will provide symptomatic relief of the pain of proctalgia fugax.

SUGGESTED READING

Waldman SD: Proctalgia fugax. In: Atlas of Uncommon Pain Syndromes, ed 2. Philadelphia, Saunders, 2008.

Osteitis Pubis

Osteitis pubis is a constellation of symptoms consisting of a localized tenderness over the symphysis pubis, pain radiating into the inner thigh, and a waddling gait. Characteristic radiographic changes consisting of erosion, sclerosis, and widening of the symphysis pubis are pathognomonic for osteitis pubis. A disease of the second through fourth decades, osteitis pubis affects females more frequently than males. Osteitis pubis occurs most commonly following bladder, inguinal, or prostate surgery and is thought to be due to hematogenous spread of infection to the relatively avascular symphysis pubis. Osteitis pubis can appear without obvious inciting factor or infection.

Signs and Symptoms

On physical examination, the patient will exhibit point tenderness over the symphysis pubis. The patient may be tender over the anterior pelvis and note that the pain radiates into the inner thigh with palpation of the symphysis pubis. Patients may adopt a waddling gait in order to avoid movement of the symphysis pubis. This dysfunctional gait may result in lower extremity bursitis and tendinitis, which may confuse the clinical picture and further increase the patient's pain and disability.

Testing

Plain radiographs are indicated in all patients who present with pain thought to be emanating from the symphysis pubis, to rule out occult bony pathology and tumor. Based on the patient's clinical presentation, additional testing including complete blood count, prostate-specific antigen, erythrocyte sedimentation rate, serum protein electrophoresis, and antinuclear antibody testing may be indicated. Magnetic resonance imaging of the pelvis is indicated if occult mass or tumor is suspected. Radionuclide bone scanning may be useful to rule out stress fractures not seen on plain radiographs.

Differential Diagnosis

A pain syndrome clinically similar to osteitis pubis can be seen in patients suffering from rheumatoid arthritis and ankylosing spondylitis but without the characteristic radiographic changes of osteitis pubis. Multiple myeloma and metastatic tumors may also mimic the pain and radiographic changes of osteitis pubis. Insufficiency fractures of the pubic rami should also be considered if generalized osteoporosis is present.

Treatment

Initial treatment of the pain and functional disability associated with osteitis pubis should include a combination of the nonsteroidal anti-inflammatory agents or cyclooxygenase-2 inhibitors and physical therapy. The local application of heat and cold may also be beneficial. For patients who do not respond to these treatment modalities, the injection of the pubic symphysis with local anesthetic and steroid may be a reasonable next step.

SUGGESTED READING

Waldman SD: Osteitis pubis. In: Atlas of Common Pain Syndromes, ed 2. Philadelphia, Saunders, 2008.

CHAPTER 184

Piriformis Syndrome

Piriformis syndrome is an entrapment neuropathy that presents as pain, numbness, paresthesias, and associated weakness in the distribution of the sciatic nerve. Piriformis syndrome is caused by compression of the sciatic nerve by the piriformis muscle as it passes through the sciatic notch. The piriformis muscle's primary function is to externally rotate the femur at the hip joint. The piriformis muscle is innervated by the sacral plexus. With internal rotation of the femur, the tendinous insertion and belly of the muscle can compress the sciatic nerve and, if this persists, cause entrapment of the sciatic nerve. These symptoms often begin as severe pain in the buttocks, which may radiate into the lower extremity and foot. Patients suffering from piriformis syndrome may develop altered gait, which may result in the development of coexistent sacroiliac, back, and hip pain, which may confuse the clinical picture. Untreated, progressive motor deficit of the gluteal muscles and lower extremity can result. The onset of symptoms of piriformis syndrome is usually after direct trauma to the sacroiliac and gluteal region and occasionally as a result of repetitive hip and lower extremity motions or repeated pressure on the piriformis muscle and underlying sciatic nerve.

Signs and Symptoms

Physical findings include tenderness over the sciatic notch. A positive Tinel's sign over the sciatic nerve as it passes beneath the piriformis muscle is often present. A positive straight leg raising test is suggestive of sciatic nerve entrapment, which may be due to piriformis syndrome. Palpation of the piriformis muscle will reveal tenderness and a swollen, indurated muscle belly. Lifting or bending at the waist and hips will increase the pain symptomatology in most patients suffering from piriformis syndrome. Weakness of affected gluteal muscles and lower extremity and ultimately muscle wasting are often seen in advanced untreated piriformis syndrome.

Testing

Electromyography will help distinguish lumbar radiculopathy from piriformis syndrome. Plain radiographs of the back, hip, and pelvis are indicated in all patients who present with piriformis syndrome to rule out occult bony pathology. Based on the patient's clinical presentation, additional testing including complete blood count, uric acid, erythrocyte sedimentation rate and antinuclear antibody testing may be indicated. Magnetic resonance imaging of the back is indicated if herniated disc, spinal stenosis, or a space-occupying lesion is suspected. Injection in the region of the sciatic nerve at this level will serve as both a diagnostic and therapeutic maneuver.

Differential Diagnosis

Piriformis syndrome is often misdiagnosed as lumbar radiculopathy or attributed to primary hip pathology. Radiographs of the hip and electromyography will help distinguish piriformis syndrome from radiculopathy or pain emanating from the hip. Most patients suffering from a lumbar radiculopathy will have back pain associated with reflex, motor, and sensory changes associated with neck pain, whereas patients with piriformis syndrome will have only secondary back pain and no reflex changes. The motor and sensory changes of piriformis syndrome will be limited to the distribution of the sciatic nerve below the sciatic notch. It should be remembered that lumbar radiculopathy and sciatic nerve entrapment may coexist as the so-called "double crush" syndrome. As mentioned, piriformis syndrome causes alteration of gait that may result in secondary back and radicular symptomatology, which may coexist with this entrapment neuropathy.

Treatment

Initial treatment of the pain and functional disability associated with piriformis syndrome should include a combination of the nonsteroidal anti-inflammatory agents or cyclooxygenase-2 inhibitors and physical therapy. The local application of heat and cold may also be beneficial. Any repetitive activity that may exacerbate the patient's symptomatology should be avoided. Nighttime splinting of the affected extremity by placing a pillow between the legs if the patient sleeps on his or her side may be beneficial. If the patient is suffering from significant paresthesias, gabapentin may be added. For patients who do not respond to these treatment modalities, injection with local anesthetic and steroid in the region of the sciatic nerve at the level of the piriformis muscle may be a reasonable next step. Rarely, surgical release of the entrapment is required to provide relief.

SUGGESTED READING

Waldman SD: Piriformis syndrome. In: Atlas of Common Pain Syndromes, ed 2. Philadelphia, Saunders, 2008.

CHAPTER 185

Arthritis Pain of the Hip

Arthritis of the hip is a common painful condition encountered in clinical practice. The hip joint is susceptible to the development of arthritis from a variety of conditions that have in common the ability to damage the joint cartilage. Osteoarthritis of the joint is the most common form of arthritis that results in hip joint pain. However, rheumatoid arthritis and post-traumatic arthritis are also common causes of hip pain secondary to arthritis. Less common causes of arthritis-induced hip pain include the collagen vascular diseases, infection, villonodular synovitis, and Lyme disease. Acute infectious arthritis will usually be accompanied by significant systemic symptoms including fever and malaise and should be easily recognized by the astute clinician and treated appropriately with culture and antibiotics, rather than injection therapy. The collagen vascular diseases will generally manifest as a polyarthropathy rather than a monoarthropathy limited to the hip joint, although hip pain secondary to collagen vascular disease responds exceedingly well to the treatment modalities described here.

Signs and Symptoms

The majority of patients presenting with hip pain secondary to arthritis of the hip joint will present with the complaint of pain that is localized around the hip and upper leg. The pain may initially present as ill-defined pain in the groin and occasionally is localized to the buttocks. Activity makes the pain worse, with rest and heat providing some relief. The pain is constant and characterized as aching in nature. The pain may interfere with sleep. Some patients will complain of a grating or popping sensation with use of the joint, and crepitus may be present on physical examination.

In addition to the pain mentioned, patients suffering from arthritis of the hip joint will often experience a gradual decrease in functional ability with decreasing hip range of motion, making simple everyday tasks such as walking, climbing stairs, and getting in and out of cars quite difficult. With continued disuse, muscle wasting may occur and a "frozen hip" due to adhesive capsulitis may develop.

Testing

Plain radiographs are indicated in all patients who present with hip pain. Based on the patient's clinical presentation, additional testing including complete blood count, erythrocyte sedimentation rate, and antinuclear antibody testing may be indicated. Magnetic resonance imaging of the hip is indicated if aseptic necrosis or occult mass or tumor is suspected.

Differential Diagnosis

Lumbar radiculopathy may mimic the pain and disability associated with arthritis of the hip. In such patients, the hip examination should be negative. Entrapment neuropathies such as meralgia paresthetica may also confuse the diagnosis, as may trochanteric bursitis, both of which may coexist with arthritis of the hip. Primary and metastatic tumors of the hip and spine may also manifest in a manner analogous to arthritis of the hip.

Treatment

Initial treatment of the pain and functional disability associated with arthritis of the hip should include a combination of the nonsteroidal anti-inflammatory agents or cyclooxygenase-2 inhibitors and physical therapy. The local application of heat and cold may also be beneficial. For patients who do not respond to these treatment modalities, an intra-articular injection of local anesthetic and steroid may be a reasonable next step.

SUGGESTED READING

Waldman SD: Arthritis of the hip. In: Atlas of Common Pain Syndromes, ed 2. Philadelphia, Saunders, 2008.

CHAPTER 186

Femoral Neuropathy

Femoral neuropathy is an uncommon cause of anterior thigh and medial calf pain that has many etiologies. Femoral neuropathy may be due to compression by tumor, retroperitoneal hemorrhage, or abscess. Stretch injuries to the femoral nerve as it passes under the inguinal ligament from extreme extension or flexion at the hip may also produce the symptoms of femoral neuropathy. Direct trauma to the nerve from surgery or during cardiac catheterization can also produce this clinical syndrome, as can diabetes, which can produce vascular lesions of the nerve itself.

The patient with femoral neuropathy presents with pain that radiates into the anterior thigh and midcalf and is associated with weakness of the quadriceps muscle. This weakness can result in significant functional deficit with the patient being unable to fully extend the knee, which can allow the knee to buckle, resulting in inexplicable falls. The patient suffering from femoral neuropathy may also experience weakness of the hip flexors, making walking up stairs quite difficult.

Signs and Symptoms

The patient with femoral neuropathy will present with pain that radiates into the anterior thigh and medial calf. This pain may be paresthetic or burning in character. The intensity is moderate to severe. Weakness of the quadriceps muscle can be quite marked, and over time atrophy of the quadriceps may occur, especially in diabetic patients. Patients with femoral neuropathy may complain of a sunburned feeling over the anterior thigh. The patient may also complain that the knee feels like it is giving way.

Testing

Electromyography can help identify the exact source of neurologic dysfunction and help clarify the differential diagnosis and thus should be the starting point of the evaluation of all patients suspected of having femoral neuropathy. Plain radiographs of the spine, hip, and pelvis are indicated in all patients who present with femoral neuropathy, to rule out occult bony pathology. Based on the patient's clinical presentation, additional testing including complete blood cell count, uric acid, erythrocyte sedimentation rate, and antinuclear antibody testing may be indicated. Magnetic resonance imaging of the spine and pelvis is indicated if tumor or hematoma is suspected. Injection of the femoral nerve at the femoral triangle serves as both a diagnostic and therapeutic maneuver.

Differential Diagnosis

It is difficult to separate femoral neuropathy from an L4 radiculopathy on purely clinical grounds. There may be subtle differences in that the L4 radiculopathy may manifest with sensory changes into the foot and weakness of the dorsiflexors of the foot. It should be remembered that intrapelvic or retroperitoneal tumor or hematoma may compress the lumbar plexus and mimic the clinical presentation of femoral neuropathy.

Treatment

Mild cases of femoral neuropathy will usually respond to conservative therapy, and surgery should be reserved for more severe cases. Initial treatment of femoral neuropathy should consist of treatment with simple analgesics, nonsteroidal anti-inflammatory agents, or cyclooxygenase-2 inhibitors. If diabetes is thought to be the etiology of the patient's femoral neuropathy, tight control of blood sugars is mandatory. Avoidance of repetitive activities thought to be responsible for the exacerbation of femoral neuropathy (e.g., repetitive hip extension and flexion) will also help ameliorate the patient's symptoms. If the patient fails to respond to these conservative measures, a next reasonable step is injection of the femoral nerve with a local anesthetic and steroid.

SUGGESTED READING

Waldman SD: Femoral neuropathy. In: Atlas of Uncommon Pain Syndromes, ed 2. Philadelphia, Saunders, 2008.

Phantom Limb Pain

Almost all patients who undergo amputation experience the sensation that the absent body part is still present. This sensation is often painful and quite distressing to the patient. The genesis of this phenomenon is not fully understood, but it is thought to be mediated in large part at the spinal cord level. Congenitally absent limbs do not seem to be subject to the same phenomenon. Patients with phantom limb pain will often describe the limb in vivid detail, albeit with the limb distorted or in abnormal position. In many patients, the sensation of a phantom limb will fade with time, but in some, phantom pain remains a distressing part of their daily life. The pain of a phantom limb is often described as a constant unpleasant, dysesthetic pain that may be exacerbated by movement or stimulation of the affected cutaneous regions. There may be sharp, shooting neuritic pain superimposed on the constant dysesthetic symptoms. Some patients suffering from phantom limb pain will also note a burning component reminiscent of reflex sympathetic dystrophy. Some investigators report that severe limb pain prior to amputation increases the incidence of phantom limb pain, but other investigators have failed to prove this correlation.

Signs and Symptoms

The phantom limb pain may take multiple forms. It most often takes the form of dysesthetic pain. Additionally, the patient with phantom limb pain may experience abnormal kinesthetic sensation (i.e., the limb is in an abnormal position). The patient may also experience abnormal kinetic sensation (i.e., that the phantom limb is moving). It has been reported that many patients with phantom limb pain experience a telescoping phenomenon (i.e., that the proximal part of the absent limb is missing). When this occurs, that patient may report that the phantom foot feels like it is attached directly to the proximal thigh. Phantom limb pain may fade over time, with younger patients more likely to experience a diminution of phantom limb symptomatology. Due to the unusual nature of phantom limb sensation and pain, a behavioral component to the pain is invariably present.

Testing

In most instances, the diagnosis of phantom limb pain is easily made on clinical grounds. Testing is generally used to identify other treatable coexisting diseases such as radiculopathy. Such testing should include basic screening laboratory testing; examination of the stump for neuroma, tumor, or occult infection; and plain radiographs and radionuclide bone scanning if fracture or osteomyelitis is suspected.

Differential Diagnosis

Careful initial evaluation, including a thorough history and physical examination, is indicated in all patients suffering from phantom limb pain if the possibility of infection or fracture is present. If the amputation was necessitated due to malignancy, the possibility of occult tumor remains ever present. Other causes of pain in the distribution of the innervation of the affected limb including radiculopathy and peripheral neuropathy should be considered.

Treatment

The first step for all clinicians caring for patients with phantom limb pain is to reassure the patient that phantom sensations and/or pain following loss of limb is normal and that these sensations are real, not imagined. This alone will often reduce the anxiety and suffering the patient is experiencing. It is the consensus of most pain specialists that the earlier in the natural course of the painful diseases that may lead to amputation (e.g., peripheral vascular insufficiency) that treatment is initiated, the less likely it is that the patient will develop phantom limb pain. In fact, many pain specialists will recommend preemptive analgesia if the viability of the limb is in doubt prior to surgical amputation whenever possible. The following treatments have been shown to be useful in the palliation of phantom limb pain.

ADJUVANT ANALGESICS

The anticonvulsant gabapentin represents a first-line treatment in the palliation of pain of phantom limb. Treatment with gabapentin should begin early in the course of the disease, and this drug may be used concurrently with neural blockade, opioid analgesics, and other adjuvant analgesics including the antidepressant compounds if care is taken to avoid central nervous system side effects. Gabapentin is started at a bedtime dose of 300 mg and is titrated upward in 300-mg increments to a maximum dose of 3600 mg given in divided doses as side effects allow.

Carbamazepine should be considered in patients suffering from severe neuritic pain who have failed to respond to nerve blocks and gabapentin. If this drug is used, rigid monitoring for hematologic parameters, especially in patients receiving chemotherapy or radiation therapy, is indicated. Phenytoin may also be beneficial to treat neuritic pain but should not be used in patients with lymphoma because the drug may induce a pseudolymphoma–like state that is difficult to distinguish from the actual lymphoma itself.

Antidepressants may also be useful adjuncts in the initial treatment of the patient suffering from phantom limb pain. On an acute basis, these drugs will help alleviate the significant sleep disturbance that is commonly seen in this setting. In addition, the antidepressants may be valuable in helping ameliorate the neuritic component of the pain, which is treated less effectively with narcotic analgesics. After several weeks of treatment, the antidepressants may exert a mood-elevating effect that may be desirable in some patients. Care must be taken to observe closely for central nervous system side effects in this patient population. These drugs may cause urinary retention and constipation.

NERVE BLOCKS

Sympathetic neural blockade with local anesthetics and steroids via either epidural nerve block or blockade of the sympathetic nerves subserving the painful area appears to be a reasonable next step if the pharmacologic modalities mentioned fail to control the pain of phantom limb. The exact mechanism of pain relief from neural blockade when treating phantom limb pain is unknown but may be related to modulation of pain transmission at the spinal cord level. In general, neurodestructive procedures have a very low success rate and should be used only after all other treatments have been optimized, if at all.

OPIOID ANALGESICS

Opioid analgesics have a limited role in the management of phantom limb pain and in the experience of this author frequently do more harm than good. Careful administration of potent, long-acting narcotic analgesics (e.g., oral morphine elixir or methadone) on a time-contingent rather than an as-needed (prn) basis may represent a beneficial adjunct to the pain relief provided by sympathetic neural blockade. Because many patients suffering from phantom limb pain are elderly or may have severe multisystem disease, close monitoring for the potential side effects of potent narcotic analgesics (e.g., confusion or dizziness, which may cause a patient to fall) is warranted. Daily dietary fiber supplementation and milk of magnesia should be started along with opioid analgesics to prevent the side effect of constipation.

ADJUNCTIVE TREATMENTS

The application of ice packs to the area affected with phantom limb pain may provide relief in some patients. Application of heat will increase pain in most patients, presumably because of increased conduction of small fibers, but is beneficial in an occasional patient and may be worth trying if application of cold is ineffective. Transcutaneous electrical nerve stimulation and vibration may also be effective in a limited number of patients. The favorable risk-to-benefit ratio of all these modalities makes them reasonable alternatives for patients who cannot or will not undergo sympathetic neural blockade or tolerate pharmacologic interventions. The topical application of capsaicin may be beneficial in some patients suffering from phantom limb pain. However, the burning associated with this drug when applied to the painful area will often limit the utility of this intervention.

SUGGESTED READING

Waldman SD: Phantom limb pain. In: Atlas of Common Pain Syndromes, ed 2. Philadelphia, Saunders, 2008.

Trochanteric Bursitis

Trochanteric bursitis is a commonly encountered pain complaint in clinical practice. The patient suffering from trochanteric bursitis will frequently complain of pain in the lateral hip that can radiate down the leg, mimicking sciatica. The pain is localized to the area over the trochanter. Often, the patient will be unable to sleep on the affected hip and may complain of a sharp, catching sensation with range of motion of the hip, especially on first arising. The patient may note that walking upstairs is becoming increasingly more difficult. Trochanteric bursitis often coexists with arthritis of the hip joint, back and sacroiliac joint disease, and gait disturbance.

The trochanteric bursa lies between the greater trochanter and the tendon of the gluteus medius and the iliotibial tract. This bursa may exist as a single bursal sac or in some patients as a multisegmented series of sacs that may be loculated in nature. The trochanteric bursa is vulnerable to injury from both acute trauma and repeated microtrauma. Acute injuries frequently take the form of direct trauma to the bursa via falls directly onto the greater trochanter or previous hip surgery as well as from overuse injuries including running on soft or uneven surfaces. If the inflammation of the trochanteric bursa becomes chronic, calcification of the bursa may occur.

Signs and Symptoms

Physical examination of the patient suffering from trochanteric bursitis will reveal point tenderness in the lateral thigh just over the greater trochanter. Passive adduction and abduction as well as active resisted abduction of the affected lower extremity will reproduce the pain.

Sudden release of resistance during this maneuver will markedly increase the pain. There should be no sensory deficit in the distribution of the lateral femoral cutaneous nerve as seen with meralgia paresthetica, which is often confused with trochanteric bursitis

Testing

Plain radiographs of the hip may reveal calcification of the bursa and associated structures consistent with chronic inflammation. Magnetic resonance imaging is indicated if occult mass or tumor of the hip or groin is suspected. Complete blood count and erythrocyte sedimentation rate are useful if infection is suspected. Electromyography will help distinguish trochanteric bursitis from meralgia paresthetica and sciatica.

Differential Diagnosis

Trochanteric bursitis frequently coexists with arthritis of the hip, which may require specific treatment in order to provide palliation of pain and return of function. Occasionally, trochanteric bursitis can be confused with meralgia paresthetica as both present with pain in the lateral thigh. The two syndromes can be distinguished in that patients suffering from meralgia paresthetica will not have pain on palpation over the greater trochanter. Electromyography will help sort out confusing clinical presentations. The clinician must consider the potential for primary or secondary tumors of the hip in the differential diagnosis of trochanteric bursitis.

Treatment

A short course of conservative therapy consisting of simple analgesics, nonsteroidal anti-inflammatory agents, or cyclooxygenase-2 inhibitors is a reasonable first step in the treatment of patients suffering from trochanteric bursitis. The patient should be instructed to avoid repetitive activity that may be responsible for the development of trochanteric bursitis, such as running on sand. If the patient does not experience rapid improvement, injection of the trochanteric bursa is a reasonable next step.

SUGGESTED READING

Waldman SD: Trochanteric bursitis. In: Atlas of Common Pain Syndromes, ed 2. Philadelphia, Saunders, 2008.

CHAPTER 189

Arthritis Pain of the Knee

Arthritis of the knee is a common painful condition encountered in clinical practice. The knee joint is susceptible to the development of arthritis from a variety of conditions that have in common the ability to damage the joint cartilage. Osteoarthritis of the joint is the most common form of arthritis that results in knee joint pain. However, rheumatoid arthritis and post-traumatic arthritis are also common causes of knee pain secondary to arthritis. Less common causes of arthritis-induced knee pain include the collagen vascular diseases, infection, villonodular synovitis, and Lyme disease. Acute infectious arthritis will usually be accompanied by significant systemic symptoms including fever and malaise and should be easily recognized by the astute clinician and treated appropriately with culture and antibiotics, rather than injection therapy. The collagen vascular diseases will generally manifest as a polyarthropathy rather than a monoarthropathy limited to the knee joint, although knee pain secondary to collagen vascular disease responds exceedingly well to the treatment modalities described in this chapter.

Signs and Symptoms

The majority of patients presenting with knee pain secondary to osteoarthritis and post-traumatic arthritis will present with the complaint of pain that is localized around the knee and distal femur. Activity makes the pain worse, with rest and heat providing some relief. The pain is constant and characterized as aching in nature. The pain may interfere with sleep. Some patients will complain of a grating or popping sensation with use of the joint, and crepitus may be present on physical examination.

In addition to the pain mentioned, patients suffering from arthritis of the knee joint will often experience a gradual decrease in functional ability, with decreasing knee range of motion making simple everyday tasks such as walking, climbing stairs, and getting in and out of cars quite difficult. With continued disuse, muscle wasting may occur and a "frozen knee" due to adhesive capsulitis may develop.

Testing

Plain radiographs are indicated in all patients who present with knee pain. Based on the patient's clinical presentation, additional testing including complete blood count, erythrocyte sedimentation rate, and antinuclear antibody testing may be indicated. Magnetic resonance imaging of the knee is indicated if aseptic necrosis or occult mass or tumor is suspected.

Differential Diagnosis

Lumbar radiculopathy may mimic the pain and disability associated with arthritis of the knee. In such patients, the knee examination should be negative. Entrapment neuropathies such as meralgia paresthetica may also confuse the diagnosis, as may bursitis of the knee, both of which may coexist with arthritis of the knee. Primary and metastatic tumors of the femur and spine may also manifest in a manner analogous to arthritis of the knee.

Treatment

Initial treatment of the pain and functional disability associated with arthritis of the knee should include a combination of the nonsteroidal anti-inflammatory agents or cyclooxygenase-2 inhibitors and physical therapy. The local application of heat and cold may also be beneficial. For patients who do not respond to these treatment modalities, an intra-articular injection of local anesthetic and steroid may be a reasonable next step.

SUGGESTED READING

Waldman SD: Arthritis pain of the knee. In: Atlas of Common Pain Syndromes, ed 2. Philadelphia, Saunders, 2008.

Baker's Cyst of the Knee

A common finding on physical examination of the knee, Baker's cyst is the result of an abnormal accumulation of synovial fluid in the medial aspect of the popliteal fossa. Overproduction of synovial fluid from the knee joint results in the formation of a cystic sac. This sac often communicates with the knee joint with a one-way valve effect, causing a gradual expansion of the cyst. Often, a tear of the medial meniscus or a tendinitis of the medial hamstring tendon is the inciting factor responsible for the development of a Baker's cyst. Patients suffering from rheumatoid arthritis are especially susceptible to the development of Baker's cysts.

Signs and Symptoms

Patients with Baker's cysts will complain of a feeling of fullness behind the knee. Often, they will notice a lump behind the knee that becomes more apparent when they flex the affected knee. The cyst may continue to enlarge and may dissect inferiorly into the calf. Patients suffering from rheumatoid arthritis are prone to this phenomenon, and the pain associated with dissection into the calf may be confused with thrombophlebitis and inappropriately treated with anticoagulants. Occasionally, the Baker's cyst may spontaneously rupture, usually after frequent squatting.

On physical examination, the patient suffering from Baker's cyst will have a cystic swelling in the medial aspect of the popliteal fossa. Baker's cysts can become quite large, especially in patients suffering from rheumatoid arthritis. Activity including squatting or walking makes the pain of Baker's cyst worse, with rest and heat providing some relief. The pain is constant and characterized as aching in nature. The pain may interfere with sleep. Baker's cyst may spontaneously rupture, and there may be rubor and color in the calf, which may mimic thrombophlebitis. Homans' sign will be negative and no cords will be palpable.

Testing

Plain radiographs are indicated in all patients who present with Baker's cyst. Based on the patient's clinical presentation, additional testing including complete blood count, erythrocyte sedimentation rate, and antinuclear antibody testing may be indicated. Magnetic resonance imaging of the knee is indicated if internal derangement or occult mass or tumor is suspected and is also useful in confirming the presence of a Baker's cyst.

Differential Diagnosis

As mentioned, Baker's cyst may rupture spontaneously and may be misdiagnosed as thrombophlebitis. Occasionally, tendinitis of the medial hamstring tendon may be confused with Baker's cyst, as may injury to the medial meniscus. Primary or metastatic tumors in the region, although rare, must be considered in the differential diagnosis.

Treatment

Although surgery is often required to successfully treat Baker's cyst, conservative therapy consisting of an elastic bandage combined with a short trial of nonsteroidal anti-inflammatory agents or cyclooxygenase-2 inhibitors is warranted. It these conservative treatments fail, injection of the Baker's cyst represents a reasonable next step.

SUGGESTED READING

Waldman SD: Baker's cyst. In: Atlas of Common Pain Syndromes, ed 2. Philadelphia, Saunders, 2008.

CHAPTER 191

Bursitis Syndromes of the Knee

Bursitis of the knee is one of the most common causes of knee pain encountered in clinical practice. The bursae of the knee are vulnerable to injury from both acute trauma and repeated microtrauma. The bursae of the knee may exist as single bursal sacs or in some patients may exist as a multisegmented series of sacs that may be loculated in nature (Fig. 191-1). Acute injuries to the bursae of the knee frequently take the form of direct trauma to the bursa via falls or blows directly to the knee or from patellar, tibial plateau, and proximal fibular fractures as well as from overuse injuries including running on soft or uneven surfaces or from jobs requiring crawling on the knees such as carpet laying. If the inflammation of the bursae of the knees becomes chronic, calcification of the bursa may occur.

Suprapatellar Bursitis

The suprapatellar bursa extends superiorly from beneath the patella under the quadriceps femoris muscle. The patient suffering from suprapatellar bursitis will frequently complain of pain in the anterior knee above the patella, which can radiate superiorly into the distal anterior thigh. Often, the patient will be unable to kneel or walk down stairs. The patient may also complain of a sharp, catching sensation with range of motion of the knee, especially on first arising. Suprapatellar bursitis often coexists with arthritis and tendinitis of the knee joint, and these other pathologic processes may confuse the clinical picture.

SIGNS AND SYMPTOMS

Physical examination may reveal point tenderness in the anterior knee just above the patella. Passive flexion as well as active resisted extension of the knee will reproduce the pain. Sudden release of resistance during this maneuver will markedly increase the pain. There may be swelling in the suprapatellar region with a boggy feeling to palpation. Occasionally the suprapatellar bursa may become infected with systemic symptoms including fever and malaise, as well as local symptoms including rubor, color, and dolor being present.

TESTING

Plain radiographs of the knee may reveal calcification of the bursa and associated structures including the quadriceps tendon consistent with chronic inflammation. Magnetic resonance imaging (MRI) is indicated if internal derangement, occult mass, or tumor of the knee is suspected. Electromyography will help distinguish suprapatellar bursitis from femoral neuropathy, lumbar radiculopathy, and plexopathy. Complete blood count, automated chemistry profile including uric acid, sedimentation rate, and antinuclear antibody testing are indicated if collagen vascular disease is suspected. If infection is considered, aspiration, Gram stain, and culture of bursal fluid are indicated on an emergent basis

DIFFERENTIAL DIAGNOSIS

Due to the unique anatomy of the region, not only the suprapatellar bursa but also the associated tendons and other bursae of the knee can become inflamed and confuse the diagnosis. The suprapatellar bursa extends superiorly from beneath the patella under the quadriceps femoris muscle and its tendon. The bursa is held in place by a small portion of the vastus intermedius muscle called the articularis genus muscle. Both the quadriceps tendon and the suprapatellar bursa are subject to the development of inflammation following overuse, misuse, or direct trauma. The quadriceps tendon is made up of fibers from the four muscles that comprise the quadriceps muscle: the vastus lateralis, the vastus intermedius, the vastus medialis, and the rectus femoris. These muscles are the primary extensors of the lower extremity at the knee. The tendons of these muscles converge and unite to form a single exceedingly strong tendon. The patella functions as a sesamoid bone within the quadriceps tendon with fibers of the tendon expanding around the patella forming the medial and lateral patellar retinacula, which help strengthen the knee joint. These fibers are called expansions and are subject to strain, and the tendon proper is subject to the development of tendinitis. The suprapatellar, infrapatellar, and prepatellar bursa may also concurrently become inflamed with dysfunction of the quadriceps tendon. It should be remembered that anything that alters the normal biomechanics of the knee can result in inflammation of the suprapatellar bursa.

TREATMENT

A short course of conservative therapy consisting of simple analgesics, nonsteroidal anti-inflammatory agents, or cyclooxygenase (COX)-2 inhibitors and a knee brace to prevent further trauma is a reasonable first step in the treatment of patients suffering from suprapatellar bursitis. If the patient does not experience rapid improvement, injection of the suprapatellar bursa is a reasonable next step. Physical therapy including the application of local heat and cold to restore function should be implemented after the acute pain and swelling have subsided following injection.

Prepatellar Bursitis

The prepatellar bursa is vulnerable to injury from both acute trauma and repeated microtrauma. The prepatellar bursa lies between the subcutaneous tissues and the patella. This bursa may exist as a single bursal sac or in some patients as a multisegmented series of sacs that may be loculated in nature. Acute injuries frequently take the form of direct trauma to the bursa via falls directly onto the knee or from patellar fractures as well as from overuse injuries including running on soft or uneven surfaces. Prepatellar bursitis may also result from jobs requiring crawling or kneeling on the knees such as carpet laying or scrubbing floors—hence, the other name for prepatellar bursitis is *housemaid's knee*. If the inflammation of the prepatellar bursa becomes chronic, calcification of the bursa may occur.

SIGNS AND SYMPTOMS

The patient suffering from prepatellar bursitis will frequently complain of pain and swelling in the anterior knee over the patella, which can radiate superiorly and inferiorly into the area surrounding the knee. Often, the patient will be unable to kneel or walk down stairs. The patient may also complain of a sharp, catching sensation with range of motion of the knee, especially on first arising. Prepatellar bursitis often coexists with arthritis and tendinitis of the knee joint, and these other pathologic processes may confuse the clinical picture.

TESTING

Plain radiographs of the knee may reveal calcification of the bursa and associated structures including the

quadriceps tendon consistent with chronic inflammation. MRI is indicated if internal derangement, occult mass, or tumor of the knee is suspected. Electromyography will help distinguish prepatellar bursitis from femoral neuropathy, lumbar radiculopathy, and plexopathy. Antinuclear antibody testing is indicated if collagen vascular disease is suspected. If infection is considered, aspiration, Gram stain, and culture of bursal fluid are indicated on an emergent basis.

DIFFERENTIAL DIAGNOSIS

Due to the unique anatomy of the region, not only the prepatellar bursa but also the associated tendons and other bursae of the knee can become inflamed and confuse the diagnosis. The prepatellar bursa lies between the subcutaneous tissues and the patella. The bursa is held in place by ligamentum patellae. Both the quadriceps tendon as well as the prepatellar bursa are subject to the development of inflammation following overuse, misuse, or direct trauma. The quadriceps tendon is made up of fibers from the four muscles that comprise the quadriceps muscle: the vastus lateralis, the vastus intermedius, the vastus medialis, and the rectus femoris. These muscles are the primary extensors of the lower extremity at the knee. The tendons of these muscles converge and unite to form a single exceedingly strong tendon. The patella functions as a sesamoid bone within the quadriceps tendon with fibers of the tendon expanding around the patella forming the medial and lateral patella retinacula, which help strengthen the knee joint. These fibers are called expansions and are subject to strain, and the tendon proper is subject to the development of tendinitis. The suprapatellar, infrapatellar, and prepatellar bursa may also concurrently become inflamed with dysfunction of the quadriceps tendon. It should be remembered that anything that alters the normal biomechanics of the knee can result in inflammation of the prepatellar bursa.

TREATMENT

A short course of conservative therapy consisting of simple analgesics, nonsteroidal anti-inflammatory agents or COX-2 inhibitors, and a knee brace to prevent further trauma is a reasonable first step in the treatment of patients suffering from prepatellar bursitis. If the patient does not experience rapid improvement, injection of the prepatellar bursa is a reasonable next step. Physical therapy including the application of local heat and cold to restore function should be implemented after the acute pain and swelling have subsided following injection.

Superficial Infrapatellar Bursitis

The superficial infrapatellar bursa is vulnerable to injury from both acute trauma and repeated microtrauma. The superficial infrapatellar bursa lies between the subcutaneous tissues and the upper part of the ligamentum patellae. The deep infrapatellar bursa lies between the ligamentum patellae and the tibia. These bursae may exist as single bursal sacs or in some patients as a multisegmented series of sacs that may be loculated in nature. Acute injuries frequently take the form of direct trauma to the bursa via falls directly onto the knee or from patellar fractures as well as from overuse injuries including running on soft or uneven surfaces. Superficial infrapatellar bursitis may also result from jobs requiring crawling on the knees or kneeling, such as carpet laying or scrubbing floors. If the inflammation of the superficial infrapatellar bursa becomes chronic, calcification of the bursa may occur.

SIGNS AND SYMPTOMS

The patient suffering from superficial infrapatellar bursitis will frequently complain of pain and swelling in the anterior knee over the patella, which can radiate superiorly and inferiorly into the area surrounding the knee. Often, the patient will be unable to kneel or walk down stairs. The patient may also complain of a sharp, catching sensation with range of motion of the knee, especially on first arising. Superficial infrapatellar bursitis often coexists with arthritis and tendinitis of the knee joint, and these other pathologic processes may confuse the clinical picture.

TESTING

Plain radiographs of the knee may reveal calcification of the bursa and associated structures including the quadriceps tendon consistent with chronic inflammation. MRI is indicated if internal derangement, occult mass, or tumor of the knee is suspected. Electromyography will help distinguish superficial infrapatellar bursitis from femoral neuropathy, lumbar radiculopathy, and plexopathy. Antinuclear antibody testing is indicated if collagen vascular disease is suspected. If infection is considered, aspiration, Gram stain, and culture of bursal fluid are indicated on an emergent basis.

DIFFERENTIAL DIAGNOSIS

Due to the unique anatomy of the region, not only the superficial infrapatellar bursa but also the associated tendons and other bursae of the knee can become inflamed and confuse the diagnosis. Both the quadriceps tendon and the superficial infrapatellar bursa are subject to the development of inflammation following overuse, misuse, or direct trauma. The quadriceps tendon is made up of fibers from the four muscles that compose the quadriceps muscle: the vastus lateralis, the vastus intermedius, the vastus medialis, and the rectus femoris. These muscles are the primary extensors of the lower extremity at the knee. The tendons of these muscles converge and unite to form a single exceedingly strong tendon. The patella functions as a sesamoid bone within the quadriceps tendon with fibers of the tendon expanding around the patella forming the medial and lateral patellar retinacula, which help strengthen the knee joint. These fibers are called expansions and are subject to strain, and the tendon proper is subject to the development of tendinitis. The suprapatellar, infrapatellar, and superficial infrapatellar bursa may also concurrently become inflamed with dysfunction of the quadriceps tendon. It should be remembered that anything that alters the normal biomechanics of the knee can result in inflammation of the superficial infrapatellar bursa.

TREATMENT

A short course of conservative therapy consisting of simple analgesics, nonsteroidal anti-inflammatory agents, or COX-2 inhibitors and a knee brace to prevent further trauma is a reasonable first step in the treatment of patients suffering from superficial infrapatellar bursitis. If the patient does not experience rapid improvement, the superficial infrapatellar technique is a reasonable next step. Physical therapy including the application of local heat and cold to restore function should be implemented after the acute pain and swelling have subsided following injection.

Pes Anserine Bursitis

The pes anserine bursa lies beneath the pes anserine tendon, which is the insertional tendon of the sartorius, gracilis, and semitendinosus muscle to the medial side of the tibia. This bursa may exist as a single bursal sac or in some patients as a multisegmented series of sacs that may be loculated in nature. Patients with pes anserine bursitis will present with pain over the medial knee joint and increased pain on passive valgus and external rotation of the knee. Activity, especially involving flexion and external rotation of the knee, will make the pain worse, with rest and heat providing some relief. Often, the patient will be unable to kneel or walk down stairs.

SIGNS AND SYMPTOMS

The pain of pes anserine bursitis is constant and characterized as aching in nature. The pain may interfere with sleep. Coexistent bursitis, tendinitis, arthritis, and/or internal derangement of the knee may confuse the clinical picture following trauma to the knee joint. Frequently, the medial collateral ligament is also involved if the patient has sustained trauma to the medial knee joint. If the inflammation of the pes anserine bursa becomes chronic, calcification of the bursa may occur.

Physical examination may reveal point tenderness in the anterior knee just below the medial knee joint at the tendinous insertion of the pes anserine. Swelling and fluid accumulation surrounding the bursa are often present. Active resisted flexion of the knee will reproduce the pain. Sudden release of resistance during this maneuver will markedly increase the pain. Rarely, the pes anserine bursa will become infected in a manner analogous to infection of the prepatellar bursa.

TESTING

Plain radiographs of the knee may reveal calcification of the bursa and associated structures including the pes anserine tendon consistent with chronic inflammation. MRI is indicated if internal derangement, occult mass, or tumor of the knee is suspected. Electromyography will help distinguish pes anserine bursitis from neuropathy, lumbar radiculopathy, and plexopathy.

DIFFERENTIAL DIAGNOSIS

The pes anserine bursa is prone to the development of inflammation following overuse, misuse, or direct trauma. The medial collateral ligament is often also involved if the medial knee has been subjected to trauma. The medial collateral ligament is a broad, flat bandlike ligament that runs from the medial condyle of the femur to the medial aspect of the shaft of the tibia where it attaches just above the grove of the semimembranosus muscle. It also attaches to the edge of the medial semilunar cartilage. The medial collateral ligament is crossed at its lower part by the tendons of the sartorius, gracilis, and semitendinosus muscles. Because of the unique anatomic relationships of the medial knee, it is often difficult on clinical grounds to accurately diagnose which anatomic structure is responsible for the patient's pain. MRI will help sort things out and rule out lesions such as tears of the medial meniscus that may require surgical intervention. It should be remembered that anything that alters the normal biomechanics of the knee can result in inflammation of the pes anserine bursa.

TREATMENT

A short course of conservative therapy consisting of simple analgesics, nonsteroidal anti-inflammatory agents, or COX-2 inhibitors and a knee brace to prevent further trauma is a reasonable first step in the treatment of patients suffering from pes anserine bursitis. If the patient does not experience rapid improvement, injection of the pes anserine bursa is a reasonable next step. The use of physical modalities including local heat and gentle range of motion exercises should be introduced several days after the injection. Vigorous exercises should be avoided because they will exacerbate the patient's symptomatology.

Complications and Pitfalls in the Treatment of Bursitis of the Knee

Coexistent bursitis, tendinitis, arthritis, and internal derangement of the knee may also contribute to the patient's pain and may require additional treatment. The simple analgesics and nonsteroidal anti-inflammatory agents are a reasonable starting place in the treatment of bursitis of the knee. If ineffective, the injection of the inflamed bursa with local anesthetic and steroid is a reasonable next step. The injection of the inflamed bursa is a generally safe procedure if careful attention is paid to the clinically relevant anatomy in the areas to be injected. The clinician should remember that failure to identify infection or primary or metastatic tumors of the distal femur, joint, or proximal tibia and fibula that may be responsible for the patient's pain may yield disastrous results.

SUGGESTED READING

Waldman SD: Bursitis of the knee. In: Physical Diagnosis of Pain: An Atlas of Signs and Symptoms. Philadelphia, Saunders, 2006.

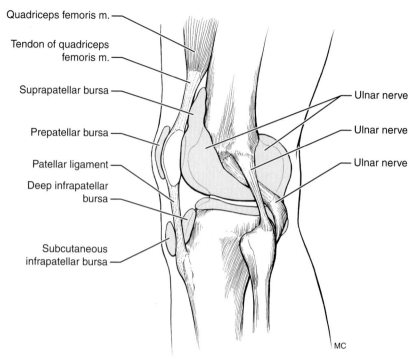

Quadriceps femoris m.

Tendon of quadriceps femoris m.

Suprapatellar bursa

Prepatellar bursa

Patellar ligament

Deep infrapatellar bursa

Subcutaneous infrapatellar bursa

Ulnar nerve

Ulnar nerve

Ulnar nerve

MC

FIGURE 191–1 The bursae of the knee.

CHAPTER 192

Anterior Tarsal Tunnel Syndrome

Anterior tarsal tunnel syndrome is caused by compression of the deep peroneal nerve as it passes beneath the superficial fascia of the ankle. The most common causes of compression of the deep peroneal nerve at this anatomic location is trauma to the dorsum of the foot. Severe, acute plantar flexion of the foot has been implicated in anterior tarsal tunnel syndrome as has the wearing of overly tight shoes or squatting and bending forward such as when planting flowers. Anterior tarsal tunnel syndrome is much less common that posterior tarsal tunnel syndrome.

Signs and Symptoms

This entrapment neuropathy presents primarily as pain, numbness, and paresthesias of the dorsum of the foot that radiates into the first dorsal web space. These symptoms may also radiate proximal to the entrapment into the anterior ankle. There is no motor involvement unless the distal lateral division of the deep peroneal nerve is involved. Nighttime foot pain analogous to the nocturnal pain of carpal tunnel syndrome is often present. The patient may report that holding the foot in the everted position may decrease the pain and paresthesias of anterior tarsal tunnel syndrome.

Physical findings include tenderness over the deep peroneal nerve at the dorsum of the foot. A positive Tinel's sign just medial to the dorsalis pedis pulse over the deep peroneal nerve as it passes beneath the fascia is usually present. Active plantar flexion will often reproduce the symptoms of anterior tarsal tunnel syndromes. Weakness of the extensor digitorum brevis may be present if the lateral branch of the deep peroneal nerve is affected.

Testing

Electromyography will help distinguish lumbar radiculopathy and diabetic polyneuropathy from anterior tarsal tunnel syndrome. Plain radiographs are indicated in all patients who present with anterior tarsal tunnel syndrome to rule out occult bony pathology. Based on the patient's clinical presentation, additional testing including complete blood count, uric acid, erythrocyte sedimentation rate, and antinuclear antibody testing may be indicated. Magnetic resonance imaging scan of the ankle and foot is indicated if joint instability or a space-occupying lesion is suspected.

Differential Diagnosis

Anterior tarsal tunnel syndrome is often misdiagnosed as arthritis of the ankle joint, lumbar radiculopathy, or diabetic polyneuropathy. Patients with arthritis of the ankle joint will have radiographic evidence of arthritis. Most patients suffering from a lumbar radiculopathy will have reflex, motor, and sensory changes associated with back pain, whereas patients with anterior tarsal tunnel syndrome will have no reflex changes and motor and sensory changes will be limited to the distal deep peroneal nerve. Diabetic polyneuropathy will generally manifest as symmetrical sensory deficit involving the entire foot rather than limited just in the distribution of the deep peroneal nerve. It should be remembered that lumbar radiculopathy and deep peroneal nerve entrapment may coexist as

the so-called "double crush" syndrome. Furthermore, because anterior tarsal tunnel syndrome is seen in patients with diabetes, it is not surprising that diabetic polyneuropathy is usually present in diabetic patients with anterior tarsal tunnel syndrome.

Treatment

Mild cases of tarsal tunnel syndrome will usually respond to conservative therapy, and surgery should be reserved for more severe cases. Initial treatment of tarsal tunnel syndrome should consist of treatment with simple analgesics, nonsteroidal anti-inflammatory agents, or cyclooxygenase-2 inhibitors and splinting of the ankle. At a minimum, the splint should be worn at night, but ideally it should be worn 24 hours a day. Avoidance of repetitive activities thought to be responsible for the evolution of tarsal tunnel syndrome, such as prolonged squatting, wearing shoes that are too tight, and so on, will also help ameliorate the patient's symptoms. If the patient fails to respond to these conservative measures, a next reasonable step is injection of the anterior tarsal tunnel with local anesthetic and steroid.

SUGGESTED READING

Waldman SD: Anterior tarsal tunnel syndrome. In: Atlas of Common Pain Syndromes, ed 2. Philadelphia, Saunders, 2008.

Posterior Tarsal Tunnel Syndrome

Posterior tarsal tunnel syndrome is caused by compression of the posterior tibial nerve as it passes through the posterior tarsal tunnel. The posterior tarsal tunnel is made up of the flexor retinaculum, the bones of the ankle, and the lacunata ligament. In addition to the posterior tibial nerve, the tunnel contains the posterior tibial artery and a number of flexor tendons that are subject to tenosynovitis. The most common causes of compression of the posterior tibial nerve at this anatomic location is trauma to ankle including fracture, dislocation, and crush injuries. Thrombophlebitis involving the posterior tibial artery has

also been implicated in the evolution of posterior tarsal tunnel syndrome. Patients with rheumatoid arthritis have a higher incidence of posterior tarsal tunnel syndrome than the general population. Posterior tarsal tunnel syndrome is much more common that anterior tarsal tunnel syndrome.

Signs and Symptoms

Posterior tarsal tunnel syndrome manifests in a manner analogous to carpal tunnel syndrome. The patient will complain of pain, numbness, and paresthesias of the sole of the foot. These symptoms may also radiate proximal to the entrapment into the medial ankle. The medial and lateral plantar divisions of the posterior tibial nerve provide motor innervation to the intrinsic muscles of the foot. The patient may note weakness of the toe flexors and instability of the foot due to weakness of the lumbrical muscles. Nighttime foot pain analogous to the nocturnal pain of carpal tunnel syndrome is often present.

Physical findings include tenderness over the posterior tibial nerve at the medial malleolus. A positive Tinel's sign just below and behind the medial malleolus over the posterior tibial nerve is usually present. Active inversion of the ankle will often reproduce the symptoms of posterior tarsal tunnel syndromes. Weakness of the flexor digitorum brevis and the lumbrical muscles may be present if the medial and lateral branches of the posterior tibial nerve are affected.

Testing

Electromyography will help distinguish lumbar radiculopathy and diabetic polyneuropathy from posterior tarsal tunnel syndrome. Plain radiographs are indicated in all patients who present with posterior tarsal tunnel syndrome, to rule out occult bony pathology. Based on the patient's clinical presentation, additional testing including complete blood count, uric acid, erythrocyte sedimentation rate, and antinuclear antibody testing may be indicated. Magnetic resonance imaging of the ankle and foot is indicated if joint instability or a space-occupying lesion is suspected.

Differential Diagnosis

Posterior tarsal tunnel syndrome is often misdiagnosed as arthritis of the ankle joint, lumbar radiculopathy, or diabetic polyneuropathy. Patients with arthritis of the ankle joint will have radiographic evidence of arthritis. Most patients suffering from a lumbar radiculopathy will have reflex, motor, and sensory changes associated with back pain, whereas patients with posterior tarsal tunnel syndrome will have no reflex changes and motor and sensory changes will be limited to the distal posterior tibial nerve. Diabetic polyneuropathy will generally manifest as symmetrical sensory deficit involving the entire foot rather than limited just in the distribution of the posterior tibial nerve. It should be remembered that lumbar radiculopathy and posterior tibial nerve entrapment may coexist as the so-called "double crush" syndrome. Furthermore, because posterior tarsal tunnel syndrome is seen in patients with diabetes, it is not surprising that diabetic polyneuropathy is usually present in diabetic patients with posterior tarsal tunnel syndrome.

Treatment

Mild cases of tarsal tunnel syndrome will usually respond to conservative therapy, and surgery should be reserved for more severe cases. Initial treatment of tarsal tunnel syndrome should consist of treatment with simple analgesics, nonsteroidal anti-inflammatory agents, or cyclooxygenase-2 inhibitors and splinting of the ankle. At a minimum, the splint should be worn at night, but ideally it should be worn 24 hours a day. Avoidance of repetitive activities thought to be responsible for the evolution of tarsal tunnel syndrome will also help ameliorate the patient's symptoms. If the patient fails to respond to these conservative measures, a next reasonable step is injection of the posterior tarsal tunnel with local anesthetic and steroid.

SUGGESTED READING

Waldman SD: Posterior tarsal tunnel syndrome. In: Atlas of Common Pain Syndromes, ed 2. Philadelphia, Saunders, 2008.

Achilles Tendinitis

Achilles tendinitis is being seen with increasing frequency in clinical practice as jogging has increased in popularity. The Achilles tendon is susceptible to the development of tendinitis both at its insertion on the calcaneus and at its narrowest part at a point approximately 5 cm above its insertion. The Achilles tendon is subject to repetitive motion that may result in microtrauma, which heals poorly owing to the tendon's avascular nature. Running is often implicated as the inciting factor of acute Achilles tendinitis. Tendinitis of the Achilles tendon frequently coexists with bursitis of the associated bursae of the tendon and ankle joint, creating additional pain and functional disability. Calcium deposition around the tendon may occur if the inflammation continues, making subsequent treatment more difficult. Continued trauma to the inflamed tendon may ultimately result in tendon rupture.

Signs and Symptoms

The onset of Achilles tendinitis is usually acute, occurring after overuse or misuse of the ankle joint. Inciting factors may include activities such as running and sudden stopping and starting such as when playing tennis. Improper stretching of the gastrocnemius and Achilles tendon before exercise has also been implicated in the development of Achilles tendinitis as well as acute tendon rupture. The pain of Achilles tendinitis is constant and severe and is localized in the posterior ankle. Significant sleep disturbance is often reported. The patient may attempt to splint the inflamed Achilles tendon by adopting a flatfooted gait to avoid plantar flexing the affected tendon. Patients with Achilles tendinitis will exhibit pain with resisted plantar flexion of the foot. A creaking or grating sensation may be palpated when passively plantar flexing the foot. As mentioned, the chronically inflamed Achilles tendon may suddenly rupture with stress or during vigorous injection procedures into the tendon itself.

Testing

Plain radiographs are indicated for all patients who present with posterior ankle pain. Based on the patient's clinical presentation, additional testing, including complete blood count, erythrocyte sedimentation rate, and antinuclear antibody testing, may be indicated. Magnetic resonance imaging of the ankle is indicated if joint instability is suspected. Radionuclide bone scanning is useful to identify stress fractures of the tibia not seen on plain radiographs.

Differential Diagnosis

Achilles tendinitis is generally easily identified on clinical grounds. Because a bursa is located between the Achilles tendon and the base of the tibia and the upper posterior calcaneus, coexistent bursitis may confuse the diagnosis. Stress fractures of the ankle may also mimic Achilles tendinitis and may be identified on plain radiographs or radionuclide bone scanning.

Treatment

Initial treatment of the pain and functional disability associated with Achilles tendinitis should include a combination of the nonsteroidal anti-inflammatory drugs or cyclooxygenase-2 inhibitors and physical therapy. The local application of heat and cold may also be beneficial. Avoidance of repetitive activities responsible for the evolution of the tendinitis, such as jogging, should be encouraged. For patients who do not respond to these treatment modalities, injection of the Achilles tendon with local anesthetic and steroid may be a reasonable next step.

SUGGESTED READING

Waldman SD: Achilles tendinitis. In: Atlas of Common Pain Syndromes, ed 2. Philadelphia, Saunders, 2008.

CHAPTER 195

Metatarsalgia

Along with sesamoiditis, metatarsalgia is another painful condition of the forefoot that is being seen with increasing frequency in clinical practice owing to the increased interest in jogging and long distance running. Metatarsalgia is characterized by tenderness and pain over the metatarsal heads. The patient often feels that he or she is walking with a stone in their shoe. The pain of metatarsalgia worsens with prolonged standing or walking for long distances and is exacerbated by improperly fitting or padded shoes. Often, the patient suffering from metatarsalgia will develop hard callus formation over the heads of the second and third metatarsal as he or she tries to shift the weight off the head of the first metatarsal to relieve the pain. This callus formation increases the pressure on the metatarsal heads and further exacerbates the patient's pain and disability.

Signs and Symptoms

On physical examination, pain can be reproduced by pressure on the metatarsal heads. Callus formation will often be present over the heads of the second and third metatarsal and can be distinguished from plantar warts by the lack of thrombosed blood vessels, which appear as small dark spots through the substance of the wart when the surface is trimmed. The patient with metatarsalgia will often exhibit an antalgic gait in an effort to reduce weight bearing during the static stance phase of walking. Ligamentous laxity and flattening of the transverse arch may also be present, giving the foot a splayed-out appearance.

Testing

Plain radiographs are indicated in all patients who present with metatarsalgia to rule out fractures and to identify sesamoid bones that may have become inflamed. Based on the patient's clinical presentation, additional testing including complete blood count, erythrocyte sedimentation rate, and antinuclear antibody testing may be indicated. Magnetic resonance imaging of the metatarsal bones is indicated if joint instability, occult mass, or tumor is suspected. Radionuclide bone scanning may be useful in identifying stress fractures that may be missed on plain radiographs of the foot.

Differential Diagnosis

Primary pathology of the foot including gout and occult fractures may mimic the pain and disability associated with metatarsalgia. Entrapment neuropathies such as tarsal tunnel syndrome may also confuse the diagnosis, as may bursitis and plantar fasciitis of the foot, both of which may coexist with sesamoiditis. Sesamoid bones beneath the heads of the metatarsal bones are present in some individuals and are subject to the development of inflammation called sesamoiditis. Sesamoiditis is another common cause of forefoot pain and may be distinguished from metatarsalgia by the fact that the pain of metatarsalgia is centered over the patient's metatarsal heads and does not move when the patient actively flexes his or her toes, as is the case with sesamoiditis. The muscles of the metatarsal joints and their attaching tendons are also susceptible to trauma and to wear and tear from overuse and misuse and may contribute to forefoot pain. Primary and metastatic tumors of the foot may also present in a manner analogous to arthritis of the midtarsal joints.

Treatment

Initial treatment of the pain and functional disability associated with metatarsalgia should include a combination of the nonsteroidal anti-inflammatory agents or cyclooxygenase-2 inhibitors and physical therapy. The local application of heat and cold may also be beneficial. Avoidance of repetitive activities that aggravate the patient's symptomatology as well as short-term immobilization of the midtarsal joint may also provide relief. For patients who do not respond to these treatment modalities, injection of the affected metatarsal heads with local anesthetic and steroid may be a reasonable next step.

SUGGESTED READING

Waldman SD: Metatarsalgia. In: Atlas of Common Pain Syndromes, ed 2. Philadelphia, Saunders, 2008.

Plantar Fasciitis

Plantar fasciitis is characterized by pain and tenderness over the plantar surface of the calcaneus. Occurring twice as commonly in women, plantar fasciitis is thought to be caused by an inflammation of the plantar fascia. This inflammation can occur alone or can be part of a systemic inflammatory condition such as rheumatoid arthritis, Reiter's syndrome, or gout. Obesity also seems to predispose to the development of plantar fasciitis, as does going barefoot or wearing house slippers for prolonged periods. High-impact aerobic exercise has also been implicated.

Signs and Symptoms

The pain of plantar fasciitis is most severe on first walking after non–weight bearing and is made worse by prolonged standing or walking. Characteristic radiographic changes are lacking in plantar fasciitis, but radionuclide bone scanning may show increased uptake at the point of attachment of the plantar fascia to the medial calcaneal tuberosity.

On physical examination, the patient will exhibit point tenderness over the plantar medial calcaneal tuberosity. The patient may also be tender along the plantar fascia as it moves anteriorly. Pain will be increased by dorsiflexing the toes, which pulls the plantar fascia taut, and then palpating along the fascia from the heel to the forefoot.

Differential Diagnosis

The pain of plantar fasciitis can often be confused with the pain of Morton's neuroma or sesamoiditis. The characteristic pain on dorsiflexion of the toes associated with plantar fasciitis should help distinguish these painful conditions of the foot. Stress fractures of the metatarsals or sesamoid bones, bursitis, and tendinitis may also confuse the clinical picture.

Testing

Plain radiographs are indicated in all patients who present with pain thought to be emanating from plantar fasciitis, to rule out occult bony pathology and tumor. Based on the patient's clinical presentation, additional testing including complete blood count, prostate-specific antigen, erythrocyte sedimentation rate, and antinuclear antibody testing may be indicated. Magnetic resonance imaging of the foot is indicated if occult mass or tumor is suspected. Radionuclide bone scanning may be useful to rule out stress fractures not seen on plain radiographs.

Treatment

Initial treatment of the pain and functional disability associated with plantar fasciitis should include a combination of the nonsteroidal anti-inflammatory agents or cyclooxygenase-2 inhibitors and physical therapy. The local application of heat and cold may also be beneficial. Avoidance of repetitive activities that aggravate the patient's symptomatology, as well as avoidance of walking barefoot or with shoes that do not provide good support, combined with short-term immobilization of the affected foot may also provide relief. For patients who do not respond to these treatment modalities, injection of the plantar fascia with local anesthetic and steroid may be a reasonable next step.

SUGGESTED READING

Waldman SD: Plantar fasciitis. In: Atlas of Common Pain Syndromes, ed 2. Philadelphia, Saunders, 2008.

CHAPTER 197

Complex Regional Pain Syndrome

Complex regional pain syndrome (CRPS) is defined by the International Association for the Study of Pain as "a variety of painful conditions following injury which appears regionally having a distal predominance of abnormal findings, exceeding in both magnitude and duration the expected clinical course of the inciting event often resulting in significant impairment of motor function, and showing variable progression over time." Whether this definition clarifies or confuses these often difficult-to-diagnose-and-treat conditions remains to be seen, but the following generalizations are useful when confronted with a patient thought to be suffering from CRPS.

Types

CRPS is divided into two types: CRPS I and CRPS II. CRPS I occurs more commonly in females and has a peak occurrence in the fourth and fifth decades. Both CRPS types I and II share a unique constellation of signs and symptoms, including allodynia, spontaneous pain, hyperalgesia, autonomic dysfunction including sudomotor and vasomotor changes, edema, and trophic changes (Table 197-1). CRPS I, which was previously known as reflex sympathetic dystrophy, is thought to occur following minor trauma, including soft tissue injuries and minor fractures. CRPS II, which was previously known as causalgia, is thought to occur following injuries that involve a major peripheral nerve.

Causes

Clinically, CRPS types I and II manifest in an analogous manner, with the common denominator being trauma as

TABLE 197–1 Common Characteristics of Complex Regional Pain Syndrome

- Allodynia
- Spontaneous pain
- Hyperalgesia
- Autonomic dysfunction
  - Sudomotor changes
  - Vasomotor changes
- Edema
- Trophic changes

a precipitating event. This trauma usually involves a distal extremity, although CRPS can occur following central nervous system disorders such as stroke or spinal cord injuries or myocardial ischemic events. In rare patients, classic CRPS can occur without demonstrable antecedent trauma.

Signs and Symptoms

Initially, the pain will manifest in a single extremity or unilateral face that the sufferer will describe as burning and distressing in nature. The complaints of pain will often seem out of proportion to the degree of trauma that the patient has sustained. Any stimulus of the affected body part will result in an exacerbation of pain with hyperalgesia (an increased response to noxious stimuli) and allodynia (a painful response from a stimulus that does not ordinarily elicit pain) is often present. This pain is nondermatomal, and it does not follow the distribution of a specific peripheral nerve. Autonomic dysfunction of the affected body part is manifested by disorders of sweating, temperature regulation, and edema. In the early stages of CRPS, the affected body part feels warmer to the examiner than the normal body part, with this temperature disparity reversing itself in the later stages of the disease (see later). Edema of the affected body part is invariably present, and placing the affected part in the dependent position will often exacerbate the patient's symptomatology.

Trophic changes such as abnormal skin appearance and hair and nail growth and osteoporosis begin early in the course of CRPS and worsen if the disease is left untreated until significant functional abnormalities, including loss of range of motion and tremor of the affected body part, result.

Stages

Traditionally, CRPS types I and II have been divided into three stages, although many clinicians find it more useful to conceptualize CRPS as a continuum of signs and symptoms that are best treated early.

- *Stage I* CRPS is characterized by the onset of pain with hyperalgesia and allodynia with early trophic skin and nail changes apparent to the careful observer. This stage is thought to last 2 to 3 months.

- *Stage II* CRPS is characterized by the pain being accompanied with more obvious trophic changes and marked edema. Early functional limitations are identified on careful manual muscle and range of motion testing. This stage is thought to last 3 to 6 months.
- *Stage III* CRPS is characterized by obvious skin, nail, and hair changes and significant functional limitations of the affected body part, including atrophy, contractures, and a spread of symptoms to adjacent tissue. Many of these changes are irreversible.

Pathophysiology

Although the exact pathophysiology responsible for CRPS is not yet elucidated, it is thought that the unique pattern of pain and sensory abnormalities are due to changes in how the somatosensory areas of the thalamus and cerebral cortex process thermal, mechanical, and pain stimuli. This alteration in processing of this information appears to lead to a central sensitization with hyperexcitability of both motor and sensory neurons. Dysregulation of the sympathetic response that is thought to be centrally mediated is postulated to be responsible for the autonomic changes observed in CRPS.

Diagnostic Testing

Although there are no diagnostic tests that are specific for CRPS, there are several diagnostic interventions that can help support or refute a diagnosis of CRPS. Because osteoporosis is a common finding associated with CRPS, three-phase bone scanning can help identify findings consistent with a diagnosis of CRPS within the first year to 18 months following the onset of symptoms. This test becomes less useful as the disease progresses. Findings suggestive of CRPS include a homogeneous unilateral hyperperfusion in the affected body part at 30 seconds post injection during the perfusion phase and at 2 minutes during the blood pool phase. The mineralization phase, which is scanned at 3 hours post injection, will most often show unilateral periarticular isotope uptake, with increased uptake in the metacarpal and metatarsal bones strengthening the diagnosis of CRPS. Later in the course of the disease, plain radiographs can provide useful diagnostic information as the trophic changes associated with the disease become more apparent. Subperiosteal and trabecular bone resorption and subchondral erosions are highly suggestive of CRPS. Quantification of temperature abnormalities of the affected body part compared with the contralateral side with digital thermography or temperature probes may also be of value.

Treatment

The successful treatment of CRPS has two requirements. First, any nidus of tissue trauma that is contributing to the ongoing sympathetic dysfunction responsible for the symptoms of CRPS must be identified and removed; second, interruption of the sympathetic innervation or sympathetic neural blockade with local anesthetics and/or steroids must be implemented immediately. Neuroaugmentation via spinal cord stimulation is also a useful modality if sympathetic blocks and adjuvant analgesics fail to control the patient's symptomatology. Occupational therapy consisting of tactile desensitization of the affected skin may also be of value. Underlying depression and sleep disturbance are best treated with a tricyclic antidepressant such as nortriptyline given as a single bedtime dose of 25 mg. Gabapentin may help palliate any component of neuritic pain. Opioid analgesics and benzodiazepines should be avoided to prevent iatrogenic chemical dependence. Underlying depression and behavioral abnormalities may require psychiatric intervention as a part of a multimodality treatment plan.

SUGGESTED READING

Baron R: Complex regional pain syndromes. In: McMahon S, Koltzenburg M (eds): Wall and Melzack's Textbook of Pain, ed. 5. Philadelphia, Churchill Livingstone, 2006.

CHAPTER 198

Rheumatoid Arthritis

Rheumatoid arthritis (RA) is the most common of the connective tissue diseases, with approximately 1.5% of the population affected. The cause of RA is unknown, but there appears to be a genetic predisposition to the development of this disease. Environmental factors may trigger the activation of RA and initiate the autoimmune response that ultimately can lead to potentially devastating multisystem disease. The possibility of an infectious etiology has gained new credence as the pathophysiologic processes behind Lyme disease are being elucidated.

The disease can occur at any age, with the juvenile variant termed *Still's disease.* Patients between the ages of 22 and 55 are most often affected, with increasing incidence with age. Women are affected 2.5 times more often than are men. Although the clinical diagnosis of RA is usually obvious in full-blown cases, the variability of presentation, severity, and progression can make the disease more difficult to diagnose. Because of the nonspecific nature of the signs and symptoms of RA, as well as the significant overlap of symptoms associated with other connective tissue diseases, the American College of Rheumatology has promulgated useful guidelines to assist the clinician in the diagnosis of RA. These guidelines are presented in Table 198-1.

TABLE 198–1 ACR Clinical Classification Criteria for Rheumatoid Arthritis

Four of the following seven must be present, with items 1 through 4 lasting at least 6 weeks.
1. Morning stiffness for at least 1 hour
2. Arthritis of three or more of the following joints: right or left PIP, MCP, wrist, elbow, knee, ankle, and MTP joints
3. Arthritis of wrist, MCP, or PIP joint
4. Symmetric involvement of joints
5. Rheumatoid nodules over bony prominences, or extensor surfaces, or in juxta-articular regions
6. Positive serum rheumatoid factor
7. Radiographic changes including erosions or bony decalcification localized in or adjacent to the involved joints

Signs and Symptoms

The onset of the disease may be subtle, with early signs and symptoms nonspecific. Easy fatigability, malaise, myalgias, anorexia, and generalized weakness are often the first symptoms the patient with RA may experience. Ill-defined morning stiffness most often will progress to symmetrical joint pain with calor, tenosynovitis, and fusiform joint effusions. The rubor accompanying many of the other inflammatory arthritides (e.g., gout, septic arthritis) is not a predominant feature of RA. The wrists, knees, ankles, fingers and bones of the feet are most often affected, although any joint can be affected. Untreated, the synovitis becomes worse, and joint effusions are common. Tendons may become inflamed and may spontaneously rupture. Ultimately, the destruction of the cartilage and supportive bone will result in severe disability and pain. Deformities of the affected joints, including flexion contractures and ulnar drift of the fingers and wrist as a result of slippage of the extensor tendons of the metacarpophalangeal joints, will ultimately occur with poorly treated or untreated disease.

Extra-articular manifestations of RA are common. Carpal tunnel syndrome is frequently associated with RA and in fact may point to diagnosis if the clinician thinks about it. Carpal tunnel syndrome and the other entrapment neuropathies such as tardy ulnar palsy are the result of proliferation and thickening of the affected connective tissue. Ruptured Baker's cysts are not uncommonly seen in patients with RA and can mimic deep vein thrombosis, leading to unnecessary anticoagulation. Other extra-articular manifestations of RA include rheumatoid nodules that are painless masses that appear under the skin and around the extensor tendons. These nodules can also occur in the lung. Ocular manifestations are common, and uveitis and iritis can be quite severe. Vasculitis and anemia can also occur and, if undiagnosed, can lead to life-threatening multisystem organ failure. Pericarditis and pleuritis herald significant extra-articular disease and must be treated aggressively.

These signs and symptoms of RA are the result of the autoimmune response associated with the disease. Immunologic abnormalities associated with RA include inflammatory immune complexes in the synovial fluid as well as antibodies that are produced by the patient's own plasma cells. Among these antibodies is a substance called rheumatoid factor (RF), which also serves as the basis of the serologic test used in the diagnosis of RA. As RA progresses, the patient's own T-helper cell lymphocytes infiltrate the synovial tissue of the joints. These T-helper cells produce cytokines that facilitate the inflammatory response and contribute to ongoing joint damage. Macrophages and their cytokines (e.g., tumor necrosis factor, granulocyte-macrophage colony-stimulating factor) are also abundant in diseased synovium. Increased adhesion molecules contribute to inflammatory cell emigration and retention in the synovial tissue. Increased macrophage-derived lining cells are prominent along with some lymphocytes and vascular changes in early disease.

Prominent immunologic abnormalities that may be important in the pathogenesis of RA include immune complexes found in joint fluid cells and in vasculitis. Plasma cells produce antibodies (e.g., RF) that contribute to these complexes. Lymphocytes that infiltrate the synovial tissue are primarily T-helper cells, which can produce proinflammatory cytokines. Macrophages are also present in the diseased synovium of the patient suffering from RA and produce additional cytokines that attract other cells involved in the inflammatory response, further perpetuating joint damage as well as setting the stage for vasculitis. These cells produce a variety of other substances that damage the joint, including fibrin, prostaglandins, collagenase, and interleukin-2. This ongoing inflammatory response leads to thickening of the synovium of the affected joints with pannus formation.

Laboratory Findings

A normochromic normocytic anemia is a common finding in patients suffering from RA with the patient's hemoglobin being mildly decreased, with levels greater than 10 g/dL usually seen unless there has been chronic bleeding from vasculitis of the stomach, kidneys, and so forth. Neutropenia can occur in a small percentage of patients with RA and is usually associated with splenomegaly, which is termed *Felty's syndrome.* Thrombocytosis and mild to moderate hypergammaglobulinemia may also be present. The erythrocyte sedimentation rate is elevated in more than 90% of patients suffering from RA, as is C-reactive protein.

Antibodies to the gamma globulins mentioned can be detected by a latex agglutination test and are called RFs. Although not pathognomonic for RA, RF titers greater than 1:160 dilution are highly suggestive of the disease, and their presence makes the diagnosis of RA one of exclusion. The RF titer is indicative of the severity of the disease, with higher titers signaling more severe disease. These titers will drop and can be used as a rough measure of the success of the various treatments available for RA.

Synovial fluid analysis of patients suffering from active RA will reveal a leukocytosis consisting of predominantly polymorphonuclear cells, with lymphocytes and monocytes also present. The viscosity is decreased, and the protein levels are increased. Unlike the crystal arthropathies, no crystals are present.

Radiographic Findings

Early in the course of the disease, the radiographic findings of RA are nonspecific and are often limited to soft tissue swelling and a suggestion of increased synovial fluid. As the disease progresses, osteochondral destruction and pannus formation become more evident. The earliest specific radiographic findings of RA are most often found in the second and third metacarpophalangeal joints and the third proximal interphalangeal joints. Fusiform soft tissue swelling, concentric loss of the joint space, and periarticular loss of bone are also seen, as are marginal erosions of the articular surfaces, which have lost their protective articular cartilage. Superficial erosions beneath inflamed tendon sheaths may also occur. With further destruction of the joint, complete loss of the articular space can be seen and a variety of deformities and deviations of the joints and bones may occur, such as boutonnière and swan neck deformities of the digits. The characteristic ulnar drift or deviation of the metacarpophalangeal joints is pathognomonic of RA, can be diagnosed by visual inspection of the affected joints, and is vividly demonstrated on plain radiographs and magnetic resonance imaging.

Differential Diagnosis

As mentioned, the nonspecific nature of many of the signs and symptoms associated with RA coupled with the significant overlap of symptoms associated with the other causes of arthritis and the connective tissue diseases may make the diagnosis of RA challenging. The American College of Rheumatology diagnostic guidelines may help decrease the confusion, but the clinician should be cautioned that more than one form of arthritis may coexist and synovial fluid analysis, which is often overlooked, may be the quickest way to sort things out.

Osteoarthritis can be difficult to distinguish from early or mild RA because nontraumatic osteoarthritis is often symmetrical, with joint swelling and pain. Like RA, rubor is not a prominent feature of osteoarthritis compared with the crystal and infectious arthropathies. Osteoarthritis preferentially affects the proximal and distal interphalangeal joints (as characterized by Heberden's and Bouchard's nodules), first carpometacarpal and first metatarsophalangeal joints, knee, shoulder joints, and spine early in the course of the disease, with RA preferentially affecting the second and third metacarpophalangeal joints and the third proximal interphalangeal joints. The absence of significantly elevated RF and erythrocyte sedimentation rates, rheumatoid nodules, and systemic symptomatology can also help distinguish RA from osteoarthritis. Evaluation of the synovial fluid in patients suffering from osteoarthritis will reveal white blood cell counts much lower than those seen in RA.

After osteoarthritis, systemic lupus erythematosus is probably the disease most commonly confused with active RA, although all of the other connective tissue diseases can at times be difficult to distinguish from RA. These diseases are discussed in greater detail next, and the diagnostic criteria presented should aid the clinician in the differential diagnosis of confusing clinical presentations of symmetrical arthritis.

In addition to the connective tissue diseases and crystal arthropathies such as gout and pseudogout, amyloidosis, celiac disease, and sarcoidosis may also mimic RA, as can acute rheumatic fever secondary to streptococcal infections. Infectious arthritis usually manifests as a monoarticular or asymmetrical arthritis, as does Lyme disease and Reiter's syndrome. Ankylosing spondylitis preferentially affects males and involves the sacroiliac joints and axial skeleton to a much greater extent than the peripheral joints.

Treatment

Although there is no cure for RA, most patients will experience good to excellent palliation of their symptoms and decrease the potential for severe disability with appropriate treatment of their disease. However, it should be noted that despite optimal treatment, 8% to 10% of patients suffering from RA will experience serious disability that will interfere with the ability to provide self-care and carry out their activities of daily living.

The initial treatment of RA should focus on two factors: (1) rest and protection of affected joints and (2) aggressive treatment of the acute inflammatory process. The failure to rest and splint the joints acutely inflamed by RA can often lead to irreversible joint damage with attendant pain and disability. Splinting may also help slow the progression of hand and feet deformities that can be so distressing and disabling to the patient suffering from RA. Aggressive treatment of the inflammatory response associated with acute RA requires skillful use of the drugs discussed later.

PHARMACOLOGIC TREATMENT WITH ANTI-INFLAMMATORY AGENTS

Acute inflammation should be treated aggressively with the nonsteroidal anti-inflammatory drugs (NSAIDs) such

as aspirin, ibuprofen, and so on. These drugs have significant renal, gastrointestinal, and hepatic side effects and must be used with caution. For patients with gastrointestinal side effects, enteric coated products or the nonacetylated salicylates such as salsalate or choline magnesium salicylate may be considered. The addition of cytoprotective drugs like misoprostol or the H_2 receptor antagonists like ranitidine may also help decrease the incidence of gastrointestinal side effects and allow the RA patient to continue to take these much-needed drugs. For patient who cannot tolerate the NSAIDs, the cyclooxygenase (COX)-2 inhibitors may be considered with an eye to their potential cardiac side effects. Fish oil supplementation may also help suppress intra-articular prostaglandins as well as promote cardiovascular health. Whether these drugs alter the ultimate course of the disease remains an area of intense debate.

Although NSAIDs are generally the first line of treatment for acute RA, it should be remembered that the corticosteroids can provide dramatic relief of the pain and disability associated with acute exacerbations of the disease. Unfortunately, there are two major problems associated with the use of corticosteroids in the treatment of acute RA: (1) the corticosteroids tend to become less effective in suppressing the acute inflammatory response over time, and this class of drugs has significant side effects with chronic use. (2) Like the NSAIDs, it is unclear whether treatment with corticosteroids will alter the ultimate course of RA in the individual patient, although the ability of this class of drugs to palliate the acute symptoms of RA is unsurpassed. In general, daily treatment of RA with corticosteroids should be limited to those patients who are unable to tolerate other treatment options or in those patients with life-threatening extra-articular manifestations of the disease, such as pericarditis, pleurisy, or nephritis. Injection of acutely inflamed and painful joints with small amounts of anti-inflammatory steroid may be useful to provide symptomatic relief and stop the inflammatory process and to allow the patient to avoid all of the side effects associated with the systemic administration of this class of drugs.

PHARMACOLOGIC TREATMENT WITH DISEASE-MODIFYING DRUGS

As mentioned, it is unclear whether the NSAIDs or corticosteroids as a sole therapeutic agent can effectively modify the course of RA. For this reason, there is a move toward the use of disease-modifying drugs such as methotrexate, hydroxychloroquine, sulfasalazine, penicillamine, and gold earlier in the course of the disease. Methotrexate is an immunosuppressive drug that is reasonably well tolerated and is increasingly becoming a first-line drug in the treatment of RA (see later).

Gold is available as a parenteral solution that is usually administered via intramuscular injection on a weekly basis as well as an oral formulation. Although effective in the treatment of RA, the gold salts are not without side effects, which include significant renal and hepatic toxicity and potentially life-threatening skin and blood dyscrasias.

If gold is ineffective or causes toxic side effects, oral penicillamine may be considered. Potentially serious side effects associated with penicillamine therapy include bone marrow suppression, renal damage, a lupus-like syndrome, Goodpasture's syndrome, and myasthenia gravis. Careful monitoring for these potentially life-threatening side effects is mandatory, and the drug should only be used by those familiar with its potential toxicity.

Hydroxychloroquine can also provide symptomatic relief for the patient suffering from mild to moderately active RA. Reasonably well tolerated, the major serious side effects of this drug include myopathy, which may be irreversible, and ophthalmologic side effects including reversible corneal opacities and potentially irreversible retinal degeneration. Both of these serious side effects require careful neurologic and ophthalmologic monitoring while the drug is being used.

Sulfasalazine, which is used primarily for ulcerative colitis, may also be used to treat RA. Less toxic than gold and penicillamine, it is slower acting but generally well tolerated. An enteric coated product has increased its tolerability. Monitoring of basic hematologic and blood chemistries to identify the relatively uncommon hematologic, renal, and hepatic side effects should be carried out in all patients treated with this drug.

PHARMACOLOGIC TREATMENT WITH IMMUNOSUPPRESSIVE DRUGS

In addition to the disease-modifying drugs mentioned, the immunosuppressive drugs including methotrexate, azathioprine, and cyclosporine are increasingly being used relatively early in the course of RA. These drugs have in common their ability to suppress active inflammation in RA. Generally well tolerated, these drugs are not without side effects. Careful monitoring for bone marrow suppression, hepatic and renal dysfunction, and pneumonitis is mandatory. The potential of the immunosuppressive drugs to trigger malignancy is of real concern, especially with prolonged use of azathioprine.

As mentioned, the immunosuppressive drug methotrexate is now being used early in the course of active RA. It can be given orally as a once-weekly dose and is generally well tolerated. Side effects include interference with folic acid metabolism, which requires concomitant folic acid replacement. Methotrexate also has significant hepatotoxicity in some patients, and any elevation of liver function tests and potentially fatal fibrosis of the liver require immediate attention and liver biopsy. Although rare, fatal pneumonitis has been reported with the use of methotrexate in the treatment of RA.

Etanercept and infliximab are new disease-modifying drugs that have shown promise when given alone or in combination with methotrexate in the management of RA. Both etanercept and infliximab block tumor necrosis factor alpha, which is a protein that the body produces during the inflammatory response. The increased amounts of tumor necrosis factor alpha seen in patients with acute RA accelerate the inflammatory response and contribute to the pain, swelling, and stiffness associated with the disease. The mechanism of action for these drugs is thought to be via the binding of free tumor necrosis factor alpha, decreasing the amounts available to promote the inflammatory response. Given via subcutaneous injection twice a week, etanercept is well tolerated with rare side effects, including neurologic dysfunction, optic neuritis, and, occasionally, pancytopenia. Infliximab is given via intravenous infusion, and these infusions are often accompanied by chills, fever, blood pressure abnormalities, and rash. These drugs should not be used in patients with active infections as even minor infections may become life threatening due to the drug's ability to suppress the inflammatory response. Reactivation of tuberculosis has also been reported following administration of these drugs when treating RA.

TREATMENT WITH PHYSICAL MODALITIES, ORTHOTICS, AND PHYSICAL AND OCCUPATIONAL THERAPY

As mentioned, the pharmacologic treatment of the pain and disability of RA is only one part of a successful treatment strategy. Just as acute inflammation must be aggressively treated to avoid further joint destruction, the aggressive use of physical modalities, orthotics, and physical and occupational therapy is paramount to modify the relentless progression of inadequately treated RA.

The use of local heat and cold can provide significant symptomatic relief for the pain, swelling, and stiffness of RA. Although conventional wisdom suggests that the application of heat should be avoided in the acutely inflamed joint, many patients suffering from RA find superficial moist heat to provide significant symptomatic relief. Other patients find the use of superficial cold to be more beneficial. Deep heating modalities such as ultrasound and diathermy should be avoided during the acute phases of RA but may be useful as part of a comprehensive rehabilitation program for joints that are no longer acutely inflamed.

The use of orthotic devices to prevent joint deformity is an integral part of the treatment of the patient with RA. The use of night splints to slow the progression of ulnar drift should be considered early in the course of the disease. The use of shoe inserts and careful fitting of shoes can also help preserve function and ease pain. Protection of the elbows and Achilles tendons during periods of bed rest will also decrease the development of rheumatoid nodules at pressure areas. As the acute inflammation is brought under control, a gentle physical therapy program that focuses on reconditioning, joint protection, and restoration of range of motion and function should be undertaken.

Perhaps nowhere else in medicine is the role of patient education and the use of assistive devices more important than in the care of the patient suffering from RA. Instruction in proper lifting techniques and joint protection strategies and training in the use of assistive devices such as jar openers and buttonhooks are paramount if preservation of joint function is to be achieved.

SURGICAL TREATMENT OPTIONS

Surgical treatment should be limited to the repair of acute joint injuries, such as subluxed joints, torn cartilage, ruptured tendons, etc. and the release of associated entrapment neuropathies. Total joint arthroplasty is indicated in those patients with severely damaged joints that are compromising the patient's ability to provide self-care and carry out his or her activities of daily living. It should be remembered that patients suffering from RA are at particular risk for C1-2 subluxations and that early surgical treatment may be required to avoid fatal spinal cord injury. Any surgical interventions should include a concurrent plan of physical medicine and rehabilitation to avoid further loss of function in the postoperative period.

SUGGESTED READING

Waldman SD: Connective tissue diseases. In: Pain Management. Philadelphia, Saunders, 2007.

CHAPTER 199

Systemic Lupus Erythematosus

The second most common connective tissue disease encountered in clinical practice, systemic lupus erythematosus (SLE) is a disease of unknown etiology. Ninety percent of patients suffering from SLE are women. There is an increased incidence of this disease among African Americans and Asians. Affecting the joints, skin, blood vessels, and major organ systems, SLE has the potential to cause much suffering and disability, although the disease is less problematic for those patients lucky enough to have a milder, less virulent form.

Signs and Symptoms

As mentioned, there is a wide spectrum of how SLE presents and ultimately manifests itself. The clinical picture can range from a mild, nonprogressive disease to an aggressive syndrome affecting multiple organ systems and producing life-threatening sequelae. SLE may manifest as an acute febrile illness with arthralgias and rash that is difficult to distinguish from the acute febrile exanthems with involvement of the central nervous system and other major organ systems, or the onset may be much more subtle and insidious leading to significant delays in diagnosis. Manifestations referable to any organ system may appear. It is either the cutaneous manifestations or the almost universal complaint of polyarthralgias that usually leads the clinician to consider the diagnosis of SLE.

Although polyarthritis is present in more than 90% of patients with SLE, in contradistinction to rheumatoid arthritis, the joint disease associated with SLE tends to be much less destructive and deforming. In rare patients, significant joint destruction and deformity resembling those seen in rheumatoid arthritis can be observed. This form of arthritis, called *Jaccoud's arthritis*, is usually seen in SLE patients who present acutely with a constellation of symptoms reminiscent of acute rheumatic fever.

The characteristic cutaneous lesion associated with SLE is the butterfly rash. A variant form of SLE, which is characterized by discoid cutaneous lesions, is known as discoid lupus erythematosus. The discoid variant of the disease tends to be milder with less systemic involvement than the systemic lupus erythematosus. Recurrent mouth ulcers and focal areas of alopecia are reasonably common, as are purpuric lesions secondary to small vessel vasculitis. Photosensitivity is reported by more than 40% of patients suffering from SLE.

In addition to those joint and dermatologic manifestations of SLE, the clinician will do well to remember that this disease can affect virtually any organ system. Table 199-1 provides some of the common extra-articular manifestations of SLE; these include vasculitis, pleuritis, pneumonitis, myocarditis, endocarditis, pericarditis, glomerulonephritis, hepatitis, splenomegaly, and generalized adenopathy. Hematologic side effects including pancytopenia, thrombocytopenia, leukopenia, and a hypercoagulable state with secondary pulmonary and coronary artery embolic phenomena and/or thrombosis can occur. Neurologic dysfunction, including headaches, seizures, confusion, and occasionally frank psychosis, can occur.

TABLE 199–1 Extra-Articular Manifestations of Systemic Lupus Erythematosus

- Dermatologic manifestations
  - Butterfly rash
  - Discoid lesions
  - Focal alopecia
  - Maculopapular lesions
- Vascular manifestations
  - Vasculitis
  - Thrombosis
- Pulmonary manifestations
  - Pleuritis
  - Pleural effusion
  - Pleurisy
  - Pulmonary embolus
- Cardiac manifestations
  - Myocarditis
  - Endocarditis
  - Pericarditis
- Renal manifestations
  - Proteinuria
  - Glomerulonephritis
- Hepatic manifestations
  - Hepatitis
- Hematologic manifestations
  - Pancytopenia
  - Leukopenia
  - Thrombocytopenia
  - Hypercoagulable state
- Neurologic manifestations
  - Headaches
  - Seizures
  - Confusion
  - Psychosis
- Generalized lymphadenopathy
- Splenomegaly

Laboratory Findings

The antinuclear antibody (ANA) test is positive in more than 98% of patients suffering from SLE. Occasional false positives occur in those patients with serology that is positive for syphilis, and positive ANA titers can occur from drug-induced lupus-like states. If the clinical diagnosis is in doubt or if a patient's presentation is highly selective for SLE but the ANA is negative, more specific testing for the presence of anti–double-stranded DNA antibody can help clarify the situation because high titers of anti–double-stranded DNA antibody are highly specific for SLE.

The erythrocyte sedimentation rate is significantly elevated in most patients suffering from SLE. In contradistinction to rheumatoid arthritis with consistently elevated C-reactive protein levels, C-reactive protein levels are surprisingly low, even in the face of active disease. As mentioned, a whole range of hematologic abnormalities, including pancytopenia, thrombocytopenia, leukopenia, and coagulopathy, may be present. The presence of high levels of anticardiolipin antibodies should alert the clinician to the significantly increased possibility of hypercoagulability.

Differential Diagnosis

SLE is obvious when a patient (particularly a young woman) is febrile with an erythematous skin rash, polyarthritis, evidence of renal disease, intermittent pleuritic pain, leukopenia, and hyperglobulinemia with anti–double-stranded DNA antibodies. Early-stage SLE can be difficult to differentiate from other connective tissue disorders and may be mistaken for rheumatoid arthritis if arthritic symptoms predominate. Mixed connective tissue disease has the clinical features of SLE with overlapping features of systemic sclerosis, rheumatoid-like polyarthritis, and polymyositis or dermatomyositis (see later).

As mentioned, there are several drugs in current clinical use that can produce a clinical syndrome that resembles SLE and can also produce a positive ANA test. These drugs include hydralazine, procainamide, and several beta blockers. The lupus-like symptoms and positive ANA generally disappear after discontinuation of the offending drug.

Treatment

In general, if SLE is diagnosed early in the course of the disease and its effects on the joints and other organ systems are appropriately treated, the long-term prognosis of this disease is much better than that for many of the other connective tissue diseases. The rational treatment of SLE is driven by the severity and extra-articular manifestations of the disease, as long-term studies have shown that much of the morbidity and, in some cases, mortality associated with SLE are iatrogenically introduced complications of treatment. For purposes of treatment, SLE is divided into mild and severe disease classifications.

Mild SLE is characterized in those patients in whom SLE is manifested by fever, arthralgias, headache, rash, and mild pericarditis. Severe SLE is characterized by the symptoms of pleural effusions, severe pericarditis, myocarditis, renal dysfunction, thrombocytopenic purpura, vasculitis, hemolytic anemia, hypercoagulable state, and significant central nervous system involvement. The patient with severe SLE must be viewed as suffering from a potentially life-threatening emergency and treated as such.

Mild SLE is treated symptomatically with an eye toward early identification of renal damage and the development of a hypercoagulable state. The nonsteroidal anti-inflammatory drugs and aspirin (especially if thrombosis is a concern) are an excellent starting point in the treatment of mild SLE. The antimalarial drugs such as chloroquine, hydroxychloroquine, or quinacrine can be added if dermatologic or joint manifestations remain problematic. It should remembered that lupus is a disease that, like multiple sclerosis, is characterized by remissions and exacerbations and, like multiple sclerosis, has an extremely unpredictable course. Failure to recognize the appearance of warning signs of increasing renal, cardiac, hematologic, or pulmonary dysfunction can have disastrous results.

The classification of a patient's lupus as severe represents a need for aggressive treatment with corticosteroids and close monitoring for occult system failure.

Prednisone at a starting dose of 60 mg/day is indicated at the first sign of trouble, although some experienced clinicians will prescribe high-dose intravenous methylprednisolone at a dosage of 1000 mg for 3 to 4 days, especially if florid central nervous system symptoms are present. The addition of immunosuppressive drugs such as azathioprine or cyclophosphamide is also useful if there is significant renal disease. The risk of thrombosis as heralded by high anticardiolipin antibodies may suggest prophylactic anticoagulation.

As severe SLE is controlled, suppression of the autoimmune and inflammatory responses is usually required. This is best accomplished with low-dose corticosteroids or low-dose immunosuppressive therapy. The effectiveness of suppressive therapy can be monitored by the subjective clinical response to the therapeutic regimen chosen and objectified by following titers of anti–double-stranded DNA antibody. The clinician should be vigilant to the possibility of exacerbation of the inflammatory and autoimmune response as the corticosteroids are tapered, and such exacerbations should be treated promptly to avoid sequelae. Intercurrent infections can be quite problematic for the patient suffering from SLE and should be treated aggressively. The clinician should also be aware that even in the face of excellent disease control, pregnancy is associated with flaring of symptoms and spontaneous abortions and late-term fetal deaths are quite common.

SUGGESTED READING

Waldman SD: Connective tissue diseases. In: Pain Management. Philadelphia, Saunders, 2007.

CHAPTER 200

Scleroderma-Systemic Sclerosis

Scleroderma is a connective tissue disease of unknown etiology that is characterized by diffuse fibrosis of the skin and connective tissue, vascular damage, arthritis, and abnormalities of the esophagus, gastrointestinal tract, kidneys, heart, and lungs. This fibrosis is the result of abnormal collagen deposition in the affected structures. The disease may be localized to the skin or a single organ system or may cause severe multisystem disease. There is

a trend to call the systemic variant of the disease *systemic sclerosis* to more accurately reflect the multisystem nature of the disease. Like systemic lupus erythematosus, the severity and course of the disease vary widely from patient to patient. Scleroderma is four times more common in women than in men, and its onset is rare before the age of 30 or after the age of 50. Exposure to contaminated cooking oils, polyvinyl chloride, and silica has also been implicated as a risk factor for the development of scleroderma.

Signs and Symptoms

Unlike rheumatoid arthritis, the onset of scleroderma can be very subtle and insidious. The initial complaints of patients suffering from scleroderma usually reflect the pain or deformity associated with swelling and loss of range of motion of the digits (sclerodactyly) and the associated Raynaud's phenomenon. Polyarthralgias and dysphagia can also be prominent initial features of the disease.

Most distressing to the patient are the cutaneous changes associated with scleroderma. Most often, it is the unsightly changes of sclerodactyly that cause the patient to initially seek medical attention. The skin changes of scleroderma tend to be symmetrical, affecting the distal upper extremities first. Untreated, the skin will become shiny and atrophic looking with a swollen, taut appearance. Hyperpigmentation and telangiectasias of the digits, face, chest, and lips may also occur. A mask-like facies may appear, which can be quite distressing to the patient and family. Subcutaneous calcifications of the fingers and over the elbows, ankles, and knees may cause further pain and deformity. Ulcerations of the skin overlying these calcifications and the fingertips due to the trophic nature of the skin and vasculitis are common.

Tendinitis and bursitis, especially of the large joints, can contribute to pain and disability and can accelerate loss of range of motion of already compromised joints. Flexion contractures of the fingers, wrists, and elbows due to fibrosis of the synovium and overlying skin can be particularly problematic and very difficult to treat once they have occurred.

Complicating the cutaneous and musculoskeletal manifestations of the disease is the almost universal complaint of dysphagia due to impaired esophageal motility. Fibrosis of the esophagus and lower esophageal sphincter can further exacerbate the problem of dysphagia as a result of acid reflux–induced distal esophageal strictures. Hypomotility of the small intestine can result in malabsorption, and diffuse fibrosis of the large intestine can further compromise gastrointestinal function.

Pulmonary fibrosis, pleurisy, and pleural effusions can compromise pulmonary function. Untreated, this fibrosis may affect the small vessels of the lung, and pulmonary hypertension with all of its attendant problems may develop. The fibrosis associated with scleroderma may also affect the muscle and conduction system of the heart. Cardiac arrhythmias may result, and compromised cardiac output secondary to myocardial fibrosis combined with pulmonary hypertension may result in treatment-refractory congestive heart failure. The onset of pulmonary and cardiac symptoms early in the course of the disease is a poor prognostic sign.

The kidneys are most often the most severely affected by scleroderma, with fibrosis of the small arteries of the kidneys resulting in the rapid deterioration of renal function and malignant hypertension. This deterioration of renal function may be exacerbated when concomitant heart failure is present. Untreated, it is the unremitting deterioration of renal function that is fatal in patients suffering from scleroderma.

Laboratory Findings

Although the diagnosis of scleroderma is most often made on clinical grounds, confirmatory laboratory testing is sometimes useful when the diagnosis is in question or if a variant of scleroderma (e.g., CREST syndrome) is being considered (see later). Antinuclear antibody (ANA) titers are elevated in more than 90% of patients suffering from scleroderma. Although by no means specific for the disease, the presence of high ANA titers at least points the clinician in the direction of connective tissue disease. If the diagnosis of scleroderma is still in question, the pattern of the ANA testing may be helpful. In patients with scleroderma, specific ANA testing will show an antinucleolar pattern, whereas patients with CREST syndrome will demonstrate an anticentromere pattern. It should be noted that approximately one third of patients suffering from scleroderma will have a positive rheumatoid factor, which may confuse the picture. The erythrocyte sedimentation rate will often be elevated in patients with scleroderma, but frequently not to the extent seen in patients with rheumatoid arthritis and systemic lupus erythematosus.

Differential Diagnosis

Due to the often subtle and insidious onset of scleroderma, the diagnosis is often delayed or confused with other connective tissue diseases or other systemic diseases of the heart, lungs, joints, skin, and kidneys. Variants of scleroderma can manifest in myriad fashion and confuse the clinical picture. CREST syndrome is one such variant. Its constellation of systems include calcinosis, Raynaud's phenomenon, esophageal dysfunction, sclerodactyly, and telangiectasia. Also known as limited cutaneous scleroderma, this variant of scleroderma has a much more benign course and infinitely better prognosis. Scleroderma that is limited to the skin and adjacent connective tissue, without multisystem involvement, can also occasionally make the diagnosis of scleroderma more difficult. Like CREST syndrome, the clinical course and prognosis of this localized variant of scleroderma are relatively benign. Mixed connective tissue disease (MCTD), which combines elements of polymyositis, systemic lupus erythematosus, and scleroderma, can also present a diagnostic dilemma. If MCTD is being considered in the differential diagnosis of scleroderma, testing for the presence of anti–nuclear ribonucleoprotein antibody will prompt the clinician to suspect that MCTD is the culprit rather than classic scleroderma.

Treatment

The treatment of scleroderma has its basis in the treatment of specific organ system dysfunction related to the disease rather than any treatment that is specifically aimed at treatment of the underlying disease itself. Early treatment of organ system dysfunction is critical if the clinician hopes to improve the quality of life and prognosis for the patient suffering from scleroderma. Nowhere is this statement more valid than when dealing with renal dysfunction. The early use of angiotensin-converting enzyme inhibitors and vasodilators such as minoxidil is indicated to control hypertension and improve renal blood flow.

The use of nonsteroidal anti-inflammatory drugs and corticosteroids in low doses to treat synovitis, arthritis, and myositis should be considered early in the course of the disease. The calcium channel blockers may help ameliorate the symptomatology associated with Raynaud's phenomenon, and there is anecdotal evidence that topical nitroglycerin ointment may also help provide symptomatic relief. Methotrexate and penicillamine may help slow the progression of fibrosis, especially of the skin and digits.

Treatment of reflux with histamine-blocking agents, use of bed blocks, and multiple small feedings may also provide symptomatic relief and help prevent lower esophageal erosions and stricture. Oral antibiotics may also be used if malabsorption secondary to bacterial overgrowth in dilated small intestine and bowel is a problem. As with the other connective tissue diseases, the rational use of occupational and physical therapy can help decrease pain and preserve and improve function.

SUGGESTED READING

Waldman SD: Connective tissue diseases. In: Pain Management. Philadelphia, Saunders, 2007.

CHAPTER 201

Polymyositis

Less common than rheumatoid arthritis, systemic lupus erythematosus, or scleroderma, polymyositis is a connective tissue disease of unknown etiology. The disease is characterized by muscle inflammation that progresses to degenerative muscle disease and atrophy. There are many variants of polymyositis, including dermatomyositis, which is, from a clinical viewpoint, simply polymyositis with significant cutaneous manifestations. Affecting women twice as frequently as men, polymyositis can overlap with basically all of the connective tissue diseases, making diagnosis on purely clinical grounds somewhat more challenging. Generally not occurring in adults before the age of 40 or after the age of 60, there is a childhood variant that carries a poor prognosis. The clinician should be aware that there is a strong correlation with the presence of malignancy in patients who present with polymyositis, and a search for underlying malignancy must be an integral part of any diagnostic workup and treatment plan of patients suspected of having

polymyositis. Whether the malignancy serves as a trigger to the autoimmune response to muscle in this disease or is simply a trigger to an unknown cascade of events has yet to be elucidated. It is interesting to note that there is a greater incidence of malignancy in those patients suffering from dermatomyositis relative to polymyositis. The type and location of tumor are not consistent, making the search for associated occult malignancy all the more difficult.

Signs and Symptoms

The onset of polymyositis is often preceded by an acute infection, often viral in nature. The onset of symptoms may be acute or may come on gradually, with the patient thinking that he or she simply has not shaken the initial febrile illness. Rash and muscle weakness are generally the presenting symptoms, with the proximal muscle groups generally affected initially more commonly than the distal muscle groups. Myalgias and polyarthralgias may be present, as may constitutional symptoms resembling polymyalgia rheumatica (see later). In some patients, the onset of profound muscle weakness may be rapid, with the patient presenting with the inability to rise from a sitting position or the complaint of the inability to raise the arms above the head to comb or curl his or her hair. In rare patients, weakness of the muscles controlling the vocal cords may cause dysphasia that may be mistaken for myasthenia gravis or a stroke. In severe cases, acute respiratory insufficiency may occur, and the association of recent febrile illness may yield the mistaken diagnosis of Guillain-Barré disease. Involvement of the gastrointestinal tract may lead to symptoms as described for scleroderma. Cardiac arrhythmias and conduction defects are seen in many patients suffering from polymyositis, as is renal failure due to acute myoglobinuria from rhabdomyolysis in acute exacerbations of the disease.

In general, the small muscles of the hands and feet are spared, as are the muscles of facial expression.

When patients with polymyositis exhibit significant cutaneous manifestations, for clinical purposes, the disease is called dermatomyositis. A heliotrope periorbital blush is pathognomonic for the disease. There may be a peeling or splitting of skin over the radial sides of the digits that is highly suggestive of dermatomyositis. A generalized maculopapular rash may also appear. Subcutaneous calcific nodules may be present in many patients with undiagnosed and untreated disease.

Laboratory Testing

There is no specific diagnostic test for polymyositis or dermatomyositis. The erythrocyte sedimentation rate is usually elevated, as is the serum muscle enzyme determinations, especially in acute disease. The monitoring of creatine kinase (CK) levels may serve as a useful guide as to the efficacy of treatment. Approximately 60% of patients with polymyositis have antibodies to thymic nuclear antigen.

Differential Diagnosis

As with the other connective tissue diseases, the overlap of symptoms can make the diagnosis of a specific disease difficult on purely clinical grounds. The findings of proximal muscle weakness, characteristic skin rash (in the case of dermatomyositis), positive electromyography, and elevated serum muscle enzymes strongly support the diagnosis of polymyositis or dermatomyositis. If the diagnosis is still in doubt, muscle biopsy may help clarify the situation as in most cases it will be diagnostic.

Treatment

Corticosteroids are the first drug of choice for acute polymyositis. A starting dose of 60 mg is usually adequate to control the acute inflammatory response and improve the clinical symptoms. The corticosteroids can be tapered based on both the clinical response to the drug and the decrease in elevated serum CK to normal. The minimum dose of corticosteroid necessary to control symptoms and depress CK should be used to avoid steroid-induced myopathy, which may confuse the clinical management and exacerbate the patient's disability. A trial of immunosuppressive drugs including methotrexate, cyclosporine, azathioprine, and cyclophosphamide may be considered if corticosteroids fail to control the disease or the side effects associated with the drug preclude its use. It should be remembered that weakness unresponsive to the therapies mentioned may be secondary to associated malignancies (e.g., paraneoplastic syndrome), and that treatment of the tumor may be required to improve the patient's weakness. The use of physical and occupational therapy to optimize function and to help the patient learn to use assistive devices is indicated early in the course of the disease.

SUGGESTED READING

Waldman SD: Connective tissue diseases. In: Pain Management. Philadelphia, Saunders, 2007.

CHAPTER 202

Polymyalgia Rheumatica

Polymyalgia rheumatica (PMR) is a connective tissue disease of unknown etiology that occurs primarily in patients older than 60 years. It occurs in females twice as commonly as in males and may be associated with temporal arteritis. PMR is characterized by a constellation of musculoskeletal symptoms that include deep, aching pain of the cervical, pectoral, and pelvic regions; morning stiffness; arthralgias; and stiffness after inactivity. Constitutional symptoms consisting of malaise, fever, anorexia, weight loss, and depression may be so severe as to mimic the cachexia and inanition of malignancy. Unlike polymyositis, there is no significant proximal muscle weakness—rather the feeling of more generalized weakness and lassitude. In contradistinction to polymyositis, muscle biopsy results and electromyography are normal.

Signs and Symptoms

The onset of PMR is variable; some patients experience a rather acute, fulminant onset of symptoms, and other patients experience a more gradual onset of symptoms, more like an influenza syndrome that just does not go away. It is often the deep muscle aching and overwhelming feeling of fatigue that lead the patient to seek medical attention. The astute physician may pick up on the gelling phenomenon (stiffness after periods of inactivity) that is very common with PMR and make the diagnosis on clinical grounds while waiting for confirmatory laboratory results (see later).

Laboratory and Radiographic Testing

The consistent finding in patients with PMR is the markedly elevated erythrocyte sedimentation rate (ESR). Values are consistently greater than 100 mm/hr. C-reactive protein is also consistently elevated in patients with untreated PMR. As mentioned, objective tests for inflammatory muscle disease are negative despite the often dramatic muscle pain that patients report with this disease.

Despite the complaint of arthralgias, plain radiographs of the joints fail to reveal significant effusions or joint destruction that are often seen with rheumatoid arthritis and some of the other connective tissue diseases.

Differential Diagnosis

PMR is most often confused with other systemic diseases such as hypothyroidism, depression, or malignancy such as multiple myeloma. It is often initially misdiagnosed as polymyositis but can be easily distinguished from polymyositis by simple electromyography, which is negative in PMR and extremely positive in polymyositis. The relative absence of acutely inflamed joints and lack of evidence of destruction on plain radiographs of the small joints, coupled with the absence of rheumatoid nodules and a negative rheumatoid factor, should point the clinician away from the diagnosis of rheumatoid arthritis.

Treatment

The mainstay of treatment of PMR is the use of prednisone at a starting dose of 15 to 20 mg/day. The symptoms of PMR will usually respond dramatically to the relatively low doses of steroids, and the drug should be tapered as the clinical situation dictates. Unlike many of the other connective tissue diseases in which the ESR serves as a useful marker as to the effectiveness of treatment, the ESR may remain significantly elevated in otherwise symptom-free patients. It should be remembered that temporal arteritis is often seen concomitantly with PMR, and if temporal arteritis is suspected, a much higher dose of prednisone in the range of 60 to 100 mg/day should be used until temporal artery biopsy can be obtained to confirm the diagnosis, to decrease the risk of blindness.

SUGGESTED READING

Waldman SD: Connective tissue diseases. In: Pain Management. Philadelphia, Saunders, 2007.

CHAPTER 203

Central Pain States

Central pain is defined as pain caused by a lesion or dysfunction in the central nervous system. This definition obviously covers a significant number of very diverse pathologic conditions that have in common the ability to cause pain. Other terms that have been used interchangeably for the more general term central pain include thalamic pain, deafferentation pain, and anesthesia dolorosa.

Pathologic processes involving the central nervous system that have been implicated in the evolution of central pain are summarized in Table 203-1. As can be seen from this list of pathologic conditions, lesions or dysfunction located anywhere in the central nervous system from the dorsal horn to the cerebral cortex, have the propensity to cause central pain. However, the majority of central pain states appear to arise from lesions of the ventroposterior thalamus, the lower portions of the brainstem, the spinothalamic pathways, and the spinal cord. In general, the location of the lesions determines the location of the pain; for example, large thalamic lesions most often cause hemibody pain, and large spinal cord lesions most often cause bilateral pain caudad to the location of the lesion.

Although there is no one characteristic type of pain associated with central pain states, some generalizations regarding the quality of the pain can be made. Constant burning

TABLE 203-1 Common Causes of Central Pain

Brain and Brainstem Lesions and Dysfunction

- Thalamic infarcts and hemorrhage
  - Especially those involving the ventroposterior portion
- Vascular malformations, infarcts, and hemorrhage of the brain and brainstem
- Traumatic brain injury
- Brain tumors
- Infections and inflammation of the brain and brainstem
- Multiple sclerosis
- Syringobulbia
- Epilepsy
- Parkinson's disease

Spinal Cord Lesions and Dysfunction

- Multiple sclerosis
- Syringomyelia
- Traumatic spinal cord injuries
- Spinal cord tumors
- Infections and inflammation of the spinal cord
- Vascular lesions of the spinal cord

TABLE 203-2 Generally Accepted Treatments for Central Pain States

Pharmacologic

- Antidepressants
- Anticonvulsants
- Analgesics
- Local anesthetics/antiarrhythmics
- Neuroleptics
- Cannabinoids?
- Adrenergic drugs
- Cholinergic drugs
- GABAergic drugs
- Glutaminergic drugs?

Neuroaugmentation

- Transcutaneous nerve stimulation
- Spinal cord stimulation
- Deep brain stimulation
- Surface stimulation of the motor cortex

Neurodestructive Approaches

- Thalamotomy
- Cordotomy
- Dorsal root entry zone lesioning

or dysesthetic pain is the most common type of pain associated with central pain states, with shooting and lancinating pain also commonly reported. The intensity of central pain can range from mild to severe, yet patients suffering from central pain almost uniformly report their pain as distressing and unpleasant, suggesting a component of suffering superimposed on the perceived pain. Allodynia, hypersensitivity, and dysesthesias are often reported, as well as a worsening of pain with strong emotional states.

The treatment of central pain is uniformly difficult, and often the pain management specialist can only provide partial ameliorations of the symptoms associated with central pain. Generally accepted treatments for central pain are listed in Table 203-2. In most patients suffering from central pain, a multimodality approach will be required to optimize results.

SUGGESTED READING

Boivie J: Central pain. In McMahon SB, Koltzenburg M (eds): Wall and Melzack's Textbook of Pain, ed 5. Philadelphia, Churchill Livingstone, 2006.

CHAPTER 204

Conversion Disorder

Conversion disorder is listed in the *Diagnostic and Statistical Manual of Mental Disorders of the American Psychiatric Association, Fourth Edition, Text Revision (DSM-IV-TR)* as a somatoform disorder. The diagnostic criteria as promulgated by the disorders in the *Diagnostic and Statistical Manual of Mental Disorders of the American Psychiatric Association (DSM-IV)* are outlined in Table 204-1.

Sigmund Freud first used the term *conversion* to refer to a subconscious substitution of a somatic symptom to replace a repressed ideation or thought. Freud suggested that this conversion was the psyche's defense against unacceptable impulses. Others have rejected Freud's explanation of how a deep-seated fear or unacceptable impulse can subconsciously create a somatic symptom and have put forth an alternative theory in which the symptoms that are "converted" are in fact a learned response to stress, albeit a pathologic one. Under this scenario, the patient receives primary gain by avoiding the activity or situation that is creating the stress and, by virtue of the somatic symptom, receives secondary gain in the form of sympathy and social acceptability from friends, coworkers, and family.

TABLE 204–1 Diagnostic Criteria for Conversion Disorder as Defined in the *DSM-IV*

One or more symptoms or deficits are present that affect voluntary motor or sensory function that suggest a neurologic or other general medical condition.

- Psychological factors are judged to be associated with the symptom or deficit because conflicts or other stressors precede the initiation or exacerbation of the symptom or deficit.
- The symptom or deficit is not intentionally produced or feigned (as in factitious disorder or malingering).
- The symptom or deficit, after appropriate investigation, cannot be explained fully by a general medical condition, the direct effects of a substance, or as a culturally sanctioned behavior or experience.
- The symptom or deficit causes clinically significant distress or impairment in social, occupational, or other important areas of functioning or warrants medical evaluation.
- The symptom or deficit is not limited to pain or sexual dysfunction, does not occur exclusively during the course of somatization disorder, and is not better accounted for by another mental disorder.

The incidence of conversion disorder varies across cultures, with this psychological disorder being quite rare in the United States. The reason for this disparity in incidence across cultures is not completely clear, but it has been suggested that the almost complete integration of Freudian concepts into American culture has rendered the conversion disorder almost too obvious to be an effective coping mechanism.

The patient suffering from a conversion disorder will generally exhibit symptoms that are severe and have the ability to interfere with the patient's normal activities of daily living or to somehow allow the patient to avoid situations that are similar to those that caused the conversion disorder to begin with. Although the symptoms of conversion disorder may resolve spontaneously and often without apparent reason, the prolonged loss of function induced by this purely subconscious psychological phenomenon can result in permanent somatic complication such as contractures or disuse atrophy.

The most common symptoms associated with conversion disorders are outlined in Table 204-2. It must be emphasized that the somatic symptoms associated with a conversion disorder are not under voluntary control and thus not subject to easy detection on physical examination by identification of features that are suggestive of voluntary control, such as inconsistency and variability of signs and symptoms, which tend to be self-limited and of relatively brief duration.

La belle indifférence has historically been thought to be highly suggestive of conversion disorder, although this neurologic finding consists of an odd or inappropriate lack of concern for the impact and severity of the "converted" somatic symptomatology and the complete denial of any psychological problems associated with the

TABLE 204–2 Somatic Signs and Symptoms Commonly Associated with Conversion Disorder

- Weakness
- Paralysis
- Blindness
- Deafness
- Aphonia
- Sensory disturbances
- Abnormal involuntary movements including tremor
- Pseudoseizures

somatic difficulties. In fact, *la belle indifférence* can be seen with a variety of other organically based neurologic disorders including right cerebral hemisphere strokes. Because of this fact, it should be remembered that conversion disorder is a diagnosis of exclusion, and a careful search for a somatic basis for the patient's unexplained signs and symptoms should be carried out before ascribing the patient's malady to a purely psychogenic basis.

SUGGESTED READING

Bond MR: Psychiatric disorders and pain. In McMahon SB, Koltzenburg M (eds): Wall and Melzack's Textbook of Pain, ed 5. Philadelphia, Churchill Livingstone, 2006.

CHAPTER 205

Munchausen Syndrome

Munchausen syndrome is a rare psychiatric disease that primarily affects males, in which the patient goes from physician to physician presenting dramatic and often textbook-perfect complaints of severe and frequently life-threatening maladies. The life-threatening nature of the patient's complaints is often reinforced by the patient inducing factitious disease by injecting infected material to cause an actual fever, using tourniquets to cause limb swelling, and so on. The worrisome nature of the patient's fictional complaints often leads to increasingly invasive diagnostic testing and treatments that in and of themselves can induce morbidity and, rarely, mortality. Cardiac symptomatology is a fertile ground for the patient suffering from Munchausen syndrome and has led to the identification of a subset of Munchausen syndrome known as *cardiopathia fantastica.*

It is important to note that in contradistinction to patients suffering from conversion disorder, in which the patient is not conscious of his or her confabulations, the patient suffering from Munchausen syndrome is fully aware that he or she is lying and is fully conscious that there is no disease. Although the exact pathophysiology responsible for Munchausen syndrome is unknown, the current thinking is that most patients suffering from this disease have an associated personality disorder. Another important distinction when comparing conversion disorder with Munchausen syndrome is that patients suffering from a conversion disorder almost always have clearly identifiable primary and secondary gains, whereas the patient suffering from Munchausen syndrome has no obvious primary or secondary gain. The patient with Munchausen syndrome consciously and actively seeks the role of patient, which apparently fulfills some deep-rooted psychological need. Munchausen patients seek this patient role and will actively undergo painful and risky diagnostic and therapeutic interventions to further this goal.

In addition to the subset of Munchausen syndrome known as cardiopathia fantastica, there is another subset of Munchausen syndrome known as Munchausen syndrome by proxy, or fabricated or induced illness, in which a caregiver actively induces illness in the patient to gain sympathy, obtain attention, or obtain other secondary gain. Munchausen syndrome by proxy has been recognized as a potential cause of elder and child abuse.

Like the associated personality disorders frequently identified in patients suffering from Munchausen syndrome, patients with this rare disease are notoriously hard to treat. Although antipsychotic drugs have been used to treat Munchausen syndrome, there is little evidence to support their effectiveness.

SUGGESTED READING

Bond MR: Psychiatric disorders and pain. In McMahon SB, Koltzenburg M (eds): Wall and Melzack's Textbook of Pain, ed 5. Philadelphia, Churchill Livingstone, 2006.

CHAPTER 206

Thermal Injuries

Thermal injuries are damage to tissue as the result of contact of the affected tissue with extreme heat or cold. When a thermal injury occurs, the most superficial areas (i.e., the skin or mucosa) are first affected with the loss of the barrier function, increasing the patient's risk for infection. As deeper layers are affected, fluid leaking from capillaries leads to fluid loss, edema, and pain.

Thermal injuries are classified according to the depth of tissue damage. The traditional three-part classification of first-, second-, and third-degree burns has been replaced by a six-part system that more accurately defines the extent of injury. Such accurate classification is necessary when formulating a treatment plan as well as for forecasting a prognosis. The six-part classification is outlined in Table 206-1.

TABLE 206–1 Classification of Thermal Injuries

- **First-degree burns** are usually limited to erythema, limited pale-white plaque formation, and mild pain at the site of injury. First-degree burns extend only into the epidermis.
- **Second-degree burns** exhibit frank fluid extravasation and blister formation. Second-degree burns involve the papillary layer of dermis and may also involve portions of the deeper reticular dermis layer.
- **Third-degree burns** additionally include charring of the skin and subcutaneous tissues and eschar formation. Destruction of the pain receptors and nerve endings render third-degree wounds less painful than second-degree burns. Hair follicles and sudoriferous glands are permanently destroyed, and significant scarring usually occurs.
- **Fourth-degree burns** are burns in which the majority of the dermis is destroyed, leaving the underlying muscle and/or bone exposed. There is no sensation in the burn area as pain receptors and nerve endings are completely destroyed. Skin grafting and radical débridement of nonviable tissue are required, and death may occur.
- **Fifth-degree burns** are burns in which the skin, subcutaneous tissue, and muscle have been destroyed, leaving the underlying bone exposed. Thermal damage to the underlying bone further complicates the care and worsens the prognosis.
- **Sixth-degree burns** are burns in which all the skin and subcutaneous tissue as well as muscle are destroyed and there is significant thermal injury to the underlying bone. Mortality associated with sixth-degree burns is extremely high.

TABLE 206–2 Rule of Nines for Assessment of Total Body Surface Area Affected by a Burn—Adult

Anatomic Structure	Surface Area
Head	9%
Anterior torso	18%
Posterior torso	18%
Each leg	18%
Each arm	9%
Perineum	1%

In addition to this classification of burns that focuses on the degree of tissue damage, the severity of thermal injury is assessed in terms of the *total body surface area* (TBSA), which is defined as the percentage of the total body affected by second-degree or greater burns. The TBSA is easily assessed by using the rule of nines, which is outlined in

TABLE 206–3 Rule of Nines for Assessment of Total Body Surface Area Affected by a Burn—Infant

Anatomic Structure	Surface Area
Head	18%
Anterior torso	18%
Posterior torso	18%
Each leg	14%
Each arm	9%
Perineum	1%

The Parkland Formula for Fluid Replacement Following Serious Thermal Injury

Fluid = 4 mL × %TBSA × weight (in kg)
Half of this fluid as lactated Ringer's solution should be given in the first 8 hours post injury and the remainder given in the subsequent 16 hours.

*Note the %TBSA excludes any first-degree burns and only counts second-degree burns or worse.

Table 206-2. It should be noted that due to the larger head size of infants relative to their body, a modified rule of nines calculation is used for infants (Table 206-3).

The first step in the treatment of all thermal injuries is to remove the offending substance to prevent further tissue damage. Such items as smoldering clothing, adherent chemicals, or ice are removed as quickly as possible. The injured areas are carefully cleaned to decrease the risk of infection, nonviable tissue is debrided, tetanus toxoid is administered, the wounds are covered with an antibiotic ointment such as silver sulfadiazine, and sterile dressings are placed. Large amounts of fluid leakage are associated with more serious burns, and immediate replacement of fluids with lactated Ringer's solution is essential to avoid dehydration and renal insufficiency. The Parkland formula is an easy way to estimate the amount of fluid that must be given, with urine output and vital signs allowing the clinician to fine-tune the patient's fluid requirements. The Parkland formula is outlined in Table 206-3. If smoke inhalation has occurred, careful attention to the patient's upper airway and respiratory status is mandatory. Intravenous opioid analgesics should be used to help palliate the patient's pain. For thermal injuries involving small surface areas, topical local anesthetics can be used with caution. For more serious burns, rapid transfer of the patient to a burn center will greatly improve the patient's prognosis.

SUGGESTED READING

Papini R: Management of burn injuries of various depths. BMJ 2004;329(7458):158-160.

CHAPTER 207

Electrical Injuries

The unique effects of supraphysiologic levels of electrical energy on human tissue create a spectrum of injuries beyond that associated with thermal injury. The three major groups of tissue injury associated with electricity are (1) low-voltage injuries, (2) high-voltage injury, and (3) injuries caused by lightning. The extent of the tissue injury induced by electricity is dependent on a number of variables, which are listed in Table 207-1. It is the interaction of each of the variables that ultimately determines the individual patient's morbidity and mortality.

In general, the greater the voltage, the greater is the amount of current that can pass through tissue assuming the resistance of the tissue remains relatively constant.

TABLE 207–1 Factors Affecting the Extent of Tissue Injury from Electricity

- Voltage
- Type of current (alternating current [AC] or direct current [DC])
- Path of the current
- Resistance or conductance of the tissue
- Contact surface area
- Duration of exposure

Because alternating current is an oscillating current in which the direction of flow rapidly changes, it is approximately three times as dangerous as an equivalent voltage of direct current (in the United States, this change in direction of flow occurs 60 times per second, or 60 cycles per second). The reason for this increased danger is thought to be related to the increased ability of alternating current to produce tetany, making it impossible for the patient to withdraw the body part making contact with the source of electricity. The phenomenon of electrical-induced tetany can occur at a threshold level of approximately 15 mA, and this threshold level is known as the let-go level. Because increases in the duration of the contact with the electrical source increase the amount of tissue damage, voltages above the let-go level are associated with significantly higher morbidity and mortality. Levels above 30 mA are associated with tetany of the cardiac muscle. Alternating current also has a greater ability to overcome the resistance of the epidermis compared with direct current, further increasing its propensity to cause tissue damage.

Because electricity tends to flow through the path of least resistance, the flow of electricity and its associated tissue damage will be in large part determined by the resistance of the tissues through which the electricity passes. This flow can be caused by either direct or indirect contact with an electrical source. Direct contact occurs when a patient actually touches a conductor of electricity. Indirect flow can occur when the patient becomes a portion of an electrical arc, when flashes from another path the electricity is taking (e.g., down a ladder or a tree), jump to the patient, and simply from blunt injury from the superheating of the surrounding air, which is known as a thermoacoustic blast. It should be noted that the temperature of arcing electricity is extremely high (i.e., 2,500 to 10,000° F) and these high temperatures can ignite clothing or melt coins and other metal objects, creating even greater thermal tissue damage.

The more resistant a tissue, the more heating of that tissue will occur. This direct transfer of electrical energy to heat is known as *joule heating* and is the major cause of thermal tissue damage associated with electrical injuries. The relative conductivity of tissue is summarized in Table 207-2, with nerves being the least resistive (most conductive) and bone being the most resistive (least conductive). Because nerves and blood vessels have a relatively low resistance to the flow of electrical current compared to muscle and bone, they can carry electrical currents without significant joule heating. Due to the higher resistance to the flow of electricity in muscle and bone, more joule heating occurs and, hence, a greater amount of thermal injury can be expected.

In most instances, a history of electrical injury is well known, although, occasionally, victims are simply found in an unconscious state with no obvious cause for their injury. In this setting, a careful search for skin surface damage indicative of electrical injury is indicated. With high-voltage injuries, the entrance and exit wounds may appear deceptively minor with well-circumscribed damages with a leather-like texture and hyperemic

TABLE 207–2 The Relative Resistance of Tissues to the Flow of Electricity

Least Resistive	Nerve
↓	Blood vessels
↓	Muscles
↓	Skin
↓	Fat
Most Resistive	Bone

borders that belie the much more serious deep tissue damage. If a flash-type injury has occurred, there may be more extensive burning present. With lightning injuries, there is a pathognomonic cutaneous sign known as the Lichtenberg figure, which is a Christmas tree–like or fern-like pattern that appears in the first few hours after a lightning strike. As mentioned, lightning strike can superheat the air, creating a thermoacoustic blast that can cause extensive blunt trauma. With low-voltage injuries, the affected skin and subcutaneous tissue will appear edematous with an areola of dry, shriveled skin surrounding the injury. Cutaneous injury from the intentional use of electricity to incapacitate individuals (e.g., taser) will also exhibit a perimeter effect that is analogous to a first-degree burn. This perimeter effect can also be seen after cardiac defibrillation or cardioversion.

SUGGESTED READING

Bingham H: Electrical burns. Clin Plast Surg 1986;13(1):75-85.

CHAPTER 208

Cancer Pain

Pain is extremely prevalent in cancer patients. It is a major impediment to an adequate quality of life and may undermine efforts to assess and treat the underlying disease. Pain severe enough to require treatment with opioids occurs in about one third of patients undergoing active treatment and in more than two thirds of those with advanced disease. Although extensive clinical experience indicates that most cancer patients can attain acceptable pain relief, there is compelling evidence that treatment is often inadequate. In a small portion of patients, this is because of the refractoriness of pain or the patient's reluctance to comply with an effective therapy; far more often, however, uncontrolled cancer pain reflects a failure of clinical management. Physicians and nurses often seem unaware of the problem of cancer pain and frequently compromise treatment with inappropriate concerns about the risks of therapy (particularly addiction) and ignorance about the assessment and treatment of pain.

A comprehensive approach to managing cancer pain can have a gratifying outcome and should be reviewed as a fundamental element in the treatment of the cancer patient. Simple pharmacologic approaches alone can provide relief in more than 70% of cancer patients with pain, while other treatment modalities, including nerve blocks and neurodestructive procedures, can help many others.

Pain

Pain assessment in the cancer patient requires understanding of the relationships among pain, nociception, and suffering. *Nociception* refers to the activity in the afferent nervous system induced by potentially tissue-damaging stimuli. A comprehensive assessment will identify a nociception lesion in most patients with cancer pain. *Pain* is the perception of nociception. It is strongly influenced by affective and cognitive processes unique to the individual. These processes may eventuate in an intensity of pain that is either greater or less than that anticipated by the degree of tissue damage. *Suffering* is a construct that refers to a more global response, which is related to unrelieved symptoms (including pain) and many perceived losses, including those related to evolving disability, social isolation, financial concerns, loss of role in the family, and fear of death. It is important for the clinician to recognize that suffering may occur in the absence of active nociception.

Clinical interventions targeted solely at the complaint of pain—particularly at the nociceptive component—are unlikely to measurably benefit patients whose complaints are an expression of a more global degree of suffering. Indeed, such treatment plans are often perceived by patient and family as uncompassionate.

Establishing a Pain Diagnosis

The goals of pain assessment in the cancer patient are to identify the underlying nociceptive lesion, clarify the various non-nociceptive contributions to the pain, and determine the degree and causes of suffering. From this information, a "pain diagnosis" can be elaborated; practically, this is a problem list that can be used to target specific problems for treatment and organize a multimodal therapeutic approach.

The first step in establishing the diagnosis is to characterize the pain complaint fully. Specific inquiries should evaluate onset, duration, severity, quality, location, radiation, temporal characteristics, provocative and palliative factors, and course. A medical history should access both previous and current use of analgesic and other drugs. The physicians should elicit any history of chronic nonmalignant pain, chronic opioid use, and/or substance abuse. The extent of disease at the time of evaluation and the patient's general medical condition should also be assessed. An integral part of this initial evaluation is the assessment of the affective, behavioral, and social disturbances related to the pain. Patients with cancer pain commonly experience anxiety and vegetative signs, such as sleep disturbances, lassitude, and anorexia.

After taking an adequate history, the physician should perform a general medical and neurologic examination. The physical examination, like the history, should attempt to clarify the specific pain syndrome to determine the extent of the disease, clarify the nature of the specific nociceptive lesions underlying the pain, and assess the degree of physical impairment (Table 208-1).

After obtaining a working clinical diagnosis from the history and physical examination, the physician should consider appropriate laboratory, electrodiagnostic, or radiographic procedures; these evaluations further clarify the nature of the nociceptive lesion presumed to underlie the pain. The primary clinician must carefully review all test results, including radiographs, to obtain clinicopathologic correlation for the pain. If there is a change in the patient's clinical status, it is important that the clinician avoid over-reliance on past test results so that incorrect diagnosis can be avoided. When in doubt, this is one clinical setting in which repeating tests will often yield important clinical information. Effective analgesic treatment should be provided to the patient throughout the evaluation, particularly during procedures; the psychological impact of the evaluation will be far less averse and the quality of tests enhanced if the patient's cooperation is not compromised by pain.

The pain diagnosis can be clarified in most patients after this comprehensive assessment is completed. The problem list may include the pain itself, physical and psychological disturbances contributing to the pain, associated symptoms, and physical impairments; any psychological disturbances contributing to the pain, associated symptoms, and physical impairments; and psychological, social, or familial problems that independently augment the patient's suffering. These problems can be prioritized according to their impact on the patient's quality of life and allow planned therapeutic interventions to be staged appropriately.

TABLE 208–1 Cancer Pain Syndromes

I. Pain Syndromes Associated with Direct Tumor Involvement		
1. *Bone*		
a. Base of skull	b. Vertebral body	c. Generalized bone pain
• Orbital • Parasellar • Sphenoidal sinus • Middle cranial fossa • Civus • Jugular foramen • Occipital condyle	• Atlantoaxial • C7 to T1 • L1 • Sacral	
2. *Nerves*		
a. Peripheral nerve syndromes	b. Leptomeningeal metastases	
• Paraspinal tumor • Chest wall tumor • Retroperitoneal tumor	c. Painful polyneuropathy	
	d. Brachial, lumbar, sacral plexopathies	
	e. Epidural spinal cord compression	
3. *Viscera*		
4. *Blood vessels*		
5. *Mucous membranes*		
II. Pain Associated with Cancer Therapy		
1. *Postoperative*	2. *Postchemotherapy*	3. *Postradiation*
a. Thoracotomy	a. Painful polyneuropathy	a. Fibrosis of brachial or lumbosacral plexus
b. Mastectomy	b. Aseptic necrosis of bone	
c. Radical surgery of the neck	c. Pseudorheumatism caused by steroids	
d. Amputation		
		b. Myelopathy
		c. Radiation-induced peripheral nerve tumors
		d. Mucositis
III. Pain Indirectly Related or Unrelated to Cancer		
1. *Myofascial pains*		
2. *Postherpetic neuralgia*		
3. *Chronic headache syndromes*		

Therapeutic Approaches to Cancer Pain Management

Antineoplastic therapies should be considered as a first step in the analgesic management of patients whose pain is a direct effect of the neoplasm. Radiotherapy provides adequate analgesia in more than half of patients treated, and pain is a common primary indication for this modality. Although toxicity and unpredictable pain relief limit the utility of chemotherapy as an analgesic intervention, some patients obtain symptom relief from the administration of chemotherapeutic drugs. The varying analgesic response and risks associated with surgical extirpation of a neoplasm limit surgery as a primary analgesic therapy. However, tumor resection performed for other indications, such as vertebral body resection for epidural spinal cord compression, may provide analgesia. Although all patients with cancer pain should be considered for antineoplastic therapy, most pain management depends on the expert application of one or more primary analgesic modalities. Pharmacotherapy is the most important of these.

Pharmacologic Approaches

Three categories of analgesic medications—nonsteroidal anti-inflammatory drugs (NSAIDs), opioid analgesics, and the so-called adjuvant analgesics—are used in the pharmacotherapy of cancer pain. The Cancer Pain Relief Program of the World Health Organization has developed guidelines for the selection of drugs from these categories. The approach, known as the "analgesic ladder," can be summarized as follows: For mild pain, an NSAID is administered and an adjuvant is added if a specific indication for one exists. If the regimen fails to control pain or the patient presents with moderate to severe pain, a so-called "weak" oral opioid is administered in combination with an NSAID; again, adjuvant analgesics (e.g., antidepressants, local anesthetics, anticonvulsants, GABA inhibitors) are added if indicated. If maximal doses of weaker opioid analgesics do not control the pain or the patient's pain is severe, a so-called "strong" opioid is administered, with or without an NSAID or adjuvant drugs.

SUGGESTED READINGS

Cherny NI: Cancer pain assessment. In McMahon SB, Koltzenburg M (eds): Wall and Melzack's Textbook of Pain, ed 5. Philadelphia, Churchill Livingstone, 2006.

De Leon-Casasola OA (ed): Cancer Pain Management. Pharmacological, Interventional, and Palliative Care Approaches. Philadelphia, Saunders, 2006.

Hoskin PJ: Cancer pain: Treatment overview. In McMahon SB, Koltzenburg M (eds): Wall and Melzack's Textbook of Pain, ed 5. Philadelphia, Churchill Livingstone, 2006.

Mantyh P: Cancer pain: Causes, consequences and therapeutic opportunities. In McMahon SB, Koltzenburg M (eds): Wall and Melzack's Textbook of Pain, ed 5. Philadelphia, Churchill Livingstone, 2006.

CHAPTER 209

Multiple Sclerosis

Multiple sclerosis is a disease of unknown etiology that is associated with idiopathic inflammatory demyelinating disease of the central nervous system. Current thinking suggests that multiple sclerosis results from the triggering of an autoimmune process by yet unproved triggering agents. Although a number of viruses and/or environmental triggers have been suggested, none have yet been conclusively proved as the factor or factors responsible for the triggering of multiple sclerosis. The autoantigen thought to be responsible for the clinical symptomatology associated with multiple sclerosis appears to be one or more of the myelin proteins with the autoimmune inflammatory cascade targeting and ultimately damaging the oligodendroglia cells and their associated membrane myelin.

There appears to be a genetic predisposition to the development of multiple sclerosis as witnessed by a 10% to 20% familial incidence and a 30% risk that a monozygous twin will develop multiple sclerosis if the other twin has it. Research has shown that the human leukocyte antigen patterns of patients with multiple sclerosis tend to differ from those of the general population.

In addition to the familial predilection to develop the disease, there is a unique geographic distribution to the disease, with the highest incidence of the disease occurring in the temperate latitudes and the Western Hemisphere. This geographic disparity in the incidence of multiple sclerosis is highlighted when comparing the U.S. incidence of multiple sclerosis of approximately 1 case per 1000 persons with the international incidence of only 1 case per 1 million persons.

Women are affected almost twice as often as are men; the symptoms of multiple sclerosis in men tend to manifest later than in women, but men more commonly suffer more severe forms of the disease. Rare in Eskimos, Native Americans, and Asians, multiple sclerosis occurs most commonly in whites, especially those who spent their first 15 years growing up in a temperate climate. The onset of multiple sclerosis is rarely seen before the second decade or after the fifth decade.

The classic central nervous system lesion associated with multiple sclerosis is the plaque. This plaque formation is thought to be the end result of repeated episodes of central nervous system autoimmune inflammation, axonal damage, and demyelination. This pathologic process tends to result in a disease in which the patient's symptoms tend to occur later in the disease and are characterized by clinical exacerbations and remissions. These plaques tend to be distributed in a multicentric pattern with skip lesions often seen. For reasons that have yet to be elucidated, the pathologic process associated with multiple sclerosis has a predilection for the optic nerve, periventricular white matter of the cerebellum, brainstem, basal ganglia, and spinal cord (Table 209-1). Multiple sclerosis plaques involving these anatomic areas are readily identified on magnetic resonance imaging, making the diagnosis of multiple sclerosis much easier than in the past. Multiple sclerosis rarely affects the peripheral nervous system.

Clinically, the classic manifestation of multiple sclerosis is that of the patient presenting with an unexplained dysfunction of the central nervous system. This dysfunction most often takes the form of optic neuritis, transverse myelitis, internuclear ophthalmoplegia, and pain and/or paresthesias (Table 209-2). Due to the nature of the pathologic process responsible for the

TABLE 209–1 Central Nervous System Tissues Most Commonly Affected with Multiple Sclerosis

- Optic nerve
- Periventricular white matter of the cerebellum
- Brainstem
- Basal ganglia
- Spinal cord

TABLE 209–2 The Most Common Clinical Presentations of Multiple Sclerosis

- Optic neuritis
- Transverse myelitis
- Internuclear ophthalmoplegia
- Pain
- Paresthesias

clinical symptoms of multiple sclerosis, the severity of symptoms can vary greatly from patient to patient as can the progression of the disease, with milder forms of the disease progressing slowly over decades and the rare, more fulminate forms of the disease progressing to serious and often permanent neurologic dysfunction (e.g., paraplegia, blindness) over a few days. More than 70% of patients suffering from multiple sclerosis are classified as having the relapsing/remitting form of the disease, which has as its hallmark acute exacerbations followed by partial or full remissions. This relapsing/remitting form of the disease carries a more favorable prognosis than do more fulminate forms of this disorder. Even with the more fulminate forms of multiple sclerosis, death is rarely directly attributable to multiple sclerosis but rather due to the disability resulting from the disease.

Symptoms most commonly associated with multiple sclerosis are outlined in Table 209-3, with optic neuritis, transverse myelitis, sensory dysfunction, and motor dysfunction most often pointing the clinician toward a diagnosis of multiple sclerosis. For the clinician confronted with a patient with optic neuritis, it should be assumed that it is most likely due to multiple sclerosis, although other causes of acute optic neuritis, including tumors, ischemic optic neuropathy, arteriovenous malformations, and infections of the anatomic region of the optic nerve, must be ruled out. The same approach should be taken with patients presenting with acute transverse myelitis without obvious etiology with abscess, tumor, aneurysm, infection, and postinfectious etiologies (e.g., Epstein-Barr virus and Lyme disease infections) being considered in the differential diagnosis.

Physical findings commonly associated with multiple sclerosis are also seen in many other disease processes, although some valid generalizations can be made. Common ocular findings in patients with acute optic neuritis include an initially normal funduscopic examination in the setting of complete visual loss. It has been said that when the patient's acute optic neuritis is due to multiple sclerosis, the patient sees nothing and the physician sees nothing. Patients may volunteer that their

TABLE 209–3 Symptoms Most Commonly Associated with Multiple Sclerosis

- Sensory Dysfunction
  - Paresthesias
  - Pain
  - Numbness
  - Trigeminal neuralgia
- Motor Dysfunction
  - Muscle cramping
  - Spasticity
  - Weakness
- Autonomic Dysfunction
  - Bladder
  - Bowel
  - Sexual dysfunction
- Spinal Cord Dysfunction
- Transverse myelitis
- Cerebellar Dysfunction
  - Dysarthria
  - Tremor
  - Ataxia
- Constitutional symptoms
  - Fatigue
  - Dizziness
  - Myalgias
- Ocular Symptoms
  - Visual disturbance
  - Blindness
  - Diplopia
  - Ocular palsies
- Impairment of Higher Functions
  - Short attention span
  - Impaired problem solving
  - Poor concentration
  - Impaired judgment
  - Poor memory
- Behavioral Changes
  - Depression
  - Dysphoria
  - Dementia
- Seizures

visual dysfunction may worsen after taking a hot bath, exercising, being exposed to high ambient temperatures, or eating a hot meal. This unique symptom is known as the Uhthoff phenomenon. As the optic neuritis persists for several weeks, optic atrophy may be seen on funduscopic examination. Examination of the extraocular muscles will often reveal bilateral internuclear ophthalmoplegia, which is the result of multiple sclerosis affecting the median longitudinal fasciculus and resulting in a weakness in adduction of the ipsilateral eye with nystagmus on abduction of the contralateral eye, an incomplete or slow abduction of the ipsilateral eye upon lateral gaze, with complete preservation of convergence. Other ocular findings associated with multiple sclerosis include pupillary dysfunction and nystagmus.

Cerebellar dysfunction associated with multiple sclerosis may result in the physical findings of truncal or limb ataxia, disequilibrium, intension tremor, saccadic dysmetria, and a pattern of scanning speech. These findings may be subtle or, in more severe acute presentations or exacerbations of the disease, quite obvious.

Spinal cord dysfunction associated with multiple sclerosis will often manifest with the constellation of findings associated with transverse myelitis (i.e., weakness, numbness, paralysis, spasticity, and hyperreflexia). Unlike Guillain-Barré, the level of spinal cord dysfunction in multiple sclerosis tends to remain constant. Decreased joint proprioception and vibratory sense and, less commonly, abnormal pain and temperature perception can also

be identified with careful neurologic examination. A positive Lhermitte sign consisting of sudden shocklike paresthesias in the trunk and extremities with flexion of the neck is often present.

Testing in patients suspected of suffering from multiple sclerosis is required for three reasons: (1) to rule out other more treatable causes of neurologic dysfunction, such as stroke, epidural abscess, and hypoglycemia; (2) to identify other abnormalities due to the disability associated with multiple sclerosis, such as dehydration, urosepsis, and so on; and (3) to confirm the diagnosis of multiple sclerosis. To accomplish these three goals, basic screening laboratory testing, including complete blood count, chemistry profile, erythrocyte sedimentation rate, electrolytes, serum thyroxine, and antinuclear antibody testing should be obtained. Magnetic resonance imaging (MRI) of the head and spine with and without gadolinium will confirm the diagnosis of multiple sclerosis in the vast majority of cases; lesions identified on MRI often presage the clinical onset of the disease by several years. Spinal fluid analysis is reserved for patients with unusual clinical presentations and/or equivocal findings on MRI.

Treatment of patients with multiple sclerosis is based on the type of multiple sclerosis the patient is suffering from and variables including the severity of symptoms and rate of progression of the disease. Relapsing/remitting multiple sclerosis is usually treated with beta interferon or glatiramer acetate (Copaxone) with the

TABLE 209–4 Diseases That May Mimic Multiple Sclerosis

- Amyotrophic lateral sclerosis
- Autoimmune disorders
- Behçet's disease
- Bell's palsy
- Brain abscess
- Brainstem tumors
- Central nervous system infections
- Cerebellar tumors
- Cervical intervertebral disc disorders
- Cervical myelopathy
- Drug-induced central nervous system dysfunction
- Friedreich's ataxia
- Guillain-Barré syndrome
- Hereditary ataxias
- HIV infection and AIDS
- Leukodystrophies
- Lumbar intervertebral disc disorders
- Pernicious anemia
- Progressive multifocal leukoencephalopathy
- Sarcoidosis
- Small vessel cerebrovascular disease
- Spinal cord arteriovenous malformations
- Spinal cord infections
- Spinal cord infarctions
- Spinal cord injuries
- Spinal cord tumors
- Stroke, hemorrhagic
- Stroke, ischemic
- Subdural hematoma
- Syphilis
- Syringomyelia
- Systemic lupus erythematosus
- Tick-borne diseases, Lyme disease
- Transient ischemic attack
- Trigeminal neuralgia
- Vasculitides
- Vitamin deficiencies
- von Recklinghausen disease
- Wilson's disease

recombinant monoclonal antibody natalizumab (Tysabri) reserved for patients refractory to interferons owing to the patient's increased risk of developing progressive multifocal leukoencephalopathy. For patients with more progressive forms of multiple sclerosis, the addition of corticosteroids, cyclophosphamide, and methotrexate may be indicated.

The differential diagnosis of patients suspected of multiple sclerosis is a long one and is outlined in Table 209-4. It is incumbent on the clinician presented with such a patient to aggressively rule out other causes of the patient's neurologic dysfunction that may be more amenable to treatment. Thus, although multiple sclerosis is not a diagnosis of exclusion, it should be thought of as a diagnosis that requires a thorough search of other diseases prior to confirming the final diagnosis of multiple sclerosis.

SUGGESTED READINGS

Campbell W: DeJong's The Neurological Examination, ed 6. Philadelphia, Lippincott Williams and Wilkins, 2005.

Goetz CG: Textbook of Clinical Neurology, ed 2. Philadelphia, Saunders, 2003.

CHAPTER 210

Post-Polio Syndrome

Post-polio syndrome refers to a constellation of signs and symptoms that appear decades after the patient was initially infected and includes new asymmetrical muscle weakness in muscles that were not originally affected by the original infection, new muscle atrophy, myalgias and arthralgias, generalized fatigue, difficulty breathing, difficulty swallowing, centrally mediated sleep disorders, and decreased tolerance to cold ambient temperatures (Table 210-1). These signs and symptoms are often worse in the early afternoon. It is estimated that between 30% and 50% of polio survivors will experience post-polio syndrome to a greater or lesser extent.

TABLE 210–1 Symptoms Associated with Post-Polio Syndrome

- New asymmetrical muscle weakness in muscles that were not originally affected by the original infection
- New muscle atrophy
- Myalgias
- Arthralgias
- Generalized fatigue
- Difficulty breathing
- Difficulty swallowing
- Centrally mediated sleep disorders
- Decreased tolerance to cold ambient temperatures

Although the exact cause of post-polio syndrome is unknown, several pathophysiologic mechanisms have been proposed that either alone or together may be responsible for the signs and symptoms of post-polio syndrome. Many experts believe that post-polio syndrome is a combination of a gradual decompensation of the normal process of nerve denervation and reinnervation and the decrease in muscle strength that occurs as part of the normal aging process. Other experts have postulated that post-polio syndrome is due to the reactivation of a latent virus in a manner analogous to the varicella zoster/ shingles mechanism. Another possibility is that post-polio syndrome is simply the result of a new infection with an enterovirus similar to polio with the patient's immune system mistaking the new virus for the old polio virus and setting up an autoimmune response that attacks nerve cells.

TABLE 210–2 Diseases That May Mimic Post-Polio Syndrome

- Amyotrophic lateral sclerosis
- Anemia
- Cervical myelopathy
- Chronic infection
- Collagen vascular disorders
- Deconditioning
- Depression
- Fibromyalgia
- Hypothyroidism
- Infectious myopathy
- Inflammatory myopathy
- Multiple sclerosis
- Myotonic dystrophy
- Myasthenia gravis
- Neurodegenerative disorders
- Polymyositis
- Weakness due to aging
- Weight gain

Risk factors that increase the probability of developing post-polio syndrome include the severity of the initial infection, with more severe infections increasing the risk; the age of onset of polio, with the younger patients more likely to develop post-polio syndrome; and the amount of physical activity the patient performs, with increased levels of physical activity increasing risk. Paradoxically, the greater the patient's recovery from his or her initial polio infection, the greater is the patient's chance of developing post-polio syndrome.

On physical examination, asymmetrical muscle weakness and atrophy may be observed in muscles that were affected initially by the poliovirus or in muscles that were not obviously affected at the time of initial infection. Fasciculations can sometimes be observed with careful examination of weakened and/or atrophied muscles.

Testing in patients suspected of suffering from post-polio syndrome is required for three reasons: (1) to rule out other more treatable causes of neurologic dysfunction, (2) to identify other abnormalities due to the disability associated with post-polio syndrome, and (3) to help confirm the diagnosis of post-polio syndrome. To accomplish these three goals, basic screening laboratory tests including complete blood count, chemistry profile, erythrocyte sedimentation rate, electrolytes, serum thyroxine, and antinuclear antibody testing should be obtained. Magnetic resonance imaging of the head and spine with and without gadolinium will help rule out other central nervous system diseases that may mimic post-polio syndrome (see later). Electromyography is highly specific in the diagnosis of anterior horn cell disease, although the test can be suggestive but not specific for polio.

Treatment of post-polio syndrome is aimed primarily at maximizing function and the relief of symptoms. Physical and occupational therapy to maintain and improve function is the cornerstone of the management of post-polio syndrome. Respiratory and speech therapy is indicated if swallowing, sleep, and/or breathing problems are present. Treatment of osteoporosis to prevent fractures is also indicated. The pain of post-polio syndrome is managed with simple analgesics, anti-inflammatory agents, topical analgesic balms, and moist heat. Opioids should be avoided if at all possible. Weakness can be managed pharmacologically with anticholinesterase agents such as pyridostigmine (Mestinon). Neuritic pain, although uncommon, can be managed with the anticonvulsants.

Failure to treat post-polio syndrome may result in loss of functional ability, an increased risk of falls due to muscle weakness, dehydration and malnutrition secondary to swallowing abnormalities, and recurrent respiratory infections due to diaphragmatic weakness. Inactivity associated with post-polio syndrome may increase the risk of osteoporosis.

Diseases that need to be considered in the differential diagnosis of post-polio syndrome are outlined in Table 210-2. Given the implications of missing the diagnosis of many of the diseases listed in Table 210-2, post-polio syndrome must be considered a diagnosis of exclusion.

SUGGESTED READINGS

Campbell W: DeJong's The Neurological Examination, ed 6. Philadelphia, Lippincott Williams and Wilkins, 2005.

Goetz CG: Textbook of Clinical Neurology, ed 2. Philadelphia, Saunders, 2003.

Waldman SD: Post-polio syndrome. In: Atlas of Common Pain Syndromes, ed 2. Philadelphia, Saunders, 2008.

CHAPTER 211

Guillain-Barré Syndrome

Classic Guillain-Barré syndrome (GBS) is an acute, auto-immune polyradiculopathy characterized by the onset of paresthesias beginning in the finger tips and toes associated with lower extremity weakness that tends to increase in severity and to ascend to affect more proximal muscles and nerves over a period of hours to days. As the weakness and sensory dysfunction ascend, respiratory difficulties combined with paralysis of the lower cranial nerves may occur. This ascending paralysis may lead to the need for ventilatory support in approximately 30% of patients suffering from GBS. Autonomic dysfunction can be severe with orthostatic hypotension and cardiac arrhythmias complicating the care of the patient with evolving acute classic GBS.

The patient presenting with classic GBS will frequently give a history of an antecedent respiratory illness approximately 2 to 4 weeks prior to the onset of the signs and symptoms of GBS. Fever is rarely a component of acute GBS, and most experts believe that if unexplained fever is present during the onset of acute classic GBS, the diagnosis is probably not GBS. Areflexia is considered to be a cardinal finding of acute classic GBS, and the finding of hyperreflexia should point the clinician toward another diagnosis, such as myelopathy, motor neuron disease, or hyperthyroidism. Other diseases that may mimic acute classic GBS are listed in Table 211-1. Bladder and bowel incontinence are not usually associated with acute classic GBS except in the most severe cases, and even in this setting, it calls the diagnosis of GBS into question. Urinary retention and/or gastroparesis due to autonomic dysfunction may be present in patients suffering from more severe acute classic GBS.

Muscle pain is also a prominent feature of acute classic GBS. This pain tends to affect muscles that are weakened by GBS more severely than unaffected muscles. The character of the pain is most often deep, ill defined, and aching. The pain of GBS may persist long after recovery of motor and sensory function has begun.

The temporal pattern of acute classic GBS generally consists of three phases: (1) the evolution phase, (2) the plateau phase, and (3) the clinical recovery phase. The evolution phase is the period of time from onset of symptoms to the nadir of symptoms. Although initial symptoms can progress rather rapidly over a period of hours to a few days, the average time for patients suffering from acute classic GBS to reach nadir is approximately 12 to 14 days. The plateau phase begins at the nadir of symptoms and continues until the clinical recovery phase begins. The plateau phase on average can last for 2 to 4 weeks before the clinical recovery phase begins. The clinical recovery phase takes place over a period of many weeks, with most patients experiencing significant recovery within 25 to 30 weeks. Approximately 85% of patients suffering from acute classic GBS can expect a full recovery of function within 6 to 9 months. The remaining 15% may suffer from permanent residual neurologic defects including foot drop, weakness, and the like. When treated in tertiary care centers, the overall mortality associated with acute classic GBS is approximately 5%, with pulmonary embolus, adult respiratory arrest syndrome, and sepsis accounting for most deaths associated with this disease.

Acute classic GBS can affect all ages; young adults and the elderly are most often affected. Rare cases of infantile acute classic GBS have also been reported. There is a slight male-to-female predominance of 1.5:1 for the risk of developing acute classic GBS. It appears that pregnancy may confer some protection against acute classic GBS, although the exact reason for this finding has not been elucidated.

TABLE 211–1 Diseases That May Be Confused with Acute Classic Guillain-Barré Syndrome

- Alcohol poisoning
- Basilar artery insufficiency
- Botulism
- Brainstem stroke
- Cauda equina syndrome
- Charcot-Marie-Tooth disease
- Chronic inflammatory demyelinating polyneuropathy
- Diphtheria
- Encephalitis
- Fish neurotoxin poisoning
- Folate deficiency
- Heavy metal intoxication
- Hereditary neuropathies
- HIV peripheral neuropathy
- Hyperglycemia
- Hypoglycemia
- Hyperkalemia
- Hypokalemia
- Hyperosmolar coma
- Hypophosphatemia
- Lyme disease
- Meningitis
- Multiple sclerosis
- Myasthenia gravis
- Organophosphate poisoning
- Polio
- Polymyositis
- Porphyria
- Sarcoid meningitis
- Spinal cord infections
- Spinal cord injuries
- Systemic lupus erythematosus
- Tetanus
- Thiamine deficiency
- Tick paralysis
- Transverse myelitis
- Vitamin B-12 deficiency
- Vitamin B-6
- West Nile encephalitis

Although most clinicians use the term *Guillain-Barré syndrome* to describe classic GBS, distinct variants of GBS exist. These include the Miller Fisher variant GBS, which manifests with acute ophthalmoplegia, ataxia, and areflexia with paralysis evolving in a *descending* pattern, in contradistinction to classic GBS, in which the paralysis is always ascending. Other variants of GBS include the Chinese paralytic syndrome, which specifically targets the nodes of Ranvier and appears seasonally primarily in China and Mexico.

Although the exact cause or causes of acute classic GBS remain elusive, antecedent bacterial and viral infections as well as, on rare occasions, vaccine administrations have been implicated as the most likely causes of the triggering of the cascade of autoimmune events that result in the onset of the signs and symptoms associated with the disease. Bacteria that have been implicated include *Campylobacter, Haemophilus influenzae,* and *Borrelia burgdorferi,* among others. *Mycoplasma pneumoniae* and Epstein-Barr virus and cytomegalovirus have also been implicated. Influenza, rabies, and polio vaccination have been associated with acute classic GBS, although no definitive link has been established.

The diagnosis of acute classic GBS is almost always made on clinical grounds. Testing that may help solidify the diagnosis of acute classic GBS includes spinal fluid analysis and magnetic resonance imaging with and without gadolinium enhancement. Finding on cerebrospinal fluid analysis includes elevated protein with normal cerebrospinal fluid cell counts. If there is a strong clinical suspicion of acute classic GBS in the presence of normal cerebrospinal fluid protein levels, serial cerebrospinal fluid analysis may reveal a trend of increasing protein levels, which is consistent with the disease. Although magnetic resonance imaging of the spinal nerves is not diagnostic for acute classic GBS, selective gadolinium enhancement of the ventral portion of the spinal nerve root is highly suggestive of classic GBS. Electromyography and nerve conduction velocity testing are abnormal but not diagnostic in the vast majority of patients suffering from acute classic GBS, and these tests may help diagnose other diseases that may mimic acute classic GBS, such as acute inflammatory muscle disease.

The treatment of acute classic GBS during the evolution phase of the disease is aimed at the management of the symptoms caused by the progressive neurologic dysfunction associated with the disease. First and foremost, careful serial evaluation of the patient's respiratory status is paramount if disaster is to be avoided. Aggressive management of impending respiratory insufficiency with endotracheal intubation and mechanical intubation should be considered sooner rather than later given the progressive nature of the disease. Careful observation for cardiac arrhythmias should also be carried out. As the disease progresses, treatment should be aimed at prevention of complications secondary to immobility, such as bed sores and thrombophlebitis, as well as avoidance of hospital-acquired infections. Aggressive physical and occupational therapy to maintain function should be an integral portion of the treatment plan. Pain should be managed with simple analgesics and nonsteroidal anti-inflammatory drugs, with narcotics being reserved for acute exacerbations or incident-related pain.

SUGGESTED READING

Shields RW Jr, Wilbourn AJ: Demyelinating disorders of the peripheral nervous system. In Goetz CG (ed): Textbook of Clinical Neurology, ed. 3. Philadelphia, Saunders, 2007.

CHAPTER 212

Sickle Cell Disease

Sickle cell disease is the name applied to a group of genetic hemoglobinopathies that have in common an abnormal hemoglobin that tends to cause a change in the shape of the red blood cell during deoxygenation. This abnormal hemoglobin has been designated as Hgb S or Hb S. These changes in the shape of the red blood cell usually take the form of a sickle shape and are due to aggregation of the hemoglobin protein. When the hemoglobin aggregates during deoxygenation, the red blood cell becomes rigid, which damages the cell membrane, causing the red blood cells to adhere to the blood vessel walls, occluding the lumen of the vessel. If this process continues unabated, tissue ischemia and ultimately infarction may occur. These ischemic episodes are called vaso-occlusive or sickle cell crises, and they occur intermittently and are associated with significant morbidity and, rarely, mortality. Although all organs are at risk for damage from vaso-occlusive crises, the long bones and spleen are particularly susceptible to damage. In many patients with more severe forms of sickle cell disease the spleen can suffer complete infarction, resulting in an autosplenectomy.

Other serious complications associated with sickle cell disease include aplastic crises and splenic sequestration crises. Aplastic crises occur when infection with parvovirus B19 causes an acute halt to erythropoiesis with resultant rapidly progressive anemia due to the significantly shortened life expectancy of red blood cells with sickle cell hemoglobin. Aplastic crises manifest themselves clinically as an acute and rapid deterioration of the patient's cardiovascular status with tachycardia, dyspnea, and extreme pallor. A rapidly decreasing reticulocyte count is highly suggestive of aplastic crises in this clinical setting. Splenic sequestration crisis is manifested clinically as an acutely painful enlargement of the spleen.

These complications of sickle cell disease mentioned can act either alone or in combination to produce significant morbidity for patients suffering from this serious disease (Table 212-1). More common problems caused by these complications include hyposplenism-associated infections, stroke, cholelithiasis, osteomyelitis, retinopathy, and nephropathy.

Sickle cell disease occurs most commonly in individuals whose ancestors hailed from sub-Saharan Africa, the Middle East, India, and the Mediterranean. The predilection

TABLE 212–1 Morbidity Associated with the Complications of Sickle Cell Disease

- Hyposplenism-associated infections
- Stroke
- Cholelithiasis
- Cholecystitis
- Osteomyelitis (especially *Salmonella* and *Staphylococcus*)
- Aseptic necrosis
- Retinopathy
- Retinal detachments
- Vitreous hemorrhages
- Nephropathy
- Priapism
- Penile infarction

for this region is thought to be the result of natural selection because although sickle cell disease is associated with a shortened life expectancy of 40 to 50 years, the presence of sickle cell hemoglobin confers resistance to malaria, which was a leading cause of death in this geographic region.

The treatment of sickle cell disease is aimed at the palliation of acute symptoms of pain and dyspnea, the correction of underlying anemia, and the treatment of underlying infections or other comorbidities that may cause an exacerbation of the patient's symptomatology. In general, the pain associated with milder vaso-occlusive crises should be treated with simple analgesics and/or nonsteroidal anti-inflammatory drugs and oxygen. More severe pain may require opioid analgesics, although the risks of chemical dependence and addiction are high in this patient population owing to the recurring nature of the crises. The administration of zinc may help stabilize the red blood cell membrane, and the administration of hydroxyurea to increase the production of fetal hemoglobin in place of sickle hemoglobin can be considered.

SUGGESTED READING

Steinberg MH: Sickle cell anemia and associated hemoglobinopathies. In Goldman L, Ausiello DA (eds): Cecil Medicine, ed 23. Philadelphia, Saunders, 2008.

CHAPTER 213

Dependence, Tolerance, and Addiction

To understand the concepts and interrelationships of *chemical dependence, tolerance,* and *addiction,* one must first clearly define these medical conditions and then use these terms strictly as terms of art, that is, as terms that have special and specific meanings from one clinician to another. Perhaps in no other area of medicine has the lack of clarity and consistency in word usage done more damage to the understanding of disease and the care of patients.

Dependence

Dependence is defined as a physiologic state in which continued intake of a substance is required to maintain homeostasis. This term is frequently confused with *addiction,* although many drugs that are not traditionally associated with addiction (e.g., antihypertensives, antidepressants, beta-blockers) can cause dependence. In general, when such drugs are abruptly discontinued, physiologic disturbances may result but without routinely inciting dysfunctional behavioral patterns usually associated with addiction. Traditionally, dependence has been divided into two subsets: (1) physiologic dependence and (2) psychological dependence. Physiologic dependence is characterized by physiologic disturbances as described earlier. Psychological dependence is characterized by behavioral abnormalities caused by the patient's psychological belief that he or she must continue to use the substance to maintain homeostasis.

Tolerance

Tolerance is a physiologic phenomenon in which the organism adapts to the effects of the drug and over time there is a diminution of one or more of the drug's actions. This diminution of the drug's actions can be limited to its beneficial therapeutic effects (e.g., decreased pain relief with a given dose of opioid) or can affect only the side effects of a drug (e.g., the dry mouth associated with the tricyclic antidepressant use).

Addiction

Addiction is a disease state that is characterized by dysfunctional behavior surrounding the use of a substance. This dysfunctional behavior can take the form of inability to control the use of the substance to the point of compulsion despite the harm to the patient's health and interpersonal relationships. It must be emphasized that addiction can involve the use of illicit or licit substances and it is the behavior surrounding the acquisition and use and/ or misuse of these drugs that is indicative of addiction.

Predicting Who Is at Risk for the Development of Dependence, Tolerance, and Addiction

Genetic, psychosocial, and environmental factors notwithstanding, the clinician can generally identify the likelihood of the development of dependence and tolerance with the use of any given drug with a reasonable degree of certainty. Unfortunately, this is not the case with addiction. As the use of opioids for the treatment of nonmalignant pain has increased, this fact has become painfully apparent. Although no laboratory or psychological test has been devised to predict with a high degree of accuracy which patients are at risk for the development of addiction, the clinical use of opioids and other substances that have been traditionally associated with addiction has led to the development of a number of warning signs that addiction is a distinct possibility that can aid the clinician in identifying the patient who is at risk for addiction (Table 213-1). Although several psychological tests have been used as predictive screening instruments, such as the Cage Inventory and the Webster Opioid Risk tool, none has gained widespread acceptance.

The Neurobiology of Addiction

Although the exact causes of addiction have not been elucidated, there is a consensus that all addictions involve the reward centers of the brain. These centers are thought

TABLE 213–1 Behaviors Suggestive That an Increased Risk of Addiction Exists

- Excessive focus on controlled substances at each visit
- After-hours telephone calls regarding need for controlled substances
- Lost prescriptions
- Requests for early refills
- Spilled prescriptions necessitating early refills
- Reports of stolen prescriptions
- Reports that pharmacy filled the wrong medication
- Forging of prescriptions
- Obtaining controlled substance from more than one provider
- Obtaining controlled substances from illicit sources
- Unauthorized drug escalations
- Frequent emergency department visits for uncontrolled symptoms
- Medication overdose
- Driving while intoxicated
- Patient from a different geographic area
- Allergic to almost all other pain medications
- Not interested in diagnosis or treatment, just drugs

to be the mesolimbic pathway that connects the ventral trigeminal area of the midbrain with the prefrontal cortex and the nucleus accumbens where dopamine is released. Dopamine plays a complex role in the reward behavior that has evolved in humans over time, including the initiation of cause-and-effect relationship between a behavior such as drug taking and the anticipated reward, the valuation of the reward relative to the behavior, and, perhaps most important, initiating signals that tell the patient just how much the reward is desired. Given that humans have evolved such systems that are able to modulate or control behavior to allow the organism to seek natural rewards such as water, food, and sex without such behaviors becoming all consuming (i.e., addictive), it appears that certain substances such as opioids have the ability to override this modulating system to lead to the behaviors we recognize as addiction.

What causes this dysfunction of the reward and modulation systems is still unknown, but several theories have been put forth to explain it. The homeostasis theory suggests that exposure to controlled substances causes a disequilibrium between the positive reward of the drug and the subsequent negative reinforcement (e.g., symptoms of physiologic withdrawal, loss of the feeling of well-being associated with the drug). The incentive salience theory suggests that sensitization of the dopaminergic reward system and dysfunction of the modulating systems change the way the patient perceives the drug's effect, causing the patient not only to like the drug but to want or crave it to the exclusion of all else. The habit theory suggests that addiction is at least in part a learned behavior, with the addiction triggered by environmental cues in the patient's subconscious that cause the addictive behavior to become automatic.

SUGGESTED READING

Hunt SP, Urch CE: Pain, opiates, and addiction. In McMahon SB, Koltzenburg M (eds): Wall and Melzack's Textbook of Pain, ed 5. Philadelphia, Churchill Livingstone, 2006.

CHAPTER 214

Placebo and Nocebo

Placebo

The term *placebo* is derived from the Latin for "I will please." The term *placebo* is the name given to the sham treatment, be it pill, injection, laying on of the hands, surgery, etc., that the patient perceives as therapeutic. The placebo response is the patient's psychological and behavioral response of analgesia following the administration of the sham treatment. It has been stated that approximately one third of patients receiving a placebo will exhibit a positive placebo response. Although this number has been more recently called into question, suffice to say that the phenomenon of placebo response is frequently encountered in clinical practice and is real.

The concept of the placebo and placebo response is hundreds of years old, but the complex neurobiologic mechanisms responsible for this phenomenon remain elusive. Although there is no doubt that the patient's belief that an effective treatment has been administered and that treatment will be beneficial can produce in the patient the perception of pain relief, it must be understood that often other variables that may be responsible for the patient's placebo response are at play. These include the normal waxing and waning of the patient's perception of pain, the patient's interaction with the practitioner administering the placebo, the patient's expectancy of pain relief, and so on.

Nocebo

The concept of the nocebo response is essentially the opposite of the placebo response. With the nocebo response, the patient's belief that the treatment administered is ineffective and will produce harm will result in the patient perceiving that the pain is worse following the sham treatment. As with the placebo response, variables other than the administration of the sham treatment may be responsible for the patient perceiving that the pain is worse.

SUGGESTED READING

Field HL, Price DD: Placebo analgesia. In McMahon SB, Koltzenburg M (eds): Wall and Melzack's Textbook of Pain, ed 5. Philadelphia, Churchill Livingstone, 2006.

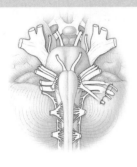

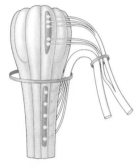

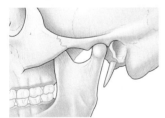

SECTION 4

Diagnostic Testing

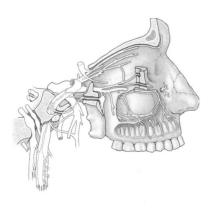

CHAPTER 215

Radiography

First described by Roentgen in 1895, x-rays have been used to aid in the diagnosis and treatment of disease by utilizing the different radiographic densities of the various tissues that make up the body to produce two-dimensional images of the body part being imaged. These radiographic densities range from bone as the most dense of body tissues, muscle being less dense than bone, fat being less dense from muscle, and air being the least dense of all.

X-rays are invisible to the human eye and reside in the spectrum of radiation energy between gamma rays and ultraviolet radiation (Fig. 215-1). X-rays used in clinical medicine are most often generated by a high voltage vacuum tube with a rotating anode (Fig. 215-2). The x-ray vacuum tube consists of a negatively charged anode that is also known as the filament and a positively charged anode known as the target. In modern x-ray vacuum tubes, the anode target is usually made of highly heat-resistant elements such as tungsten combined with other elements such as rhenium.

When the x-ray vacuum tube is energized, the filament is heated to a very high temperature within the vacuum, which causes electrons from its surface to boil away from the filament and coalesce in a negatively charged cloud known as a space charge. This phenomenon was first described by Edison during his seminal work on the electric incandescent light bulb and is also known as the Edison effect. These negatively charged electrons within the space charge are amenable to attraction and acceleration toward the positively charged anode or target when it is energized with high voltage. In modern x-ray equipment in common clinical use, these high voltages range from 70 to 100 kV.

When the negatively charged electrons from the space charge are accelerated toward the positively charged anode, two interactions can occur. The first interaction, which has limited utility in medical imaging, occurs when the negatively charged rapidly accelerating electron interacts directly with an electron in an orbital shell of a tungsten atom of the anode target displacing the orbital electron, creating an orbital gap. This orbital gap is immediately filled by an electron from a more distant orbital shell. This displacement and filling create an energy disequilibrium resulting in the radiation of an x-photon with energy characteristics that are unique to the specific element from which the electron was displaced, as well as the specific orbital shell from which it was previously

displaced. As mentioned, the specific energy characteristics of the x-photon produced by this displacement of an electron from the anode targets orbital shell limit its clinical utility in medical imaging.

The second interaction that can occur when the negatively charged, rapidly accelerating electron interacts directly with an electron in an orbital shell of a tungsten atom of the anode target has much greater utility in medical imaging and is termed the *braking radiation effect* or *Bremsstrahlung*. This braking radiation effect occurs when the rapidly accelerating negatively charged electrode passes in close proximity to a nucleus of a tungsten atom of the anode target. The positively charged nucleus alters the path of the accelerating negatively charged electron and reverses the direction of the electron's path. This change in direction results in a dissipation of the kinetic energy of the electron, with the difference in the kinetic energy before and after being subjected to the braking forces of the nucleus radiated as an x-photon of varying energy. The modern x-ray tubes are able to produce specific x-photon spikes, which can be used to produce consistent x-rays suitable for medical imaging.

It should be noted that almost of all of the electrical energy input applied to the x-ray vacuum tube required to produce x-ray photons is not converted into x-ray photons but is converted to heat. In even the most efficient x-ray vacuum tubes, only about 1% of the electrical energy input is actually converted to x-ray photons. The amount of heat converted from electrical energy input is significant, and mechanisms to dissipate the heat before it damages the anode target are required to produce clinically useful medical x-rays. This heat dissipation is accomplished by using substances that will rapidly conduct heat away from the anode target, such as molybdenum and cooling oil, and by rotating the anode target so that the area that is being heated is constantly changing as the anode target spins.

As mentioned, the tissues that make up the human body have different radiographic densities, and modern x-ray equipment has been designed to improve the contrast between these differing densities to optimize the diagnostic capabilities of radiographic imaging. This is done primarily by altering three variables that can be adjusted to produce the desired radiograph: (1) the kV (kilovoltage) potential, (2) the mA (milliamperage), and (3) the exposure time in seconds.

363

By increasing the kV potential, the difference in the potential between the cathode and the anode is increased, which increases the energy of the x-ray beam. The more the energy of the beam increases, the greater is the penetrating power of the beam; this, however, occurs at the expense of contrast, as the more powerful the beam, the less effect the variations in the tissue density will have in attenuating the beam.

By increasing the mA, more current is allowed to flow through the filament of the cathode side of the tube, which increases the number of electrons that boil off the filament into the space charge. This results in a larger number of negatively charged electrons from the space charge available to be accelerated toward the anode target. This increase in electrodes speeding toward and interacting with the nucleus of the atoms of the anode target material will produce a concomitant increase in the number of x-photons available to produce the x-ray image. The more x-ray photons impinging on the x-ray film, the greater is the exposure and the blacker the film will be.

The third variable that can be altered to produce clinically useful x-ray images is the exposure time. By increasing the exposure time in seconds, there will be a greater number of photons available to impinge on the x-ray film, thus making the film blacker. It should be noted that as a practical matter the interrelationship between mA and the exposure time in seconds is linear. Thus, to produce a given exposure, you could double the mA and cut the exposure time in seconds by half, or double the exposure time in seconds and cut the mA by half.

Traditional radiography systems use a system of film and cassette composed of one or two image-intensifying screens known as a film-screen system. The film of the typical film-screen system is a Mylar sheet that has been coated with a silver halide emulsion on each side that will react to light. The cassette of the typical film-screen system is impervious to visible light but has a radiolucent panel on the side, which admits x-ray photons as well as an image-intensifying screen adjacent to each side of the emulsion-coated film. These image-intensifying screens convert the invisible x-ray photons to visible photons from the blue end of the visible light radiation spectrum. This system allows for the more efficient exposure of the emulsion-coated x-ray film, thus reducing the amount of x-ray exposure to the patient.

SUGGESTED READING

Hon DD, Carrino JA: Radiography. In: Waldman SD: Pain Management. Philadelphia, Saunders, 2007.

SPECTRUM OF RADIATION ENERGY

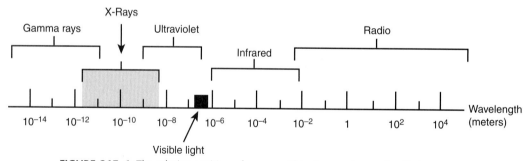

FIGURE 215–1 The relative position of x-rays within the spectrum of radiation energy.

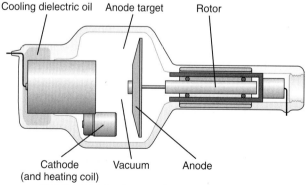

FIGURE 215–2 The typical x-ray vacuum tube.

Nuclear Scintigraphy

Nuclear scintigraphy uses the unique properties of certain radioactive elements, which are combined with other biologically active substances known as radiopharmaceuticals to provide both physiologic and anatomic information about specific tissues in the body. By matching the specific properties of a given radiopharmaceutical with the normal or abnormal biologic process that takes place at a cellular and subcellular level in a specific tissue, nuclear scintigraphy can aid in the diagnosis of a variety of pathologic conditions.

It should be noted that unlike other medical imaging tests that provide primarily anatomic information, medical scintigraphy provides primarily physiologic information with clinical anatomic information inferred as the result of abnormal physiology that may cause and increase or decrease in the distribution of a radiopharmaceutical in the tissue being imaged. These images are obtained through the detection of radionuclide emissions by a gamma camera or, more recently, positron emission tomography. New hybrid systems combine a camera capable of detecting radionuclide emissions with a computed tomographic scanner or magnetic resonance imaging camera to produce computer-generated images that provide better physiologic and anatomic diagnostic information by superimposing the images obtained by each imaging modality. The process is known as *image fusion*.

To image specific tissues, radionuclides are attached to a special pharmaceutical known as a tracer to create radiopharmaceuticals that interact with that tissue in a consistent way in health and disease. By taking into account the different ways a specific radiopharmaceutical is handled by the tissue in question when affected by a specific disease process, a diagnosis can often be made. For example, the increased blood flow and metabolic activity associated with a bony metastasis of the femur will consistently cause an increased uptake of the tracer methylenediphosphonate. By attaching the radionuclide technetium-99 to the methylenediphosphonate, an increased concentration of the methylenediphosphonate–technetium-99 radiopharmaceutical will be taken up by the metastasis. This will result in an increased emission of gamma rays from the technetium, which will appear as a hot spot on the scintigraph, alerting the clinician to the fact that bony pathology exists. It should be noted that some disease processes produce decreased uptake of the trace–radionuclide complex and scintigraphy will reveal a cold spot suggesting pathology involving that specific tissue.

Although most scintigraphic studies involve the injection of a radiopharmaceutical, some studies require inhalation or ingestion of the radionuclide or the use of the patient's own red or white blood cells as a tracer to which to attach the radionuclide. Some radionuclides are produced by the process of fission or fusion in nuclear reactors, whereas others are produced in cyclotrons. Some of the radionuclides that are more commonly used in clinical medicine are listed in Table 216-1.

TABLE 216–1 Commonly Used Radionuclides in Clinical Medicine

Most Commonly Used Intravenous Radionuclides
• Technetium-99m
• Gallium-67
• Chromium-51
• Iodine-123
• Iodine-131
• Oxygen-15
• Krypton-81
• Nitrogen-13
• Thallium-201
• Fluorine-18 fluorodeoxyglucose
• Indium-111–labeled leukocytes
• Indium-111–labeled erythrocytes
Most Commonly Used Gaseous/Aerosol Radionuclides
• Xenon-133
• Krypton-81m
• Technetium-99m
• Technetium-99m DTPA
Most Commonly Used Oral Radionuclides
• Technetium-99m colloid
• Selenium-75
• Iodine-123
• Iodine-131
• Indium-111

Each of these radionuclides exposes both the patient and, in many instances, their caregivers and family to a dose of radiation. Although the total dose of radiation for most commonly used scintigraphic studies is small, they present a risk to the patient and those around them.

SUGGESTED READING

Hon DD, Carrino JA: Nuclear medicine techniques. In: Waldman SD (ed): Pain Management. Philadelphia, Saunders, 2007.

CHAPTER 217

Computed Tomography

The process of producing images with computed tomography (CT) is based on the same fundamental principles that are applied to radiography (i.e., that various types of tissues have different densities when exposed to x-ray photons) (see Chapter 215). Although the number of x-ray tubes and digital detectors and how the x-ray photon beam or body part moves relative to the x-ray photon detectors as CT scanners have evolved since their introduction to clinical medicine in 1972, all modern CT scanners utilize the basic concept of tomography in which sequential thin slicelike images of a specific body part are obtained using x-ray photons and then processed by a computer using complex algorithms to produce an image. It is the ability of these complex computer algorithms to reconstruct the data obtained in a variety of ways that allows CT to provide the clinician with high-resolution images that can be manipulated to maximize their diagnostic potential. This is done by dividing each slice of tissue scanned into small volumetric boxes known as voxels. The computer then analyzes a number of variables for each voxel and assigns it a number based on the voxel's mean tissue radiodensity relative to the constants of air and water. These numbers are measured in Hounsfield units, which are named in honor of the inventor of the CT scanner, Sir Godfrey Hounsfield. These density numbers are in essence a way to provide an "apples to apples" comparison of the relative radiodensities of adjacent tissues and translate these densities into a diagnostic image. By convention, water has been assigned a Hounsfield unit attenuation value of 0 and air is assigned a −1000 Hounsfield unit attenuation value.

In a manner analogous to radiography, tissues with less radiodensity such as air and fat will appear black on the reconstructed CT image, and more radiodense tissues such as bone and metallic implants will appear white. Tissues such as muscle that have a relative radiodensity between that of air and of bone will appear in a shade of gray that corresponds to that tissue's assigned Hounsfield unit attenuation value. This gray scale representation of each voxel produces a two-dimensional digital image that is read in a manner analogous to a radiograph. Further computer repossessing of this digital gray-scale two-dimensional image using volume-rendering algorithms can produce a three-dimensional representation of the body part being imaged.

Continued improvements in CT technology combined with more powerful computers and more robust software have resulted in CT scanners that boast much greater spatial resolution, acquisition times in seconds rather than minutes, and more sophisticated data reconstructions. These advances have also allowed cine applications to assess blood flow, blood volume, and transit times, as well as the use of gated studies that allow cardiac CT imaging.

SUGGESTED READING

Nielsen JA, Carrino JA: Computed tomography. In: Waldman SD (ed): Pain Management. Philadelphia, Saunders, 2007.

Magnetic Resonance Imaging

Unlike radiography, nuclear medicine, and computed tomography, which all rely on ionizing radiation to produce images, magnetic resonance imaging (MRI) produces clinically useful images by recording and processing alterations in the absorption and emission of energy that occur when powerful magnetic and radiofrequency forces are applied directly onto the nucleus of hydrogen atoms that are an intrinsic part of the body tissues being imaged. To understand how MRI works, it is first necessary to understand how this precise application of magnetic and radiofrequency forces at the submolecular level affects the hydrogen atom, which makes up approximately 63% of the human body.

Under ambient conditions, these hydrogen atoms are randomly spinning or precessing like a top around a vertical axis in all directions (Fig. 218-1). By virtue of the hydrogen's large magnetic moment, when a hydrogen atom is placed in a strong magnetic field, the proton that makes up the hydrogen atom's nucleus tends to line up with the direction of the magnetic field. When a patient is placed inside the magnetic field produced by an MRI scanner, the body part being imaged is placed in the isocenter of the magnetic field. The magnetic field causes the protons of each hydrogen atom's nucleus to align with either the patient's head or feet (Fig. 218-2). For the purposes of producing an image using MRI, these aligned protons cancel each other out. However, there are a tiny number of hydrogen protons that are not canceled out, and it is these hydrogen protons that are used to create magnetic resonance images.

Because these few non–canceled-out hydrogen protons are spinning or precessing around their axis in a random manner, they are susceptible to manipulation by subjecting them to large amounts of energy. This energy is applied in the form of an intense radiofrequency (RF) pulse that is delivered by a powerful RF generator made up of an RF synthesizer, a signal amplifier, and a specialized transmitting coil. To optimize the delivery of the strong RF signal to the hydrogen protons that reside within the body part being imaged, the RF coils are designed to fit or wrap around the body part being imaged.

When this RF system is turned on, a pulse of RF energy causes the noncanceled hydrogen protons to all spin or precess in the same direction. The RF energy pulse also causes these hydrogen protons to all spin at a particular frequency. When this strong RF pulse of energy is turned off, the noncanceled hydrogen protons that were brought into resonance with the delivery of the RF pulse "relax" and begin to return to their normal random alignment and release the energy that was previously absorbed from the strong RF pulse. The RF receiver portion of the MRI system, which is made up of an RF receiver, preamplifier, and signal processing system, detects this release of energy and transmits it to the MRI scanner's computer processing software to produce a clinical usable image. By exploiting the relationship of the time required for a certain percentage of the relaxing hydrogen protons to return to their natural state after the RF pulse is turned off, the MRI scanner's processing computer can isolate certain time constants during the relaxation process that allow fine-tuning of the images produced. Examples of more commonly used techniques that exploit these time constants during the relaxation process include T1 and T2 images. To further enhance images obtained from MRI, specialized image acquisition techniques such as fat suppression imaging or the administration of a contrast agent can be considered. The most commonly used contrast agent in MRI is the paramagnetic element gadolinium, which enhances tissues and fluids, making it useful in the detection of tumors. Although gadolinium-based contrast agents are reasonably safe, they should be used with caution in patients with renal failure.

SUGGESTED READING

Chou ET, Carrino JA: Magnetic resonance imaging. In: Waldman SD (ed): Pain Management. Philadelphia, Saunders, 2007.

Main magnetic field

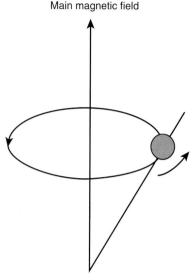

FIGURE 218–1 The nucleus of the hydrogen atom spinning or precessing around its access.

Main magnetic field

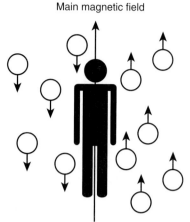

FIGURE 218–2 The orientation of the protons of the nucleus of the hydrogen atoms of a patient placed in an MRI scanner's magnetic field.

CHAPTER 219

Discography

Discography is indicated as a diagnostic maneuver in a carefully selected subset of patients suffering from pain that is thought to be discogenic in nature. Patients who may benefit from discography include (1) those patients with persistent neck, cervical radicular, thoracic, back, and/or lumbar radicular pain in whom traditional diagnostic modalities (e.g., magnetic resonance imaging [MRI], computed tomographic [CT] scanning, and electromyography) have failed to clearly delineate a cause of the pain; (2) those patients in whom equivocal findings such as bulging lumbar discs are identified on traditional diagnostic imaging modalities, to determine whether such abnormalities are in fact responsible for the patient's pain; (3) those patients who are to undergo lumbar fusion, where discography may help identify which levels need to be fused; (4) those patients who have previously undergone fusion of the lumbar spine, where discography may help identify whether levels above and below the fusion are responsible for persistent pain; and (5) those patients in whom recurrent disc herniation cannot be separated from scar tissue with traditional imaging techniques.

In each of these patient populations, the clinician must correlate the data obtained from the injection itself, the provocation of pain on injection, the radiographic appearance of the discogram obtained, and, in selected patients, the relief of pain after the disc is injected with local anesthetic. Failure to carefully correlate all of this diagnostic information in the context of the patient's clinical presentation may lead the clinician to erroneously interpret the results of discography and adversely influence subsequent clinical decision making.

Complications directly related to discography are generally self-limited, although occasionally, even with the best technique, severe complications can occur. The most common severe complication after discography is infection of the disc, which is commonly referred to as discitis. Because of the limited blood supply of the disc, such infections can be extremely hard to eradicate. Discitis usually manifests as an increase in spine pain several days to a week after discography. Acutely, there will be no change in the patient's neurologic examination as a result of disc infection.

Epidural abscess, which can rarely occur after discography, generally manifests within 24 to 48 hours. Clinically, the signs and symptoms of epidural abscess are high fever, spine pain, and progressive neurologic deficit. If either discitis or epidural abscess is suspected, blood and urine cultures should be taken, antibiotics started, and emergent MRI scan of the spine obtained to allow identification and drainage of any abscess formation to prevent irreversible neurologic deficit.

In addition to infectious complications, pneumothorax may occur after lumbar discography. This complication should rarely occur if CT guidance is used during needle placement. Small pneumothorax after lumbar discography can often be treated conservatively, and tube thoracostomy can be avoided. Trauma to retroperitoneal structures, including the kidney, may also occur if CT guidance is not used to avoid and localize these structures.

Direct trauma to the nerve roots and the spinal cord can occur if the needle is allowed to traverse the entire disc or is placed too laterally. These complications should rarely occur if incremental CT scans are taken while advancing the needle. Such needle-induced trauma to the lower lumbar spinal cord and cauda equina can result in deficits, including cauda equina syndrome and paraplegia.

SUGGESTED READING

Waldman SD: Lumbar discography. In: Atlas of Interventional Pain Management, ed 2. Philadelphia, Saunders, 2004.

CHAPTER 220

Electromyography and Nerve Conduction Studies

Electromyography (EMG) and nerve conduction studies (NCS) can provide the clinician with invaluable diagnostic information regarding neuromuscular disease when combined with information obtained from the targeted history and physical examination, laboratory testing, and diagnostic imaging. For the clinician to optimize the information obtained from EMG and NCS, two important concepts relative to these important neurophysiologic tests must be understood. First, EMG and NCS are primarily tests of nerve and muscle function, meaning that they provide different but complementary information from diagnostic imaging testing and are for the most part tests based on anatomy. Second, there is a delay between the onset of neuromuscular symptoms and the point at which EMG and NCS will be positive. In the case of EMG, a period of 10 to 21 days must pass between the onset of symptoms before the test becomes abnormal and can aid in the diagnosis of the patient's problem. Although in the setting of complete nerve transactions, NCS are positive immediately, it takes 4 to 7 days following severe nerve injury for NCS to become positive and aid in the diagnosis of the patient's problem.

The Role of Electromyography and Nerve Conduction Studies in the Diagnosis of Central Nervous System Disease

EMG and NCS are useful in the diagnosis of certain disorders affecting the cranial nerves, especially the trigeminal, facial, spinal accessory, and hypoglossal nerves. These disorders include trigeminal neuralgia, Raeder's paratrigeminal neuralgia, Bell's palsy, multiple sclerosis, Wallenberg's syndrome, and many of the polyneuropathies that affect the cranial nerves. Diseases that affect primarily the brain are less amenable to diagnosis by EMG and NCS, and diagnostic imaging studies such as magnetic resonance imaging (MRI) will generally provide much more accurate diagnostic information.

The Role of Electromyography and Nerve Conduction Studies in the Diagnosis of Spinal Cord Disease

Disorders of the spinal cord amenable to diagnosis with EMG include diseases that affect the motor neurons and their associated axons, including amyotrophic lateral sclerosis, syringomyelia, spinal cord tumors, spinal cord infarcts, infections, polio, and severe myelopathy. It should be noted that patients exhibiting significant neurologic symptoms secondary to midline herniated intervertebral disc and/or myelopathy may have relatively normal EMG and NCS and the clinical correlation of the physical examination and the results of diagnostic imaging is crucial to avoid clinical disaster.

The Role of Electromyography and Nerve Conduction Studies in the Diagnosis of Motor Neuron Disease

A variety of diseases affect the motor neurons and will produce the characteristic findings on EMG and, to a much lesser extent, on NCS. These changes include diffuse changes of denervation including fibrillations, positive sharp waves, neuropathy motor unit potentials, and reduced motor unit potential recruitment patterns. Diseases that affect the motor neurons are listed in Table 220-1. It is important that the clinician remember that cervical spondylosis and syringomyelia may masquerade clinically as motor neuron disease and must be carefully ruled out by including diagnostic imaging such as MRI whenever the diagnosis of motor neuron disease is being considered.

The Role of Electromyography and Nerve Conduction Studies in the Diagnosis of Spinal Nerve Root Disorders

EMG is abnormal in more than 90% of patients suffering from clinically significant spinal nerve root disorders. Herniated intervertebral disc and spondylitic disease including neuroforaminal stenosis are common causes of positive EMG findings in the setting of spinal nerve root disorders. Pathologic processes that cause a slower compromise of the spinal nerve roots, such as spinal stenosis or midline herniated discs, which may cause compression

only of the spinal cord, may not cause significant EMG abnormalities. With most diseases involving only the spinal nerve roots, NCS findings may be mild and nonspecific. It should be noted that although EMG is highly diagnostic for the presence of spinal nerve root disorders, pathologic lesions affecting only a portion of the affected myotome may produce equivocal EMG findings and clinical correlation with physical findings and diagnostic imaging is essential to avoid misdiagnosis.

The Role of Electromyography and Nerve Conduction Studies in the Diagnosis of Plexus Lesions

Brachial and lumbar plexopathies are amenable to diagnosis by the skilled electromyographer. Accurate EMG diagnosis of plexus lesions requires an intimate knowledge of the complex anatomy of the plexus being evaluated as well as a clear understanding of how a lesion affecting a discrete portion of the plexus appears on both EMG and clinical examination. Common diseases causing plexus abnormalities on EMG are listed in Table 220-2 and include idiopathic inflammatory plexitis such as Parsonage-Turner syndrome; space-occupying lesions such as Pancoast's tumor; infection and hematoma; plexus trauma ranging from stretch lesions associated with sports injuries, thoracic outlet syndrome, and childbirth to complete avulsions of portions of the plexus from the spinal cord following motor vehicle accidents; and radiation-induced plexopathy that occurs as a side effect of cancer treatment.

The Role of Electromyography and Nerve Conduction Studies in the Diagnosis of Peripheral Nerve Disease

Common disorders of the peripheral nerves that are associated with NCS abnormalities include the peripheral

TABLE 220–1 Diseases That Affect the Motor Neurons

- Amyotrophic lateral sclerosis
- Poliomyelitis
- Human immunodeficiency virus
- Herpes zoster
- Lyme disease
- Primary lateral sclerosis
- Shy-Drager syndrome
- Paraneoplastic motor neuron disorders
- Progressive bulbar palsy

TABLE 220–2 Disorders Associated with EMG Abnormalities Affecting the Cervical, Lumbar, and Hypogastric Plexus

- Idiopathic inflammatory plexitis
- Infectious plexitis
- Space-occupying lesions
  - Pancoast's tumor
  - Retroperitoneal tumors
  - Hematoma
  - Abscess
- Trauma
  - Stretch injuries
  - Avulsion injuries
- Radiation-induced plexopathy

neuropathies, traumatic nerve lesions, and the entrapment neuropathies. The extent of nerve damage will in general correlate with the degree of abnormality on NCS testing. In the setting of trauma, the degree of damage inflicted on the nerve being evaluated will be reflected not only in the NCS/EMG findings but in the physical examination as well. This degree of damage also correlates with the prognosis of a given traumatic nerve lesion.

The mildest form of nerve trauma is called neuropraxia, which is associated with conduction loss without associated structural damage to the axon and is commonly seen in patients suffering from entrapment neuropathies such as carpal tunnel syndrome. With removal of the compression causing the neuropraxia, the numbness and weakness associated with the nerve entrapment will generally resolve over a period of weeks.

If there is actual structural damage to the axon and myelin sheath, a more severe form of nerve trauma called axonotmesis will result in more profound clinical symptoms and a poorer prognosis compared with neuropraxia. Since the neural tube consisting of the endoneurium, perineurium, and epineurium is intact in axonotmesis, the axon has the potential to regenerate. If the neural tube and axons, myelin sheath, and neural tube are completely disrupted, the most severe form of neural injury, neurotmesis, exists. In the absence of surgical reanastomosis of the transected nerve ends, complete nerve regeneration is unlikely.

Causes of nontraumatic neuropathies are listed in Table 220-3. Nontraumatic neuropathies are generally associated with abnormal NCS findings consisting of slowing of nerve conduction velocities and the temporal dispersion of evoked responses. Although pure demyelinating or pure axonal neuropathies exist, they are much less common than mixed pattern neuropathies. These neuropathies can present as mononeuropathies such as mononeuritis monoplex, affecting only a single peripheral nerve, or polyneuropathies, affecting multiple peripheral nerves. The clinical presentation of mononeuropathies is sensory and/or motor deficit in the distribution of a single nerve. The clinical presentation of polyneuropathies is that of dysesthesias that initially appear distally in a classic stocking-and-glove distribution. Unless there is significant axonal degeneration, significant EMG abnormalities are usually absent in the setting of peripheral neuropathies.

Entrapment neuropathies are another common cause of peripheral nerve abnormalities on NCS and, to a lesser extent, on EMG. In the absence of predisposing factors such as occupation or another concomitant disease associated with peripheral neuropathy such as diabetes, entrapment neuropathies generally present as mononeuropathies. The most common entrapment neuropathy is carpal tunnel syndrome, which is an entrapment of the median nerve at the wrist. Clinically, patients with entrapment neuropathies will complain of dysesthesias, numbness, pain, and, in more severe cases, weakness in the distribution of the peripheral nerve being compressed. The classic NCS finding of an entrapment neuropathy is slowing of the nerve conduction velocity across the area of entrapment. Left untreated, EMG abnormalities in the muscles that are supplied by the portion of the peripheral nerve distal to the site of entrapment will be present.

The Role of Electromyography and Nerve Conduction Studies in the Diagnosis of Myopathies

Although much less common than the peripheral neuropathies, myopathies can be extremely debilitating. Common causes of myopathies associated with abnormalities on EMG are listed in Table 220-4.

TABLE 220–3 Common Causes of Peripheral Neuropathies

- Trauma or compression of nerves
- Diabetes
- Infectious etiologies including leprosy
- Vitamin deficiencies
- Alcoholism
- Autoimmune diseases
- Renal disease
- Hepatic disease
- Endocrinopathies including hypothyroidism
- Amyloidosis
- HIV/AIDS
- Toxic exposure including heavy metals, chemicals, and chemotherapy
- Inherited disorders including Charcot-Marie-Tooth disease

TABLE 220–4 Common Causes of Myopathies Associated with EMG Abnormalities

- Collagen vascular diseases including polymyositis and dermatomyositis
- Drug induced including the steroids, statins, colchicine, cocaine, etc.
- Sarcoidosis
- Acute alcoholic myopathy
- Infectious etiologies including trichinosis, cysticercosis, toxoplasmosis, HIV, Lyme disease, etc.
- Endocrinopathies including Cushing's disease, hypothyroidism, hyperthyroiditis, hyperparathyroidism
- Familial periodic paralysis
- Muscular dystrophy
- Malignant hyperthermia

Myopathy presents clinically as symmetrical weakness of the proximal muscles associated with fever, malaise, muscle aching, and a normal sensory examination.

SUGGESTED READINGS

Campbell W: DeJong's The Neurological Examination, ed 6. Philadelphia, Lippincott Williams and Wilkins, 2005.

Goetz CG: Textbook of Clinical Neurology, ed 2. Philadelphia, Saunders, 2003.

Waldman SD: Carpal tunnel syndrome. In: Atlas of Common Pain Syndromes, ed 2. Philadelphia, Saunders, 2008.

Waldman SD: Parsonage-Turner syndrome. In: Atlas of Uncommon Pain Syndromes, ed 2. Philadelphia, Saunders, 2008.

CHAPTER 221

Evoked Potential Testing

Evoked potentials (EPs) are a useful diagnostic test to help identify abnormalities of the peripheral and central nervous system that may help explain why the patient is having pain or functional disability. EP testing is also useful in helping prove the absence of neural pathway abnormalities in the patient who complains of otherwise unexplained visual or hearing loss and/or unexplained numbness. Such information is extremely useful when there is a clinical impression of behavioral issues influencing a patient's pain response.

EPs are electrophysiologic responses of the nervous system to externally applied sensory stimuli. EP testing can provide information on the peripheral and the central sensory nervous system pathways that is unobtainable by electromyography (EMG) and magnetic stimulation evaluations. EP testing provides objective and reproducible data to delineate sensory system lesions that are unsuspected or are clinically ambiguous on the basis of history and physical examination findings alone. EP testing can provide information on the anatomic location of nervous system lesions and help to monitor progression or regression.

EP responses are of very low amplitude (0.1 to 20 μV) and are obscured by random electrical "noise" such as muscle artifact, electroencephalographic activity, and interference from surrounding electrical devices. Extraction of the EP response is accomplished by computer averaging. This technique summates the EP response, which is "time-locked" to the applied sensory stimuli, and minimizes unwanted noise interference.

A variety of stimuli may elicit EPs, but the most commonly used are visual, auditory, and somatosensory. These three stimuli give rise to visual evoked potentials (VEPs), brainstem auditory evoked potentials (BAEPs), and somatosensory evoked potentials (SEPs), which evaluate functions of their respective sensory systems. EP responses consist of a sequence of peaks and waves characterized by latency, amplitude, configuration, and interval between individual peaks (interpeak latency). In this manner, EP responses are similar to conventional NCS responses and magnetically stimulated motor EP. There is a standardized nomenclature for the individual peaks and waves of the various EP responses. The peaks and waves may be identified by positive or negative polarity, the latency period, and by the anatomic site where the response was recorded (e.g., Erb's point). Normal values for EP responses are generally established by each electrophysiology laboratory, using 2.5 or 3.0 standard deviations from mean values as the upper limits of normal.

EP equipment, like that for EMG, is a biologic amplifier. In its most basic form, EP equipment consists of recording electrodes attached to specific areas over the scalp, spine, and extremities. Input from the electrodes is routed to an amplifier, which filters, averages, displays, and records data. Recording electrodes are placed on the scalp in a manner analogous to conventional electroencephalography. The configuration of electrode placement for a specific test is referred to as a *montage*.

Visual Evoked Potentials

VEPs are used to evaluate pathology affecting the visual pathways. They are primarily generated in the visual cortex and, therefore, may be affected by pathology anywhere along the visual pathways, from the corneas to the visual cortex. A reversing checkerboard pattern projected through a video monitor is most often used to stimulate the visual pathways (pattern-reversal VEP). Each eye is tested individually to localize abnormalities to the affected side. Generally, 100 pattern reversals (trials) are required to obtain a clearly defined response. The test is repeated to confirm reproducibility of responses. The resultant VEP consists of three peaks: The primary peak of interest in VEP testing occurs at approximately 100 msec, has positive polarity, and is thus referred to as the *P100 peak*.

VEP testing is useful in the diagnosis of many conditions that affect the visual pathways but is most often used in the diagnosis of multiple sclerosis (MS). The demyelination of the optic nerve that occurs in MS has the same effect as demyelination in peripheral nerves (i.e., slowing of conduction velocity), resulting in increased response latency. If axonal loss also occurs, response amplitude is also reduced. These abnormalities correspond to the changes seen in demyelination and axonopathy found in conventional NCS. In MS patients, the most common abnormalities are increased P100 latency and increased interocular latencies. Reduction of P100 amplitude may also occur, although this is generally associated with compressive or ischemic lesions. In patients suspected to have MS, VEP abnormality rates are approximately 63%, and they approach 85% in patients with confirmed MS. VEP abnormalities may antedate typical changes of MS seen on magnetic resonance imaging. MS may also produce abnormalities of BAEP and SEP; therefore, testing all three may improve the diagnostic yield over that of VEP alone.

Ocular disorders, tumors, inflammatory conditions, and ischemia of the optic pathways may be associated with VEP abnormalities. VEP abnormalities have also been reported in a variety of cerebral degenerative disorders and neuropathies with CNS involvement. There are a few reports of VEP abnormalities in patients with migraine headaches. VEP testing has been used for visual screening of infants and persons who are suspected of having visual pathway disease but are unable to respond to or comply with conventional ophthalmologic or optometric testing.

BRAINSTEM AUDITORY EVOKED POTENTIALS

In the manner that visual stimuli are used to evaluate visual pathways, auditory stimuli are used to assess the auditory pathways. The auditory pathway extends from the middle ear structures through the eighth cranial nerve and brainstem to the auditory cortex. Auditory stimuli presented to each ear individually produce the BAEP, which consists of a series of waves that correspond closely to these auditory pathway structures. BAEP evaluation, therefore, allows relatively specific localization of auditory pathway pathology. BAEP responses are recorded from electrodes placed on the scalp, near or on each ear.

The most commonly used auditory stimulus is brief, electrical pulses, referred to as *clicks*, which are presented to each ear through audiologic earphones. (Earphones that fit *into* the auditory canal can also be used.) These click stimuli may be varied in frequency, intensity, and rate. A well-defined BAEP response generally requires 1000 to 2000 stimuli.

The typical BAEP response consists of a sequence of seven positive waves, of which the first five are used clinically. They are numbered sequentially by Roman numerals I through V and occur within the first 10 msec after presentation of auditory stimuli. Each wave closely corresponds to structures along the auditory pathway that are believed to generate it. Wave I is thought to be generated by cranial nerve (CN) VIII; wave II by CN VIII and the cochlear nucleus; wave III by the lower pons; and waves IV and V by the upper pons and lower midbrain. Diagnosis of the anatomic site of pathology is based on which wave or waves demonstrate increased latency or are absent. Determination of interpeak latency is important, because disorders such as peripheral hearing loss may increase the latency of the entire BAEP response but do not change the interpeak latency relationships. Severe hearing loss may render recording of the BAEP impossible owing to degradation of the response. BAEP response amplitudes vary considerably among normal subjects. To reduce intersubject variability, the ratio of wave I–to–wave V amplitudes is calculated. If the wave V amplitude is reduced in comparison to wave I, an intrinsic brainstem impairment is implied. A reduction of wave I–to–wave V amplitude ratio suggests possible hearing impairment.

BAEPs may aid in the diagnosis of a variety of diseases affecting the auditory pathways. The BAEP may be abnormal in 32% to 64% of persons with MS, although it is less sensitive than either VEP or SEP testing. BAEPs are particularly useful in the diagnosis of cerebellopontine angle tumors such as acoustic neuromas. BAEP testing has been found to be superior to routine audiometry and computed tomography in the diagnosis of cerebellopontine angle tumors. BAEP are also useful in (1) the evaluation of strokes and tumors involving the auditory pathways, (2) the evaluation of, and as a predictor of outcome for, comatose and head-injured persons, and (3) the diagnosis of a variety of neurodegenerative disorders, such as Friedreich's ataxia, in which the responses are abnormal. BAEP abnormalities have been reported in association with Arnold-Chiari malformations, postconcussion syndrome, vertebrobasilar transient ischemic attacks, basilar migraines, and spasmodic torticollis. These responses are used in audiometric screening of infants and of patients with mental deficiency who are unable to undergo routine audiometric testing.

SOMATOSENSORY EVOKED POTENTIALS

SEPs assess the function of somatosensory pathways by stimulation of sensory nerves. SEPs may be recorded by stimulation of mixed or pure sensory nerves in the upper and lower extremities, in dermatomal areas of the skin, and from some cranial nerves with sensory function. The somatosensory pathway consists of the peripheral nerve, dorsal columns of the spinal cord, medial lemniscus, ventroposterior lateral thalamus, and primary sensory cortex. SEPs appear to be related to the senses of joint position, touch, vibration, and stereognosis but are not related to pain and temperature sensation.

Typically, SEPs are obtained through electrical stimulation of a peripheral nerve after recording electrodes are placed at sites along the somatosensory pathway. In upper and lower extremity SEPs, stimulation is generally applied at the more distal portion of major nerves, with recording sites along the extremity, over certain spinous processes, and on the scalp over regions that correspond to the somatosensory cortex. In SEP evaluation of dermatomal sensory areas, stimulation is performed over an area of skin that is innervated by a given dermatome (e.g., lateral foot for the S1 dermatome), and recording is usually limited to the scalp.

SEP responses consist of a group of waveforms, each corresponding to the anatomic site of the recording electrode (e.g., Erb's point). Abnormalities are manifested as increased latency, reduced amplitude, or absence of a given wave. The anatomic site of the lesion is determined by the point at which the abnormality is seen in a wave corresponding to recording electrode sites along the somatosensory pathway. The SEP is analogous to conventional nerve conduction testing, in which the site of the NCS abnormality corresponds to the site of disease. Because peripheral nerve disorders may prolong response latencies along the entire length of the somatosensory pathway, interpeak latency determinations are important. Additionally, conventional nerve conduction testing of the peripheral portions of the nerve can help to exclude peripheral neuropathy.

SEPs are often abnormal in persons with MS. SEP testing is frequently performed in conjunction with VEP and BAEP testing to enhance diagnostic sensitivity, with SEPs being the most sensitive of the three modalities. SEP abnormalities are more often seen in MS patients with sensory symptoms and are more common in the lower extremities. Generally, conventional NCS are used in evaluation of sensory disturbances of the peripheral nerve, although SEPs may be recordable from the scalp (owing to amplification effects of the cerebral cortex) when sensory nerve action potentials (SNAPs) are unrecordable. This amplification effect may be particularly useful in evaluating some entrapment neuropathies, such as meralgia paresthetica, in which recording of the response from the peripheral nerve is technically difficult or impossible. SEPs are useful in the diagnosis of brachial plexus lesions and may be complementary to conventional EMG. SEPs may help to confirm axonal continuity and to determine whether lesions are preganglionic or postganglionic. Ulnar nerve SEP may be useful in the diagnosis of thoracic outlet syndrome and appear to be complementary to EMG testing.

The use of SEPs in the diagnosis of radiculopathy has been controversial. Many studies using SEP of peripheral nerves in the diagnosis of radiculopathy have found the test to be of limited utility. This limitation was attributed to "overshadowing" of abnormalities in a single nerve root by contributions from uninvolved nerve roots that supply the same peripheral nerve. Recording of SEP from a dermatomal area supplied by a single nerve root (e.g., the webbed space between the great and first toes innervated by the L5 nerve root) represents an attempt to circumvent this problem. Dermatomal SEPs have been generally found to improve diagnostic yield; however, EMG testing remains the most sensitive electrodiagnostic test for radiculopathy.

SEPs are frequently abnormal in patients with myelopathy, and they may be abnormal in the presence of normal EMG evaluation. Serial SEPs have been found useful in determining the extent of spinal cord trauma and may help to determine prognosis for recovery.

SEPs recorded from the trigeminal nerve have been reported to be abnormal in persons with MS-related trigeminal neuralgia and with parasellar and cerebellopontine angle tumors affecting the trigeminal nerve. Alterations of trigeminal SEPs also relate well to successful treatment of trigeminal neuralgia by retrogasserian injection of glycerol and thermocoagulation-induced lesions. Trigeminal SEPs generally have not been found useful in the diagnosis of "idiopathic" trigeminal neuralgia.

Other uses of SEP are in the evaluation of spinal cord syndromes such as transverse myelitis, syringomyelia, and spinal cord ischemia and of tumors, infarctions, and hemorrhages involving the somatosensory pathways of the brainstem and cortex. Some neurodegenerative disorders, such as Huntington's chorea, and some neuropathies involving the central somatosensory pathways may also be associated with SEP abnormalities.

COGNITIVE EVOKED POTENTIALS

Cognitive EPs, or endogenous event-related potentials, are long-latency EPs related to cognitive processing. Testing consists of random presentations of infrequent or rare stimuli interdispersed with different, more frequently occurring common stimuli. The subject is instructed to attend to the infrequent stimuli only. Normal persons produce a P300 response with a latency of approximately

300 msec and positive polarity. The P300 response latency may be abnormally prolonged or reduced in amplitude in disorders that impair cognition, such as dementias, autism, schizophrenia, and Huntington's chorea.

Summary

EMG and EP testing are essential tools in the diagnosis of neuromuscular disorders. They provide reliable and reproducible information on function of the nervous system that would not be obtainable through other means. They provide an extension of the clinical examination and are complementary to laboratory, radiologic, and other evaluations. Development of new techniques and improvements in old ones continue to expand the clinical utility of these tests. For example, the addition of transcranial magnetic stimulation has allowed evaluation of central motor pathways that had not been possible with EMG or other EP testing. Further refinements in cognitive EP testing may allow greater understanding of the nature and complexity of cognitive processing. The clinical neurophysiology laboratory is an increasingly important part of the total clinical milieu. With this thought in mind, the prudent practitioner will find greater utility and put more reliance on these tests for evaluation of patients, now and in the future.

SUGGESTED READINGS

Campbell W (ed): DeJong's The Neurological Examination, ed 6. Philadelphia, Lippincott Williams and Wilkins, 2005.

Goetz CG (ed): Textbook of Clinical Neurology, ed 2. Philadelphia, Saunders, 2003.

Waldman HJ: Evoked potential testing. In Waldman SD (ed): Pain Management. Philadelphia, Saunders, 2007.

Waldman SD: Parsonage-Turner syndrome. Atlas of Uncommon Pain Syndromes, ed 2. Philadelphia, Saunders, 2008.

Waldman SD: Trigeminal neuralgia. In: Atlas of Common Pain Syndromes, ed 2. Philadelphia, Saunders, 2008.

CHAPTER 222

Pain Assessment Tools for Adults

The Joint Commission on Accreditation of Healthcare Organizations (JCAHO) has stated that the assessment of pain is a required part of patient care and went on to say that pain should be considered the fifth vital sign. As has been aptly pointed out by many, pain is neither vital nor is it a sign. Having said that, there are few who would not agree that the ongoing assessment of a patient's pain is a worthwhile endeavor. However, given that pain is a subjective response that is registered as a conscious experience unique to the patient, objectification presents a variety of problems. A complete solution for these problems awaits discovery of a method to objectively measure pain the way we objectively measure a patient's blood pressure or pulse, however, several assessment tools have been developed to allow the clinician to try to quantify the patient's subjective pain experience.

Single-Dimension Pain Assessment Tools

VISUAL ANALOG SCALE

The most commonly used pain assessment tool is the visual analog scale (VAS), which is unidimensional measurement tool that allows the patient to assign a number to their subjective pain experience (Fig. 222-1). The typical VAS is composed of a 10-cm straight line with the left end of the line labeled "no pain" and the right end of the line labeled "worst pain imaginable." The patient is then instructed to mark where on the VAS he or she believes the pain being experienced at that point in time is located. The distance from the left end of the line is then measured, and a numerical value from 1 to 10 or 1 to 100 is assigned. Research has shown the VAS to be a sensitive measure of variations in the patient's pain in response to treatment and procedures and reproducible over time for the individual patient. Shortcomings of the VAS include the fact that the VAS attempts to assign a single unidimensional value to the complex multidimensional pain experience. Furthermore, if the patient has to decide if the pain he or she is having is the worst pain imaginable, even the patient may have no concept of what the worst pain imaginable is like. If the patient decides that the current pain they are experiencing is in fact the worst pain imaginable and at a later point in time they perceive their pain as worse than the previous pain that they described as the worst pain imaginable, there is no mechanism for the patient to document the change.

NUMERICAL PAIN INTENSITY SCALE

Like the VAS, the Numerical Pain Intensity Scale (NPIS) assigns a value of "no pain" on the left end of the scale and a value of "worst pain imaginable" to the right end of the scale (Fig. 222-2). Instead of a simple line without gradations or numbers as is found on the VAS, numbers from 0 to 10 are spaced evenly along the line from left to right. The patient is shown the NPIS and asked to circle a number that corresponds to the level of pain that he or she is currently having. The NPIS has the advantage that it requires no measurements and is self-scoring, making it easier to use than the VAS. Like the VAS, the NPIS suffers from the same unidimensional measurement limitation of the patient's complex multidimensional pain experience. Patients may also tend to assign the pain level they are experiencing a number off the scale (e.g., "my pain is a 100!").

VERBAL DESCRIPTOR SCALE

The verbal descriptor scale (VDS) is another unidimensional pain assessment tool that uses descriptive words rather than numbers to allow the patient to assign a value to his or her current pain experience (Fig. 222-3). Like the NPIS, the VDS is self-scoring, making it easy to use at the bedside. Like all of the unidimensional pain assessment tools, it fails to measure the multidimensional aspects of the patient's pain experience. Another disadvantage of the VDS is that it forces the patient to use someone else's words to describe his or her pain, which may lead to misinterpretation.

Multidimensional Pain Assessment Tools

As mentioned, pain is a complex, subjective, multidimensional conscious experience that is unique to the individual patient. Multidimensional pain assessment tools attempt to overcome some of the shortcomings of unidimensional pain assessment tools by attempting to measure the various dimensions that make up the pain experience. Examples of multidimensional pain assessment tools include the various forms of the McGill Pain Questionnaire, the Brief Pain Inventory, the Memorial Pain Assessment Card, and the Multidimensional Affect and Pain Survey.

McGILL PAIN QUESTIONAIRE

The McGill Pain Questionnaire (MPQ) is a three-part pain assessment tool that measures several dimensions of the patient's pain experience (Fig. 222-4). The first part consists of an anatomic drawing of the human form on which the patient marks where his or her

pain is located. The second part of the MPQ is a VDS that allows the patient to record the intensity level of his or her current pain experience. The third part of the MPQ is a pain verbal descriptor inventory consisting of 72 descriptive adjectives. The patient is asked to review this list of pain descriptors and circle the ones that serve to best describe his or her current pain experience. Each part or dimension of the MPQ is individually scored and a cumulative total score is also recorded.

Although the length of time required for the patient to correctly complete the MPQ is a major limitation to this multidimensional pain assessment tool, extensive clinic experience with the MPQ has shown that it is a reliable and valid way to quantify an individual patient's conscious pain experience. The MPQ may also aid the clinician in identifying the specific type of pain syndrome, such as neuropathic, that the patient suffers from.

BRIEF PAIN INVENTORY

Like the MPQ, the Brief Pain Inventory (BPI) uses an anatomic drawing of the human form on which the patient marks where his or her pain is located (Fig. 222-5).

The BPI also includes a number of questions about their pain treatment in the past 24 hours as well as 11 different numerical pain intensity scales that ask the patient to rank various aspects of his or her current pain experience and the effect that pain is having on the patient's activities of daily living. While a valid and reliable multidimensional pain assessment tool, the BPI is reasonably time consuming for the patient to fill out, which may limit its utility in many clinical settings.

MULTIDIMENSIONAL AFFECT AND PAIN SURVEY

Like the MPQ and the BPI, the Multidimensional Affect and Pain Survey (MAPS) suffers from the disadvantage of complexity and the length of time it takes to administer this pain assessment tool. The MAPS is made up of an extensive list of descriptor adjectives that encompass the pain and emotional experience. This descriptor list is subdivided into clusters, with the patient required to answer a question about each descriptor to further refine the assessment.

MEMORIAL PAIN ASSESSMENT CARD

Designed in part to address the time-consuming nature of the MPI and the BPI, the Memorial Pain Assessment Card (MPAC) is a multidimensional pain assessment tool that is very quick to administer (Fig. 222-6). Designed initially for use in the assessment of very ill inpatients suffering from pain of malignant origin, the MPAC is now used in a variety of pain settings. Its ease of use makes it ideally suited in clinical situations such as acute pain management, where frequent repeated assessments are desirable.

SUGGESTED READING

Correll DJ: The measurement of pain: Objectifying the subjective. In Waldman SD (ed): Pain Management. Philadelphia, Saunders, 2007.

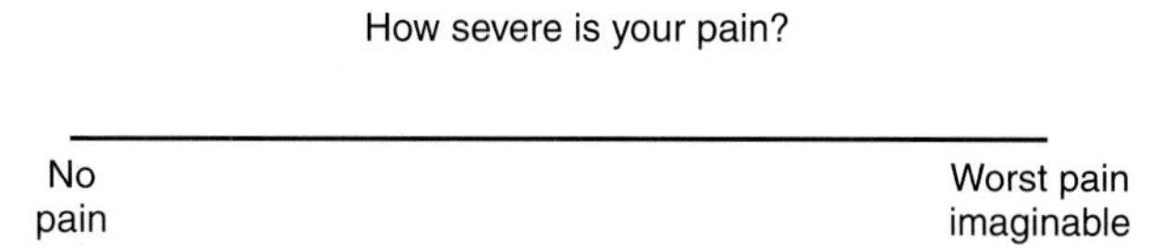

How severe is your pain?
No pain
Worst pain imaginable

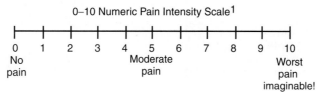

FIGURE 222–1 Example of a visual analog scale for the assessment of pain.

0–10 Numeric Pain Intensity Scale[1]
0
1
2
3
4
5
6
7
8
9
10
No pain
Moderate pain
Worst pain imaginable!
[1]If used as a graphic rating scale, a 10 cm baseline is recommended.

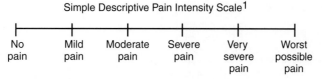

FIGURE 222–2 Example of a numerical pain intensity scale for the assessment of pain.

Simple Descriptive Pain Intensity Scale[1]
No pain
Mild pain
Moderate pain
Severe pain
Very severe pain
Worst possible pain
[1]If used as a graphic rating scale, a 10 cm baseline is recommended.

FIGURE 222–3 Example of a verbal descriptor scale for the assessment of pain.

McGill Pain Questionnaire

Patient's Name _____ Date _____ Time _____ am/pm

PRI: S _____ A _____ E _____ M _____ PRI(T) _____ PPI _____
      (1-10)   (11-15)   (16)   (17-20)   (1-20)

1 FLICKERING ____	11 TIRING ____	BRIEF ____ RHYTHMIC ____ CONTINUOUS ____
QUIVERING ____	EXHAUSTING ____	MOMENTARY ____ PERIODIC ____ STEADY ____
PULSING ____		TRANSIENT ____ INTERMITTENT ____ CONSTANT ____

1 FLICKERING ____
QUIVERING ____
PULSING ____
THROBBING ____
BEATING ____
POUNDING ____

2 JUMPING ____
FLASHING ____
SHOOTING ____

3 PRICKING ____
BORING ____
DRILLING ____
STABBING ____
LANCINATING ____

4 SHARP ____
CUTTING ____
LACERATING ____

5 PINCHING ____
PRESSING ____
GNAWING ____
CRAMPING ____
CRUSHING ____

6 TUGGING ____
PULLING ____
WRENCHING ____

7 HOT ____
BURNING ____
SCALDING ____
SEARING ____

8 TINGLING ____
ITCHY ____
SMARTING ____
STINGING ____

9 DULL ____
SORE ____
HURTING ____
ACHING ____
HEAVY ____

10 TENDER ____
TAUT ____
RASPING ____
SPLITTING ____

11 TIRING ____
EXHAUSTING ____

12 SICKENING ____
SUFFOCATING ____

13 FEARFUL ____
FRIGHTFUL ____
TERRIFYING ____

14 PUNISHING ____
GRUELLING ____
CRUEL ____
VICIOUS ____
KILLING ____

15 WRETCHED ____
BLINDING ____

16 ANNOYING ____
TROUBLESOME ____
MISERABLE ____
INTENSE ____
UNBEARABLE ____

17 SPREADING ____
RADIATING ____
PENETRATING ____
PIERCING ____

18 TIGHT ____
NUMB ____
DRAWING ____
SQUEEZING ____
TEARING ____

19 COOL ____
COLD ____
FREEZING ____

20 NAGGING ____
NAUSEATING ____
AGONIZING ____
DREADFUL ____
TORTURING ____

PPI
0 NO PAIN ____
1 MILD ____
2 DISCOMFORTING ____
3 DISTRESSING ____
4 HORRIBLE ____
5 EXCRUCIATING ____

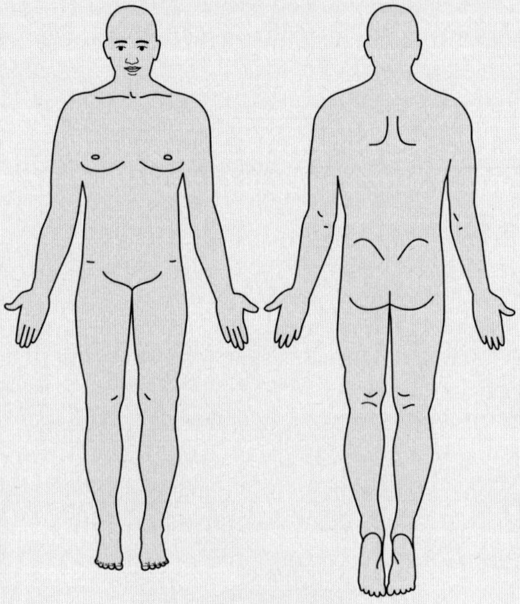

E = EXTERNAL
I = INTERNAL

COMMENTS:

FIGURE 222–4 The McGill Pain Questionnaire. (From Melzack R: The McGill Pain Questionnaire: Major properties and scoring methods. Pain 1975; 1:277-299.)

Brief Pain Inventory (Short Form)

Study ID#_____ Hospital#_____
Do not write above this line.

Date: _____

Time: _____

Name: _____
　　　　Last　　　　　First　　　　Middle initial

1) Throughout our lives, most of us have had pain from time to time (such as minor headaches, sprains, and toothaches). Have you had pain other than these everyday kinds of pain today?

　　　　　1. yes　　　2. no

2) On the diagram, shade in the areas where you feel pain. Put an X on the area that hurts the most.

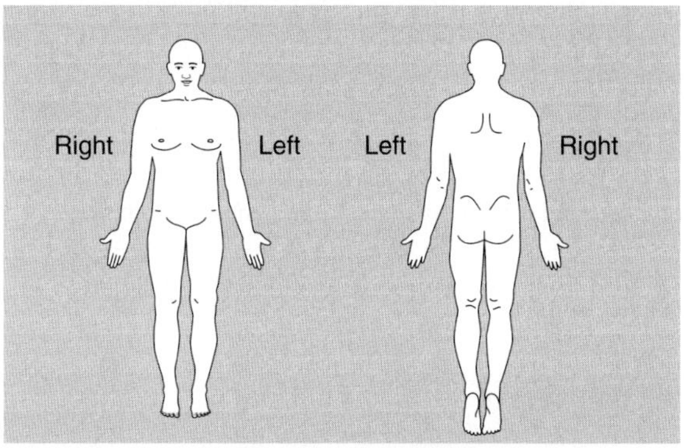

3) Please rate your pain by circling the one number that best describes your pain at its **WORST** in the past 24 hours.

0　1　2　3　4　5　6　7　8　9　10
No　　　　　　　　　　　　　Pain as bad as
Pain　　　　　　　　　　　　you can imagine

4) Please rate your pain by circling the one number that best describes your pain at its **LEAST** in the past 24 hours.

0　1　2　3　4　5　6　7　8　9　10
No　　　　　　　　　　　　　Pain as bad as
Pain　　　　　　　　　　　　you can imagine

5) Please rate your pain by circling the one number that best describes your pain on the **AVERAGE.**

0　1　2　3　4　5　6　7　8　9　10
No　　　　　　　　　　　　　Pain as bad as
Pain　　　　　　　　　　　　you can imagine

6) Please rate your pain by circling the one number that tells how much pain you have **RIGHT NOW.**

0　1　2　3　4　5　6　7　8　9　10
No　　　　　　　　　　　　　Pain as bad as
Pain　　　　　　　　　　　　you can imagine

7) What treatments or medications are you receiving for your pain?

_____

8) In the past 24 hours, how much **RELIEF** have pain treatments or medications provided? Please circle the one percentage that most shows how much relief you have received.

0% 10% 20% 30% 40% 50% 60% 70% 80% 90% 100%
No　　　　　　　　　　　　　　　　　　　　　Complete
Relief　　　　　　　　　　　　　　　　　　　　Relief

9) Circle the one number that describes how, during the past 24 hours **PAIN HAS INTERFERED** with your:

A. General Activity:

0　1　2　3　4　5　6　7　8　9　10
Does not　　　　　　　　　　　　Completely
interfere　　　　　　　　　　　　interferes

B. Mood

0　1　2　3　4　5　6　7　8　9　10
Does not　　　　　　　　　　　　Completely
interfere　　　　　　　　　　　　interferes

C. Walking Ability

0　1　2　3　4　5　6　7　8　9　10
Does not　　　　　　　　　　　　Completely
interfere　　　　　　　　　　　　interferes

D. Normal work (includes both work outside the home and housework)

0　1　2　3　4　5　6　7　8　9　10
Does not　　　　　　　　　　　　Completely
interfere　　　　　　　　　　　　interferes

E. Relation with other people

0　1　2　3　4　5　6　7　8　9　10
Does not　　　　　　　　　　　　Completely
interfere　　　　　　　　　　　　interferes

F. Sleep

0　1　2　3　4　5　6　7　8　9　10
Does not　　　　　　　　　　　　Completely
interfere　　　　　　　　　　　　interferes

G. Enjoyment of life

0　1　2　3　4　5　6　7　8　9　10
Does not　　　　　　　　　　　　Completely
interfere　　　　　　　　　　　　interferes

FIGURE 222–5 The Brief Pain Inventory multidimensional pain assessment tool. (From Cleeland CS, Ryan KM: Pain assessment: Global use of the Brief Pain Inventory. Ann Acad Med Singapore 1994; 23:129-138.)

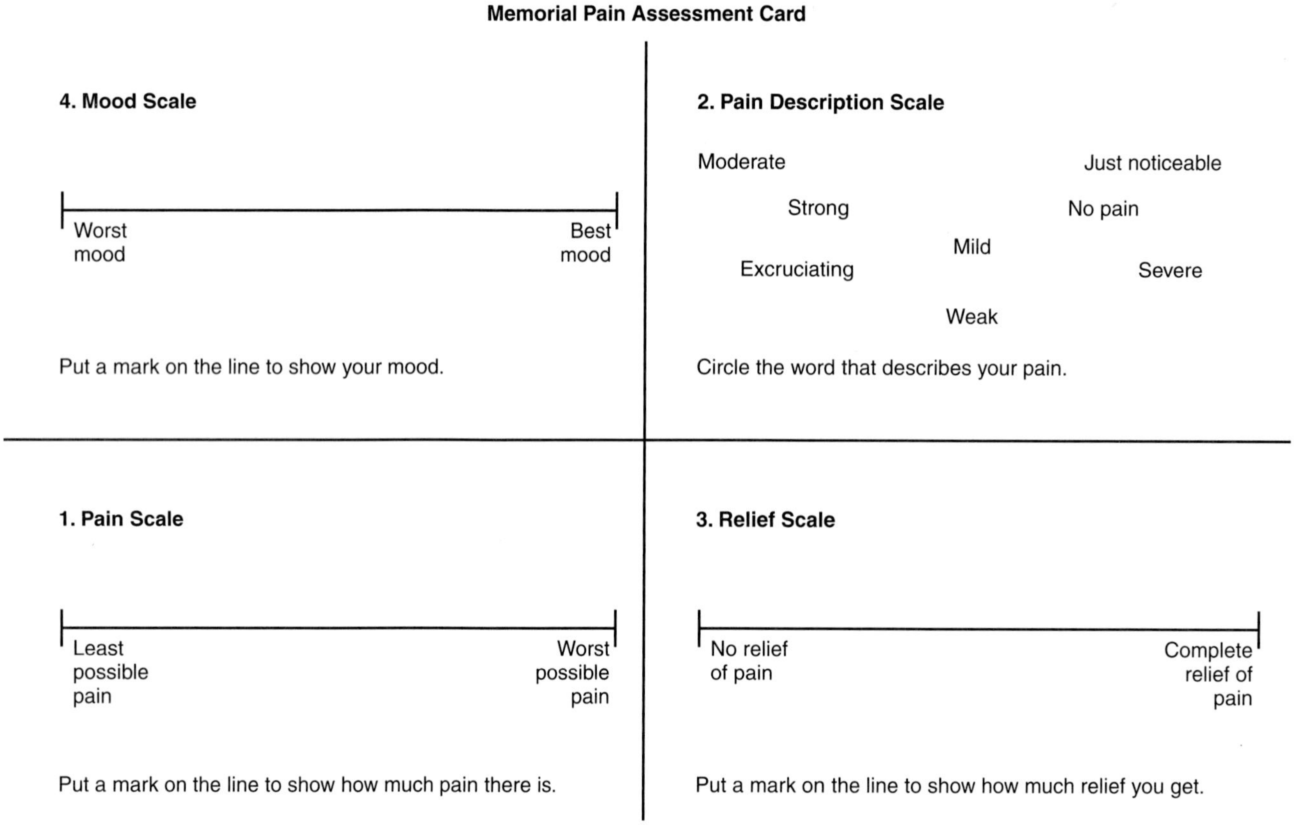

Memorial Pain Assessment Card

4. Mood Scale

|————————————————————————|
Worst   Best
mood   mood

Put a mark on the line to show your mood.

2. Pain Description Scale

Moderate   Just noticeable

Strong   No pain

Mild

Excruciating   Severe

Weak

Circle the word that describes your pain.

1. Pain Scale

|————————————————————————|
Least   Worst
possible   possible
pain   pain

Put a mark on the line to show how much pain there is.

3. Relief Scale

|————————————————————————|
No relief   Complete
of pain   relief of
pain

Put a mark on the line to show how much relief you get.

FIGURE 222–6 The Memorial Pain Assessment Card. (From Fishman B, Pasternak S, Wallenstein SL, et al: The Memorial Pain Assessment Card. A valid instrument for the evaluation of cancer pain. Cancer 1987; 60:1151-1158.)

CHAPTER 223

Pain Assessment Tools for Children and the Elderly

The assessment of pain in children and the elderly is a difficult but necessary part of the care of these special patient populations. In both of these patient populations, problems in the patient's ability to comprehend and verbalize their pain symptomatology make many of the traditional pain assessment tools used in adults less useful. In very young children, infants, and those elderly patients with diminished mental capacity, the available pain assessment tools are based primarily on the observations of the clinician rather than on input from the patient. Examples of such observational pain assessment tools include the COMFORT Scale and a tool specially designed to assess neonatal pain called CRIES (Figs. 223-1 and 223-2).

For children more than 3 years of age, some degree of patient self-assessment is actually possible using a specially designed numerical pain intensity scale known as the Wong-Baker Faces Scale (Fig. 223-3). This pain assessment tool uses a 6-point scale with corresponding line drawings of faces that exhibit emotions from smiling to crying. Some experts have criticized this pain assessment tool because it may confuse the child into thinking that even though the pain is severe, they may not choose the corresponding face that is crying because the child in pain is not actually crying at the time of the assessment. Other pain assessment tools that have been validated for use in children over 3 years of age include the Faces Pain

Scale and the Oucher Scale, which is available in specialized versions that are race specific featuring Caucasian, African American, and Asian children.

Sensory and cognitive impairments may make some standard pain assessment tools used in adults less useful than others. Studies of standard unidimensional and multidimensional pain assessment tools in the elderly have revealed some interesting findings. In general, unless sensory or cognitive impairments are severe, most elderly patients can easily understand and use a traditional numerical pain intensity scale. Pain assessment tools that rely on faces tied to a numerical pain intensity scale may lead to erroneous assessment as some elderly patients may read too much of the affective component of pain (i.e., anger, anxiety, boredom) into the faces. In general, pain scales that rely on verbal descriptors provide the most accurate and reproducible pain assessment in elderly patients in the absence of severe sensory or cognitive impairment.

SUGGESTED READING

Correll DJ: The measurement of pain: Objectifying the subjective. In Waldman SD (ed): Pain Management. Philadelphia, Saunders, 2007.

		DATE/TIME						
ALERTNESS	1 - Deeply asleep 2 - Lightly asleep 3 - Drowsy 4 - Fully awake and alert 5 - Hyper alert							
CALMNESS	1 - Calm 2 - Slightly anxious 3 - Anxious 4 - Very anxious 5 - Panicky							
RESPIRATORY DISTRESS	1 - No coughing and no spontaneous respiration 2 - Spontaneous respiration with little or no response to ventilation 3 - Occasional cough or resistance to ventilation 4 - Actively breathes against ventilator or coughs regularly 5 - Fights ventilator; coughing or choking							
CRYING	1 - Quiet breathing, no crying 2 - Sobbing or gasping 3 - Moaning 4 - Crying 5 - Screaming							
PHYSICAL MOVEMENT	1 - No movement 2 - Occasional, slight movement 3 - Frequent, slight movement 4 - Vigorous movement 5 - Vigorous movements including torso and head							
MUSCLE TONE	1 - Muscles totally relaxed; no muscle tone 2 - Reduced muscle tone 3 - Normal muscle tone 4 - Increased muscle tone and flexion of fingers and toes 5 - Extreme muscle rigidity and flexion of fingers and toes							
FACIAL TENSION	1 - Facial muscles totally relaxed 2 - Facial muscle tone normal; no facial muscle tension evident 3 - Tension evident in some facial muscles 4 - Tension evident throughout facial muscles 5 - Facial muscles contorted and grimacing							
BLOOD PRESSURE (MAP) BASELINE	1 - Blood pressure below baseline 2 - Blood pressure consistently at baseline 3 - Infrequent elevations of 15% or more above baseline (1-3 during 2 minutes observation) 4 - Frequent elevations of 15% or more above baseline (>3 during 2 minutes observation) 5 - Sustained elevations of 15% or more							
HEART RATE BASELINE	1 - Heart rate below baseline 2 - Heart rate consistently at baseline 3 - Infrequent elevations of 15% or more above baseline (1-3 during 2 minutes observation) 4 - Frequent elevations of 15% or more above baseline (>3 during 2 minutes observation) 5 - Sustained elevations of 15% or more							
		TOTAL SCORE						

FIGURE 223–1 The COMFORT scale. (From Ambuel B, Hamlett KW, Marx CM, Blumer JL: Assessing distress in pediatric intensive care environments: The COMFORT scale. J Pediatr Psychol 1992; 17:95-109.)

	DATE/TIME						
Crying - Characteristic cry of pain is high pitched. 0 – No cry or cry that is not high pitched 1 – Cry high pitched but baby is easily consolable 2 – Cry high pitched and baby is inconsolable							
Requires O₂ for Sao₂ <95% - Babies experiencing pain manifest decreased oxygenation. Consider other causes of hypoxemia, e.g., oversedation, atelectasis, pneumothorax 0 – No oxygen required 1 – <30% oxygen required 2 – >30% oxygen required							
Increased vital signs (BP* and HR*) - Take BP last as this may awaken child, making other assessments difficult 0 – Both HR and BP unchanged or less than baseline 1 – HR or BP increased but increase is <20% of baseline 2 – HR or BP is increased >20% over baseline							
Expression - The facial expression most often associated with pain is a grimace. A grimace may be characterized by brow lowering, eyes squeezed shut, deepening nasolabial furrow, or open lips and mouth. 0 – No grimace present 1 – Grimace alone is present 2 – Grimace and non-cry vocalization grunt is present							
Sleepless - Scored based upon the infant's state during the hour preceding this recorded score. 0 – Child has been continuously asleep 1 – Child has awakened at frequent intervals 2 – Child has been awake constantly							
TOTAL SCORE							

*Use baseline preoperative parameters from a nonstressed period. Multiply baseline HR by 0.2 and then add to baseline HR to determine the HR that is 20% over baseline. Do the same for BP and use the mean BP.

Indications: For neonates (0–6 months)

Instructions:
Each of the five (5) categories is scored from 0-2, which results in a total score between 0 and 10.
The interdisciplinary team in collaboration with the patient/family (if appropriate) can determine appropriate interventions in response to CRIES Scale scores.

FIGURE 223–2 CRIES. (From Krechel SW, Bildner J: CRIES: A new neonatal postoperative pain measurement score. Initial testing of validity and reliability. Paediatr Anaesth 1995; 5:53-61.)

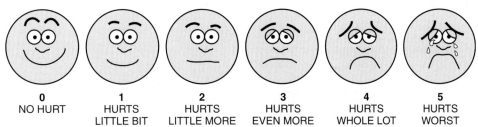

0	1	2	3	4	5
NO HURT	HURTS LITTLE BIT	HURTS LITTLE MORE	HURTS EVEN MORE	HURTS WHOLE LOT	HURTS WORST

FIGURE 223–3 Wong-Baker Faces Scale. (From Wong DL, Baker CM: Pain in children: Comparison of assessment scales. Pediatr Nurs 1988; 14:9-17.)

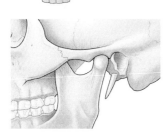

Nerve Blocks, Therapeutic Injections, and Advanced Interventional Pain Management Techniques

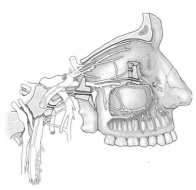

CHAPTER 224

Atlanto-Occipital Block Technique

The atlanto-occipital joint is dissimilar from the functional units of the lower cervical spine. The joint is not a true facet joint because it lacks posterior articulations characteristic of a true zygapophyseal joint. The atlanto-occipital joint allows the head to nod forward and backward with an isolated range of motion of approximately 35 degrees. This joint is located anterior to the posterolateral columns of the spinal cord. Neither the atlas nor the axis has intervertebral foramen to accommodate the first or second cervical nerves. These nerves are primarily sensory, and after leaving the spinal canal, they travel through muscle and soft tissue laterally and then superiorly to contribute fibers to the greater and lesser occipital nerves. The atlanto-occipital joint is susceptible to arthritic changes and trauma secondary to acceleration-deceleration injuries. Such damage to the joint results in pain secondary to synovial joint inflammation and adhesions.

To perform atlanto-occipital block, the patient is placed in a prone position. Pillows are placed under the chest to allow the cervical spine to be moderately flexed without discomfort to the patient. The forehead is allowed to rest on a folded blanket. If fluoroscopy is used, the beam is rotated in a sagittal plane from an anterior to a posterior position, which allows identification and visualization of the foramen magnum. Just lateral to the foramen magnum is the atlanto-occipital joint. A total of 5 mL of contrast medium suitable for intrathecal use is drawn up in a sterile 12-mL syringe. Then, 3 mL of preservative-free local anesthetic is drawn up in a separate 5-mL sterile syringe. When treating pain thought to be secondary to an inflammatory process, a total of 40 mg of depot steroid is added to the local anesthetic with the first block and 20 mg of depot steroid is added with subsequent blocks.

After preparation of the skin with antiseptic solution, a skin wheal of local anesthetic is raised at the site of needle insertion. An 18-gauge, 1-inch needle is inserted at the insertion site to serve as an introducer. The fluoroscopy beam is aimed directly through the introducer needle, which will appear as a small point on the fluoroscopy screen. The introducer needle is then repositioned under fluoroscopic guidance until this small point is visualized over the posterolateral aspect of the atlanto-occipital joint. This lateral placement avoids trauma to the vertebral artery, which lies medial to the joint at this level.

A 25-gauge, 3½-inch styletted spinal needle is then inserted through the 18-gauge introducer. If bony contact is made, the spinal needle is withdrawn and the introducer needle repositioned over the lateral aspect of the joint. The 25-gauge spinal needle is then re-advanced until a pop is felt, indicating placement within the atlanto-occipital join (Fig. 224-1). It is essential to then confirm fluoroscopically that the needle is actually in the joint, which is anterior to the posterior lateral aspect of the spinal cord. This is accomplished by rotating the C-arm to the horizontal plane and confirming needle placement within the joint (Fig. 224-2). If intra-articular placement cannot be confirmed, the needle should be withdrawn.

After confirmation of needle placement within the atlanto-occipital joint, the stylet is removed from the 25-gauge spinal needle, and the hub is observed for blood or cerebrospinal fluid. If neither is present, gentle aspiration of the needle is carried out, and if no blood or cerebrospinal fluid is seen, 1 mL of contrast medium is slowly injected under fluoroscopy. An arthrogram of the normal atlanto-occipital joint reveals a bilateral concavity representing the intact joint capsule. However, if the joint has been traumatized, it is not unusual to see contrast medium flow freely from the torn joint capsule into the cervical epidural space. If the contrast medium is seen to rapidly enter the venous plexus rather than outline the joint, the needle is almost always not within the joint space. If this occurs, the needle should be repositioned into the joint prior to injection. If the contrast medium remains within the joint or if it outlines the joint and a small amount leaks into the epidural space, 1 to 1.5 mL of the local anesthetic and steroid is slowly injected through the spinal needle.

Side Effects and Complications

The proximity to the brainstem and spinal cord makes it imperative that this procedure be carried out only by those well versed in the regional anatomy and experienced in performing interventional pain management techniques. Fluoroscopic guidance is recommended for most practitioners because neural trauma is a possibility even in the most experienced hands. The proximity to the vertebral artery combined with the vascular nature of this anatomic region makes the potential for intravascular injection high. Even small amounts of injection of local anesthetic into the vertebral arteries will result in seizures. Given the proximity of the brain and brainstem, ataxia after atlanto-occipital block due to vascular uptake of local anesthetic is not an uncommon occurrence.

SUGGESTED READING

Waldman SD: Atlanto-occipital block technique. In: Atlas of Interventional Pain Management, ed 2. Philadelphia, Saunders, 2004.

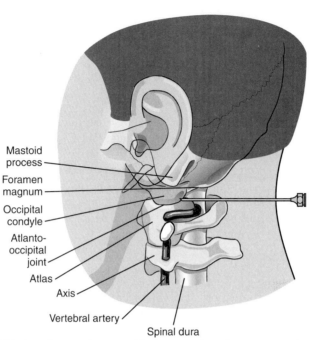

Mastoid
process
Foramen
magnum
Occipital
condyle
Atlanto-
occipital
joint
Atlas
Axis
Vertebral artery
Spinal dura

FIGURE 224–1 Atlanto-occipital block technique. (From Waldman SD: Atlas of Interventional Pain Management, ed 2. Philadelphia, Saunders, 2004.)

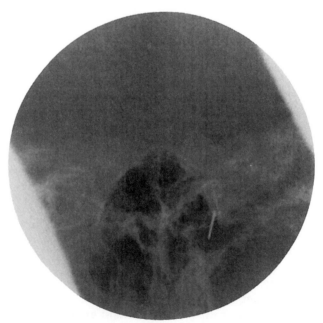

FIGURE 224–2 Fluoroscopic confirmation of needle positioning in the atlanto-occipital joint. (From Waldman SD: Atlas of Interventional Pain Management, ed 2. Philadelphia, Saunders, 2004.)

Atlantoaxial Block

The atlantoaxial joint is dissimilar from the functional units of the lower cervical spine. The joint is not a true facet joint because it lacks posterior articulations characteristic of a true zygapophyseal joint. Furthermore, there is no true disc or intervertebral foramen between atlas and axis. The atlantoaxial joint allows the greatest degree of motion of all the joints of the neck in that it not only allows the head to flex and extend approximately 10 degrees but it allows more than 60 degrees of rotation in the horizontal plane. The integrity and stability of the atlantoaxial joint is almost entirely ligamentous in nature. Even minor injury of the ligaments due to trauma can result in joint dysfunction and pain. Severe disruption of the ligaments has the same effect as a fracture of the odontoid process and can result in paralysis and death.

Atlantoaxial block is usually done under fluoroscopic guidance because of the proximity to the spinal cord and vertebral artery, although some pain specialists have gained sufficient familiarity with the procedure to perform it safely without fluoroscopy. The patient is placed in a prone position. Pillows are placed under the chest to allow the cervical spine to be moderately flexed without discomfort to the patient. The forehead is allowed to rest on a folded blanket.

If fluoroscopy is used, the beam is rotated in a sagittal plane from an anterior to a posterior position, which allows identification and visualization of the foramen magnum and atlas. Just lateral and inferior to the atlas and to the foramen magnum is the atlantoaxial joint. A total of 5 mL of contrast medium suitable for intrathecal use is drawn up in a sterile 12-mL syringe. Then, 3 mL of preservative-free local anesthetic is drawn up in a separate 5-mL sterile syringe. When treating pain thought to be secondary to an inflammatory process, a total of 40 mg of depot steroid is added to the local anesthetic with the first block and 20 mg of depot steroid is added with subsequent blocks.

After preparation of the skin with antiseptic solution, a skin wheal of local anesthetic is raised at the site of needle insertion. An 18-gauge, 1-inch needle is placed at the insertion site to serve as an introducer. The fluoroscopy beam is aimed directly through the introducer needle, which will appear as a small point on the fluoroscopy screen. The introducer needle is then repositioned under fluoroscopic guidance until this small point is visualized over the posterolateral aspect of the atlantoaxial joint. This lateral placement avoids trauma to the spinal cord, which lies medial to the joint at this level. It should be remembered that the vertebral artery is lateral to the atlantoaxial joint, and care must be taken to avoid arterial trauma or inadvertent intra-arterial injection.

A 25-gauge, 3½-inch styletted spinal needle is then inserted through the 18-gauge introducer. If bony contact is made, the spinal needle is withdrawn and the introducer needle repositioned over the lateral aspect of the joint. The 25-gauge spinal needle is then re-advanced until a pop is felt, indicating placement within the atlantoaxial joint (Fig. 225-1). It is essential to then confirm that the needle is actually in the joint, which is anterior to the posterior lateral aspect of the spinal cord. This is accomplished by rotating the C-arm to the horizontal plane and confirming needle placement within the joint. If intra-articular placement cannot be confirmed, the needle should be withdrawn.

After confirmation of needle placement within the atlantoaxial joint, the stylet is removed from the 25-gauge spinal needle, and the hub is observed for blood or cerebrospinal fluid. If neither is present, gentle aspiration of the needle is carried out, and if no blood or cerebrospinal fluid is seen, 1 mL of contrast medium is slowly injected under fluoroscopy. An arthrogram of the normal atlantoaxial joint reveals a bilateral concavity representing the intact joint capsule. However, if the joint has been traumatized, it is not unusual to see contrast medium flow freely from the torn joint capsule into the cervical epidural space. If the contrast medium is seen to rapidly enter the venous plexus rather than outline the joint, the needle is almost always not within the joint space. If this occurs, the needle should be repositioned into the joint prior to injection. If the contrast medium remains within the joint or if it outlines the joint and a small amount leaks into the epidural space, 1 to 1.5 mL of the local anesthetic and steroid is slowly injected through the spinal needle.

The proximity to the brainstem and spinal cord makes it imperative that this procedure be carried out only by those well versed in the regional anatomy and experienced in performing interventional pain management techniques. Fluoroscopic guidance is recommended for most practitioners because neural trauma is a possibility even in the most experienced hands. The proximity to the vertebral artery combined with the vascular nature of this anatomic region makes the potential for intravascular injection high. Even small amounts of injection of local anesthetic into the vertebral arteries will result in seizures. Given the proximity of the brain and brainstem, ataxia after atlantoaxial block due to vascular uptake of local anesthetic is not an uncommon occurrence. Many patients also complain of a transient increase in headache and cervicalgia after injection of the joint.

SUGGESTED READING

Waldman SD: Atlantoaxial block technique. In: Atlas of Interventional Pain Management, ed 2. Philadelphia, Saunders, 2004.

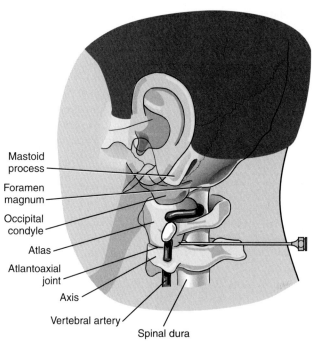

Mastoid process

Foramen magnum

Occipital condyle

Atlas

Atlantoaxial joint

Axis

Vertebral artery

Spinal dura

FIGURE 225–1 Atlantoaxial block technique. (From Waldman SD: Atlas of Interventional Pain Management, ed 2. Philadelphia, Saunders, 2004.)

Sphenopalatine Ganglion Block

The sphenopalatine ganglion (pterygopalatine, nasal, or Meckel's ganglion) is located in the pterygopalatine fossa, posterior to the middle nasal turbinate. It is covered by a 1- to 1.5-mm layer of connective tissue and mucous membrane. This 5-mm triangular structure sends major branches to the gasserian ganglion, trigeminal nerves, carotid plexus, facial nerve, and the superior cervical ganglion. The sphenopalatine ganglion can be blocked by topical application of local anesthetic or by injection.

Transnasal Approach

Sphenopalatine ganglion block via the transnasal approach is accomplished by the application of suitable local anesthetic to the mucous membrane overlying the ganglion. The patient is placed in the supine position, and the anterior nares are inspected for polyps, tumors, and foreign body. Three millimeters of either 2% viscous lidocaine or 10% cocaine hydrochloride is drawn up in a 5-mL sterile syringe. The tip of the nose is then drawn upward as if to place a nasogastric tube, and 0.5 mL of local anesthetic is injected into each nostril. The patient is asked to sniff vigorously to draw the local anesthetic posteriorly, which serves the double function of lubricating the nasal mucosa as well as providing topical anesthesia.

Two 3½-inch cotton-tipped applicators are soaked in the local anesthetic chosen, and one applicator is advanced along the superior border of the middle turbinate of each nostril until the tip comes into contact with the mucosa overlying the sphenopalatine ganglion (Fig. 226-1). Then 1 mL of local anesthetic is instilled over each cotton-tipped applicator. The applicator acts as a tampon that allows the local anesthetic to remain in contact with the mucosa overlying the ganglion. The applicators are removed after 20 minutes. Because of the highly vascular nature of the nasal mucosa, epistaxis is the major complication of this technique. This vascularity can lead to significant systemic absorption of local anesthetic with resultant local anesthetic toxicity, especially when cocaine is used. The patient's blood pressure, pulse, and respirations are monitored for untoward side effects.

Greater Palatine Approach

Sphenopalatine ganglion block via the greater palatine foramen approach is accomplished by the injection of local anesthetic onto the ganglion. The patient is placed in the supine position with the cervical spine extended over a foam wedge. The greater palatine foramen is identified just medial to the gumline of the third molar on the posterior portion of the hard palate. A dental needle with a 120-degree angle is advanced approximately 2.5 cm through the foramen in a superior and slightly posterior trajectory (Fig. 226-2). The maxillary nerve is just superior to the ganglion, and if the needle is advanced too deep, a paresthesia may be elicited. After careful gentle aspiration, 2 mL of local anesthetic is slowly injected.

Lateral Approach

Sphenopalatine ganglion block via the lateral approach is accomplished by the injection of local anesthetic onto the ganglion via a needle placed through the coronoid notch. The patient is placed in the supine position with the cervical spine in the neutral position. The coronoid notch is identified by asking the patient to open and close the mouth several times and palpating the area just anterior and slightly inferior to the acoustic auditory meatus. After the notch is identified, the patient is asked to hold his or her mouth open in the neutral position.

A total of 2 mL of local anesthetic is drawn up in a 3-mL sterile syringe. Some pain management specialists empirically add a small amount of depot steroid preparation to the local anesthetic. After the skin overlying the coronoid notch is prepared with antiseptic solution, a 22-gauge, 3½-inch styletted needle is inserted just below the zygomatic arch directly in the middle of the coronoid notch. The needle is advanced approximately 1.5 to 2 inches in a plane perpendicular to the skull until the lateral pterygoid plate is encountered. At this point, the needle is withdrawn slightly and redirected slightly superior and anterior, with the goal of placing the needle just above the lower aspect of the lateral pterygoid plate so it can enter the pterygopalatine fossa below the maxillary nerve and in close proximity to the sphenopalatine ganglion (Fig. 226-3). If this procedure is performed under fluoroscopy, the needle tip will be visualized just under the lateral nasal mucosa and position can be confirmed by injecting 0.5 mL of contrast medium. Additional confirmation of needle position can be obtained by needle stimulation at 50 Hz. If the needle is in correct position, the patient will experience a buzzing sensation just behind the nose with no stimulation into the distribution of other areas innervated by the maxillary nerve.

After correct needle placement is confirmed, careful aspiration is carried out, and 2 mL of solution is injected in incremental doses. During the injection procedure, the patient must be observed carefully for signs of local anesthetic toxicity. Because of the proximity of the maxillary nerve, the patient may also experience partial blockade of the maxillary nerve.

SUGGESTED READINGS

Waldman SD: Sphenopalatine ganglion block—greater palatine approach. In: Atlas of Interventional Pain Management, ed 2. Philadelphia, Saunders, 2004.

Waldman SD: Sphenopalatine ganglion block—lateral approach. In: Atlas of Interventional Pain Management, ed 2. Philadelphia, Saunders, 2004.

Waldman SD: Sphenopalatine ganglion block—transnasal approach. In: Atlas of Interventional Pain Management, ed 2. Philadelphia, Saunders, 2004.

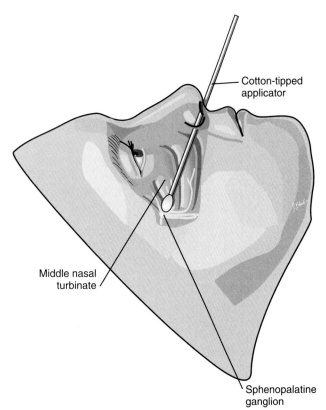

FIGURE 226–1 Sphenopalatine ganglion block: transnasal approach. (From Waldman SD: Atlas of Interventional Pain Management, ed 2. Philadelphia, Saunders, 2004, p 12.)

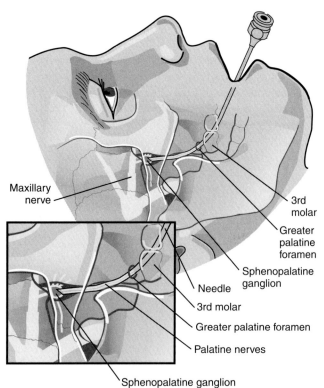

FIGURE 226–2 Sphenopalatine ganglion block: greater palatine foramen approach. (From Waldman SD: Atlas of Interventional Pain Management, ed 2. Philadelphia, Saunders, 2004, p 16.)

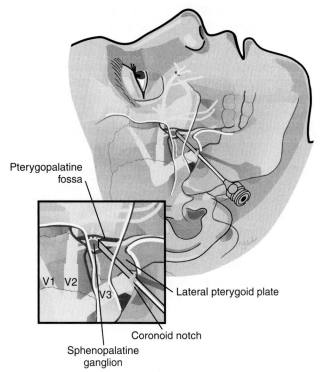

Pterygopalatine
fossa

V1 V2

V3

Lateral pterygoid plate

Coronoid notch

Sphenopalatine
ganglion

FIGURE 226–3 Sphenopalatine ganglion block: lateral approach. (From Waldman SD: Atlas of Interventional Pain Management, ed 2. Philadelphia, Saunders, 2004, p 19.)

CHAPTER 227

Greater and Lesser Occipital Nerve Block

The greater occipital nerve arises from fibers of the dorsal primary ramus of the second cervical nerve and to a lesser extent from fibers of the third cervical nerve. The greater occipital nerve pierces the fascia just below the superior nuchal ridge along with the occipital artery. It supplies the medial portion of the posterior scalp as far anterior as the vertex.

The lesser occipital nerve arises from the ventral primary rami of the second and third cervical nerves. The lesser occipital nerve passes superiorly along the posterior border of the sternocleidomastoid muscle, dividing into cutaneous branches that innervate the lateral portion of the posterior scalp and the cranial surface of the pinna of the ear.

Technique

The patient is placed in a sitting position with the cervical spine flexed and the forehead on a padded bedside table. A total of 8 mL of local anesthetic is drawn up in a 12-mL sterile syringe. When treating occipital neuralgia or other painful conditions involving the greater and lesser occipital nerves, a total of 80 mg of depot steroid is added to the local anesthetic with the first block and 40 mg of depot steroid is added with subsequent blocks.

The occipital artery is then palpated at the level of the superior nuchal ridge. After preparation of the skin with antiseptic solution, a 22-gauge, 1½-inch needle is inserted just medial to the artery and is advanced perpendicularly until the needle approaches the periosteum of the underlying occipital bone. A paresthesia may be elicited and the patient should be warned of such. The needle is then redirected superiorly, and after gentle aspiration, 5 mL of solution is injected in a fanlike distribution with care being taken to avoid the foramen magnum, which is located medially (Fig. 227-1).

The lesser occipital nerve and a number of superficial branches of the greater occipital nerve are then blocked by directing the needle laterally and slightly inferiorly. After gentle aspiration, an additional 3 to 4 mL of solution is injected (see Fig. 227-1).

The scalp is highly vascular, and this coupled with the fact that both nerves are in close proximity to arteries means that the pain specialist should carefully calculate the total milligram dosage of local anesthetic that may be safely given, especially if bilateral nerve blocks are being performed. This vascularity and the proximity to the arterial supply give rise to an increased incidence of postblock ecchymosis and hematoma formation.

These complications can be decreased if manual pressure is applied to the area of the block immediately after injection. Despite the vascularity of this anatomic region, this technique can be safely performed in the presence of anticoagulation by using a 25- or 27-gauge needle, albeit at increased risk of hematoma, if the clinical situation dictates a favorable risk-to-benefit ratio. Application of cold packs for 20-minute periods after the block will also decrease the amount of postprocedure pain and bleeding the patient may experience. Care must be taken to avoid inadvertent needle placement into the foramen magnum, because the subarachnoid administration of local anesthetic in this region will result in an immediate total spinal anesthetic.

SUGGESTED READING

Waldman SD: Greater and lesser occipital nerve block. In: Atlas of Interventional Pain Management, ed 2. Philadelphia, Saunders, 2004.

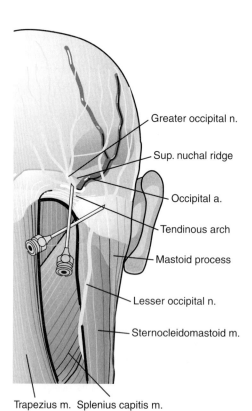

FIGURE 227–1 Injection technique for greater and lesser occipital nerve block. (From Waldman SD: Atlas of Interventional Pain Management, ed 2. Philadelphia, Saunders, 2004, p 25.)

Gasserian Ganglion Block

The gasserian ganglion is formed from two roots that exit the ventral surface of the brainstem at the midpontine level. These roots pass in a forward and lateral direction in the posterior cranial fossa across the border of the petrous bone. They then enter a recess called Meckel's cave, which is formed by an invagination of the surrounding dura mater into the middle cranial fossa. The dural pouch that lies just behind the ganglion is called the trigeminal cistern and contains cerebrospinal fluid.

The gasserian ganglion is canoe shaped, with the three sensory divisions—the ophthalmic (V1), the maxillary (V2), and the mandibular (V3)—exiting the anterior convex aspect of the ganglion (Fig. 228-1). A small motor root joins the mandibular division as it exits the cranial cavity via the foramen ovale.

Technique

The patient is placed in the supine position with the cervical spine extended over a rolled towel. Approximately 2.5 cm lateral to the corner of the mouth (Fig. 228-2), the skin is prepared with antiseptic solution and sterile drapes are placed. The skin and subcutaneous tissues are then anesthetized with 1% lidocaine with epinephrine.

A 20-gauge, 13-cm styletted needle is advanced through the anesthetized area, traveling perpendicular to the pupil of the eye (when the eye is looking straight ahead). The trajectory of the needle is cephalad toward the acoustic auditory meatus. The needle is advanced until contact is made with the base of the skull. The needle is withdrawn slightly and is "walked" posteriorly into the foramen ovale (Fig. 228-3). Paresthesia of the mandibular nerve will probably be elicited as the needle enters the foramen ovale, and the patient should be warned of such.

After the needle enters the foramen ovale, the needle stylet is removed. A free flow of cerebrospinal fluid (CSF) is usually observed. If no CSF is observed, the needle tip is probably anterior to the trigeminal cistern but may still be within Meckel's cave. Needle position can be confirmed by injection of 0.1-mL increments of preservative-free 1% lidocaine and observing the clinical response. Alternatively, 0.1 to 0.4 mL of contrast medium suitable for central nervous system use may be administered under fluoroscopic guidance prior to injection of the neurolytic substance. Sterile glycerol, 6.5% phenol in glycerin, and

absolute alcohol all have been successfully used for neurolysis of the gasserian ganglion. The neurolytic agent should be administered in 0.1-mL increments, with time allotted between additional increments to allow for observation of the clinical response. If hyperbaric neurolytic solutions such as glycerol or phenol in glycerin are used, the patient should be moved to the sitting position with the chin on the chest prior to injection. This will ensure that the solution is placed primarily around the maxillary and mandibular divisions and avoids the ophthalmic division. The patient should be left in the supine position if absolute alcohol is used. This same approach to the gasserian ganglion block may be used to place radiofrequency needles, cryoprobes, compression balloons, and stimulating electrodes.

Side Effects and Complications

Because of the highly vascular nature of the pterygopalatine space as well as its proximity to the middle meningeal artery, significant hematoma of the face and subscleral hematoma of the eye are common sequelae to gasserian ganglion block. The ganglion lies within the central nervous system, and small amounts of local anesthetic injected into the CSF may lead to total spinal anesthesia. For this reason, it is imperative that small, incremental doses of local anesthetic be injected, with time allowed after each dose to observe the effect of prior doses.

Because of the potential for anesthesia of the ophthalmic division with its attendant corneal anesthesia, corneal sensation should be tested with a cotton wisp after gasserian ganglion block with either local anesthetic or neurolytic solution. If corneal anesthesia is present, sterile ophthalmic ointment should be used and the affected eye patched to avoid damage to the anesthetic cornea. This precaution must be continued for the duration of corneal anesthesia. Ophthalmologic consultation is advisable should persistent corneal anesthesia occur.

Postprocedure dysesthesia occurs in approximately 6% of patients who undergo neurodestructive procedures of the gasserian ganglion. These dysesthesias can range from mild pulling or burning sensations to severe postprocedure pain called *anesthesia dolorosa*. These postprocedure symptoms are thought to be due to incomplete destruction of the ganglion. Sloughing of skin in the area of anesthesia may also occur.

In addition to disturbances of sensation, blockade or destruction of the gasserian ganglion may result in abnormal motor function, including weakness of the muscles of mastication and facial asymmetry. Horner's syndrome may also occur as a result of block of the parasympathetic trigeminal fibers. The patient should be warned that all of these complications may occur.

SUGGESTED READING

Waldman SD: Gasserian ganglion block. In: Atlas of Interventional Pain Management, ed 2. Philadelphia, Saunders, 2004.

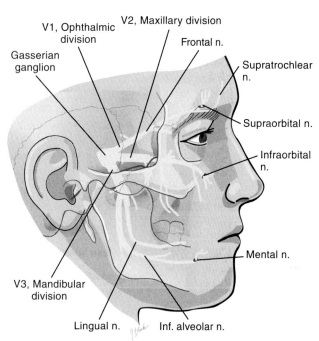

FIGURE 228–1 Gasserian ganglion: clinically relevant anatomy. (From Waldman SD: Atlas of Interventional Pain Management, ed 2. Philadelphia, Saunders, 2004, p 28.)

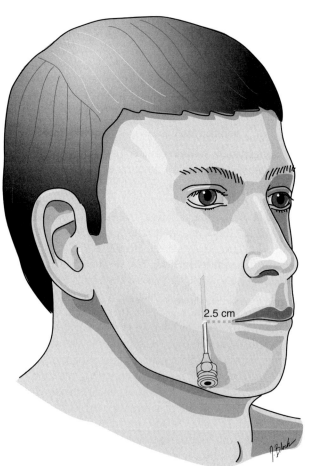

FIGURE 228–2 Approximately 2.5 cm lateral to the corner of the mouth is the needle insertion point for the gasserian ganglion block. (From Waldman SD: Atlas of Interventional Pain Management, ed 2. Philadelphia, Saunders, 2004, p 28.)

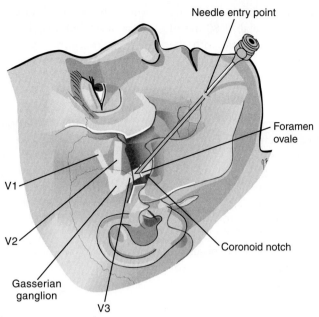

FIGURE 228–3 Gasserian ganglion block technique. (From Waldman SD: Atlas of Interventional Pain Management, ed 2. Philadelphia, Saunders, 2004, p 30.)

Trigeminal Nerve Block—Coronoid Approach

The maxillary division (V2) of the trigeminal nerve is a pure sensory nerve. It exits the middle cranial fossa via the foramen rotundum and crosses the pterygopalatine fossa. Passing through the inferior orbital fissure, it enters the orbit, emerging on the face via the infraorbital foramen. The maxillary nerve can be selectively blocked by placing a needle just above the anterior margin of the lateral pterygoid plate.

The maxillary nerve provides sensory innervation for the dura of the middle cranial fossa, the temporal and lateral zygomatic region, and the mucosa of the maxillary sinus. The nerve also provides sensory innervation for the upper molars, premolars, incisors, canines, and associated oral gingiva as well as the mucous membranes of the cheek. The nasal cavity, lower eyelid, skin of the side of the nose, and the upper lip are also subserved by the maxillary nerve.

The mandibular division (V3) is composed of a large sensory root and smaller motor root. Both leave the middle cranial fossa together via the foramen ovale and join to form the mandibular nerve. Branches of the mandibular nerve provide sensory innervation to portions of the dura mater and the mucosal lining of the mastoid sinus. Sensory innervation to the skin overlying the muscles of mastication, the tragus and helix of the ear, the posterior temporomandibular joint, chin, and dorsal aspect of the anterior two thirds of the tongue and associated mucosa of the oral cavity is also provided by the mandibular nerve. The smaller motor branch provides innervation to the masseter, external pterygoid, and temporalis muscles.

To perform trigeminal nerve block via the coronoid approach, the patient is placed in the supine position with the cervical spine in the neutral position. The coronoid notch is identified by asking the patient to open and close the mouth several times and palpating the area just anterior and slightly inferior to the acoustic auditory meatus. After the notch is identified, the patient is asked to hold his or her mouth in the neutral position.

A total of 7 mL of local anesthetic is drawn up in a 12-mL sterile syringe. When treating trigeminal neuralgia, atypical facial pain, or other painful conditions involving the maxillary and mandibular nerve, a total of 80 mg of depot steroid is added to the local anesthetic with the first block and 40 mg of depot steroid is added with subsequent blocks.

After the skin overlying the coronoid notch is prepared with antiseptic solution, a 22-gauge, 3½-inch styletted needle is inserted just below the zygomatic arch directly in the middle of the coronoid notch. The needle is advanced approximately 1.5 to 2 inches in a plane perpendicular to the skull until the lateral pterygoid plate is encountered (Fig. 229-1). At this point, if blockade of both the maxillary and mandibular nerves is desired, the needle is withdrawn slightly. After careful aspiration, 7 to 8 mL of solution is injected in incremental doses. During the injection procedure, the patient must be observed carefully for signs of local anesthetic toxicity. The coronoid approach to blockade of the trigeminal nerve may be used to place radiofrequency needles, cryoprobes, and stimulating electrodes.

Because of the highly vascular nature of the pterygopalatine fossa, significant facial hematoma may occur after trigeminal nerve block via the coronoid approach. This vascularity means that the pain specialist should use small, incremental doses of local anesthetic to avoid local anesthetic toxicity.

Postprocedure dysesthesia may occur in a small number of patients who undergo neurodestructive procedures of the branches of the trigeminal nerve. These dysesthesias can range from mild pulling or burning sensations to severe postprocedure pain called *anesthesia dolorosa*. These postprocedure symptoms are thought to be due to incomplete destruction of the neural structures. Sloughing of skin in the area of anesthesia may also occur.

In addition to disturbances of sensation, blockade or destruction of the branches of the trigeminal nerve may result in abnormal motor function, including weakness of the muscles of mastication and secondary facial asymmetry due to muscle weakness or loss of proprioception. The patient should be warned that all of these complications may occur.

SUGGESTED READING

Waldman SD: Trigeminal nerve block—coronoid approach. In: Atlas of Interventional Pain Management, ed 2. Philadelphia, Saunders, 2004.

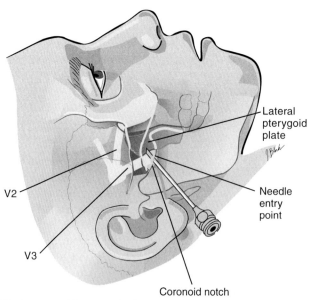

FIGURE 229–1 Trigeminal nerve block—coronoid approach. (From Waldman SD: Atlas of Interventional Pain Management, ed 2. Philadelphia, Saunders, 2004, p 36.)

Supraorbital Nerve Block

The supraorbital nerve arises from fibers of the frontal nerve, which is the largest branch of the ophthalmic nerve. The frontal nerve enters the orbit via the superior orbital fissure and passes anteriorly beneath the periosteum of the roof of the orbit. The frontal nerve gives off a larger lateral branch, the supraorbital nerve, and a smaller medial branch, the supratrochlear nerve. Both exit the orbit anteriorly. The supraorbital nerve sends fibers all the way to the vertex of the scalp and provides sensory innervation to the forehead, upper eyelid, and anterior scalp.

To perform supraorbital nerve block, the patient is placed in a supine position. A total of 3 mL of local anesthetic is drawn up in a 10-mL sterile syringe. When treating supraorbital neuralgia, acute herpes zoster, postherpetic neuralgia, or other painful conditions involving the supraorbital nerve, a total of 80 mg of depot steroid is added to the local anesthetic with the first block and 40 mg of depot steroid is added with subsequent blocks.

The supraorbital notch on the affected side is then identified by palpation. The skin overlying the notch is prepared with antiseptic solution, with care being taken to avoid spillage into the eye. A 25-gauge, 1½-inch needle is inserted at the level of the supraorbital notch and is advanced medially approximately 15 degrees off the perpendicular to avoid entering the foramen. The needle is advanced until it approaches the periosteum of the underlying bone (Fig. 230-1). A paresthesia may be elicited and the patient should be warned of such. The needle should not enter the supraorbital foramen, and should this occur, the needle should be withdrawn and redirected slightly more medially.

Because of the loose alveolar tissue of the eyelid, a gauze sponge should be used to apply gentle pressure on the upper eyelid and supraorbital tissues before injection of solution to prevent the injectate from dissecting inferiorly into these tissues. This pressure should be maintained after the procedure to avoid periorbital hematoma and ecchymosis.

After gentle aspiration, 3 mL of solution is injected in a fanlike distribution. If blockade of the supratrochlear nerve is also desired, the needle is then redirected medially, and after careful aspiration, an additional 3 mL of solution is injected in a fanlike manner.

The forehead and scalp are highly vascular, and the pain specialist should carefully calculate the total milligram dosage of local anesthetic that may be safely given, especially if bilateral nerve blocks are being performed. This vascularity gives rise to an increased incidence of post-block ecchymosis and hematoma formation. Despite the vascularity of this anatomic region, this technique can safely be performed in the presence of anticoagulation by using a 25- or 27-gauge needle, albeit at increased risk of hematoma, if the clinical situation dictates a favorable risk-to-benefit ratio. These complications can be decreased if manual pressure is applied to the area of the block immediately after injection. Application of cold packs for 20-minute periods after the block also decreases the amount of postprocedure bleeding.

SUGGESTED READING

Waldman SD: Supraorbital nerve block. In: Atlas of Interventional Pain Management, ed 2. Philadelphia, Saunders, 2004.

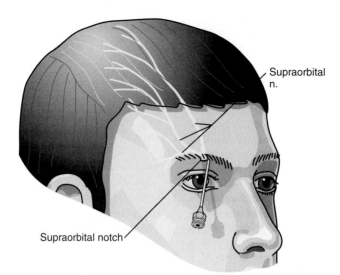

FIGURE 230–1 Supraorbital nerve block. (From Waldman SD: Atlas of Interventional Pain Management, ed 2. Philadelphia, Saunders, 2004, p 40.)

CHAPTER 231

Supratrochlear Nerve Block

The supratrochlear nerve arises from fibers of the frontal nerve, which is the largest branch of the ophthalmic nerve. The frontal nerve enters the orbit via the superior orbital fissure and passes anteriorly beneath the periosteum of the roof of the orbit. The frontal nerve gives off a larger lateral branch, the supraorbital nerve, and a smaller medial branch, the supratrochlear nerve. Both exit the orbit anteriorly. The supratrochlear nerve sends fibers to provide sensory innervation to the inferomedial section of the forehead, the bridge of the nose, and the medial portion of the upper eyelid.

To perform supratrochlear nerve block, the patient is placed in a supine position. A total of 3 mL of local anesthetic is drawn up in a 10-mL sterile syringe. When treating supratrochlear neuralgia, acute herpes zoster, postherpetic neuralgia, or other painful conditions involving the supratrochlear nerve, a total of 80 mg of depot steroid is added to the local anesthetic with the first block and 40 mg of depot steroid is added with subsequent blocks.

The supraorbital ridge on the affected side is then identified by palpation. The skin at the point where the bridge of the nose abuts the supraorbital ridge is prepared with antiseptic solution, with care being taken to avoid spillage into the eye. A 25-gauge, 1½-inch needle is inserted just lateral to the junction of the bridge of the nose and the supraorbital ridge and is advanced medially into the subcutaneous tissue (Fig. 231-1). A paresthesia may be elicited, and the patient should be warned of such. Because of the loose alveolar tissue of the eyelid, a gauze sponge should be used to apply gentle pressure on the upper eyelid and supratrochlear tissues before injection of solution to prevent the injectate from dissecting inferiorly into these tissues. This pressure should be maintained after the procedure to avoid periorbital hematoma and ecchymosis. After gentle aspiration, 3 mL of solution is injected in a fanlike distribution.

The forehead and scalp are highly vascular, and the pain specialist should carefully calculate the total milligram dosage of local anesthetic that may be safely given, especially if bilateral nerve blocks are being performed. This vascularity gives rise to an increased incidence of post-block ecchymosis and hematoma formation. Despite the vascularity of this anatomic region, this technique can safely be performed in the presence of anticoagulation by using a 25- or 27-gauge needle, albeit at increased risk of hematoma, if the clinical situation dictates a favorable risk-to-benefit ratio. These complications can be decreased if manual pressure is applied to the area of the block immediately after injection. Application of cold packs for 20-minute periods after the block also decreases the amount of postprocedure pain and bleeding the patient may experience.

SUGGESTED READING

Waldman SD: Supratrochlear nerve block. In: Atlas of Interventional Pain Management, ed 2. Philadelphia, Saunders, 2004.

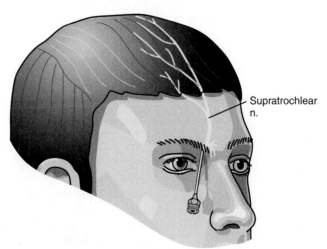

Supratrochlear n.

FIGURE 231–1 Supratrochlear nerve block. (From Waldman SD: Atlas of Interventional Pain Management, ed 2. Philadelphia, Saunders, 2004, p 42.)

CHAPTER 232

Infraorbital Nerve Block

The infraorbital nerve arises from fibers of the maxillary nerve. The infraorbital nerve enters the orbit via the inferior orbital fissure and passes along the floor of the orbit in the infraorbital groove. The nerve exits the orbit via the infraorbital foramen and provides cutaneous branches that innervate the lower eyelid, lateral naris, and upper lip. The superior alveolar branch of the infraorbital nerve provides sensory innervation to the upper incisor, canine, and associated gingiva.

Extraoral Approach

The patient is placed in a supine position. A total of 3 mL of local anesthetic is drawn up in a 10-mL sterile syringe. When treating infraorbital neuralgia, facial trauma, or other painful conditions involving the infraorbital nerve, a total of 80 mg of depot steroid is added to the local anesthetic with the first block and 40 mg of depot steroid is added with subsequent blocks.

The infraorbital notch on the affected side is then identified by palpation. The skin overlying the notch is prepared with antiseptic solution, with care being taken to avoid spillage into the eye. A 25-gauge, 1½-inch needle is inserted at the level of the infraorbital notch and is advanced medially approximately 15 degrees off the perpendicular to avoid entering the foramen. The needle is advanced until it approaches the periosteum of the underlying bone (Fig. 232-1). A paresthesia may be elicited, and the patient should be warned of such. The needle should not enter the infraorbital foramen, and should this occur, the needle should be withdrawn and redirected slightly more medially. Because of the loose alveolar tissue of the eyelid, a gauze sponge should be used to apply gentle pressure on the lower eyelid and infraorbital tissues before injection of solution to prevent the injectate from dissecting upward into these tissues. This pressure should be maintained after the procedure to avoid periorbital hematoma and ecchymosis. After gentle aspiration, 3 mL of solution is injected in a fanlike distribution.

Intraoral Approach

The patient is placed in a supine position. A total of 3 mL of local anesthetic is drawn up in a 10-mL sterile syringe. When treating infraorbital neuralgia, facial trauma, or other painful conditions involving the infraorbital nerve, a total of 80 mg of depot steroid is added to the local anesthetic with the first block and 40 mg of depot steroid is added with subsequent blocks.

The infraorbital notch on the affected side is then identified by palpation. The upper lip is then pulled backward, and a cotton ball soaked in 10% cocaine solution or 2% viscous lidocaine is placed in the alveolar sulcus, just inferior to the infraorbital foramen. After adequate topical anesthesia of the mucosa is obtained, a 25-gauge, 1½-inch needle is advanced through the anesthetized mucosa toward the infraorbital foramen (Fig. 232-2). A paresthesia may be elicited, and the patient should be warned of such. Because of the loose alveolar tissue of the eyelid, a gauze sponge should be used to apply gentle pressure on the lower eyelid and infraorbital tissues before injection of solution to prevent the injectate from dissecting upward into these tissues. This pressure should be maintained after the procedure to avoid periorbital hematoma and ecchymosis. After gentle aspiration, 3 mL of solution is injected in a fanlike distribution.

The face is highly vascular, and the pain specialist should carefully calculate the total milligram dosage of local anesthetic that may be safely given, especially if bilateral nerve blocks are being performed. This vascularity gives rise to an increased incidence of postblock ecchymosis and hematoma formation. Despite the vascularity of this anatomic region, this technique can safely be performed in the presence of anticoagulation by using a 25- or 27-gauge needle, albeit at increased risk of hematoma, if the clinical situation dictates a favorable risk-to-benefit ratio. These complications can be decreased if manual pressure is applied to the area of the block immediately after injection. Application of cold packs for 20-minute periods after the block also decreases the amount of postprocedure pain and bleeding the patient may experience.

The clinician should avoid inserting the needle directly into the infraorbital foramen because the nerve may be damaged as solution is injected into the bony canal, resulting in a compression neuropathy.

SUGGESTED READINGS

Waldman SD: Infraorbital nerve block: Extraoral approach. Atlas of Interventional Pain Management, ed 2. Philadelphia, Saunders, 2004.

Waldman SD: Infraorbital nerve block: Intraoral approach. In: Atlas of Interventional Pain Management, ed 2. Philadelphia, Saunders, 2004.

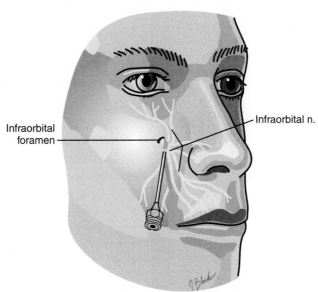

FIGURE 232–1 Infraorbital nerve block: extraoral approach. (From Waldman SD: Atlas of Interventional Pain Management, ed 2. Philadelphia, Saunders, 2004, p 46.)

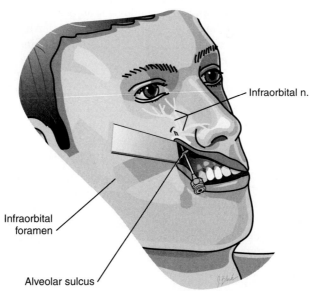

FIGURE 232–2 Infraorbital nerve block: intraoral approach. (From Waldman SD: Atlas of Interventional Pain Management, ed 2. Philadelphia, Saunders, 2004, p 48.)

CHAPTER 233

Mental Nerve Block

The mental nerve arises from fibers of the mandibular nerve. The mental nerve exits the mandible via the mental foramen at the level of the second premolar, where it makes a sharp turn superiorly. The nerve provides cutaneous branches that innervate the lower lip, chin, and corresponding oral mucosa.

Extraoral Approach

The patient is placed in a supine position. A total of 3 mL of local anesthetic is drawn up in a 10-mL sterile syringe. When treating mental neuralgia, facial trauma, or other painful conditions involving the mental nerve, a total of 80 mg of depot steroid is added to the local anesthetic with the first block and 40 mg of depot steroid is added with subsequent blocks.

The mental notch on the affected side is then identified by palpation. The skin overlying the notch is prepared with antiseptic solution. A 25-gauge, 1½-inch needle is inserted at the level of the mental notch and is advanced medially approximately 15 degrees off the perpendicular to avoid entering the foramen. The needle is advanced until it approaches the periosteum of the underlying bone (Fig. 233-1). A paresthesia may be elicited, and the patient should be warned of such. The needle should not enter the mental foramen, and should this occur, the needle should be withdrawn and redirected slightly more medially. After gentle aspiration, 3 mL of solution is injected in a fanlike distribution.

The face is highly vascular, and the pain specialist should carefully calculate the total milligram dosage of local anesthetic that may be safely given, especially if bilateral nerve blocks are being performed. This vascularity gives rise to an increased incidence of postblock ecchymosis and hematoma formation. Despite the vascularity of this anatomic region, this technique can safely be performed in the presence of anticoagulation by using a 25- or 27-gauge needle, albeit at increased risk of hematoma, if the clinical situation dictates a favorable risk-to-benefit ratio. These complications can be decreased if manual pressure is applied to the area of the block immediately after injection. Application of cold packs for 20-minute periods after the block also decreases the amount of postprocedure pain and bleeding the patient may experience.

The pain management specialist should avoid inserting the needle directly into the mental foramen because the nerve may be damaged as solution is injected into the bony canal, resulting in a compression neuropathy.

Intraoral Approach

The patient is placed in a supine position. A total of 3 mL of local anesthetic is drawn up in a 10-mL sterile syringe. When treating mental neuralgia, facial trauma, or other painful conditions involving the mental nerve, a total of 80 mg of depot steroid is added to the local anesthetic with the first block and 40 mg of depot steroid is added with subsequent blocks.

The mental notch on the affected side is then identified by palpation. The lower lip is then pulled downward, and a cotton ball soaked in 10% cocaine solution or 2% viscous lidocaine is placed in the alveolar sulcus, just above the mental foramen. After adequate topical anesthesia of the mucosa is obtained, a 25-gauge, 1½-inch needle is advanced through the anesthetized mucosa toward the mental foramen (Fig. 233-2). A paresthesia may be elicited, and the patient should be warned of such. After gentle aspiration, 3 mL of solution is injected in a fanlike distribution.

SUGGESTED READINGS

Waldman SD: Mental nerve block: Extraoral approach. In: Atlas of Interventional Pain Management, ed 2. Philadelphia, Saunders, 2004.

Waldman SD: Mental nerve block: Intraoral approach. In: Atlas of Interventional Pain Management, ed 2. Philadelphia, Saunders, 2004.

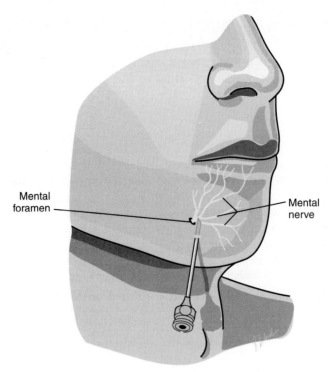

FIGURE 233–1 Mental nerve block: extraoral approach. (From Waldman SD: Atlas of Interventional Pain Management, ed 2. Philadelphia, Saunders, 2004, p 52.)

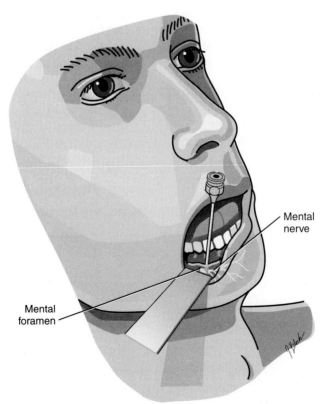

FIGURE 233–2 Mental nerve block: intraoral approach. (From Waldman SD: Atlas of Interventional Pain Management, ed 2. Philadelphia, Saunders, 2004, p 54.)

CHAPTER 234

Temporomandibular Joint Injection

The temporomandibular joint is a true joint that is divided into an upper and lower synovial cavity by a fibrous articular disc. Internal derangement of this disc may result in pain and temporomandibular joint dysfunction, but extracapsular causes of temporomandibular joint pain are much more common. The joint space between the mandibular condyle and the glenoid fossa of the zygoma may be injected with small amounts of local anesthetic and steroid. The temporomandibular joint is innervated by branches of the mandibular nerve. The muscles involved in temporomandibular joint dysfunction often include the temporalis, masseter, and external pterygoid and internal pterygoid and may include the trapezius and sternocleidomastoid. Trigger points may be identified when palpating these muscles.

To perform injection of the temporomandibular joint, the patient is placed in the supine position with the cervical spine in the neutral position. The temporomandibular joint is identified by asking the patient to open and close his or her mouth several times and palpating the area just anterior and slightly inferior to the acoustic auditory meatus. After the joint is identified, the patient is asked to hold his or her mouth in a neutral position.

A total of 0.5 mL of local anesthetic is drawn up in a 3-mL sterile syringe. When treating temporomandibular joint dysfunction, internal derangement of the temporomandibular joint, arthritis pain of the temporomandibular joint, or other painful conditions involving the temporomandibular joint, a total of 20 mg of depot steroid is added to the local anesthetic with the first block and 10 mg of depot steroid is added to the local anesthetic with subsequent blocks.

After the skin overlying the temporomandibular joint is prepared with antiseptic solution, a 25-gauge, 1-inch styletted needle is inserted just below the zygomatic arch directly in the middle of the joint space. The needle is advanced approximately ½ to ¾ inch in a plane perpendicular to the skull until a pop is felt that indicates the joint space has been entered (Fig. 234-1). After careful aspiration, 1 mL of solution is slowly injected. Injection of the joint may be repeated in 5- to 7-day intervals if the symptoms persist.

This anatomic region is highly vascular. This vascularity and proximity to major blood vessels also give rise to an increased incidence of postblock ecchymosis and hematoma formation, and the patient should be warned of such. Despite the vascularity of this anatomic region, this technique can be performed safely in the presence of anticoagulation by using a 25- or 27-gauge needle, albeit at increased risk of hematoma, if the clinical situation dictates a favorable risk-to-benefit ratio. These complications can be decreased if manual pressure is applied to the area of the block immediately following injection. Application of cold packs for 20-minute periods following the block will also decrease the amount of postprocedure pain and bleeding the patient may experience.

Additional side effects that occur with sufficient frequency include inadvertent block of the facial nerve with associated facial weakness. When this occurs, protection of the cornea with sterile ophthalmic lubricant and patching is mandatory.

SUGGESTED READING

Waldman SD: Temporomandibular joint injection. In: Atlas of Pain Management Injection Techniques, ed. 2. Philadelphia, Saunders, 2007.

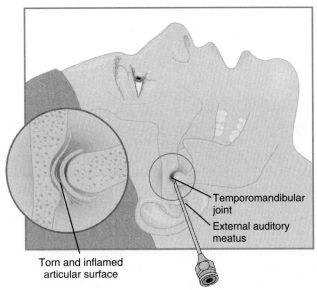

FIGURE 234–1 Temporomandibular joint injection. (From Waldman SD: Atlas of Pain Management Injection Techniques, ed. 2. Philadelphia, Saunders, 2007, p 5.)

CHAPTER 235

Glossopharyngeal Nerve Block

The glossopharyngeal nerve contains both motor and sensory fibers. The motor fibers innervate the stylopharyngeus muscle. The sensory portion of the nerve innervates the posterior third of the tongue, palatine tonsil, and the mucous membranes of the mouth and pharynx. Special visceral afferent sensory fibers transmit information from the taste buds of the posterior third of the tongue. Information from the carotid sinus and body that helps control blood pressure, pulse, and respiration is carried via the carotid sinus nerve, which is a branch of the glossopharyngeal nerve. Parasympathetic fibers pass via the glossopharyngeal nerve to the otic ganglion. Postganglionic fibers from the ganglion carry secretory information to the parotid gland.

The glossopharyngeal nerve exits from the jugular foramen in proximity to the vagus and accessory nerves and the internal jugular vein. All three nerves lie in the groove between the internal jugular vein and internal carotid artery.

The key landmark for extraoral glossopharyngeal nerve block is the styloid process of the temporal bone. This osseous process represents the calcification of the cephalad end of the stylohyoid ligament. Although usually easy to identify, the styloid process may be difficult to locate with the exploring needle if ossification is limited.

Extraoral Approach

To perform glossopharyngeal nerve block using the extraoral approach, the patient is placed in the supine position. An imaginary line is visualized running from the mastoid process to the angle of the mandible. The styloid process should lie just below the midpoint of this line. The skin is prepped with antiseptic solution. A 22-gauge, 1½-inch needle attached to a 10-mL syringe is advanced at this midpoint location in a plane perpendicular to the skin. The styloid process should be encountered within 3 cm. After contact is made, the needle is withdrawn and walked off the styloid process posteriorly (Fig. 235-1). As soon as bony contact is lost and careful aspiration reveals no blood or cerebrospinal fluid, 7 mL of 0.5% preservative-free lidocaine combined with 80 mg of methylprednisolone is injected in incremental doses. Subsequent daily nerve blocks are carried out in a similar manner, substituting 40 mg of methylprednisolone for the initial 80-mg dose. This approach may also be used for breakthrough pain in patients who previously experienced adequate pain control with oral medications.

Intraoral Approach

To perform glossopharyngeal nerve block using the intraoral approach, the patient is placed in the supine position. The tongue is anesthetized with 2% viscous lidocaine. The patient opens the mouth wide, and the tongue is then retracted inferiorly with a tongue depressor or laryngoscope blade. A 22-gauge, 3½-inch spinal needle that has been bent approximately 25 degrees is inserted through the mucosa at the lower lateral portion of the posterior tonsillar pillar (Fig. 235-2). The needle is advanced approximately 0.5 cm. After careful aspiration for blood and cerebrospinal fluid, 7 mL of 0.5% preservative-free lidocaine combined with 80 mg of methylprednisolone is injected in incremental doses. Subsequent daily nerve blocks are carried out in a similar manner, substituting 40 mg of methylprednisolone for the initial 80-mg dose.

The major complications associated with glossopharyngeal nerve block are related to trauma to the internal jugular vein and carotid artery. Hematoma formation and intravascular injection of local anesthetic with subsequent toxicity are not uncommon complications of glossopharyngeal nerve block. Blockade of the motor portion of the glossopharyngeal nerve can result in dysphagia secondary to weakness of the stylopharyngeus muscle. If the vagus nerve is inadvertently blocked, as is often the case during glossopharyngeal nerve block, dysphonia secondary to paralysis of the ipsilateral vocal cord may occur. A reflex tachycardia secondary to vagal nerve block is also observed in some patients. Inadvertent block of the hypoglossal and spinal accessory nerves during glossopharyngeal nerve block results in weakness of the tongue and trapezius muscle.

A small percentage of patients who undergo chemical neurolysis or neurodestructive procedures of the glossopharyngeal nerve experience postprocedure dysesthesias in the area of anesthesia. These symptoms range from a mildly uncomfortable burning or pulling sensation to severe pain. When this severe postprocedure pain occurs, it is called *anesthesia dolorosa*. Anesthesia dolorosa can be worse than the patient's original pain complaint and is often harder to treat. Although uncommon, infection remains an ever-present possibility, especially in the immunocompromised cancer patient. Early detection of infection is crucial to avoid potentially life-threatening sequelae.

SUGGESTED READINGS

Waldman SD: Glossopharyngeal nerve block: Extraoral Approach. In: Atlas of Interventional Pain Management, ed 2. Philadelphia, Saunders, 2004.

Waldman SD: Glossopharyngeal nerve block: Intraoral Approach. In: Atlas of Interventional Pain Management, ed 2. Philadelphia, Saunders, 2004.

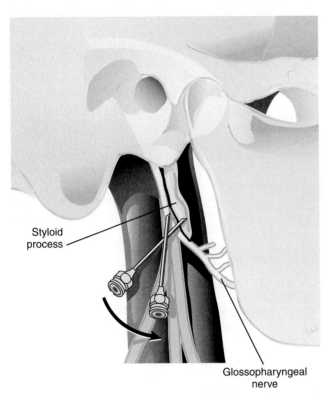

FIGURE 235–1 Glossopharyngeal nerve block: extraoral approach. (From Waldman SD: Atlas of Interventional Pain Management, ed 2. Philadelphia, Saunders, 2004, p 71.)

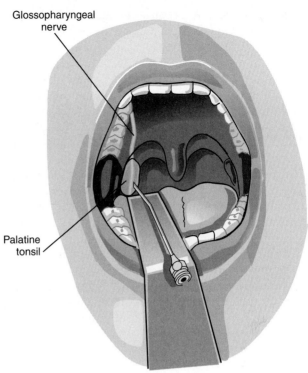

FIGURE 235–2 Glossopharyngeal nerve block: intraoral approach. (From Waldman SD: Atlas of Interventional Pain Management, ed 2. Philadelphia, Saunders, 2004, p 74.)

CHAPTER 236

Vagus Nerve Block

The vagus nerve contains both motor and sensory fibers. The motor fibers innervate the pharyngeal muscle and provide fibers for the superior and recurrent laryngeal nerves. The sensory portion of the nerve innervates the dura mater of the posterior fossa, the posterior aspect of the external auditory meatus, the inferior aspect of the tympanic membrane, and the mucosa of the larynx below the vocal cords. The vagus nerve also provides fibers to the intrathoracic contents, including the heart, lungs, and major vasculature.

The vagus nerve exits from the jugular foramen in close proximity to the spinal accessory nerve. The vagus nerve lies just caudad to the glossopharyngeal nerve and is superficial to the internal jugular vein. The vagus nerve courses downward from the jugular foramen within the carotid sheath along with the internal jugular vein and internal carotid artery.

Blockade of the vagus nerve is carried out in a manner analogous to glossopharyngeal nerve block. The key landmark for vagus nerve block is the styloid process of the temporal bone. This osseous process represents the calcification of the cephalad end of the stylohyoid ligament. Although usually easy to identify, the styloid process may be difficult to locate with the exploring needle if ossification is limited.

To perform vagus nerve block, the patient is placed in the supine position. An imaginary line is visualized running from the mastoid process to the angle of the mandible. The styloid process should lie just below the midpoint of this line. The skin is prepared with antiseptic solution. A 22-gauge, 1½-inch needle attached to a 10-mL syringe is advanced at this midpoint location in a plane perpendicular to the skin. The styloid process should be encountered within 3 cm (Fig. 236-1). After contact is made, the needle is withdrawn and "walked off" the styloid process posteriorly and in a slightly inferior trajectory. The needle is advanced approximately 0.5 cm past the depth at which the styloid process was identified. If careful aspiration reveals no blood or cerebrospinal fluid, 5 mL of 0.5% preservative-free lidocaine combined with 80 mg of methylprednisolone is injected in incremental doses. Subsequent daily nerve blocks are carried out in a similar manner, substituting 40 mg of methylprednisolone for the initial 80-mg dose. This approach may also be used for breakthrough pain in patients who previously experienced adequate pain control with oral medications.

The major complications associated with vagus nerve block are related to trauma to the internal jugular vein and carotid artery. Hematoma formation and intravascular injection of local anesthetic with subsequent toxicity are not uncommon after vagus nerve block. Blockade of the motor portion of the vagus nerve can result in dysphonia and difficulty coughing due to blockade of the superior and recurrent laryngeal nerves. A reflex tachycardia secondary to vagal nerve block is also observed in some patients. Inadvertent block of the glossopharyngeal, hypoglossal, and spinal accessory nerves during vagus nerve block will result in weakness of the tongue and trapezius muscle and numbness in the distribution of the glossopharyngeal nerve.

Although uncommon, infection remains an ever-present possibility, especially in the immunocompromised cancer patient. Early detection of infection is crucial to avoid potentially life-threatening sequelae.

SUGGESTED READING

Waldman SD: Vagus nerve block. In: Atlas of Interventional Pain Management, ed 2. Philadelphia, Saunders, 2004.

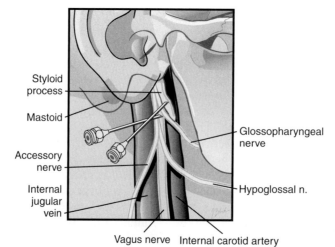

FIGURE 236–1 Vagus nerve block. (From Waldman SD: Atlas of Interventional Pain Management, ed 2. Philadelphia, Saunders, 2004, p 77.)

Spinal Accessory Nerve Block

The spinal accessory nerve arises from the nucleus ambiguus. The nerve has two roots, which leave the cranium together along with the vagus nerve via the jugular foramen. The fibers of the spinal root pass inferiorly and posteriorly to provide motor innervation to the superior portion of the sternocleidomastoid muscle. The spinal accessory exits the posterior border of the sternocleidomastoid muscle in the upper third of the muscle. The nerve, in combination with the cervical plexus, provides innervation to the trapezius muscle.

To perform spinal accessory nerve block, the patient is placed in a supine position with the head turned away from the side to be blocked. A total of 10 mL of local anesthetic is drawn up in a 20-mL sterile syringe. When treating conditions that are mediated via the spinal accessory nerve that are thought to have an inflammatory component, a total of 80 mg of depot steroid is added to the local anesthetic with the first block and 40 mg of depot steroid is added with subsequent blocks.

The patient is then asked to raise his or her head against the resistance of the pain specialist's hand to aid in identification of the posterior border of the sternocleidomastoid muscle. The posterior border of the upper third of the muscle is then identified. At a point just behind the posterior border of the upper third of the sternocleidomastoid muscle, after preparation of the skin with antiseptic solution, a 1½-inch needle is inserted with a slightly anterior trajectory (Fig. 237-1). After inserting the needle to a depth of approximately ¾ inch, gentle aspiration is carried out to identify blood or cerebrospinal fluid. If the aspiration test is negative and no paresthesia into the brachial plexus is elicited, 10 mL of solution is slowly injected in a fanlike manner, with close monitoring of the patient for signs of local anesthetic toxicity or inadvertent subarachnoid injection.

The proximity to the external jugular vein and other large vessels suggests the potential for inadvertent intravascular injection and/or local anesthetic toxicity from intravascular absorption. The pain specialist should carefully calculate the total milligram dosage of local anesthetic that may be safely given. This vascularity also gives rise to an increased incidence of postblock ecchymosis and hematoma formation. Despite the vascularity of this anatomic region, this technique can safely be performed in the presence of anticoagulation by using a 25- or 27-gauge needle, albeit at increased risk of hematoma, if the clinical situation dictates a favorable risk-to-benefit ratio. These complications can be decreased if manual pressure is applied to the area of the block immediately after injection. Application of cold packs for 20-minute periods after the block will also decrease the amount of postprocedure pain and bleeding the patient may experience.

In addition to the potential for complications involving the vasculature, the proximity of the spinal accessory nerve to the central neuraxial structures and the phrenic nerve can result in side effects and complications. If the needle is placed too deep, the potential for inadvertent epidural, subdural, or subarachnoid injection is a possibility. If the volume of local anesthetic used for this block is accidentally placed in any of these spaces, significant motor and sensory block will result. Unrecognized, these complications could be fatal. Blockade of the phrenic nerve may occur during blockade of the spinal accessory nerve. In the absence of significant pulmonary disease, unilateral phrenic nerve block should rarely create respiratory embarrassment. However, blockade of the recurrent laryngeal nerve with its attendant vocal cord paralysis combined with paralysis of the diaphragm may make the clearing of pulmonary and upper airway secretions difficult. Additionally, blockade of the vagus and glossopharyngeal nerves may also occur when performing spinal accessory nerve block.

SUGGESTED READING

Waldman SD: Spinal accessory nerve block. In: Atlas of Interventional Pain Management, ed 2. Philadelphia, Saunders, 2004.

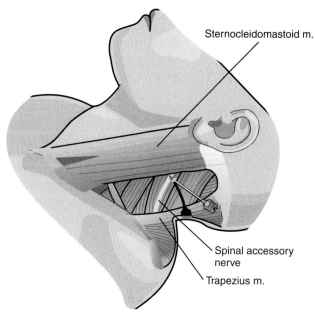

Sternocleidomastoid m.

Spinal accessory nerve

Trapezius m.

FIGURE 237–1 Spinal accessory nerve block. (From Waldman SD: Atlas of Interventional Pain Management, ed 2. Philadelphia, Saunders, 2004, p 79.)

CHAPTER 238

Phrenic Nerve Block

The phrenic nerve arises from fibers of the primary ventral ramus of the fourth cervical nerve, with contributions from the third and fifth cervical nerves. The phrenic nerve passes inferiorly between the omohyoid and sternocleidomastoid muscles. They exit the root of the neck between the subclavian artery and vein to enter the mediastinum. The right phrenic nerve follows the course of the vena cava to provide motor innervation to the right hemidiaphragm. The left phrenic nerve descends to provide motor innervation to the left hemidiaphragm in a course parallel to that of the vagus nerve.

To perform phrenic nerve block, the patient is placed in a supine position with the head turned away from the side to be blocked. A total of 10 mL of local anesthetic is drawn up in a 20-mL sterile syringe. When treating painful conditions associated with inflammation that are mediated via the phrenic nerve, a total of 80 mg of depot steroid is added to the local anesthetic with the first block and 40 mg of depot steroid is added with subsequent blocks.

The patient is then asked to raise his or her head against the resistance of the pain specialist's hand to aid in identification of the posterior border of the sternocleidomastoid muscle. In most patients, a groove between the posterior border of the sternocleidomastoid muscle and the anterior scalene muscle can be palpated. At a point 1 inch above the clavicle, at this groove or just slightly behind the posterior border of the sternocleidomastoid muscle, after preparation of the skin with antiseptic solution, a 1½-inch needle is inserted with a slightly anterior trajectory (Fig. 238-1). After inserting the needle to a depth of approximately 1 inch, gentle aspiration is carried out to identify blood or cerebrospinal fluid. If the aspiration test is negative and no paresthesia into the brachial plexus is elicited, 10 mL of solution is slowly injected in a fanlike manner, with close monitoring of the patient for signs of local anesthetic toxicity or inadvertent subarachnoid injection.

The proximity to the external jugular vein and other large vessels suggests the potential for inadvertent intravascular injection and/or local anesthetic toxicity from intravascular absorption. The pain specialist should carefully calculate the total milligram dosage of local anesthetic that may be safely given. This vascularity also gives rise to an increased incidence of postblock ecchymosis and hematoma formation. Despite the vascularity of this anatomic region, this technique can safely be performed in the presence of anticoagulation by using a 25- or 27-gauge needle, albeit at increased risk of hematoma, if the clinical situation dictates a favorable risk-to-benefit ratio. These complications can be decreased if manual pressure is applied to the area of the block immediately after injection. Application of cold packs for 20-minute periods after the block will also decrease the amount of postprocedure pain and bleeding the patient may experience.

In addition to the potential for complications involving the vasculature, the proximity of the phrenic nerve to the central neuraxial structures and the spinal accessory nerve can result in side effects and complications. If the needle is placed too deep, the potential for inadvertent epidural, subdural, or subarachnoid injection is a possibility. If the volume of local anesthetic used for this block is accidentally placed in any of these spaces, significant motor and sensory block will result. Unrecognized, these complications could be fatal. In the absence of significant pulmonary disease, unilateral phrenic nerve block should rarely create respiratory embarrassment. However, blockade of the recurrent laryngeal nerve with its attendant vocal cord paralysis combined with paralysis of the diaphragm may make the clearing of pulmonary and upper airway secretions difficult.

SUGGESTED READING

Waldman SD: Phrenic nerve block. In: Atlas of Interventional Pain Management, ed 2. Philadelphia, Saunders, 2004.

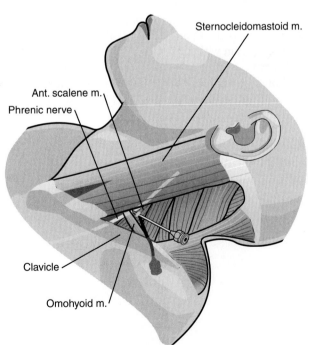

FIGURE 238–1 Phrenic nerve block. (From Waldman SD: Atlas of Interventional Pain Management, ed 2. Philadelphia, Saunders, 2004, p 82.)

CHAPTER 239

Facial Nerve Block

The facial nerve provides both motor and sensory fibers to the head. The facial nerve arises from the brainstem at the inferior margin of the pons. The sensory portion of the facial nerve is called the *nervus intermedius*. As it leaves the pons, the nervus intermedius is susceptible to compression producing a "trigeminal neuralgia–like" syndrome called *geniculate neuralgia*. After leaving the pons, the fibers of the facial nerve travel across the subarachnoid space and enter the internal auditory meatus to pass through the petrous temporal bone. The nerve then exits the base of the skull via the stylomastoid foramen. It passes downward and then turns forward to pass through the parotid gland, where it divides into fibers that provide innervation to the muscles of facial expression.

To perform facial nerve block, the patient is placed in a supine position with the head turned away from the side to be blocked to allow easy access to the mastoid process on the affected side. A total of 3 mL of local anesthetic is drawn up in a 12-mL sterile syringe. When treating geniculate neuralgia, herpes zoster, or other painful conditions involving the facial nerve, a total of 80 mg of depot steroid is added to the local anesthetic with the first block and 40 mg of depot steroid is added with subsequent blocks.

The mastoid process on the affected side is then identified by palpation. After preparation of the skin with antiseptic solution, a 22-gauge, 1½-inch needle is inserted at the anterior border of the mastoid process immediately below the external auditory meatus and at the level of the middle of the ramus of the mandible. The needle is then advanced perpendicularly until the needle approaches the periosteum of the underlying mastoid bone. The needle is then redirected slightly more anteriorly until it slides past the anterior border of the mastoid. The needle is slowly advanced approximately ½ inch beyond the edge of the mastoid (Fig. 239-1). This places the needle in proximity to the point at which the facial nerve exits the stylomastoid foramen. After gentle aspiration for blood and cerebrospinal fluid, 3 to 4 mL of solution is injected in incremental doses.

This anatomic region is highly vascular, and because of the proximity to major vessels, the pain specialist should carefully observe the patient for signs of local anesthetic toxicity during injection. This vascularity and proximity to major blood vessels also give rise to an increased incidence of postblock ecchymosis and hematoma formation, and the patient should be warned of such. Despite the vascularity of this anatomic region, this technique can be safely performed in the presence of anticoagulation by using a 25- or 27-gauge needle, albeit at increased risk of hematoma, if the clinical situation dictates a favorable risk-to-benefit ratio. These complications can be decreased if manual pressure is applied to the area of the block immediately after injection. Application of cold packs for 20-minute periods after the block will also decrease the amount of postprocedure pain and bleeding the patient may experience.

Because of the proximity to the spinal column, it is also possible to inadvertently inject the local anesthetic into the epidural, subdural, or subarachnoid space. At this level, even small amounts of local anesthetic placed into subarachnoid space may result in a total spinal anesthetic.

SUGGESTED READING

Waldman SD: Facial nerve block. In: Atlas of Interventional Pain Management, ed 2. Philadelphia, Saunders, 2004.

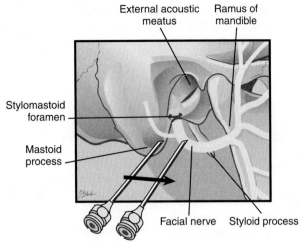

External acoustic meatus

Ramus of mandible

Stylomastoid foramen

Mastoid process

Facial nerve   Styloid process

FIGURE 239–1 Facial nerve block. (From Waldman SD: Atlas of Interventional Pain Management, ed 2. Philadelphia, Saunders, 2004, p 87.)

CHAPTER 240

Superficial Cervical Plexus Block

The superficial cervical plexus arises from fibers of the primary ventral rami of the first, second, third, and fourth cervical nerves. Each nerve divides into an ascending and a descending branch providing fibers to the nerves above and below, respectively. This collection of nerve branches makes up the cervical plexus, which provides both sensory and motor innervation. The most important motor branch is the phrenic nerve, with the plexus also providing motor fibers to the spinal accessory nerve and to the paravertebral and deep muscles of the neck. Each nerve, with the exception of the first cervical nerve, provides significant cutaneous sensory innervation. These nerves converge at the midpoint of the sternocleidomastoid muscle at its posterior margin to provide sensory innervation to the skin of the lower mandible, neck, and supraclavicular fossa. Terminal sensory fibers of the superficial cervical plexus contribute to nerves including the greater auricular and lesser occipital nerves.

To perform superficial cervical plexus block, the patient is placed in a supine position with the head turned away from the side to be blocked. A total of 15 mL of local anesthetic is drawn up in a 20-mL sterile syringe. When treating painful conditions involving the superficial cervical plexus, a total of 80 mg of depot steroid is added to the local anesthetic with the first

block and 40 mg of depot steroid is added with subsequent blocks.

The midpoint of the posterior border of the sternocleidomastoid muscle is identified by careful palpation. After preparation of the skin with antiseptic solution, a 22-gauge, 1½-inch needle is inserted at this point and is advanced just past the sternocleidomastoid muscle (Fig. 240-1). After gentle aspiration, 5 mL of solution is slowly injected. The needle is then redirected in a line that would pass just behind the lobe of the ear. After gentle aspiration, an additional 5 mL of solution is injected in a fanlike distribution. The needle is then redirected inferiorly toward the ipsilateral nipple, and after careful aspiration, the remaining 5 to 6 mL of solution is injected in a fanlike manner.

The proximity to the external jugular vein and other large vessels suggests the potential for inadvertent intravascular injection and/or local anesthetic toxicity from intravascular absorption. The pain specialist should carefully calculate the total milligram dosage of local anesthetic that may be safely given, especially if bilateral nerve blocks are being performed. This vascularity also gives rise to an increased incidence of postblock ecchymosis and hematoma formation. Despite the vascularity of this anatomic region, this technique can be safely performed in the presence of anticoagulation by using a 25- or 27-gauge needle, albeit at increased risk of hematoma, if the clinical situation dictates a favorable risk-to-benefit ratio. These complications can be decreased if manual pressure is applied to the area of the block immediately after injection. Application of cold packs for 20-minute periods after the block will also decrease the amount of postprocedure pain and bleeding the patient may experience.

In addition to the potential for complications involving the vasculature, the proximity of the superficial cervical plexus to the central neuraxial structures and the phrenic nerve can result in side effects and complications. If the needle is placed too deep, the potential for inadvertent epidural, subdural, or subarachnoid injection is a possibility. If the volume of local anesthetic used for this block is accidentally placed in any of these spaces, significant motor and sensory block will result. Unrecognized, these complications could be fatal. Additionally, blockade of the phrenic nerve occurs commonly after superficial cervical plexus block. In the absence of significant pulmonary disease, unilateral phrenic nerve block should rarely create respiratory embarrassment. However, if bilateral block is used for surgical indications, respiratory complications can occur.

SUGGESTED READING

Waldman SD: Superficial cervical plexus block. In: Atlas of Interventional Pain Management, ed 2. Philadelphia, Saunders, 2004.

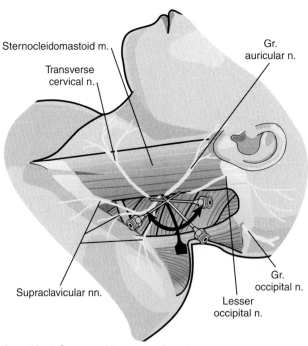

FIGURE 240–1 Superficial cervical plexus block. (From Waldman SF: Atlas of Interventional Pain Management, ed 2. Philadelphia, Saunders, 2004, p 89.)

Deep Cervical Plexus Block

The deep cervical plexus arises from fibers of the primary ventral rami of the first, second, third, and fourth cervical nerves. Each nerve divides into an ascending and descending branch providing fibers to the nerves above and below, respectively. This collection of nerve branches makes up the cervical plexus, which provides both sensory and motor innervation. The most important motor branch of the cervical plexus is the phrenic nerve. The plexus also provides motor fibers to the spinal accessory nerve and to the paravertebral and deep muscles of the neck. Each nerve, with the exception of the first cervical nerve, provides significant cutaneous sensory innervation. Terminal sensory fibers of the deep cervical plexus contribute fibers to the greater auricular and lesser occipital nerves.

To perform deep cervical plexus block, the patient is placed in a supine position with the head turned away from the side to be blocked. A total of 15 mL of local anesthetic is drawn up in a 20-mL sterile syringe. When treating painful conditions involving the deep cervical plexus, a total of 80 mg of depot steroid is added to the local anesthetic with the first block and 40 mg of depot steroid is added with subsequent blocks.

A line is drawn between the mastoid process and the posterior aspect of the insertion of the sternocleidomastoid muscle at the clavicle. A point approximately 2 inches below the mastoid process is then identified (Fig. 241-1). After preparation of the skin with antiseptic solution, a 22-gauge, 1½-inch needle is inserted at approximately ½ inch in front of the previously identified point on the line. This places the needle at the C3 or C4 level and allows a single needle to be used to block the deep cervical plexus. The needle is advanced to a depth of approximately 1 inch in a slightly anterior and caudad direction to avoid entering a neural foramen or slipping between the transverse process and entering the vertebral artery. Paresthesia will usually be elicited, and the patient should be warned of such. If paresthesia is not elicited, the needle should be withdrawn and redirected in a slightly anterior trajectory. Once paresthesia is obtained and gentle aspiration reveals no evidence of blood or cerebrospinal fluid, 15 mL of solution is slowly injected in incremental doses, with monitoring of the patient for signs of local anesthetic toxicity or inadvertent subarachnoid injection.

The proximity to the external jugular vein and other large vessels suggests the potential for inadvertent intravascular injection and/or local anesthetic toxicity from intravascular absorption. The pain specialist should carefully calculate the total milligram dosage of local anesthetic that may be safely given, especially if bilateral nerve blocks are being performed. This vascularity also gives rise to an increased incidence of postblock ecchymosis and hematoma formation. Despite the vascularity of this anatomic region, this technique can safely be performed in the presence of anticoagulation by using a 25- or 27-gauge needle, albeit at increased risk of hematoma, if the clinical situation dictates a favorable risk-to-benefit ratio. These complications can be decreased if manual pressure is applied to the area of the block immediately after injection. Application of cold packs for 20-minute periods after the block will also decrease the amount of postprocedure pain and bleeding the patient may experience.

In addition to the potential for complications involving the vasculature, the proximity of the deep cervical plexus to the central neuraxial structures and the phrenic nerve can result in side effects and complications. If the needle is placed too deep, the potential for inadvertent epidural, subdural, or subarachnoid injection is a possibility. If the volume of local anesthetic used for this block is accidentally placed in any of these spaces, significant motor and sensory block will result. Unrecognized, these complications could be fatal. Additionally, blockade of the phrenic nerve occurs commonly after deep cervical plexus block. In the absence of significant pulmonary disease, unilateral phrenic nerve block should rarely create respiratory embarrassment. However, if bilateral block is used for surgical indications, respiratory complications can occur.

SUGGESTED READING

Waldman SD: Deep cervical plexus block. In: Atlas of Interventional Pain Management, ed 2. Philadelphia, Saunders, 2004.

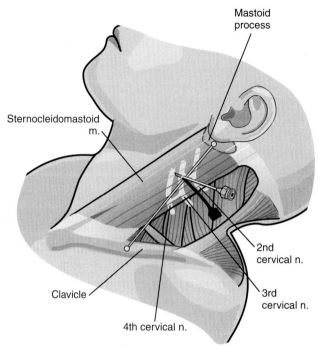

FIGURE 241–1 Deep cervical plexus block. (From Waldman SD: Atlas of Interventional Pain Management, ed 2. Philadelphia, Saunders, 2004, p 92.)

CHAPTER 242

Recurrent Laryngeal Nerve Block

The recurrent laryngeal nerves arise from the vagus nerve. The right and left nerves follow different paths to reach the larynx and trachea. The right recurrent laryngeal nerve loops underneath the innominate artery and then ascends in the lateral groove between the trachea and esophagus to enter the inferior portion of the larynx. The left recurrent laryngeal nerve loops below the arch of the aorta and then ascends in the lateral groove between the trachea and esophagus to enter the inferior portion of the larynx. These nerves provide the innervation to all the intrinsic muscles of the larynx except the cricothyroid muscle as well as providing the sensory innervation for the mucosa below the vocal cords.

To perform recurrent laryngeal nerve block, the patient is placed in a supine position with the head turned slightly away from the side to be blocked. A total of 4 mL of local anesthetic is drawn up in a 20-mL sterile syringe. When treating conditions that are mediated via the recurrent laryngeal nerve that are thought to have an inflammatory component, including pain of malignant origin, a total of 80 mg of depot steroid is added to the local anesthetic with the first block and 40 mg of depot steroid is added with subsequent blocks. Neurolytic blocks may be performed with small, incremental doses of 6.5% aqueous phenol or absolute alcohol.

The medial border of the sternocleidomastoid muscle is identified at the level of the first tracheal ring (Fig. 242-1). At this point, after preparation of the skin with antiseptic solution, a 25-gauge, ⅝-inch needle is inserted perpendicular to the skin. After inserting the needle to a depth of approximately ½ inch, gentle aspiration is carried out to identify blood or air that would indicate intratracheal placement. If the aspiration test is negative, 2 mL of solution is slowly injected, with close monitoring of the patient for signs of local anesthetic toxicity.

The proximity to the carotid artery, external jugular vein, and other vessels suggests the potential for inadvertent intravascular injection and/or local anesthetic toxicity from intravascular absorption. The pain specialist should carefully calculate the total milligram dosage of local anesthetic that may be safely given. This vascularity also gives rise to an increased incidence of postblock ecchymosis and hematoma formation. Despite the vascularity of this anatomic region, this technique can safely be performed in the presence of anticoagulation by using a 25- or 27-gauge needle, albeit at increased risk of hematoma, if the clinical situation dictates a favorable risk-to-benefit ratio. These complications can be decreased if manual pressure is applied to the area of the block immediately after injection. Application of cold packs for 20-minute periods after the block will also decrease the amount of postprocedure pain and bleeding the patient may experience.

Because the recurrent laryngeal nerves provide the innervation to all the intrinsic muscles of the larynx except the cricothyroid muscle, bilateral recurrent laryngeal nerve block is reserved for those patients who have undergone laryngectomy and/or tracheostomy, because the resulting bilateral vocal cord paralysis could result in airway obstruction.

SUGGESTED READING

Waldman SD: Recurrent laryngeal nerve block. In: Atlas of Interventional Pain Management, ed 2. Philadelphia, Saunders, 2004.

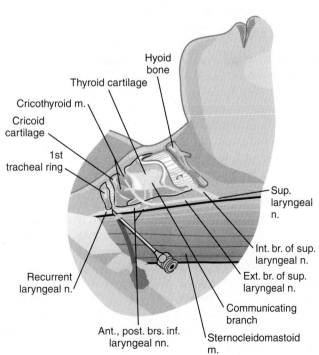

FIGURE 242–1 Recurrent laryngeal nerve block. (From Waldman SD: Atlas of Interventional Pain Management, ed 2. Philadelphia, Saunders, 2004, p 99.)

CHAPTER 243

Stellate Ganglion Block

The stellate ganglion is located on the anterior surface of the longus colli muscle. This muscle lies just anterior to the transverse processes of the seventh cervical and first thoracic vertebrae. The stellate ganglion is made up of the fused portion of the seventh cervical and first thoracic sympathetic ganglia. The stellate ganglion lies anteromedial to the vertebral artery and is medial to the common carotid artery and jugular vein. The stellate ganglion is lateral to the trachea and esophagus.

Anterior Approach

To perform blockade of the stellate ganglion using the anterior approach, the patient is placed in the supine position with the cervical spine in neutral position. From 7 to 10 mL of local anesthetic without preservative is drawn into a 12-mL sterile syringe. For disease processes that have a component of inflammation, such as acute herpes zoster, or disease processes with associated edema, such as reflex sympathetic dystrophy, 80 mg of methylprednisolone is added for the first block and 40 mg of methylprednisolone is added for subsequent blocks.

The medial edge of the sternocleidomastoid muscle is identified at the level of the cricothyroid notch (C6). The sternocleidomastoid muscle is then displaced laterally with two fingers, and the tissues overlying the transverse process of C6 (Chassaignac's tubercle) are compressed. The pulsations of the carotid artery are then identified under the palpating fingers (Fig. 243-1). The skin medial to the carotid pulsation is prepared with antiseptic solution, and a 22-gauge, 1½-inch needle is advanced until contact is made with the transverse process of C6 (Fig. 243-2). If bony contact is not made with needle insertion to a depth of 1 inch, the needle is probably between the transverse processes of C6 and C7. If this occurs, the needle should be withdrawn and re-inserted with a more cephalad trajectory. After bony contact is made, the needle is then withdrawn approximately 2 mm to bring the needle tip out of the body of the longus colli muscle. Careful aspiration is carried out, and 7 to 10 mL of solution is then injected.

Vertebral Body Approach

To perform blockade of the stellate ganglion utilizing the vertebral body approach, the patient is placed in the supine position with the cervical spine in neutral position. From 3 to 5 mL of local anesthetic is drawn into a 12-mL sterile syringe. For disease processes that have a component of inflammation, such as acute herpes zoster, or disease processes with associated edema, such as reflex sympathetic dystrophy, 80 mg of methylprednisolone is added for the first block and 40 mg of methylprednisolone is added for subsequent blocks. For neurolytic blocks, 3 to 5 mL of absolute alcohol or 6.5% aqueous phenol given in incremental doses is used. Neurolytic blocks should be done under computed tomography or fluoroscopic guidance unless the clinical situation dictates that the block be done at the bedside.

If radiographic guidance is used, the junction of the C7 transverse process with the vertebral body is identified. If a blind technique is used, the medial edge of the sternocleidomastoid muscle is identified at the level of the inferior margin of the cricoid cartilage, which is at the level of C7. The sternocleidomastoid muscle is then displaced laterally with two fingers, and the tissues overlying the transverse process of C7 are compressed. The pulsations of the carotid artery are then identified under the palpating fingers. The skin medial to the carotid pulsation is prepared with antiseptic solution, and a 22-gauge, 3½-inch spinal needle is advanced in a slightly inferior and medial trajectory until contact is made with the junction of the transverse process of C7 with the vertebral body (Fig. 243-3). If bony contact is not made with needle insertion to a depth of 1½ inches, the needle is probably either too lateral or has slid between the transverse processes of C7 and T1. If this occurs, the needle should be withdrawn and re-inserted with a more medial and inferior trajectory. After bony contact is made, the needle is then withdrawn slightly to bring the needle tip out of the periosteum of the junction of the transverse process and the vertebral body (see Fig. 243-2). Careful aspiration is carried out, and 3 to 5 mL of local anesthetic and/or steroid is injected. If neurolytic solution is being used, small incremental doses are injected with time between doses given to allow for the adequate assessment of clinical response. To obtain adequate destruction of the stellate ganglion and associated sympathetic nerves, additional increments of neurolytic solution may have to be injected at the middle of the C7 transverse process and at a point 1 cm inferior on the anteromedial margin of the vertebral body. Radiofrequency lesioning or cryoneurolysis may represent safer alternatives to destruction of the stellate ganglion.

This anatomic region is highly vascular, and because of the proximity of major vessels, the pain specialist should carefully observe the patient for signs of local anesthetic toxicity during injection. This vascularity and proximity to major blood vessels also give rise to an increased incidence of postblock ecchymosis and hematoma formation, and the patient should be warned of such. Despite the vascularity of this anatomic region, this technique can safely be performed in the presence of anticoagulation by using a 25- or 27-gauge needle, albeit at increased risk of hematoma, if the clinical situation dictates a favorable risk-to-benefit ratio. These complications can be decreased if manual pressure is applied to the area of the block immediately after injection. Application of cold packs for 20-minute periods after the block will also decrease the amount of postprocedure pain and bleeding the patient may experience.

Because of the proximity to the spinal column, it is also possible to inadvertently inject the local anesthetic solution into the epidural, subdural, or subarachnoid space. At this level, even small amounts of local anesthetic placed into the subarachnoid space may result in a total spinal anesthetic. If needle placement is too inferior, pneumothorax is possible, because the dome of the lung lies at the level of the C7-T1 interspace.

Additional side effects associated with stellate ganglion block include inadvertent block of the recurrent laryngeal nerve with associated hoarseness, dysphagia, difficulty coughing, and the sensation that there is a lump in the throat when swallowing. Horner's syndrome occurs when the superior cervical sympathetic ganglion is also blocked during stellate ganglion block. The patient should be forewarned of the possibility of these complications prior to stellate ganglion block.

SUGGESTED READINGS

Waldman SD: Stellate ganglion block: Anterior approach. In: Atlas of Interventional Pain Management, ed 2. Philadelphia, Saunders, 2004.

Waldman SD: Stellate ganglion block: Posterior approach. In: Atlas of Interventional Pain Management, ed 2. Philadelphia, Saunders, 2004.

Waldman SD: Stellate ganglion block: Vertebral body approach. In: Atlas of Interventional Pain Management, ed 2. Philadelphia, Saunders, 2004.

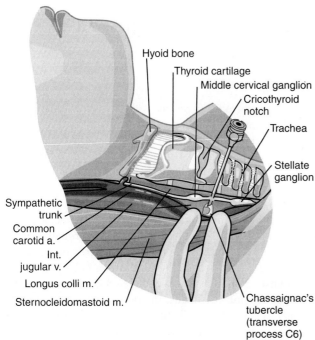

FIGURE 243–1 Identification of anatomic landmarks for stellate ganglion block. (From Waldman SD: Atlas of Interventional Pain Management, ed 2. Philadelphia, Saunders, 2004, p 101.)

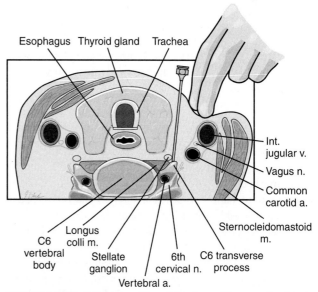

FIGURE 243–2 Correct needle position for stellate ganglion block. (From Waldman SD: Atlas of Interventional Pain Management, ed 2. Philadelphia, Saunders, 2004, p 101.)

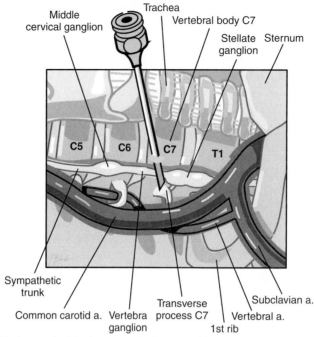

FIGURE 243–3 Stellate ganglion block: vertebral body approach. (From Waldman SD: Atlas of Interventional Pain Management, ed 2. Philadelphia, Saunders, 2004, p 110.)

CHAPTER 244

Radiofrequency Lesioning of the Stellate Ganglion

To perform radiofrequency lesioning of the stellate ganglion, the patient is placed in the supine position with the cervical spine in a slightly extended position. Then 3 mL of local anesthetic combined with 3.0 mL of water-soluble contrast media is drawn into a 12-mL sterile syringe. Using computed tomographic or fluoroscopic guidance, the junction of the C7 transverse process with the vertebral body is identified and the skin marked with a gentian violet marker. The palpating index and ring fingers of the nondominant hand should then identify the medial edge of the sternocleidomastoid muscle at the level of the inferior margin of the cricoid cartilage, which is at the level of C7. The sternocleidomastoid muscle is then displaced laterally with two fingers, and the tissues overlying the transverse process of C7 are compressed. The pulsations of the carotid artery are then identified under the palpating fingers. The skin medial to the carotid pulsation is prepared with antiseptic solution and anesthetized with local anesthetic. Using intermittent fluoroscopic guidance,

a 16-gauge introducer needle is directed toward the previously identified junction of the C7 transverse process with the vertebral body. A 20-gauge, curved, 54-cm radiofrequency needle with a 4-mm active tip is guided through the introducer and is advanced in a slightly inferior and medial trajectory until contact is made with the junction of the transverse process of C7 with the vertebral body (Fig. 244-1). If bony contact is not made with needle insertion to a depth of 1½ inches, the needle is probably either too lateral or has slid between the transverse processes of C7 and T1. If this occurs, the needle should be withdrawn and reinserted with a more medial and inferior trajectory. After bony contact is made, the needle is then withdrawn slightly to bring the needle tip out of the periosteum of the junction of the transverse process and the vertebral body. Careful aspiration is carried out, and 3 to 5 mL of the mixture of local anesthetic and contrast is injected. The contrast and local anesthetic should spread anterior to the vertebra in a cephalad and caudad direction.

No epidural, subdural, subarachnoid, intramuscular, or intravascular contrast spread should be observed. A trial stimulation of both the sensory nerves at 50 Hz, 0.9 V and motor nerves at 2 Hz, 2 V should be carried out owing to proximity of the phrenic and recurrent laryngeal nerves.

Stimulation of the phrenic nerve suggests that the needle placement is too lateral, and stimulation of the recurrent laryngeal nerve suggests that the needle is too anterior and medial. Having the patient phonate with a prolonged "ee" during stimulation will help identify stimulation of these neural structures.

After satisfactory needle placement has been confirmed, a radiofrequency lesion is made by heating at 80° C for 60 seconds or pulsed RF at 45° C to 50° C for a longer duration. The stimulating needle is then redirected in the same plane to the most medial aspect of the transverse process and both motor and sensory trial stimulation is repeated as described (see Fig. 244-1). If no evidence of stimulation of motor or sensory nerves is observed, a second lesion is made. The needle is then redirected to the uppermost portion of the junction of the C7 transverse process and the vertebral body. If trial stimulation fails to reveal stimulation of motor or sensory nerves, a third lesion is made. The stimulating needle is removed and gentle pressure is placed on the site to decrease the incidence of ecchymosis and hematoma formation.

Because of the proximity to the spinal canal, it is also possible to unintentionally inject the local anesthetic or neurolytic solution into the epidural, subdural, or subarachnoid space. At this level, even small amounts of local anesthetic placed into the subarachnoid space may result in a total spinal anesthetic. Radiofrequency lesioning of the neuraxial structures at this level can result in significant neurologic dysfunction, including quadriparesis. Unintentional lesioning of the phrenic nerve can result in diaphragmatic paralysis and respiratory embarrassment. Inadvertent lesioning of recurrent laryngeal nerve can result in prolonged or permanent hoarseness. A permanent Horner's syndrome may occur when the superior cervical sympathetic ganglion is damaged during this procedure.

Because of the more inferior needle placement with the vertebral body approach to stellate ganglion block, pneumothorax is a distinct possibility, especially on the right. All of the complications mentioned can be decreased with the use of careful trial stimulation and the use of radiographic guidance.

This anatomic region is highly vascular, and because of the proximity of major vessels, the pain specialist should carefully observe the patient for signs of local anesthetic toxicity during injection. This vascularity and proximity to major blood vessels also give rise to an increased incidence of postblock ecchymosis and hematoma formation, and the patient should be warned of such. These complications can be disastrous if neurolytic solution is used. The patient should be forewarned of the possibility of all of these complications before radiofrequency lesioning of the stellate ganglion is attempted.

SUGGESTED READING

Waldman SD: Stellate ganglion block—Radiofrequency lesioning. In: Atlas of Interventional Pain Management, ed 2. Philadelphia, Saunders, 2004.

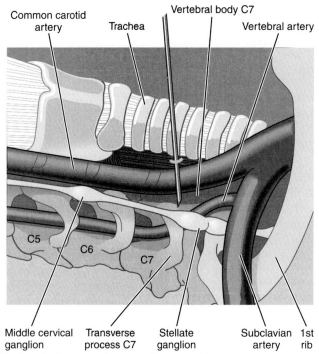

FIGURE 244–1 Stellate ganglion block: radiofrequency lesioning. (From Waldman SD: Atlas of Interventional Pain Management, ed 2. Philadelphia, Saunders, 2004, p 112.)

CHAPTER 245

Cervical Facet Block

The cervical facet joints are formed by the articulations of the superior and inferior articular facets of adjacent vertebrae. Except for the atlanto-occipital and atlantoaxial joints, the remaining cervical facet joints are true joints in that they are lined with synovium and possess a true joint capsule. This capsule is richly innervated and supports the notion of the facet joint as a pain generator. The cervical facet joint is susceptible to arthritic changes and trauma caused by acceleration-deceleration injuries. Such damage to the joint results in pain secondary to synovial joint inflammation and adhesions.

Each facet joint receives innervation from two spinal levels. Each joint receives fibers from the dorsal ramus at the same level as the vertebra as well as fibers from the dorsal ramus of the vertebra above. This fact has clinical import in that it provides an explanation for the ill-defined nature of facet-mediated pain and also explains why the dorsal nerve from the vertebra above the

offending level must often also be blocked to provide complete pain relief.

At each level, the dorsal ramus provides a medial branch that wraps around the convexity of the articular pillar of its respective vertebra. This location is constant for the C4-7 nerves and allows a simplified approach for treatment of cervical facet syndrome.

Medial Branch Technique

Cervical facet block using the medial branch technique is the preferred route of treating cervical facet syndrome. It may be done either blind or under fluoroscopic guidance. The patient is placed in a prone position. Pillows are placed under the chest to allow the cervical spine to be moderately flexed without discomfort to the patient. The forehead is allowed to rest on a folded blanket.

BLIND TECHNIQUE

If a blind technique is used, the spinous process at the level to be blocked is identified by palpation. A point slightly inferior and 2.5 cm lateral to the spinous process is then identified as the site of needle insertion. After preparation of the skin with antiseptic solution, a skin wheal of local anesthetic is raised at the site of needle insertion. Then 3 mL of preservative-free local anesthetic is drawn up in a 5-mL sterile syringe. When treating pain thought to be secondary to an inflammatory process, a total of 80 mg of depot steroid is added to the local anesthetic with the first block and 40 mg of depot steroid is added with subsequent blocks.

An 18-gauge, 1-inch needle is inserted through the skin and into the subcutaneous tissue at the previously identified insertion site to serve as an introducer. The introducer needle is then repositioned with a slightly superior and medial trajectory, pointing directly toward the posterior aspect of the articular pillar at the level to be blocked. A 25-gauge, 3½-inch styletted spinal needle is then inserted through the 18-gauge introducer and directed toward the articular pillar. After bony contact is made, the depth of the contact is noted and the spinal needle is withdrawn. The introducer needle is then repositioned aiming toward the lateralmost aspect of the articular pillar. The 25-gauge spinal needle is then readvanced until it impinges on the lateralmost aspect of the border of the articular pillar (Fig. 245-1). Should the spinal needle "walk off" the lateral aspect of the articular pillar, it is withdrawn and redirected slightly medially and carefully advanced to the depth of the previous bony contact (Fig. 245-2).

After the needle is felt to be in satisfactory position, the stylet is removed from the 25-gauge spinal needle and the hub is observed for blood or cerebrospinal fluid (CSF). If neither is present, gentle aspiration of the needle is carried out. If the aspiration test is negative, 1.5 mL of solution is injected through the spinal needle.

FLUOROSCOPIC TECHNIQUE

If fluoroscopy is used, the beam is rotated in a sagittal plane from anterior to posterior position, which allows identification and visualization of the articular pillars of the respective vertebrae. After preparation of the skin with antiseptic solution, a skin wheal of local anesthetic is raised at the site of needle insertion. An 18-gauge, 1-inch needle is inserted at the insertion site to serve as an introducer. The fluoroscopy beam is aimed directly through the introducer needle, which will appear as a small point on the fluoroscopy screen. The introducer needle is then repositioned under fluoroscopic guidance until this small point is visualized pointing directly toward the posterior aspect of the articular pillar at the level to be blocked.

A total of 5 mL of contrast medium suitable for intrathecal use is drawn up in a sterile 12-mL syringe. Then, 3 mL of preservative-free local anesthetic is drawn up in a separate 5-mL sterile syringe. When treating pain thought to be secondary to an inflammatory process, a total of 80 mg of depot steroid is added to the local anesthetic with the first block and 40 mg of depot steroid is added with subsequent blocks.

A 25-gauge, 3½-inch styletted spinal needle is then inserted through the 18-gauge introducer and directed toward the articular pillar. After bony contact is made, the spinal needle is withdrawn and the introducer needle repositioned toward the lateralmost aspect of the articular pillar. The 25-gauge spinal needle is then re-advanced until it impinges on the lateralmost aspect of the border of the articular pillar.

After confirmation of needle placement by biplanar fluoroscopy, the stylet is removed from the 25-gauge spinal needle and the hub is observed for blood or CSF. If neither is present, gentle aspiration of the needle is carried out. If the aspiration test is negative, 1 mL of contrast medium is slowly injected under fluoroscopic guidance to reconfirm needle placement. After correct needle placement is confirmed, 1.5 mL of local anesthetic with or without steroid is injected through the spinal needle.

Intra-articular Technique

BLIND TECHNIQUE

If a blind technique is used, the spinous process at the level to be blocked is identified by palpation. A point two spinal levels lower and 2.5 cm lateral to the spinous process is then identified as the site of needle insertion. Then 3 mL of preservative-free local anesthetic is drawn up in a 5-mL sterile syringe. After preparation of the skin with antiseptic solution, a skin wheal of local anesthetic is raised at the site of needle insertion. When treating pain thought to be secondary to an inflammatory process, a total of 80 mg of depot steroid is added to the local anesthetic with the first block and 40 mg of depot steroid is added with subsequent blocks.

An 18-gauge, 1-inch needle is inserted through the skin and into the subcutaneous tissues at the previously identified insertion site to serve as an introducer. The introducer needle is then repositioned with a superior and ventral trajectory, pointing directly toward the inferior margin of the facet joint at the level to be blocked. The angle of the needle from the skin is approximately 35 degrees. A 25-gauge, 3½-inch styletted spinal needle is then inserted through the 18-gauge introducer and directed toward the articular pillar just below the joint to be blocked. Care must be taken to be sure the trajectory of the needle does not drift either laterally or medially. Medial drift can allow the needle to enter the epidural, subdural, or subarachnoid space and to traumatize the dorsal root or spinal cord. Lateral drift can allow the needle to pass beyond the lateral border of the articular pillar and traumatize the vertebral artery or exiting nerve roots.

After bony contact is made, the depth of the contact is noted and the spinal needle is withdrawn. The introducer needle is then redirected slightly more superiorly. The spinal needle is then advanced through the introducer needle until it impinges on the bone of the articular pillar. This maneuver is repeated until the spinal needle slides into the facet joint (Fig. 245-3). A pop is often felt as the needle slides into the joint cavity.

After the needle is felt to be in satisfactory position, the stylet is removed from the 25-gauge spinal needle and the hub is observed for blood or CSF. If neither is present, gentle aspiration of the needle is carried out. If the aspiration test is negative, 1 mL of solution is injected slowly through the spinal needle. Rapid or forceful injection may rupture the joint capsule and exacerbate the patient's pain.

FLUOROSCOPIC TECHNIQUE

If fluoroscopy is used, the beam is rotated in a sagittal plane from anterior to posterior position, which allows identification and visualization of the articular pillars of the respective vertebrae and the adjacent facet joints. After preparation of the skin with antiseptic solution, a skin wheal of local anesthetic is raised at the site of needle insertion. An 18-gauge, 1-inch needle is inserted at the insertion site to serve as an introducer. The fluoroscopy beam is aimed directly through the introducer needle, which will appear as a small point on the fluoroscopy screen. The introducer needle is then repositioned under fluoroscopic guidance until this small point is visualized pointing directly toward the inferior aspect of the facet joint to be blocked.

A total of 5 mL of contrast medium suitable for intrathecal use is drawn up in a sterile 12-mL syringe. Then, 2 mL of preservative-free local anesthetic is drawn up in a separate 5-mL sterile syringe. When treating pain thought to be secondary to an inflammatory process, a total of 80 mg of depot steroid is added to the local anesthetic with the first block and 40 mg of depot steroid is added with subsequent blocks.

A 25-gauge, 3½-inch styletted spinal needle is then inserted through the 18-gauge introducer and directed toward the articular pillar just below the joint to be blocked. After bony contact is made, the spinal needle is withdrawn and the introducer needle repositioned superiorly, aiming toward the facet joint itself. The 25-gauge spinal needle is then re-advanced through the introducer needle until it enters the target joint.

After confirmation of needle placement by biplanar fluoroscopy, the stylet is removed from the 25-gauge spinal needle and the hub is observed for blood or CSF. If neither is present, gentle aspiration of the needle is carried out. If the aspiration test is negative, 1 mL of contrast medium is slowly injected under fluoroscopic guidance to reconfirm needle placement. After correct needle placement is confirmed, 1 mL of local anesthetic with or without steroid is slowly injected through the spinal needle. Rapid or forceful injection may rupture the joint capsule and exacerbate the patient's pain.

The proximity to the spinal cord and exiting nerve roots makes it imperative that this procedure be carried out only by those well versed in the regional anatomy and experienced in performing interventional pain management techniques. The proximity to the vertebral artery combined with the vascular nature of this anatomic region makes the potential for intravascular injection high. Even small amounts of injection of local anesthetic into the vertebral arteries will result in seizures. Given the proximity of the brain and brainstem, ataxia due to vascular uptake of local anesthetic is not an uncommon occurrence after cervical facet block. Many patients also complain of a transient increase in headache and cervicalgia after injection into the joint.

SUGGESTED READINGS

Waldman SD: Cervical facet block—Medial branch technique. In: Atlas of Interventional Pain Management, ed 2. Philadelphia, Saunders, 2004.

Waldman SD: Cervical facet block—Intra-articular technique. In: Atlas of Interventional Pain Management, ed 2. Philadelphia, Saunders, 2004.

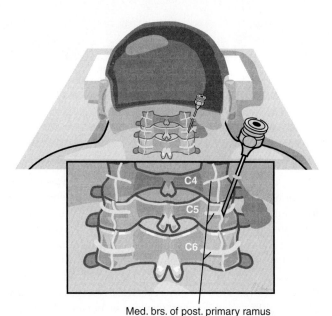

FIGURE 245–1 Cervical facet block: medial branch technique. (From Waldman SD: Atlas of Interventional Pain Management, ed 2. Philadelphia, Saunders, 2004, p 117.)

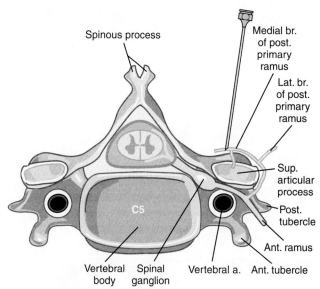

FIGURE 245–2 Correct needle position for cervical facet block. (From Waldman SD: Atlas of Interventional Pain Management, ed 2. Philadelphia, Saunders, 2004, p 117.)

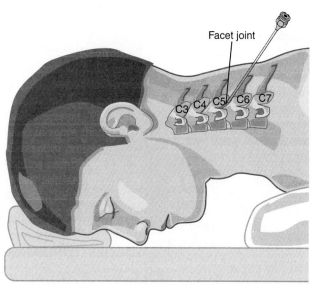

FIGURE 245–3 Cervical facet block: intra-articular technique. (From Waldman SD: Atlas of Interventional Pain Management, ed 2. Philadelphia, Saunders, 2004, p 127.)

CHAPTER 246

Radiofrequency Lesioning of the Cervical Medial Branch

Radiofrequency lesioning of the cervical facet joints by disrupting the corresponding medial branches of the affected cervical facet joints is the preferred route of denervating the cervical facet joints. This technique is best performed under fluoroscopic or computed tomographic guidance.

Posterior Approach

The patient is placed in a prone position. Pillows are placed under the chest to allow the cervical spine to be moderately flexed without discomfort to the patient. The forehead is allowed to rest on a folded blanket.

To properly position the radiofrequency cannula, the fluoroscopy beam is rotated in order to obtain a lateral view. The center of the neural arch at the targeted level is then identified. After preparation of the skin with antiseptic solution, a skin wheal of local anesthetic is raised at the site of needle insertion. A 22-gauge 2-inch needle is then inserted using "tunnel vision" so as to contact bone at the centroid of the neural arch. The fluoroscope beam is then rotated to provide a clear anteroposterior view of the waist of the articular pillar.

A 22-gauge, 4-mm active tip radiofrequency needle is then inserted through the skin and directed under anteroposterior fluoroscopic guidance toward the needle previously placed at the center of the neural arch. The needle should be noted to lie at the waist of the vertebra on anteroposterior view, just posterior to the foramen on the foraminal view, and covering the centroid, and therefore in close proximity to the medial branch in the lateral view (Fig. 246-1).

Foraminal Approach

The patient is positioned in the supine position. The skin overlying the anterior and ipsilateral region overlying the target vertebra is prepared with antiseptic solution. A lateral view is obtained with the fluoroscope and then rotated to demonstrate the foramen in its largest diameter. The fluoroscope beam is then moved caudally until the foramen is seen in its maximal dimension, which will place the beam parallel to the exiting nerve root. The targeted level is again confirmed, and the skin is anesthetized with local anesthetic over an area two times the width of the neural arch to a point even with the lower third of the foramen. A radiofrequency cannula is then inserted and advanced so as to contact bone one fourth to one third the distance between the foramen and the posterior border of the articular pillar. An anteroposterior view will confirm the cannula tip as lying at the waist of the articular column. After confirmation of proper needle placement, stimulation at 50 Hz is carried out with the patient reporting stimulation between 0.1 and 0.5 V. This should reproduce the patient's pain pattern, although the quality may not be perceived as identical by the patient. Motor stimulation of the radiofrequency cannula at 2 to 3 V at 2 Hz is increased slowly. There should be no stimulation of the upper extremity at 2½ to 3 times the voltage required for the patient to perceive sensory stimulation. If motor stimulation of the upper extremity is identified, the radiofrequency needle must be repositioned away from the cervical nerve root. After injection of local anesthetic, a radiofrequency lesion is then made at 80 degrees for 60 to 90 seconds. The needle is then repositioned superiorly or inferiorly 2 to 3 mm and a second lesion is repeated. This technique is repeated at each targeted level with care being taken to complete trial stimulation each time the radiofrequency electrode is repositioned.

The proximity to the spinal cord, exiting nerve roots, and vascular structures make it imperative that this procedure be carried out only by those well versed in the regional anatomy and experienced in performing interventional pain management techniques. The proximity to the vertebral artery combined with the vascular nature of this anatomic region makes the potential for intravascular injection or trauma to the vessel high. Even small amounts of injection of local anesthetic into the vertebral arteries will result in seizures. Given the proximity of the brain and brainstem, ataxia due to vascular uptake of local anesthetic is not an uncommon occurrence after cervical facet block. Many patients also complain of a transient increase in headache and cervicalgia after radiofrequency lesioning of these structures, and the routine injection of methylprednisolone or other steroids during or after radiofrequency lesioning may decrease the frequency of the annoying side effect.

SUGGESTED READING

Waldman SD: Cervical facet neurolysis: Radiofrequency lesioning of the cervical medial branch. In: Atlas of Interventional Pain Management, ed 2. Philadelphia, Saunders, 2004.

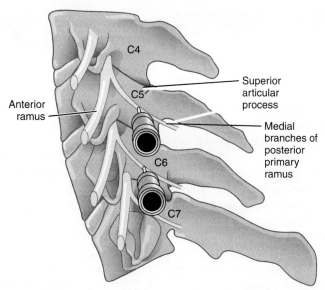

FIGURE 246–1 Radiofrequency lesioning of the cervical medial branch: posterior approach. (From Waldman SD: Atlas of Interventional Pain Management, ed 2. Philadelphia, Saunders, 2004, p 122.)

Cervical Epidural Nerve Block—Translaminar Approach

The superior boundary of the cervical epidural space is the fusion of the periosteal and spinal layers of dural at the foramen magnum. It should be recognized that these structures will allow drugs injected into the cervical epidural space to travel beyond their confines if the volume of injectate is large enough. This fact probably explains many of the early problems associated with the use of cervical epidural nerve block for surgical anesthesia when the large volumes of local anesthetics in vogue at the time were injected.

The epidural space continues inferiorly to the sacrococcygeal membrane. The cervical epidural space is bounded anteriorly by the posterior longitudinal ligament and posteriorly by the vertebral laminae and the ligamentum flavum. It should be noted that the ligamentum flavum is relatively thin in the cervical region, thickening as it continues inferiorly to the lumbar spine. This fact has direct clinical implications in that the loss of resistance when performing cervical epidural nerve block is more subtle than when performing the loss-of-resistance technique in the lumbar or lower thoracic region.

The vertebral pedicles and intervertebral foramina form the lateral limits of the epidural space. The degenerative changes and narrowing of the intervertebral foramina associated with aging may be marked in the cervical region. This results in a decreased leakage of local anesthetic out of the foramina, accounting in part for the decreased local anesthetic dosage requirements in the elderly when performing cervical epidural nerve block.

The distance between the ligamentum flavum and dura is greatest at the L2 interspace measuring 5 to 6 mm in the adult. Because of the enlargement of the cervical spinal cord corresponding to the neuromeres serving the upper extremities, this distance is decreased to 1.5 to 2.0 mm at the seventh cervical vertebra. It should be noted that flexion of the neck moves this cervical enlargement superiorly, resulting in a widening of the epidural space to 3.0 to 4.0 mm at the C7-T1 interspace. This fact has important clinical implications if cervical epidural block is performed in the lateral or prone positions.

Contents of the Epidural Space

FAT

The epidural space is filled with fatty areolar tissue. The amount of epidural fat varies in direct proportion to the amount of fat stored elsewhere in the body. The epidural fat is relatively vascular and appears to change to a denser consistency with aging. This change in consistency may account for the significant variations in required drug dosage in adults especially when utilizing the caudal approach to the epidural space. The epidural fat appears to perform two functions: (1) it serves as a shock absorber for the other contents of the epidural space as well as the dura and the contents of the dural sac; and (2) it serves as a depot for drugs injected into the cervical epidural space. This second function has direct clinical implications when choosing opioids for cervical epidural administration.

EPIDURAL VEINS

The epidural veins are concentrated primarily in the anterolateral portion of the epidural space. These veins are valveless and hence transmit both the intrathoracic and intra-abdominal pressures. As pressures in either of these body cavities increase because of Valsalva or compression of the inferior vena cava by the gravid uterus or tumor mass, the epidural veins distend and decrease the volume of the epidural space. This decrease in volume can directly affect the volume of drug needed to obtain a given level of neural blockade. Because this venous plexus serves the entire spinal column, it serves as a ready conduit for the spread of hematogenous infection.

EPIDURAL ARTERIES

The arteries that supply the bony and ligamentous confines of the cervical epidural space as well as the cervical spinal cord enter the cervical epidural space via two routes: (1) the intervertebral foramina, and (2) direct anastomoses from the intracranial portions of the vertebral arteries. There are significant anastomoses between the epidural arteries. The epidural arteries lie primarily in the lateral portions of the epidural space. Trauma to the epidural arteries can result in epidural hematoma formation and/or compromise of the blood supply of the spinal cord itself.

LYMPHATICS

The lymphatics of the epidural space are concentrated in the region of the dural roots where they remove foreign material from the subarachnoid and epidural space.

Structures Encountered During Midline Insertion of a Needle Into the Cervical Epidural Space

After traversing the skin and subcutaneous tissues, the styletted epidural needle will impinge on the supraspinous ligament, which runs vertically between the apices of the spinous processes (Fig. 247-1). The supraspinous ligament offers some resistance to the advancing needle. This ligament is dense enough to hold a needle in position even when the needle is released.

The interspinous ligament, which runs obliquely between the spinous processes, is next encountered offering additional resistance to needle advancement. Because the interspinous ligament is contiguous with the ligamentum flavum, the pain management specialist may perceive a "false" loss of resistance when the needle tip enters the space between the interspinous ligament and the ligamentum flavum. This phenomenon is more pronounced in the cervical region than in the lumbar, owing to the less well-defined ligaments.

A significant increase in resistance to needle advancement signals that the needle tip is impinging on the dense ligamentum flavum. Because the ligament is made up almost entirely of elastin fibers, there is a continued increase in resistance as the needle traverses the ligamentum flavum due to the drag of the ligament on the needle (Fig. 247-2). A sudden loss of resistance occurs as the needle tip enters the epidural space (Fig. 247-3). There should be essentially no resistance to drugs injected into the normal epidural space.

PITFALLS IN NEEDLE PLACEMENT

Although a comprehensive discussion of the pitfalls in needle placement when performing cervical epidural block is beyond the scope of this chapter, suffice to say that careful attention must be paid to the site of needle entry, needle trajectory, and end point of the needle tip, or a failed block may result. Trauma to the nerves, arteries, veins, the dural sac and its contents may also occur, with the potential for disastrous results.

Technique of Cervical Epidural Nerve Block

All equipment, including the needles and supplies for nerve block, the drugs, resuscitation equipment, oxygen supply, and suction, must be assembled and checked prior to beginning cervical epidural nerve block. Informed consent is obtained prior to implementation of cervical epidural nerve block.

POSITIONING OF THE PATIENT

Cervical epidural nerve block may be carried out in the sitting, lateral, or prone position. Each position has its own advantages and disadvantages.

The sitting position is easier for the patient and pain management specialist alike. This position not only enhances the operator's ability to identify the midline, it ensures that the cervical spine is flexed resulting in a widening of the lower cervical epidural space. The sitting position avoids the problem of rotation of the spine inherent in the use of the lateral position, which makes identification of the epidural space difficult.

The use of the sitting position may be limited because of the patient's inability to assume the sitting position (i.e., patients with acute vertebral compression fractures). A history of vasovagal syncope with previous needle punctures precludes the use of this position. In such patients, the lateral position is preferred.

As mentioned, the lateral position is preferred in those patients who cannot assume the sitting position or who are prone to vasovagal attacks. For reasons of patient comfort, the lateral position is more suitable for placement of tunneled epidural catheters or other implantable devices with an epidural terminus. If the lateral position is chosen, care must be taken to ensure that there is no rotation of the patient's spine, which will make epidural nerve block exceedingly difficult if not impossible. Furthermore, flexion of the cervical spine is mandatory to maximize the width of the epidural space.

The prone position is used primarily for placement of tunneled epidural catheters and spinal stimulator electrodes. As with other approaches to the cervical epidural space, care must be taken to flex the cervical spine to widen the epidural space. The prone position should be avoided if sedation is required because access to the airway is limited should problems occur.

Preblock Preparation

After the patient is placed in optimal position, the skin is prepped with an antiseptic solution such as povidone-iodine so that all of the surface landmarks can be palpated aseptically. A fenestrated sterile drape is placed to avoid contamination of the palpating fingers.

The interspace suitable for the intended epidural block is identified. At the level of this interspace, the operator's middle and index fingers are placed on each side of the spinous processes. The position of the interspace is reconfirmed with palpation using a rocking motion in the superior and inferior planes. The midline of the selected interspace is identified by palpating the spinous processes above and below the interspace using a lateral rocking motion to ensure that the needle entry site is exactly in the midline. Failure to accurately identify the midline is

the most common reason for difficulty in performing cervical epidural nerve block.

Choice of Needle

The 3½-inch 18-gauge Hustead or Tuohy needle is suitable for cervical epidural block for the vast majority of adult patients; however, the sharper Tuohy needle may result in an increased incidence of dural punctures. Many centers are now using sharper smaller-gauge needles (e.g., 22-gauge spinal needles) with equally good results. These smaller needles decrease the amount of procedure-related and postprocedure pain.

Identification of the Epidural Space

The choice of technique used to identify the epidural space is usually based on the pain management specialist's previous training and personal experience rather than on scientific data. It is the consensus of most experts that the loss-of-resistance technique for the identification of the epidural space has significant advantages over the hanging-drop technique. Because the hanging-drop method is associated with a 2.0% failure rate as compared with less than 0.5% rate for the loss-of-resistance technique, the hanging-drop technique cannot be recommended.

THE LOSS-OF-RESISTANCE TECHNIQUE

After careful identification of the midline at the chosen interspace using the technique described earlier, 1 mL of local anesthetic is utilized to infiltrate the skin, subcutaneous tissues, and the supraspinous and interspinous ligament. Large amounts of local anesthetic should be avoided because they disrupt the ligamentous fibers contributing to postprocedure pain.

The styletted needle is inserted exactly in the midline in the previously anesthetized area through the supraspinous ligament into the interspinous ligament. The needle stylet is removed, and a well-lubricated 5-mL glass syringe filled with preservative-free sterile saline is attached. Because saline is incompressible, it provides better tactile feedback than air. Additionally, saline avoids the risk of air embolism via the cervical epidural veins.

The right-handed physician holds the epidural needle firmly at the hub with his or her left thumb and index finger. The left hand is placed firmly against the patient's neck to ensure against uncontrolled needle movements should the patient unexpectedly move. The right hand holds the syringe with the thumb, exerting continuous firm pressure on the plunger. The needle should never be advanced without simultaneous pressure on the plunger. Ballottement of the plunger as advocated by some clinicians should not be used because it will increase the incidence of inadvertent dural puncture.

With constant pressure being applied to the plunger of the syringe with the thumb of the right hand, the needle and syringe are continuously advanced in a slow and deliberate manner with the left hand. As soon as the needle bevel passes through the ligamentum flavum and enters the epidural space, there will be a sudden loss of resistance to injection and the plunger will effortlessly surge forward. This loss of resistance provides the operator with visual as well as tactile feedback that the needle bevel has entered the epidural space. The syringe is gently removed from the needle.

An air or saline acceptance test is carried out by injecting 0.5 to 1.0 mL of air or sterile preservative-free saline with a well-lubricated sterile glass syringe to help confirm that the needle is within the epidural space. The force required for injection should not exceed that necessary to overcome the resistance of the needle. Any significant pain or sudden increases in resistance during injection suggest incorrect needle placement, and one should stop injecting immediately and reassess the position of the needle.

INJECTION OF DRUGS

When satisfactory needle position is confirmed, a syringe containing the drugs to be injected is carefully attached to the needle. Gentle aspiration is carried out to identify cerebrospinal fluid or blood. Inadvertent dural puncture can occur in the best of hands, and careful observation for spinal fluid is mandatory. If cerebrospinal fluid is aspirated, the epidural block may be repeated at a different interspace. In this situation, drug dosages should be adjusted accordingly, because subarachnoid migration of drugs through the dural rent can occur.

Aspiration of blood can be due either to damage to veins during insertion of the needle into the cervical epidural space or, less commonly, due to intravenous placement of the needle. If aspiration of blood occurs, the needle should be rotated slightly and the aspiration test repeated. If no blood is present, incremental doses of local anesthetic and other drugs may be administered while monitoring the patient carefully for signs of local anesthetic toxicity or untoward reactions to the other drugs injected.

CHOICE OF LOCAL ANESTHETIC

The spread of drugs injected into the cervical epidural space is dependent on the volume and speed of injection, the anatomic variations of the epidural space, the degree of dilatation of the epidural veins, and the position, age, and height of the patient. The pregnant patient will require a significantly lower volume to achieve the same level of blockade compared with nongravid control subjects.

Local anesthetics capable of producing adequate sensory block of the cervical nerve roots when administered via the cervical epidural route include 1.0% lidocaine, 0.25% bupivacaine, 2% 2-chloroprocaine, and 1.0% mepivacaine. Increasing the concentration of drug will increase the amount of motor block and speed the onset of action. The addition of epinephrine will decrease the amount of systemic absorption and slightly increase the duration of action. A 5- to 7-mL volume of the drugs mentioned will generally be adequate for most pain management applications in the adult population. Significant intrapatient variability exists, however, and additional incremental doses of local anesthetic may have to be administered to ensure adequate anesthesia in some adult patients. All local anesthetics administered via the cervical epidural route should be formulated for epidural use.

For diagnostic and prognostic blocks, 1.0% preservative-free lidocaine is a suitable local anesthetic. For therapeutic blocks, 0.25% preservative-free bupivacaine in combination with 80 mg of depot methylprednisolone is injected. Subsequent nerve blocks are carried out in a similar manner substituting 40 mg of methylprednisolone for the initial 80-mg dose. Daily cervical epidural nerve blocks with local anesthetic and/or steroid may be required to treat the acute painful conditions mentioned. Chronic conditions such as cervical radiculopathy, tension-type headaches, and diabetic polyneuropathy are treated on an every-other-day basis to a once-a-week basis or as the clinical situation dictates.

If the cervical epidural route is chosen for administration of opioids, 0.5 mg of morphine sulfate formulated for epidural use is a reasonable initial dose in opioid-tolerant patients. More lipid-soluble opioids such as fentanyl must be delivered by continuous infusion via a cervical epidural catheter. All opioids administered via the cervical epidural route should be formulated for epidural use.

SUGGESTED READING

Waldman SD: Cervical epidural block: Translaminar approach. In: Atlas of Interventional Pain Management, ed 2. Philadelphia, Saunders, 2004.

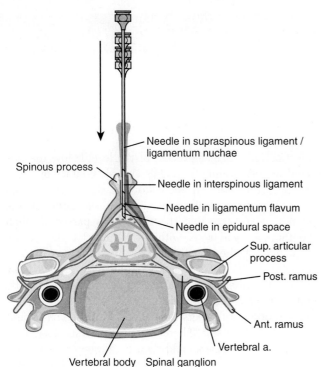

FIGURE 247–1 label text:

Spinous process

Needle in supraspinous ligament / ligamentum nuchae

Needle in interspinous ligament

Needle in ligamentum flavum

Needle in epidural space

Sup. articular process

Post. ramus

Ant. ramus

Vertebral a.

Vertebral body   Spinal ganglion

FIGURE 247–1 Correct needle position for translaminar cervical epidural block. (From Waldman SD: Atlas of Interventional Pain Management, ed 2. Philadelphia, Saunders, 2004, p 132.)

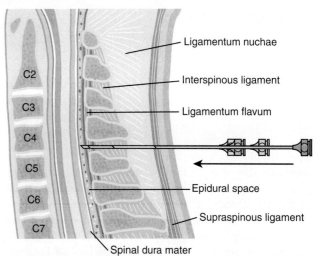

FIGURE 247–2 label text:

C2, C3, C4, C5, C6, C7

Ligamentum nuchae

Interspinous ligament

Ligamentum flavum

Epidural space

Supraspinous ligament

Spinal dura mater

FIGURE 247–2 Correct needle position for translaminar cervical epidural block shown in another plane. (From Waldman SD: Atlas of Interventional Pain Management, ed 2. Philadelphia, Saunders, 2004, p 133.)

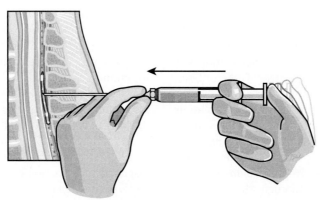

FIGURE 247–3 Needle insertion technique for translaminar cervical epidural block. (From Waldman SD: Atlas of Interventional Pain Management, ed 2. Philadelphia, Saunders, 2004, p 134.)

CHAPTER 248

Cervical Selective Nerve Root Block

The superior boundary of the cervical epidural space is the fusion of the periosteal and spinal layers of dura at the foramen magnum. The epidural space continues inferiorly to the sacrococcygeal membrane. The cervical epidural space is bounded anteriorly by the posterior longitudinal ligament and posteriorly by the vertebral laminae and the ligamentum flavum. The vertebral pedicles and intervertebral foramina form the lateral limits of the epidural space. The cervical epidural space is 3 to 4 mm at the C7-T1 interspace with the cervical spine flexed. The cervical epidural space contains a small amount of fat, veins, arteries, lymphatics, and connective tissue. The nerve roots exit their respective neural foramina and move anteriorly and inferiorly away from the cervical spine. The vertebral artery lies ventral to the neural foramen at the level of the uncinate process. Care must be taken to avoid this structure.

When performing selective nerve root block of the cervical nerve roots, the goal is to place the needle just outside the neural foramen of the affected nerve root with precise application of local anesthetic. As mentioned, placement of the needle within the neural foramina may change how the information obtained from this diagnostic maneuver should be interpreted.

Selective nerve root block of the cervical nerve roots is carried out in a manner analogous to a cervical epidural block using the transforaminal approach. The patient is placed in the supine or lateral position. With the patient in the supine or lateral position on the fluoroscopy table, the fluoroscopy beam is rotated from a lateral to oblique position to allow visualization of the affected neural foramina at its largest diameter. The fluoroscopy beam is then slowly moved from a cephalad to more caudad position to also allow visualization of the affected neural foramina. When this is accomplished, the beam should be parallel to the targeted nerve root with the nerve in the approximate center of the inferior aspect of the foramen.

The skin is then prepared with an antiseptic solution, and a skin wheal of local anesthetic is placed at a point overlying the posterior aspect of the foramen just over the tip of the superior articular process at the level below the affected neural foramen. A 25-gauge blunt or sharp 2-inch needle is then placed through the previously anesthetized area and advanced until the tip rests against

the superior articular process of the level below the targeted neural foramen (Fig. 248-1). This contact provides the operator with an indication of the depth of the neural foramina. Failure to impinge on bone at the point may indicate that the needle has passed through the foramen and rests within the neural canal or the substance of the spinal cord. Failure to identify this problem can lead to disastrous results. After this bony landmark is identified, the needle is withdrawn slightly and redirected caudally and ventrally to impinge on the nerve root just as it exits the neural foramen. The patient is then asked to say "There!" when he or she feels paresthesia. The needle should then be advanced very carefully because paresthesia will be elicited as the needle touches the nerve root. Great care must be taken to stay dorsal to the uncinate process with the target being the center of the foramen. After paresthesia is elicited in the distribution of the targeted nerve root and the needle bevel directed laterally, a fluoroscopic image is then obtained to confirm that the needle tip is at or near the lateral margin of the lateral mass. A solution containing 0.3 mL of a contrast medium suitable for subarachnoid use is then gently injected under continuous fluoroscopic guidance. The contrast should be seen to flow around the nerve root but should not flow proximally into the epidural, subdural, or subarachnoid space. A neurogram outlining the affected nerve root should be seen. Less than 0.5 mL of 4% lidocaine without preservative is then slowly injected under fluoroscopic guidance. The local anesthetic should be seen to flow into the nerve root canal. The injection of contrast and local anesthetic should be stopped immediately if the patient complains of significant pain on injection, although mild pressure paresthesia is common. After satisfactory injection of the local anesthetic and contrast, the needle is removed, and pressure is placed on the injection site.

Basically, the potential side effects and complications associated with selective nerve root block are the same as those associated with transforaminal approach to the cervical epidural space. As mentioned, flow of local anesthetic into the neural foramina reduces the specificity of diagnostic information obtained with selective nerve root block of the cervical nerve roots. Placement of the needle into the neural foramen may result in inadvertent injection into the spinal cord with resultant quadriplegia and/or death. Ventral needle placement may result in damage to vertebral artery, with the possibility of local anesthetic toxicity and, rarely, stroke.

Because of the potential for hematogenous spread via Batson's plexus, local infection and sepsis represent absolute contraindications to this technique. Anticoagulation and coagulopathy represent absolute contraindications to selective nerve root block of the cervical nerve roots because of the risk of neuraxial hematoma.

Inadvertent dural puncture occurring during selective nerve root block of the cervical nerve roots should rarely occur if attention is paid to the technical aspects of this procedure. However, failure to recognize an unintentional dural or subdural injection can result in immediate total spinal anesthesia with associated loss of consciousness, hypotension, and apnea. This can be disastrous with the patient in the prone position. It is also possible to inadvertently place the needle into the subdural or subarachnoid space with the potential for significant motor or sensory block.

This anatomic region is relatively vascular. If intravascular placement is unrecognized, injection of local anesthetic directly into a vessel could result in significant local anesthetic toxicity. Damage or injection to the segmental artery can occur with increased incidence when performing the selective nerve root block of the C5-7 nerve roots on the right.

Needle trauma to the epidural veins may result in self-limited bleeding, which may cause postprocedure pain.

Uncontrolled bleeding into the epidural space may result in compression of the spinal cord with the rapid development of neurologic deficit. Although significant neurologic deficit secondary to epidural hematoma following selective nerve root block should be exceedingly rare, this devastating complication should be considered whenever there is rapidly developing neurologic deficit after cervical epidural nerve block.

Neurologic complications after selective nerve root block are uncommon if proper technique is used and excessive sedation is avoided. Direct trauma to the spinal cord and/or nerve roots is usually accompanied by pain. If significant pain occurs during placement of the needle or during the injection of contrast and local anesthetic, the physician should immediately stop and ascertain the cause of the pain to avoid the possibility of additional neural trauma.

Although uncommon, infection in the epidural space remains an ever-present possibility, especially in the immunocompromised AIDS or cancer patient. If epidural abscess occurs, emergent surgical drainage to avoid spinal cord compression and irreversible neurologic deficit is usually required. Early detection and treatment of infection are crucial to avoid potentially life-threatening sequelae.

SUGGESTED READING

Waldman SD: Cervical selective nerve root block. In: Atlas of Interventional Pain Management, ed 2. Philadelphia, Saunders, 2004.

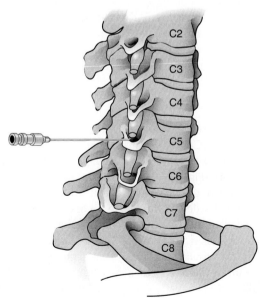

FIGURE 248–1 Cervical selective nerve root block. (From Waldman SD: Atlas of Interventional Pain Management, ed 2. Philadelphia, Saunders, 2004, p 145.)

CHAPTER 249

Brachial Plexus Block

The brachial plexus is formed by the fusion of the anterior rami of the C5, C6, C7, C8, and T1 spinal nerves. There may also be a contribution of fibers from C4 and T2 spinal nerves. The nerves that make up the plexus exit the lateral aspect of the cervical spine and pass downward and laterally in conjunction with the subclavian artery. The nerves and artery run between the anterior scalene and middle scalene muscles, passing inferiorly behind the middle of the clavicle and above the top of the first rib to reach the axilla. The scalene muscles are enclosed in an extension of prevertebral fascia, which helps contain drugs injected into this region.

Interscalene Approach

To perform brachial plexus block using the interscalene approach, the patient is placed in a supine position with the head turned away from the side to be blocked. A total of 20 to 30 mL of local anesthetic is drawn up in a 30-mL sterile syringe. When treating painful or inflammatory conditions that are mediated via the brachial plexus, a total of 80 mg of depot steroid is added to the local anesthetic with the first block and 40 mg of depot steroid is added with subsequent blocks.

The patient is then asked to raise his or her head against the resistance of the pain specialist's hand to aid in identification of the posterior border of the sternocleidomastoid muscle. In most patients, a groove between the posterior border of the sternocleidomastoid muscle and the anterior scalene muscle can be palpated. Identification of the interscalene groove can be facilitated by having the patient inhale strongly against a closed glottis. The skin overlying this area is then prepared with antiseptic solution. At the level of the cricothyroid notch (C6) at the interscalene groove, a 25-gauge, 1½-inch needle is inserted with a slightly caudad and inferior trajectory (Fig. 249-1). If the interscalene groove cannot be identified, the needle is placed just slightly behind the posterior border of the sternocleidomastoid muscle. The needle should be advanced quite slowly because paresthesia is almost always encountered when the needle tip impinges on the brachial plexus as it traverses the interscalene space at almost a right angle to the needle tip. The patient should be warned that a paresthesia will occur and asked to say "There!" as soon as paresthesia is felt.

Paresthesia should be encountered at a depth of approximately ¾ to 1 inch. After paresthesia is elicited, gentle aspiration is carried out to identify blood or cerebrospinal fluid. If the aspiration test is negative and no persistent paresthesia into the distribution of the brachial plexus remains, 20 to 30 mL of solution is slowly injected, with close monitoring of the patient for signs of local anesthetic toxicity or inadvertent subarachnoid injection. If surgical anesthesia is required for forearm or hand procedures, additional local anesthetic may have to be placed in a more caudad position along the brachial plexus to obtain adequate anesthesia of the lower portion of the brachial plexus. Alternatively, specific nerves may be blocked more distally if augmentation of the interscalene brachial plexus block is desired.

Supraclavicular Approach

To perform brachial plexus block using the supraclavicular approach, the patient is placed in a supine position with the head turned away from the side to be blocked. A total of 10 mL of local anesthetic is drawn up in a 20-mL sterile syringe. When treating painful conditions that are mediated via the brachial plexus, a total of 80 mg of depot steroid is added to the local anesthetic with the first block and 40 mg of depot steroid is added with subsequent blocks.

The patient is then asked to raise his or her head against the resistance of the pain specialist's hand to aid in identification of the posterior border of the sternocleidomastoid muscle. The point at which the lateral border of the sternocleidomastoid attaches to the clavicle is then identified. At this point, just above the clavicle, after preparation of the skin with antiseptic solution, a 1½-inch needle is inserted directly perpendicular to the table top (Fig. 249-2). The needle should be advanced quite slowly because a paresthesia is almost always encountered at a depth of approximately ¾ to 1 inch. The patient should be warned that a paresthesia will occur and asked to say "There!" as soon as the paresthesia is felt. If paresthesia is not elicited after the needle has been slowly advanced to a depth of 1 inch, the needle should be withdrawn and re-advanced with a slightly more cephalad trajectory. This maneuver should be repeated until a paresthesia is elicited. If the first rib is encountered before obtaining a paresthesia, the needle should be "walked" laterally along the first rib until a paresthesia is elicited. The needle should never be directed in a more medial trajectory, or pneumothorax is likely to occur.

After paresthesia is elicited, gentle aspiration is carried out to identify blood or cerebrospinal fluid. If the aspiration test is negative and no persistent paresthesia into the distribution of the brachial plexus remains, 10 mL of solution is slowly injected, with close monitoring of the patient for signs of local anesthetic toxicity or inadvertent neuraxial injection.

Axillary Approach

To successfully perform brachial plexus block using the axillary approach, a clear understanding of the clinically relevant anatomy is crucial. The nerves that make up the plexus exit the lateral aspect of the cervical spine and pass downward and laterally in conjunction with the subclavian artery. The nerves and artery run between the anterior scalene and middle scalene muscles, passing inferiorly behind the middle of the clavicle and above the top of the first rib to reach the axilla. The sheath that encloses the axillary artery and nerves is less consistent than that which encloses the brachial plexus at the level at which interscalene and supraclavicular brachial plexus blocks are performed, making a single injection technique less satisfactory. The median, radial, ulnar, and musculocutaneous nerves surround the artery within this imperfect sheath. David Brown has suggested that the position of these nerves relative to the axillary artery can best be visualized by placing them in the quadrants as represented on the face of a clock, with the axillary artery being at the center of the clock (Fig. 249-3). The median nerve is found in the 12 o'clock–to–3 o'clock quadrant, the ulnar nerve is found in the 3 o'clock–to–6 o'clock quadrant, the radial nerve in the 6 o'clock–to–9 o'clock quadrant, and the musculocutaneous nerve in the 9 o'clock–to–12 o'clock quadrant. To ensure adequate block of these nerves, drugs must be injected in each quadrant to place medication in proximity to each of these nerves.

To perform brachial plexus block using the axillary approach, the patient is placed in a supine position with the arm abducted 85 to 90 degrees and the fingertips resting just behind the ear. A total of 30 to 40 mL of local anesthetic is drawn up in a 50-mL sterile syringe. When treating painful or inflammatory conditions that are thought to be mediated via the brachial plexus, a total of 80 mg of depot steroid is added to the local anesthetic with the first block and 40 mg of depot steroid is added with subsequent blocks.

The pain specialist then identifies the pulsations of the axillary artery with the middle and index fingers of the nondominant hand and then traces the course of the artery distally by following the pulsations. After preparation of the skin with antiseptic solution, a 25-gauge, 1-inch needle is inserted just below the arterial pulsations (Fig. 249-4). The needle should be advanced quite slowly because paresthesia is almost always encountered as the needle tip impinges on the radial or ulnar nerve. The patient should be warned that a paresthesia will occur and asked to say "There!" as soon as the paresthesia is felt. Paresthesia should be encountered at a depth of approximately ½ to ¾ inch. After paresthesia is elicited and its distribution identified, gentle aspiration is carried out to identify blood or cerebrospinal fluid. If the aspiration test is negative and no persistent paresthesia into the distribution of the brachial plexus remains, 8 to 10 mL of solution is slowly injected, with close monitoring of the patient for signs of local anesthetic toxicity or inadvertent subarachnoid injection. If a radial paresthesia was elicited, the needle is withdrawn slightly into the 3 o'clock–to–6 o'clock quadrant, which contains the ulnar nerve, and after negative aspiration, an additional 8 to 10 mL of solution is injected. If an ulnar paresthesia was elicited, the needle is withdrawn and then slowly re-advanced in a slightly more superior direction into the 6 o'clock–to–9 o'clock quadrant, which contains the radial nerve, and the aspiration and injection technique is repeated. The needle is then withdrawn and redirected above the arterial pulsation to the 12 o'clock–to–3 o'clock quadrant, which contains the median nerve. If aspiration is negative, 8 to 10 mL of solution is then injected. The needle is then directed to the 9 o'clock–to–12 o'clock quadrant, which contains the musculocutaneous nerve. If aspiration is negative, the remaining local anesthetic is injected. Alternatively, the musculocutaneous nerve can be blocked by infiltrating the solution into the mass of the coracobrachialis muscle.

The proximity of the brachial plexus to the subclavian artery and vein as well as the median, radial, and ulnar nerves as they pass in proximity to the axillary artery suggests the potential for inadvertent intravascular injection and/or local anesthetic toxicity from intravascular absorption. Given the large doses of local anesthetic required for brachial plexus block, the clinician should carefully calculate the total milligram dosage of local anesthetic that may be safely given. This vascularity also gives rise to an increased incidence of postblock ecchymosis and hematoma formation. Despite the vascularity of this anatomic region, this technique can safely be performed in the presence of anticoagulation by using a 25- or 27-gauge needle, albeit at increased risk of hematoma, if the clinical situation dictates a favorable risk-to-benefit ratio. These complications can be decreased if manual pressure is applied to the area of the block immediately after injection. Application of cold packs for 20-minute periods after the block will also decrease the amount of postprocedure pain and bleeding the patient may experience.

In addition to the potential for complications involving the vasculature, the proximity of the brachial plexus to the central neuraxial structures and the phrenic nerve can result in side effects and complications. If the needle is placed too deep when utilizing the intrascalene or supraclavicular approach, the potential for inadvertent epidural, subdural, or subarachnoid injection is a possibility. If the volume of local anesthetic used for this block is accidentally placed in any of these spaces, significant motor and sensory block will result. Unrecognized, these complications could be fatal. It should be assumed that the phrenic nerve will also be blocked when performing brachial plexus block using the interscalene approach. In the absence of significant pulmonary disease, unilateral phrenic nerve block should rarely create respiratory embarrassment. However, blockade of the recurrent laryngeal nerve with its attendant vocal cord paralysis combined with paralysis of the diaphragm may make the clearing of pulmonary and upper airway secretions difficult. Although less likely than with the supraclavicular approach to brachial plexus block, pneumothorax when performing brachial plexus block using the intrascalene approach remains a possibility.

The distance of the median, radial, and ulnar nerves within the axilla from the neuraxis and phrenic nerve makes the complications associated with injection of drugs onto these structures highly unlikely, which is an advantage of the axillary approach compared with the interscalene and supraclavicular approaches to brachial plexus block. Because paresthesias are elicited when performing brachial plexus block using the axillary approach, the potential for postblock persistent paresthesia is a possibility and the patient should be so advised.

SUGGESTED READINGS

Brown DL: Atlas of Regional Anesthesia, ed 3. Philadelphia, Saunders, 2006.

Waldman SD: Brachial plexus block—interscalene approach. In: Atlas of Interventional Pain Management, ed 2. Philadelphia, Saunders, 2004.

Waldman SD: Brachial plexus block—supraclavicular approach. In: Atlas of Interventional Pain Management, ed 2. Philadelphia, Saunders, 2004.

Waldman SD: Brachial plexus block—axillary approach. In: Atlas of Interventional Pain Management, ed 2. Philadelphia, Saunders, 2004.

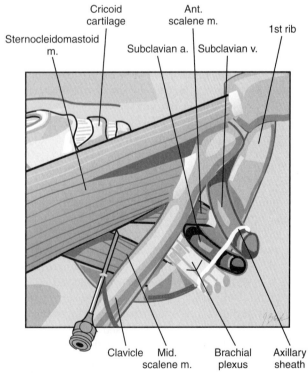

FIGURE 249–1 Brachial plexus block: interscalene approach. (From Waldman SD: Atlas of Interventional Pain Management, ed 2. Philadelphia, Saunders, 2004, p 153.)

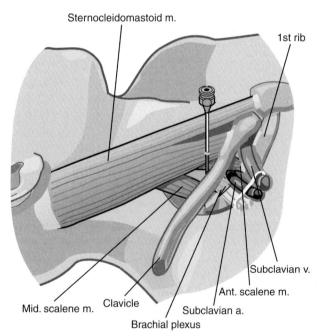

FIGURE 249–2 Brachial plexus block: supraclavicular approach. (From Waldman SD: Atlas of Interventional Pain Management, ed 2. Philadelphia, Saunders, 2004, p 156.)

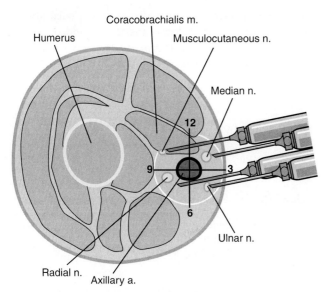

FIGURE 249–3 Quadrant approach to the location of the median, radial, ulnar, and musculocutaneous nerves relative to the axillary artery. (From Waldman SD: Atlas of Interventional Pain Management, ed 2. Philadelphia, Saunders, 2004, p 160.)

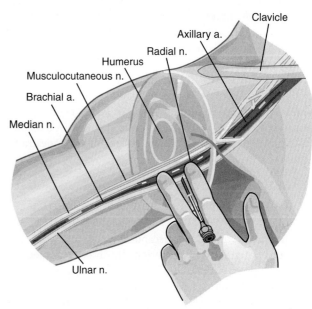

FIGURE 249–4 Brachial plexus block: axillary approach. (From Waldman SD: Atlas of Interventional Pain Management, ed 2. Philadelphia, Saunders, 2004, p 162.)

CHAPTER 250

Suprascapular Nerve Block

The suprascapular nerve is formed from fibers originating from the C5 and C6 nerve roots of the brachial plexus with some contribution of fibers from the C4 root in most patients. The nerve passes inferiorly and posteriorly from the brachial plexus to pass underneath the coracoclavicular ligament through the suprascapular notch. The suprascapular artery and vein accompany the nerve through the suprascapular notch. The suprascapular nerve provides much of the sensory innervation to the shoulder joint and provides innervation to two of the muscles of the rotator cuff and the supraspinatus and infraspinatus muscles.

To perform suprascapular nerve block, the patient is placed in the sitting position with the arms hanging loosely at the patient's side. A total of 10 mL of local anesthetic is drawn up in a 20-mL sterile syringe. When treating painful conditions that are mediated via the suprascapular nerve, a total of 80 mg of depot steroid is added to the local anesthetic with the first block and 40 mg of depot steroid is added with subsequent blocks.

The spine of the scapula is identified, and the pain specialist then palpates along the length of the scapular spine laterally to identify the acromion. At the point at which the thicker acromion fuses with the thinner scapular spine, the skin is prepared with antiseptic solution. At this point, the skin and subcutaneous tissues are anesthetized using a 1½-inch needle. After adequate anesthesia is obtained, a 25-gauge, 3½-inch needle is inserted in an inferior trajectory toward the body of the scapula (Fig. 250-1). The needle should make contact with the body of the scapula at a depth of about 1 inch. The needle is then gently "walked" superiorly and medially until the needle tip walks off the scapular body into the suprascapular notch. If the notch is not identified, the same maneuver is repeated directing the needle superiorly and laterally until the needle tip walks off the scapular body into the suprascapular notch. A paresthesia is often encountered as the needle tip enters the notch, and the patient should be warned of such. If a paresthesia is not elicited after the needle has entered the suprascapular notch, advance the needle an additional ½ inch to place the needle tip beyond the substance of the coracoclavicular ligament. The needle should never be advanced deeper, or pneumothorax is likely to occur.

After paresthesia is elicited or the needle has been advanced into the notch as described here, gentle aspiration is carried out to identify blood or air. If the aspiration test is negative, 10 mL of solution is slowly injected, with close monitoring of the patient for signs of local anesthetic toxicity.

Side Effects and Complications

The proximity to the suprascapular artery and vein suggests the potential for inadvertent intravascular injection and/or local anesthetic toxicity from intravascular absorption. Injection of the local anesthetic and/or steroid should be gentle to avoid trauma to the nerve. The clinician should carefully calculate the total milligram dosage of local anesthetic that may be safely given when performing suprascapular nerve block. Because of the proximity of the lung, if the needle is advanced too deeply through the suprascapular notch, pneumothorax is a possibility.

SUGGESTED READING

Waldman SD: Suprascapular block—Supraclavicular approach. In: Atlas of Interventional Pain Management, ed 2. Philadelphia, Saunders, 2004.

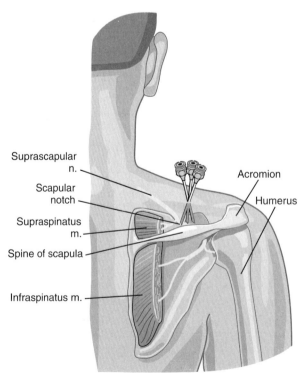

FIGURE 250–1 Suprascapular nerve block. (From Waldman SD: Atlas of Interventional Pain Management, ed 2. Philadelphia, Saunders, 2004, p 165.)

Radial Nerve Block at the Elbow

The radial nerve is made up of fibers from C5-T1 spinal roots. The nerve lies posterior and inferior to the axillary artery in the 6 o'clock–to–9 o'clock quadrant. Exiting the axilla, the radial nerve passes between the medial and long heads of the triceps muscle. As the nerve curves across the posterior aspect of the humerus, it supplies a motor branch to the triceps. Continuing its downward path, it gives off a number of sensory branches to the upper arm. At a point between the lateral epicondyle of the humerus and the musculospiral groove, the radial nerve divides into its two terminal branches. The superficial branch continues down the arm along with the radial artery and provides sensory innervation to the dorsum of the wrist and the dorsal aspects of a portion of the thumb and index and middle fingers. The deep branch provides the majority of the motor innervation to the extensors of the forearm.

Technique

The patient is placed in a supine position with the arm fully abducted at the patient's side and the elbow slightly flexed with the dorsum of the hand resting on a folded towel. A total of 7 to 10 mL of local anesthetic is drawn up in a 12-mL sterile syringe. When treating painful or inflammatory conditions that are mediated via the radial nerve, a total of 80 mg of depot steroid is added to the local anesthetic with the first block and 40 mg of depot steroid is added with subsequent blocks.

The pain specialist then identifies the lateral margin of the biceps tendon at the crease of the elbow. After preparation of the skin with antiseptic solution, a 25-gauge, 1½-inch needle is inserted just lateral to the biceps tendon at the crease and slowly advanced in a slightly medial and cephalad trajectory (Fig. 251-1). As the needle approaches the humerus, strong paresthesia in the distribution of the radial nerve will be elicited. If no paresthesia is elicited and the needle contacts bone, the needle is withdrawn and redirected slightly more medial until paresthesia is elicited. The patient should be warned that paresthesia will occur and asked to say "There!" as soon as the paresthesia is felt. After paresthesia is elicited and its distribution identified, gentle aspiration is carried out to identify blood. If the aspiration test is negative and no persistent paresthesia into the distribution of the radial nerve remains, 7 to 10 mL of solution is slowly injected, with close monitoring of the patient for signs of local anesthetic toxicity.

Radial nerve block at the elbow is a relatively safe block, with the major complications being inadvertent intravascular injection and persistent paresthesia secondary to needle trauma to the nerve. This technique can safely be performed in the presence of anticoagulation by using a 25- or 27-gauge needle, albeit at increased risk of hematoma, if the clinical situation dictates a favorable risk-to-benefit ratio. These complications can be decreased if manual pressure is applied to the area of the block immediately after injection. Application of cold packs for 20-minute periods after the block will also decrease the amount of postprocedure pain and bleeding the patient may experience.

SUGGESTED READING

Waldman SD: Radial nerve block at the elbow. In: Atlas of Interventional Pain Management, ed 2. Philadelphia, Saunders, 2004.

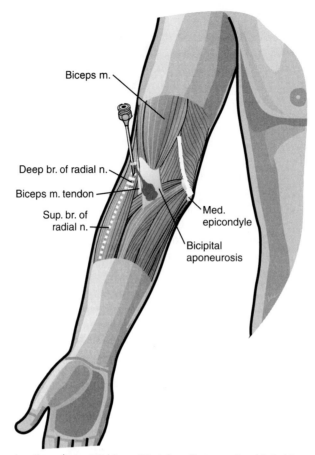

FIGURE 251–1 Radial nerve block at the elbow. (From Waldman SD: Atlas of Interventional Pain Management, ed 2. Philadelphia, Saunders, 2004, p 178.)

CHAPTER 252

Median Nerve Block at the Elbow

The median nerve is made up of fibers from C5-T1 spinal roots. The nerve lies anterior and superior to the axillary artery in the 12 o'clock–to–3 o'clock quadrant. Exiting the axilla, the median nerve descends into the upper arm along with the brachial artery. At the level of the elbow, the brachial artery is just medial to the biceps muscle. At this level, the median nerve lies just medial to the brachial artery. As the median nerve proceeds downward into the forearm, it gives off numerous branches that provide motor innervation to the flexor muscles of the forearm. These branches are susceptible to nerve entrapment by aberrant ligaments, muscle hypertrophy, and direct trauma. The nerve approaches the wrist overlying the radius. It lies deep and between the tendons of the palmaris longus muscle and the flexor carpi radialis muscle at the wrist. The terminal branches of the median nerve provide sensory innervation to a portion of the palmar surface of the hand as well as the palmar surface of the thumb, index and middle fingers, and the radial portion of the ring finger (Fig. 252-1). The median nerve also provides sensory innervation to the distal dorsal surface of the index and middle fingers and the radial portion of the ring finger.

To perform median nerve block at the elbow, the patient is placed in a supine position with the arm fully adducted at the patient's side and the elbow slightly flexed with the dorsum of the hand resting on a folded towel. A total of 5 to 7 mL of local anesthetic is drawn up in a 12-mL sterile syringe. When treating painful or inflammatory conditions that are mediated via the median nerve, a total of 80 mg of depot steroid is added to the local anesthetic with the first block and 40 mg of depot steroid is added with subsequent blocks.

The pain specialist then identifies the pulsations of the brachial artery at the crease of the elbow. After preparation of the skin with antiseptic solution, a 25-gauge, 1½-inch needle is inserted just medial to the brachial artery at the crease and slowly advanced in a slightly medial and cephalad trajectory. As the needle advances approximately ½ to ¾ inch, strong paresthesia in the distribution of the median nerve will be elicited. If no paresthesia is elicited and the needle contacts bone, the needle is withdrawn and redirected slightly more medially until a paresthesia is elicited. The patient should be warned that paresthesia will occur and asked to say "There!" as soon as the paresthesia is felt. After paresthesia is elicited and its distribution identified, gentle aspiration is carried out to identify blood. If the aspiration test is negative and no persistent paresthesia into the distribution of the median nerve remains, 5 to 7 mL of solution is slowly injected, with close monitoring of the patient for signs of local anesthetic toxicity. If no paresthesia can be elicited, a similar amount of solution is injected in a fanlike manner just medial to the brachial artery, with care being taken not to inadvertently inject into the artery.

Median nerve block at the elbow is a relatively safe block, with the major complications being inadvertent intravascular injection and persistent paresthesia secondary to needle trauma to the nerve. This technique can safely be performed in the presence of anticoagulation by using a 25- or 27-gauge needle, albeit at increased risk of hematoma, if the clinical situation dictates a favorable risk-to-benefit ratio. These complications can be decreased if manual pressure is applied to the area of the block immediately after injection. Application of cold packs for 20-minute periods after the block will also decrease the amount of postprocedure pain and bleeding the patient may experience.

SUGGESTED READING

Waldman SD: Median nerve block at the elbow. In: Atlas of Interventional Pain Management, ed 2. Philadelphia, Saunders, 2004.

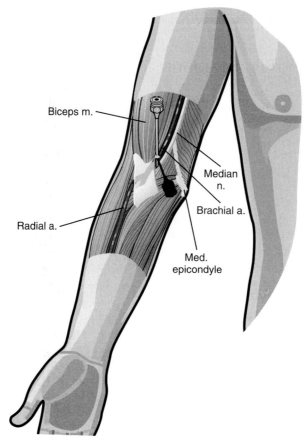

FIGURE 252–1 Median nerve block at the elbow (From Waldman SD: Atlas of Interventional Pain Management, ed 2. Philadelphia, Saunders, 2004, p 183.)

CHAPTER 253

Ulnar Nerve Block at the Elbow

The ulnar nerve is made up of fibers from C6-T1 spinal roots. The nerve lies anterior and inferior to the axillary artery in the 3 o'clock–to–6 o'clock quadrant. Exiting the axilla, the ulnar nerve descends into the upper arm along with the brachial artery. At the middle of the upper arm, the nerve courses medially to pass between the olecranon process and medial epicondyle of the humerus. The nerve then passes between the heads of the flexor carpi ulnaris muscle continuing downward, moving radially along with the ulnar artery. At a point approximately 1 inch proximal to the crease of the wrist, the ulnar nerve divides into the dorsal and palmar branches. The dorsal branch provides

sensation to the ulnar aspect of the dorsum of the hand and the dorsal aspect of the little finger and the ulnar half of the ring finger. The palmar branch provides sensory innervation to the ulnar aspect of the palm of the hand and the palmar aspect of the little finger and the ulnar half of the ring finger.

To perform ulnar nerve block at the elbow, the patient is placed in a supine position with the arm abducted 85 to 90 degrees and the dorsum of the hand resting against a folded towel. A total of 5 to 7 mL of local anesthetic is drawn up in a 12-mL sterile syringe. When treating painful or inflammatory conditions that are mediated via the ulnar nerve, a total of 80 mg of depot steroid is added to the local anesthetic with the first block and 40 mg of depot steroid is added with subsequent blocks.

The pain specialist then identifies the olecranon process and the median epicondyle of the humerus. The ulnar nerve sulcus between these two bony landmarks is then identified. After preparation of the skin with antiseptic solution, a 25-gauge, ⅝-inch needle is inserted just proximal to the sulcus and is slowly advanced in a slightly cephalad trajectory (Fig. 253-1). As the needle advances approximately ½ inch, strong paresthesia in the distribution of the ulnar nerve will be elicited. The patient should be warned that paresthesia will occur and asked to say "There!" as soon as the paresthesia is felt. After paresthesia is elicited and its distribution identified, gentle aspiration is carried out to identify blood. If the aspiration test is negative and no persistent paresthesia into the distribution of the ulnar nerve remains, 5 to 7 mL of solution is slowly injected, with close monitoring of the patient for signs of local anesthetic toxicity. If no paresthesia can be elicited, a similar amount of solution is slowly injected in a fanlike manner just proximal to the notch, with care being taken to avoid intravascular injection.

Ulnar nerve block at the elbow is a relatively safe block, with the major complications being inadvertent intravascular injection into the ulnar artery and persistent paresthesia secondary to needle trauma to the nerve. Because the nerve is enclosed by a dense fibrous band as it passes through the ulnar nerve sulcus, care should be taken to slowly inject just proximal to the sulcus to avoid additional compromise of the nerve. This technique can safely be performed in the presence of anticoagulation by using a 25- or 27-gauge needle, albeit at increased risk of hematoma, if the clinical situation dictates a favorable risk-to-benefit ratio. These complications can be decreased if manual pressure is applied to the area of the block immediately after injection. Application of cold packs for 20-minute periods after the block will also decrease the amount of postprocedure pain and bleeding the patient may experience.

SUGGESTED READING

Waldman SD: Ulnar nerve block at the elbow. In: Atlas of Interventional Pain Management, ed 2. Philadelphia, Saunders, 2004.

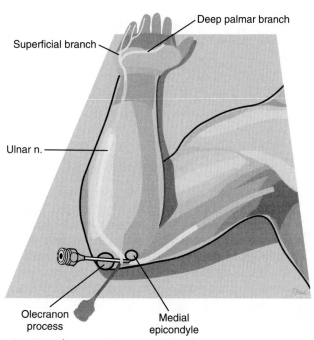

FIGURE 253–1 Ulnar nerve block at the elbow. (From Waldman SD: Atlas of Interventional Pain Management, ed 2. Philadelphia, Saunders, 2004, p 188.)

CHAPTER 254

Radial Nerve Block at the Wrist

The radial nerve is made up of fibers from C5-T1 spinal roots. The nerve lies posterior and inferior to the axillary artery in the 6 o'clock–to–9 o'clock quadrant. Exiting the axilla, the radial nerve passes between the medial and long heads of the triceps muscle. As the nerve curves across the posterior aspect of the humerus, it supplies a motor branch to the triceps. Continuing its downward path, it gives off a number of sensory branches to the upper arm. At a point between the lateral epicondyle of the humerus and the musculospiral groove, the radial nerve divides into its two terminal branches. The superficial branch continues down the arm along with the radial artery and provides sensory innervation to the dorsum of the wrist and the dorsal aspects of a portion of the thumb and index and middle fingers. The deep branch provides the majority of the motor innervation to the extensors of the forearm. The major portion of the superficial branch passes between the flexor carpi radialis tendon and the radial artery. However, there are a significant number of small branches that ramify to provide sensory innervation of the dorsum of the hand. These small branches must also be blocked to provide complete blockade of the radial nerve.

To perform radial nerve block at the wrist, the patient is placed in a supine position with the arm fully adducted at the patient's side and the elbow slightly flexed with the dorsum of the hand resting on a folded towel. A total of 7 to 8 mL of local anesthetic is drawn up in a 12-mL sterile syringe. When treating painful or inflammatory conditions that are mediated via the radial nerve, a total of 80 mg of depot steroid is added to the local anesthetic with the first block and 40 mg of depot steroid is added with subsequent blocks.

The patient is instructed to flex his or her wrist to allow the pain specialist to identify the flexor carpi radialis tendon. The distal radial prominence is then identified. After preparation of the skin with antiseptic solution, a 25-gauge, 1½-inch needle is inserted in a perpendicular trajectory just lateral to the flexor carpi radialis tendon and just medial to the radial artery at the level of the distal radial prominence (Fig. 254-1). The needle is slowly advanced. As the needle approaches the radius, strong paresthesia in the distribution of the radial nerve will be elicited. The patient should be warned that paresthesia will occur and asked to say "There!" as soon as the paresthesia is felt. After paresthesia is elicited and its distribution identified, gentle aspiration is carried out to identify blood. If the aspiration test is negative and no persistent paresthesia into the distribution of the radial nerve remains, 3 to 4 mL of solution is slowly injected, with close monitoring of the patient for signs of local anesthetic toxicity. If no paresthesia is elicited and the needle contacts bone, the needle is withdrawn out of the periosteum, and after careful aspiration, 3 to 4 mL of solution is injected.

The patient is then asked to pronate the arm, and additional 3 to 4 mL of solution is injected in a subcutaneous bead, starting at the anatomic snuff box and carrying the injection subcutaneously to just past the midline of the dorsum of the wrist.

Radial nerve block at the wrist is a relatively safe block, with the major complications being inadvertent intravascular injection and persistent paresthesia secondary to needle trauma to the nerve. This technique can be safely performed in the presence of anticoagulation by using a 25- or 27-gauge needle, albeit at increased risk of hematoma, if the clinical situation dictates a favorable risk-to-benefit ratio. These complications can be decreased if manual pressure is applied to the area of the block immediately after injection. Application of cold packs for 20-minute periods after the block will also decrease the amount of postprocedure pain and bleeding the patient may experience.

SUGGESTED READING

Waldman SD: Radial nerve block at the wrist. In: Atlas of Interventional Pain Management, ed 2. Philadelphia, Saunders, 2004.

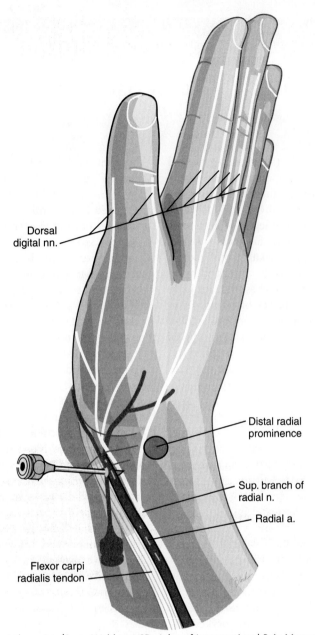

FIGURE 254–1 Radial nerve block at the wrist. (From Waldman SD: Atlas of Interventional Pain Management, ed 2. Philadelphia, Saunders, 2004, p 192.)

CHAPTER 255

Median Nerve Block at the Wrist

The median nerve is made up of fibers from C5-T1 spinal roots. The nerve lies anterior and superior to the axillary artery in the 12 o'clock–to–3 o'clock quadrant. Exiting the axilla, the median nerve descends into the upper arm along with the brachial artery. At the level of the elbow, the brachial artery is just medial to the biceps muscle. At this level, the median nerve lies just medial to the brachial artery. As the median nerve proceeds downward into the forearm, it gives off numerous branches that provide motor innervation to the flexor muscles of the forearm. These branches are susceptible to nerve entrapment by aberrant ligaments, muscle hypertrophy, and direct trauma. The nerve approaches the wrist overlying the radius. It lies deep to and between the tendons of the palmaris longus muscle and the flexor carpi radialis muscle at the wrist. The median nerve then passes beneath the flexor retinaculum and through the carpal tunnel, with the nerve's terminal branches providing sensory innervation to a portion of the palmar surface of the hand as well as the palmar surface of the thumb, index and middle fingers, and the radial portion of the ring finger. The median nerve also provides sensory innervation to the distal dorsal surface of the index and middle fingers and the radial portion of the ring finger.

To perform median nerve block at the wrist, the patient is placed in a supine position with the arm fully adducted at the patient's side and the elbow slightly flexed with the dorsum of the hand resting on a folded towel. A total of 3 to 5 mL of local anesthetic is drawn up in a 12-mL sterile syringe. When treating painful or inflammatory conditions that are mediated via the median nerve, a total of 80 mg of depot steroid is added to the local anesthetic with the first block and 40 mg of depot steroid is added with subsequent blocks.

The clinician then has the patient make a fist and at the same time flex his or her wrist to aid in identification of the palmaris longus tendon. After preparation of the skin with antiseptic solution, a 25-gauge, $^5/_8$-inch needle is inserted just medial to the tendon and just proximal to the crease of the wrist (Fig. 255-1). The needle is slowly advanced in a slightly cephalad trajectory. As the needle advances beyond the tendon at a depth of approximately $^1/_2$ inch, strong paresthesia in the distribution of the median nerve will be elicited. The patient should be warned that paresthesia will occur and asked to say "There!" as soon as the paresthesia is felt. After paresthesia is elicited and its distribution identified, gentle aspiration is carried out to identify blood. If the aspiration test is negative and no persistent paresthesia into the distribution of the median nerve remains, 3 to 5 mL of solution is slowly injected, with close monitoring of the patient for signs of local anesthetic toxicity. If no paresthesia is elicited and the needle tip hits bone, the needle is withdrawn out of the periosteum, and after careful aspiration, 3 to 5 mL of solution is slowly injected.

Median nerve block at the wrist is a relatively safe block, with the major complications being inadvertent intravascular injection and persistent paresthesia secondary to needle trauma to the nerve. This technique can safely be performed in the presence of anticoagulation by using a 25- or 27-gauge needle, albeit at increased risk of hematoma, if the clinical situation dictates a favorable risk-to-benefit ratio. These complications can be decreased if manual pressure is applied to the area of the block immediately after injection. Application of cold packs for 20-minute periods after the block will also decrease the amount of postprocedure pain and bleeding the patient may experience.

SUGGESTED READING

Waldman SD: Median nerve block at the wrist. In: Atlas of Interventional Pain Management, ed 2. Philadelphia, Saunders, 2004.

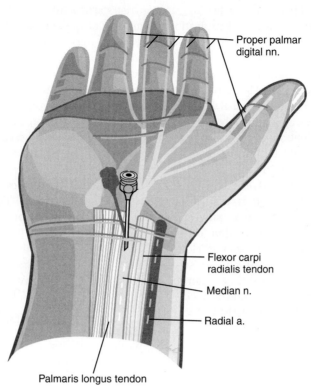

FIGURE 255–1 Median nerve block at the wrist. (From Waldman SD: Atlas of Interventional Pain Management, ed 2. Philadelphia, Saunders, 2004, p 197.)

Ulnar Nerve Block at the Wrist

The ulnar nerve is made up of fibers from C6-T1 spinal roots. The nerve lies anterior and inferior to the axillary artery in the 3 o'clock–to–6 o'clock quadrant. Exiting the axilla, the ulnar nerve descends into the upper arm along with the brachial artery. At the middle of the upper arm, the nerve courses medially to pass between the olecranon process and medial epicondyle of the humerus. The nerve then passes between the heads of the flexor carpi ulnaris muscle continuing downward, moving radially along with the ulnar artery. At a point approximately 1 inch proximal to the crease of the wrist, the ulnar divides into the dorsal and palmar branches. The dorsal branch provides sensation to the ulnar aspect of the dorsum of the hand and the dorsal aspect of the little finger and the ulnar half of the ring finger (Fig. 256-1). The palmar branch provides sensory innervation to the ulnar aspect of the palm of the hand and the

palmar aspect of the little finger and the ulnar half of the ring finger.

Technique

To perform ulnar nerve block at the wrist, the patient is placed in a supine position with the arm fully adducted at the patient's side and the wrist slightly flexed with the dorsum of the hand resting on a folded towel. A total of 5 to 7 mL of local anesthetic is drawn up in a 12-mL sterile syringe. When treating painful or inflammatory conditions that are mediated via the ulnar nerve, a total of 80 mg of depot steroid is added to the local anesthetic with the first block and 40 mg of depot steroid is added with subsequent blocks.

The clinician then has the patient make a fist and at the same time flex his or her wrist to aid in identification of the flexor carpi ulnaris tendon. After preparation of the skin with antiseptic solution, a 25-gauge, ⅝-inch needle is inserted on the radial side of the tendon at the level of the styloid process (see Fig. 256-1). The needle is slowly advanced in a slightly cephalad trajectory. As the needle advances approximately ½ inch, strong paresthesia in the distribution of the ulnar nerve will be elicited. The patient should be warned that paresthesia will occur and asked to say "There!" as soon as paresthesia is felt. After paresthesia is elicited and its distribution identified, gentle aspiration is carried out to identify blood. If the aspiration test is negative and no persistent paresthesia into the distribution of the ulnar nerve remains, 3 to 5 mL of solution is slowly injected, with close monitoring of the patient for signs of local anesthetic toxicity. If no paresthesia can be elicited, a similar amount of solution is slowly injected in a fanlike manner just proximal to the notch, with care being taken to avoid intravascular injection.

To ensure complete block of the dorsal branch of the ulnar nerve, it may be necessary to inject a bead of local anesthetic subcutaneously around the ulnar aspect of the wrist starting from the flexor carpi ulnaris tendon to the midline of the dorsum of the hand.

Ulnar nerve block at the wrist is a relatively safe block, with the major complications being inadvertent intravascular injection into the ulnar artery and persistent paresthesia secondary to needle trauma to the nerve. Like the carpal tunnel, Guyon's canal is a closed space, therefore, care should be taken to inject slowly to avoid additional compromise of the nerve. This technique can be safely performed in the presence of anticoagulation by using a 25- or 27-gauge needle, albeit at increased risk of hematoma, if the clinical situation dictates a favorable risk-to-benefit ratio. These complications can be decreased if manual pressure is applied to the area of the block immediately after injection. Application of cold packs for 20-minute periods after the block will also decrease the amount of postprocedure pain and bleeding the patient may experience.

SUGGESTED READING

Waldman SD: Ulnar nerve block at the wrist. In: Atlas of Interventional Pain Management, ed 2. Philadelphia, Saunders, 2004.

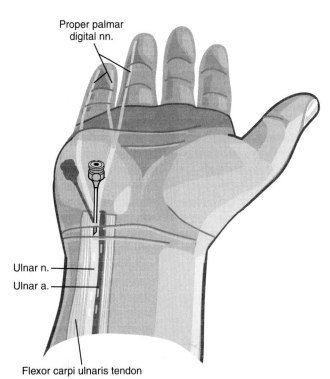

Proper palmar
digital nn.

Ulnar n.

Ulnar a.

Flexor carpi ulnaris tendon

FIGURE 256–1 Ulnar nerve block at the wrist. (From Waldman SD: Atlas of Interventional Pain Management, ed 2. Philadelphia, Saunders, 2004, p 201.)

CHAPTER 257

Metacarpal and Digital Nerve Block

The common digital nerves arise from fibers of the median and ulnar nerves. The thumb also has contributions from superficial branches of the radial nerve. The common digital nerves pass along the metacarpal bones and divide as they reach the distal palm. The volar digital nerves supply the majority of sensory innervation to the fingers and run along the ventrolateral aspect of the finger beside the digital vein and artery. The smaller dorsal digital nerves contain fibers from the ulnar and radial nerves and supply the dorsum of the fingers as far as the proximal joints.

Technique

To perform metacarpal or digital nerve block, the patient is placed in a supine position with the arm fully abducted and the elbow slightly flexed with the palm of the hand resting on a folded towel. A total of 3 mL per digit of non–epinephrine-containing local anesthetic is drawn up in a 12-mL sterile syringe.

METACARPAL NERVE BLOCK

After preparation of the skin with antiseptic solution, at a point proximal to the metacarpal head, a 25-gauge, 1½-inch needle is inserted on each side of the metacarpal bone to be blocked (Fig. 257-1). While the anesthetic is slowly injected, the needle is advanced from the dorsal surface of the hand toward the palmar surface. The common digital nerve is situated on the dorsal side of the flexor retinaculum, and thus the needle will have to be advanced almost to the palmar surface of the hand in order to obtain satisfactory anesthesia. The needle is removed, and pressure is placed on the injection site to avoid hematoma formation.

DIGITAL NERVE BLOCK

To perform digital nerve block, the patient is placed in a supine position with the arm fully abducted and the

elbow slightly flexed with the palm of the hand resting on a folded towel. A total of 3 mL per digit of non–epinephrine-containing local anesthetic is drawn up in a 12-mL sterile syringe.

After preparation of the skin with antiseptic solution, at a point at the base of the finger, a 25-gauge, 1½-inch needle is inserted on each side of the bone of the digit to be blocked (Fig. 257-2). While the anesthetic is slowly injected, the needle is advanced from the dorsal surface of the hand toward the palmar surface. The same technique can be used to block the thumb. The needle is removed, and pressure is placed on the injection site to avoid hematoma formation.

Because of the confined nature of the soft tissue surrounding the metacarpals and digits, the potential for mechanical compression of the blood supply after injection of solution must be considered. The pain specialist must avoid rapidly injecting large volumes of solution into these confined spaces, or vascular insufficiency and gangrene may occur. Furthermore, epinephrine-containing solutions should never be used to avoid ischemia and possible gangrene.

This technique can safely be performed in the presence of anticoagulation by using a 25- or 27-gauge needle, albeit at increased risk of hematoma, if the clinical situation dictates a favorable risk-to-benefit ratio. These complications can be decreased if manual pressure is applied to the area of the block immediately after injection. Application of cold packs for 10-minute periods after the block will also decrease the amount of postprocedure pain and bleeding the patient may experience.

SUGGESTED READING

Waldman SD: Metacarpal and digital nerve block. In: Atlas of Interventional Pain Management, ed 2. Philadelphia, Saunders, 2004.

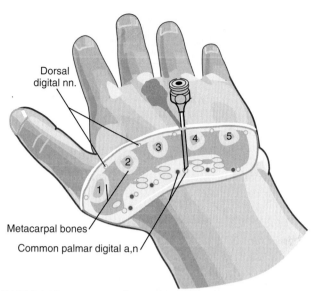

FIGURE 257–1 Metacarpal nerve block. (From Waldman SD: Atlas of Interventional Pain Management, ed 2. Philadelphia, Saunders, 2004, p 203.)

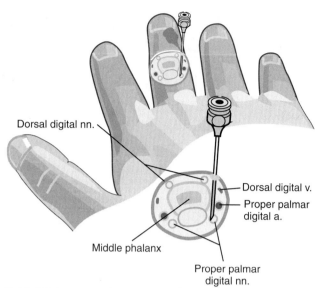

FIGURE 257–2 Digital nerve block. (From Waldman SD: Atlas of Interventional Pain Management, ed 2. Philadelphia, Saunders, 2004, p 203.)

CHAPTER 258

Intravenous Regional Anesthesia

Intravenous regional anesthesia is used primarily in two clinical situations: (1) to provide surgical anesthesia for surgical procedures on the distal extremities and (2) to administer drugs intravenously to treat painful conditions such as reflex sympathetic dystrophy that are limited to a specific extremity.

The peripheral nerves of the extremities receive their blood supply from the blood vessels that accompany them. By administering drugs intravenously and sequestering them in the extremity by use of a tourniquet, the drugs administered can then diffuse into the soft tissues and nerves. The limiting factor for this technique is the total amount of local anesthetic that can be safely administered and the length of time that the circulation of the extremity can be occluded by the tourniquet.

To perform intravenous regional anesthesia, the patient is placed in the supine position. An intravenous catheter is placed in the extremity to be treated. The affected extremity is elevated to drain excess blood (Fig. 258-1). The area underneath the tourniquet is wrapped with cotton cast padding, and a double tourniquet is placed tightly around the affected extremity. An Esmarch bandage is used to exsanguinate the extremity only if the surgeon requires a bloodless field. The upper portion of the double tourniquet is then inflated to a pressure of 100 mm Hg above the patient's systolic blood pressure (Fig. 258-2). Lidocaine 0.5% without preservative in a volume of 30 to 50 mL is used for surgical anesthesia. For pain management applications, water-soluble steroid methylprednisolone, reserpine, or bretylium is administered in solution with similar volumes of more dilute concentrations of preservative-free lidocaine.

After the solution has been injected for approximately 10 minutes, the lower tourniquet is inflated over the anesthetized area, and after ascertaining that the lower tourniquet is adequately inflated, the upper tourniquet is deflated (Fig. 258-3). The lower tourniquet is left inflated for an additional 10 to 15 minutes. The cuff is then deflated to just below the systolic pressure for a few seconds and then reinflated while the patient is observed closely for signs of local anesthetic toxicity. This maneuver is performed repeatedly while gradually decreasing the cuff pressure to allow the local anesthetic to slowly wash out. At the first sign of local anesthetic toxicity, the cuff should be reinflated for at least an additional 5 minutes or until all signs of local anesthetic toxicity have abated. After the tourniquet is completely deflated, the tourniquet and intravenous cannula are then removed.

The major side effect of intravenous regional anesthesia is phlebitis at the injection site and proximal vein. This problem occurs more frequently with the ester-type local anesthetics and with the administration of drugs in addition to local anesthetics. Patients taking aspirin may experience petechial hemorrhages distal to the tourniquet and should be warned of such. The major complication of intravenous regional anesthesia is local anesthetic toxicity secondary to tourniquet failure or improper technique. For this reason, intravenous regional anesthesia should never be performed unless equipment and personnel for resuscitation are available.

SUGGESTED READING

Waldman SD: Intravenous regional anesthesia. In: Atlas of Interventional Pain Management, ed 2. Philadelphia, Saunders, 2004.

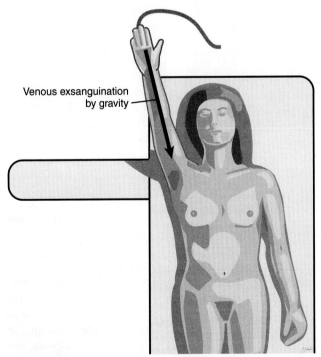

FIGURE 258–1 Intravenous regional anesthesia: venous exsanguination by gravity. (From Waldman SD: Atlas of Interventional Pain Management, ed 2. Philadelphia, Saunders, 2004, p 206.)

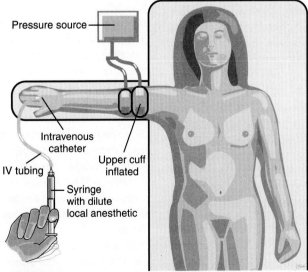

FIGURE 258–2 Intravenous regional anesthesia: inflation of the upper portion of the double tourniquet. (From Waldman SD: Atlas of Interventional Pain Management, ed 2. Philadelphia, Saunders, 2004, p 207.)

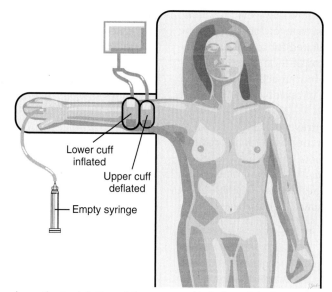

FIGURE 258–3 Intravenous regional anesthesia: deflation of the upper and inflation of the lower tourniquet. (From Waldman SD: Atlas of Interventional Pain Management, ed 2. Philadelphia, Saunders, 2004, p 207.)

CHAPTER 259

Injection Technique for Intra-articular Injection of the Shoulder

The rounded head of the humerus articulates with the pear-shaped glenoid fossa of the scapula. The articular surface is covered with hyaline cartilage, which is susceptible to arthritis. The rim of the glenoid fossa is composed of a fibrocartilaginous layer called the glenoid labrum, which is susceptible to trauma should the humerus be subluxed or dislocated. The joint is surrounded by a relatively lax capsule that allows the wide range of motion of the shoulder joint at the expense of decreased joint stability. The joint capsule is lined with a synovial membrane, which attaches to the articular cartilage. This membrane gives rise to synovial tendon sheaths and bursae, which are subject to inflammation. The shoulder joint is innervated by the axillary and suprascapular nerves.

The major ligaments of the shoulder joint are the glenohumeral ligaments in front of the capsule, the transverse humeral ligament between the humeral tuberosities, and the coracohumeral ligament, which stretches from the coracoid process to the greater tuberosity of the humerus. Along with the accessory ligaments

of the shoulder, these major ligaments provide strength to the shoulder joint. The strength of the shoulder joint also is dependent on short muscles that surround the joint: the subscapularis, the supraspinatus, the infraspinatus, and the teres minor. These muscles and their attaching tendons are susceptible to trauma and to wear and tear from overuse and misuse.

To perform intra-articular injection of the shoulder joint, the patient is placed in the supine position and proper preparation with antiseptic solution of the skin overlying the shoulder, subacromial region, and joint space is carried out. A sterile syringe containing 2.0 mL of 0.25% preservative-free bupivacaine and 40 mg of methylprednisolone is attached to a 1½-inch, 25-gauge needle using strict aseptic technique. With strict aseptic technique, the midpoint of the acromion is identified and, at a point approximately 1 inch below the midpoint, the shoulder joint space is identified. The needle is then carefully advanced through the skin and subcutaneous tissues and through the joint capsule into the joint (Fig. 259-1).

If bone is encountered, the needle is withdrawn into the subcutaneous tissues and redirected superiorly and slightly more medial. After entering the joint space, the contents of the syringe are gently injected. There should be little resistance to injection. If resistance is encountered, the needle is probably in a ligament or tendon and should be advanced slightly into the joint space until the injection proceeds without significant resistance. The needle is then removed and a sterile pressure dressing and ice pack are placed at the injection site.

The major complication of intra-articular injection of the shoulder is infection. This complication should be exceedingly rare if strict aseptic technique is adhered to. Approximately 25% of patients complain of a transient increase in pain following intra-articular injection of the shoulder joint; the patient should be warned of this.

SUGGESTED READING

Waldman SD: Intra-articular injection of the shoulder joint. In: Atlas of Pain Management Injection Techniques, ed. 2. Philadelphia, Saunders, 2007.

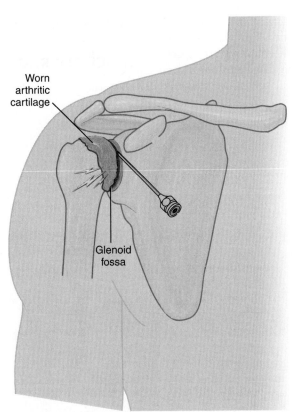

FIGURE 259–1 Intra-articular injection of the shoulder. (From Waldman SD: Atlas of Pain Management Injection Techniques, ed. 2. Philadelphia, Saunders, 2007, p 58.)

CHAPTER 260

Injection Technique for Subdeltoid Bursitis Pain

The acromial arch covers the superior aspect of the shoulder joint and articulates with the clavicle at the acromioclavicular joint. The acromioclavicular joint is formed by the distal end of the clavicle and the anterior and medial aspect of the acromion. The strength of the joint is due to the dense coracoclavicular ligament, which attaches the bottom of the distal end of the clavicle to the coracoid process. The superior portion of the joint is covered by the superior acromioclavicular ligament, which attaches the distal clavicle to the upper surface of the acromion. The inferior portion of the joint is covered by the inferior acromioclavicular ligament, which attaches the inferior portion of the distal clavicle to the acromion. The subdeltoid bursa lies primarily under the acromion extending laterally between the deltoid muscle and joint capsule.

To perform injection of the subdeltoid bursa, the patient is placed in the supine position and proper preparation with antiseptic solution of the skin overlying the superior shoulder, acromion, and distal clavicle is carried out. A sterile syringe containing 4.0 mL of 0.25% preservative-free bupivacaine and 40 mg of methylprednisolone is attached to a 1½-inch 25-gauge needle using strict aseptic technique. With strict aseptic technique, the lateral edge of the acromion is identified, and at the midpoint of the lateral edge, the injection site is identified. At this point, the needle is then carefully advanced in a slightly cephalad trajectory through the skin and subcutaneous tissues beneath the acromion capsule into the bursa (Fig. 260-1). If bone is encountered, the needle is withdrawn into the subcutaneous tissues and redirected slightly more inferiorly. After entering the bursa, the contents of the syringe are gently injected while the needle is slowly withdrawn. There should be minimal resistance to injection unless calcification of the bursal sac is present. Calcification of the bursal sac will be identified as a resistance to needle advancement with an associated gritty feel. Significant calcific bursitis may ultimately require surgical excision to effect complete relief of symptoms. The needle is then removed, and a sterile pressure dressing and ice pack are placed at the injection site.

The major complication of injection of the subdeltoid bursa is infection. This complication should be exceedingly rare if strict aseptic technique is adhered to. Approximately 25% of patients will complain of a transient increase in pain following injection of the subdeltoid bursa and should be warned of such.

SUGGESTED READING

Waldman SD: Subdeltoid bursitis pain. In: Atlas of Pain Management Injection Techniques. Philadelphia, Saunders, 2007.

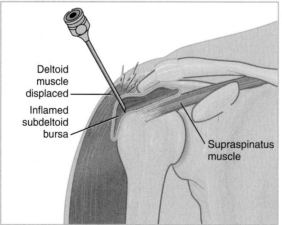

FIGURE 260–1 Injection technique for subdeltoid bursitis pain. (From Waldman SD: Atlas of Pain Management Injection Techniques. Philadelphia, Saunders, 2007, p 110.)

Injection Technique for Intra-articular Injection of the Elbow

The elbow joint is a synovial, hinge-type joint that serves as the articulation between the humerus, radius, and ulna. The joint's primary function is to position the wrist to optimize hand function. The joint allows flexion and extension at the elbow, as well as pronation and supination of the forearm. The joint is lined with synovium, and the resultant synovial space allows intra-articular injection. The entire joint is covered by a dense capsule that thickens medially to form the ulnar collateral ligament and laterally to form the radial collateral ligaments. These dense ligaments, coupled with the elbow joint's deep bony socket, make this joint extremely stable and relatively resistant to subluxation and dislocation. The anterior and posterior joint capsule is less dense and may become distended if there is a joint effusion. The olecranon bursa lies in the posterior aspect of the elbow joint and may become inflamed as a result of direct trauma or overuse of the joint. Bursae susceptible to the development of bursitis also exist between the insertion of the biceps and the head of the radius, as well as in the antecubital and cubital area.

The elbow joint is innervated primarily by the musculocutaneous and radial nerves, with the ulnar and median nerves providing varying degrees of innervation. At the middle of the upper arm, the ulnar nerve courses medially to pass between the olecranon process and medial epicondyle of the humerus. The nerve is susceptible to entrapment and trauma at this point. At the elbow, the median nerve lies just medial to the brachial artery and occasionally is damaged during brachial artery cannulation for blood gases.

To perform intra-articular injection of the elbow, the patient is placed in a supine position with the arm fully adducted at the patient's side and the elbow flexed with the dorsum of the hand resting on a folded towel. A total of 5 mL of local anesthetic and 40 mg of methylprednisolone is drawn up in a 12-mL sterile syringe.

After sterile preparation of skin overlying the posterolateral aspect of the joint, the head of the radius is identified. Just superior to the head of the radius is an indentation that represents the space between the radial head and humerus. Using strict aseptic technique, a 1-inch, 25-gauge needle is inserted just above the superior aspect of the head of the radius through the skin, subcutaneous tissues, and joint capsule into the joint (Fig. 261-1). If bone is encountered, the needle is withdrawn into the subcutaneous tissues and redirected superiorly. After entering the joint space, the contents of the syringe are gently injected. There should be little resistance to injection. If resistance is encountered, the needle is probably in a ligament or tendon and should be advanced slightly into the joint space until the injection proceeds without significant resistance. The needle is then removed, and a sterile pressure dressing and ice pack are placed at the injection site.

The major complication of intra-articular injection of the elbow is infection, which should be exceedingly rare if strict aseptic technique is adhered to. As mentioned, the ulnar nerve is especially susceptible to damage at the elbow. Approximately 25% of patients complain of a transient increase in pain after intra-articular injection of the elbow joint; the patient should be warned of this.

SUGGESTED READING

Waldman SD: Intra-articular injection of the elbow joint. In: Atlas of Pain Management Injection Techniques, ed. 2. Philadelphia, Saunders, 2007.

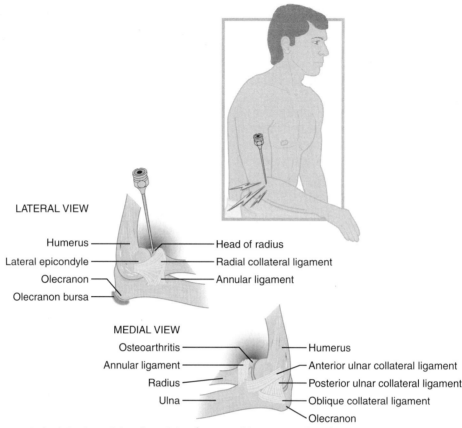

FIGURE 261–1 Intra-articular injection of the elbow joint. (From Waldman SD: Atlas of Pain Management Injection Techniques, ed. 2. Philadelphia, Saunders, 2007, p 131.)

CHAPTER 262

Injection Technique for Tennis Elbow

The most common nidus of pain from tennis elbow is the bony origin of the extensor tendon of extensor carpi radialis brevis at the anterior facet of the lateral epicondyle. Less commonly, tennis elbow pain can originate from the origin of the extensor carpi radialis longus at the supracondylar crest or, rarely, more distally at the point where the extensor carpi radialis brevis overlies the radial head. Bursitis may accompany tennis elbow. The olecranon bursa lies in the posterior aspect of the elbow joint and may also become inflamed as a result of direct trauma or overuse of the joint. Other bursae susceptible to the development of bursitis exist between the insertion of the biceps and the head of the radius, as well as in the antecubital and cubital area.

To inject tennis elbow, the patient is placed in a supine position with the arm fully adducted at the patient's side and the elbow flexed with the dorsum of the hand resting on a folded towel to relax the affected tendons. A total of 1 mL of local anesthetic and 40 mg of methylprednisolone is drawn up in a 5-mL sterile syringe.

After sterile preparation of skin overlying the posterolateral aspect of the joint, the lateral epicondyle is identified. Using strict aseptic technique, a 1-inch, 25-gauge needle is inserted perpendicular to the lateral epicondyle through the skin and into the subcutaneous tissue overlying the affected tendon (Fig. 262-1). If bone is encountered, the needle is withdrawn back into the subcutaneous tissue. The contents of the syringe are then gently injected. There should be little resistance to injection. If resistance is encountered, the needle is probably in the tendon and should be withdrawn back until the injection proceeds without significant resistance. The needle is then removed and a sterile pressure dressing and ice pack are placed at the injection site.

The major complications associated with this injection technique are related to trauma to the inflamed and previously damaged tendons. Such tendons may rupture if directly injected, and needle position should be confirmed outside the tendon prior to injection in order to avoid this complication. Another complication of this injection technique is infection, which should be exceedingly rare if strict aseptic technique is adhered to. The ulnar nerve is especially susceptible to damage at the elbow and care must be taken to avoid this nerve when injecting in this anatomic region. Approximately 25% of patients complain of a transient increase in pain after this injection technique; the patient should be warned of this.

SUGGESTED READING

Waldman SD: Tennis elbow syndrome. In: Atlas of Pain Management Injection Techniques, ed. 2. Philadelphia, Saunders, 2007.

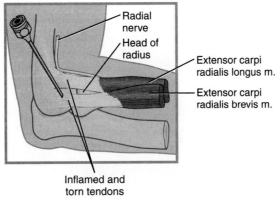

FIGURE 262–1 Injection technique for tennis elbow. (From Waldman SD: Atlas of Pain Management Injection Technique, ed. 2. Philadelphia, Saunders, 2007, p 143.)

CHAPTER 263

Injection Technique for Golfer's Elbow

The most common nidus of pain from golfer's elbow is the bony origin of the flexor tendon of the flexor carpi radialis and the humeral heads of the flexor carpi ulnaris and pronator teres at the medial epicondyle of the humerus. Less commonly, golfer's elbow pain can originate from the ulnar head of the flexor carpi ulnaris at the medial aspect of the olecranon process. Bursitis may accompany golfer's elbow. The olecranon bursa lies in the posterior aspect of the elbow joint and also may become inflamed as a result of direct trauma or overuse of the joint. Other bursae susceptible to the development of bursitis exist between the insertion of the biceps and the head of the radius, as well as in the antecubital and cubital area.

To perform an injection of golfer's elbow, the patient is placed in a supine position with the arm fully adducted at the patient's side and the elbow fully extended with the dorsum of the hand resting on a folded towel to relax the affected tendons. A total of 1 mL of local anesthetic and 40 mg of methylprednisolone is drawn up in a 5-mL sterile syringe.

After sterile preparation of skin overlying the medial aspect of the joint, the medial epicondyle is identified. Using strict aseptic technique, a 1-inch, 25-gauge needle is inserted perpendicular to the medial epicondyle through the skin and into the subcutaneous tissue overlying the affected tendon (Fig. 263-1). If bone is encountered, the needle is withdrawn back into the subcutaneous tissue.

The contents of the syringe are then gently injected. There should be little resistance to injection. If resistance is encountered, the needle is probably in the tendon and should be withdrawn back until the injection proceeds without significant resistance. The needle is then removed, and a sterile pressure dressing and ice pack are placed at the injection site.

The major complications associated with this injection technique are related to trauma to the inflamed and previously damaged tendons. Such tendons may rupture if directly injected and needle position should be confirmed outside the tendon prior to injection in order to avoid this complication. Another complication of this injection technique is infection, which should be exceedingly rare if strict aseptic technique is adhered to. The ulnar nerve is especially susceptible to damage at the elbow and care must be taken to avoid this nerve when injecting the elbow. Approximately 25% of patients complain of a transient increase in pain after this injection technique; the patient should be warned of this.

SUGGESTED READING

Waldman SD: Golfer's elbow syndrome. In: Atlas of Pain Management Injection Techniques, ed. 2. Philadelphia, Saunders, 2007.

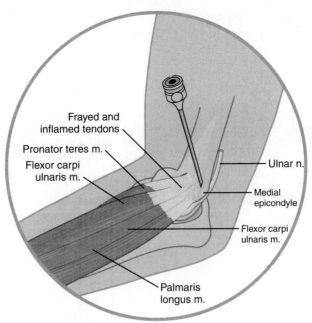

FIGURE 263–1 Injection technique for golfer's elbow. (From Waldman SD: Atlas of Pain Management Injection Techniques, ed. 2. Philadelphia, Saunders, 2007, p 150.)

CHAPTER 264

Injection Technique for Olecranon Bursitis Pain

The elbow joint is a synovial, hinge-type joint that serves as the articulation between the humerus, radius, and ulna. The joint's primary function is to position the wrist in order to optimize hand function. The joint allows flexion and extension at the elbow, as well as pronation and supination of the forearm. The joint is lined with synovium. The entire joint is covered by a dense capsule that thickens medially to form the ulnar collateral ligament and laterally to form the radial collateral ligaments. These dense ligaments, coupled with the elbow joint's deep bony socket, make this joint extremely stable and relatively resistant to subluxation and dislocation. The anterior and posterior joint capsule is less dense and may become distended if there is a joint effusion. The olecranon bursa lies in the posterior aspect of the elbow joint between the olecranon process of the ulna and the overlying skin. The olecranon bursa may become inflamed as a result of direct trauma or overuse of the joint.

The elbow joint is innervated primarily by the musculocutaneous and radial nerves, with the ulnar and median nerves providing varying degrees of innervation. At the middle of the upper arm, the ulnar nerve courses medially to pass between the olecranon process and medial epicondyle of the humerus. The nerve is susceptible to entrapment and trauma at this point. At the elbow, the median nerve lies just medial to the brachial artery and occasionally is damaged during brachial artery cannulation for blood gases.

To inject the olecranon bursa, the patient is placed in a supine position with the arm fully adducted at the patient's side and the elbow flexed with the palm of the hand resting on the patient's abdomen. A total of 2 mL of local anesthetic and 40 mg of methylprednisolone is drawn up in a 5-mL sterile syringe.

After sterile preparation of the skin overlying the posterior aspect of the joint, the olecranon process and overlying bursa are identified. Using strict aseptic technique, a 1-inch, 25-gauge needle is inserted through the skin and subcutaneous tissues directly into the bursa in the midline (Fig. 264-1). If bone is encountered, the needle is withdrawn back into the bursa. After entering the bursa, the contents of the syringe are gently injected. There should be little resistance to injection. The needle is then removed, and a sterile pressure dressing and ice pack are placed at the injection site.

The major complication of injection of the olecranon bursa is infection, which should be exceedingly rare if strict aseptic technique is adhered to. As mentioned, the ulnar nerve is especially susceptible to damage at the elbow. Approximately 25% of patients complain of a transient increase in pain after injection of the olecranon bursa; the patient should be warned of this.

SUGGESTED READING

Waldman SD: Injection technique for olecranon bursitis pain. In: Atlas of Pain Management Injection Techniques. Philadelphia, Saunders, 2007.

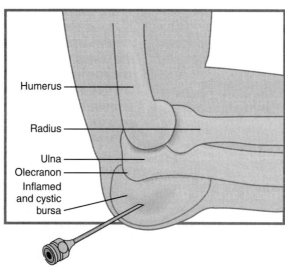

FIGURE 264–1 Injection technique for olecranon bursitis pain. (From Waldman SD: Atlas of Pain Management Injection Techniques. Philadelphia, Saunders, 2007, p 181.)

Injection Technique for Cubital Bursitis Pain

The cubital fossa lies in the anterior aspect of the elbow joint and is bounded laterally by the brachioradialis muscle, medially by the pronator teres, and contains the median nerve, which is susceptible to irritation and compression from a swollen, inflamed cubital bursa. The elbow joint is innervated primarily by the musculocutaneous and radial nerves, with the ulnar and median nerves providing varying degrees of innervation. At the middle of the upper arm, the ulnar nerve courses medially to pass between the olecranon process and medial epicondyle of the humerus. The nerve is susceptible to entrapment and trauma at this point. At the elbow, the median nerve lies just medial to the brachial artery and occasionally is damaged during brachial artery cannulation for blood gases. The median nerve also may be injured during injection of the cubital bursa.

To perform injection for cubital bursitis, the patient is placed in a supine position with the arm fully adducted at the patient's side and the elbow extended with the dorsum of the hand resting on a folded towel. A total of 2 mL of local anesthetic and 40 mg of methylprednisolone is drawn up in a 5-mL sterile syringe.

After sterile preparation of skin overlying the anterior aspect of the joint, the clinician then identifies the pulsations of the brachial artery at the crease of the elbow. After preparation of the skin with antiseptic solution, a 1-inch, 25-gauge needle is inserted just lateral to the brachial artery at the crease and slowly advanced in a slightly medial and cephalad trajectory through the skin and subcutaneous tissues (Fig. 265-1). If bone is encountered, the needle is withdrawn back into the subcutaneous tissue. The contents of the syringe are then gently injected. There should be little resistance to injection. If resistance is encountered, the needle is probably in the tendon and should be withdrawn back until the injection proceeds without significant resistance. The needle is then removed, and a sterile pressure dressing and ice pack are placed at the injection site.

Injection of the cubital bursa at the elbow is a relatively safe block, with the major complications being inadvertent intravascular injection and persistent paresthesia secondary to needle trauma to the median nerve. This technique can be safely performed in the presence of anticoagulation by using a 25- or 27-gauge needle, albeit at increased risk of hematoma, if the clinical situation dictates a favorable risk-to-benefit ratio. These complications can be decreased if manual pressure is applied to the area of the block immediately after injection. Application of cold packs for 20-minute periods following the block also decreases the amount of postprocedure pain and bleeding the patient may experience.

SUGGESTED READING

Waldman SD: Injection technique for cubital bursitis pain. In: Atlas of Pain Management Injection Techniques, ed. 2. Philadelphia, Saunders, 2007.

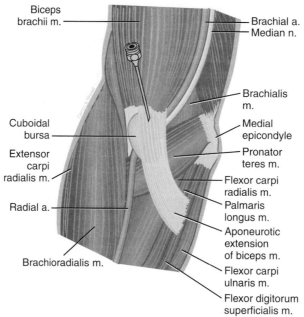

Biceps brachii m.

Brachial a.

Median n.

Brachialis m.

Medial epicondyle

Cuboidal bursa

Pronator teres m.

Extensor carpi radialis m.

Flexor carpi radialis m.

Palmaris longus m.

Radial a.

Aponeurotic extension of biceps m.

Flexor carpi ulnaris m.

Brachioradialis m.

Flexor digitorum superficialis m.

FIGURE 265–1 Injection technique for cubital bursitis pain. (From Waldman SD: Atlas of Pain Management Injection Techniques, ed. 2. Philadelphia, Saunders, 2007, p 184.)

CHAPTER 266

Technique for Intra-articular Injection of the Wrist Joint

The wrist joint is a biaxial, ellipsoid-type joint that serves as the articulation between the distal end of the radius and the articular disc above and the scaphoid, lunate, and triquetral bones below. The joint's primary role is to optimize hand function. The joint allows flexion and extension as well as abduction, adduction, and circumduction. The joint is lined with synovium, and the resultant synovial space allows intra-articular injection, although septum within the synovial space may limit the flow of injectate. The entire joint is covered by a dense capsule that is attached above to the distal ends of the radius and ulna and below to the proximal row of metacarpal bones. The anterior and posterior joint is strengthened by the anterior and posterior ligaments, with the medial and lateral ligaments strengthening the medial and lateral joint, respectively. The wrist joint also may become inflamed as a result of direct trauma or overuse of the joint.

The wrist joint is innervated primarily by the deep branch of the ulnar nerve, as well as by the anterior and posterior interosseous nerves. Anteriorly, the wrist is bounded by the flexor tendons and the median and ulnar nerves. Posteriorly, the wrist is bounded by the extensor tendons. Laterally, the radial artery can be found. The dorsal branch of the ulnar nerve runs medial to the joint; frequently this nerve is damaged when the distal ulna is fractured.

To perform intra-articular injection of the wrist, the patient is placed in a supine position with the arm fully adducted at the patient's side and the elbow slightly flexed with the palm of the hand resting on a folded towel. A total of 1.5 mL of local anesthetic and 40 mg of methylprednisolone are drawn up in a 5-mL sterile syringe. After sterile preparation of skin overlying the dorsal joint, the midcarpus proximal to the indentation of the capitate bone is identified. Just proximal to the capitate bone is an indentation that allows easy access to the wrist joint. Using strict aseptic technique, a 1-inch, 25-gauge needle is inserted in the center of the midcarpal indentation through the skin, subcutaneous tissues, and joint capsule into the joint (Fig. 266-1). If bone is encountered, the needle is withdrawn into the subcutaneous tissues and redirected superiorly. After entering the joint space, the contents of the syringe are injected gently. There should be little resistance to injection. If resistance is encountered, the needle is probably in a ligament or tendon and should be advanced slightly into the joint space until the injection proceeds without significant resistance. The needle is then removed, and a sterile pressure dressing and ice pack are placed at the injection site.

The major complication of intra-articular injection of the wrist is infection, which should be exceedingly rare if strict aseptic technique is adhered to. As mentioned, the ulnar nerve is especially susceptible to damage at the wrist. Care must be taken to avoid inadvertent intravascular injection. Approximately 25% of patients complain of a transient increase in pain following intra-articular injection of the wrist joint; the patient should be warned of this.

SUGGESTED READING

Waldman SD: Intra-articular injection of the wrist joint. In: Atlas of Pain Management Injection Techniques, ed. 2. Philadelphia, Saunders, 2007.

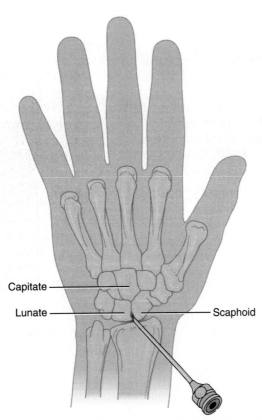

FIGURE 266–1 Technique for intra-articular injection of the wrist joint. (From Waldman SD: Atlas of Pain Management Injection Techniques, ed. 2. Philadelphia, Saunders, 2007, p 211.)

CHAPTER 267

Technique for Intra-articular Injection of the Inferior Radioulnar Joint

The radioulnar joint is a synovial, pivot-type joint that serves as the articulation between the rounded head of the ulna and the ulnar notch of the radius. The joint's primary role is to optimize hand function. The joint allows pronation and supination of the forearm. The joint is lined with synovium, and the resultant synovial space allows intra-articular injection. The entire joint is covered by a relatively weak capsule that surrounds the entire joint.

The radioulnar joint also may become inflamed as a result of direct trauma or overuse of the joint. The radioulnar joint is innervated primarily by the anterior and posterior interosseous nerves. Anteriorly, the radioulnar joint is bounded by the flexor digitorum profundus and posteriorly by the extensor digiti minimi.

To perform intra-articular injection of the inferior radioulnar joint, the patient is placed in a supine position with the arm fully adducted at the patient's side and the elbow slightly flexed with the palm of the hand resting on a folded towel. A total of 1.5 mL of local anesthetic and 40 mg of methylprednisolone are drawn up in a 5-mL sterile syringe.

After sterile preparation of skin overlying the dorsal joint, the ulnar styloid is identified. Medially, the radioulnar joint lies approximately one third of the way across the wrist. The joint can be more easily identified by gliding the distal radius and ulna together. Using strict aseptic technique, a 1-inch, 25-gauge needle is inserted in the center of the joint through the skin, subcutaneous tissues, and joint capsule into the joint (Fig. 267-1). If bone is encountered, the needle is withdrawn into the subcutaneous tissues and redirected medially. After entering the joint space, the contents of the syringe are gently injected. There should be little resistance to injection. If resistance is encountered, the needle is probably in a ligament or tendon and should be advanced slightly into the joint space until the injection proceeds without significant resistance. The needle is then removed, and a sterile pressure dressing and ice pack are placed at the injection site.

The major complication of intra-articular injection of the radioulnar joint is infection, which should be exceedingly rare if strict aseptic technique is adhered to. Approximately 25% of patients complain of a transient increase in pain after intra-articular injection of the radioulnar joint; the patient should be warned of this.

SUGGESTED READING

Waldman SD: Intra-articular injection of the inferior radioulnar joint. In: Atlas of Pain Management Injection Techniques, ed. 2. Philadelphia, Saunders, 2007.

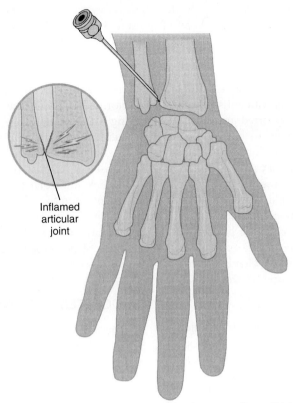

Inflamed
articular
joint

FIGURE 267–1 Technique for intra-articular injection of the inferior radioulnar joint. (From Waldman SD: Atlas of Pain Management Injection Techniques, ed. 2. Philadelphia, Saunders, 2007, p 206.)

CHAPTER 268

Injection Technique for Carpal Tunnel Syndrome

The median nerve is made up of fibers from C5-T1 spinal roots. The nerve lies anterior and superior to the axillary artery in the 12 o'clock–to–3 o'clock quadrant. Exiting the axilla, the median nerve descends into the upper arm along with the brachial artery. At the level of the elbow, the brachial artery is just medial to the biceps muscle. At this level, the median nerve lies just medial to the brachial artery. As the median nerve proceeds downward into the forearm, it gives off numerous branches that provide motor innervation to the flexor muscles of the forearm. These branches are susceptible to nerve entrapment by aberrant ligaments, muscle hypertrophy, and direct trauma. The nerve approaches the wrist overlying the radius. It lies deep to and between the tendons of the palmaris longus muscle and the flexor carpi radialis muscle at the wrist.

The median nerve then passes beneath the flexor retinaculum and through the carpal tunnel, with the nerve's terminal branches providing sensory innervation to a portion of the palmar surface of the hand as well as the palmar surface of the thumb, index, middle, and the radial portion of the ring finger. The median nerve also provides sensory innervation to the distal dorsal surface of the index and middle finger and the radial portion of the ring finger. The carpal tunnel is bounded on three sides by the carpal bones and is covered by the transverse carpal ligament. In addition to the median nerve, it contains a number of flexor tendon sheaths, blood vessels, and lymphatics.

To inject the carpal tunnel, the patient is placed in a supine position with the arm fully adducted at the patient's side and the elbow slightly flexed with the dorsum of the hand resting on a folded towel. A total of 3 mL of local anesthetic and 40 mg of methylprednisolone are drawn up in a 5-mL sterile syringe. The clinician then has the patient make a fist and at the same time flex his or her wrist to aid in identification of the palmaris longus tendon. After preparation of the skin with antiseptic solution, a ⅝-inch, 25-gauge needle is inserted just medial to the tendon and just proximal to the crease of the wrist at a 30-degree angle (Fig. 268-1). The needle is slowly advanced until the tip is just beyond the tendon. Paresthesia in the distribution of the median nerve is often elicited, and the patient should be warned of this. The patient should be told that should paresthesia occur, he or she is to say "There!" as soon as the paresthesia is felt. If paresthesia is elicited, the needle is withdrawn slightly away from the median nerve. Gentle aspiration is then carried out to identify blood. If the aspiration test is negative and no persistent paresthesia into the distribution of the median nerve remains, 3 mL of solution is slowly injected, with the patient being monitored closely for signs of local anesthetic toxicity. If no paresthesia is elicited and the needle tip hits bone, the needle is withdrawn out of the periosteum and, after careful aspiration, 3 mL of solution is slowly injected.

Injection of the carpal tunnel is a relatively safe technique, with the major complications being inadvertent intravascular injection and persistent paresthesia secondary to needle trauma to the nerve. This technique can be performed safely in the presence of anticoagulation by using a 25- or 27-gauge needle, albeit at increased risk of hematoma, if the clinical situation dictates a favorable risk-to-benefit ratio. These complications can be decreased if manual pressure is applied to the area of the block immediately after injection. There may be a transient increase in the patient's symptoms following this injection technique. Application of cold packs for 20-minute periods following the block also decreases the amount of postprocedure pain and bleeding the patient may experience.

SUGGESTED READING

Waldman SD: Injection technique for carpal tunnel syndrome. In: Atlas of Pain Management Injection Techniques. Philadelphia, Saunders, 2007.

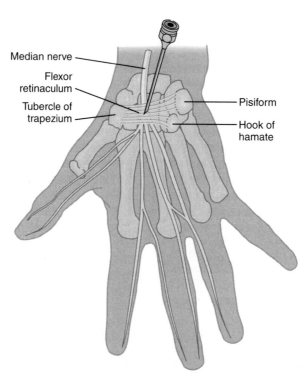

Median nerve

Flexor retinaculum

Tubercle of trapezium

Pisiform

Hook of hamate

FIGURE 268–1 Injection technique for carpal tunnel syndrome. (From Waldman SD: Atlas of Pain Management Injection Techniques. Philadelphia, Saunders, 2007, p 256.)

Injection Technique for Ulnar Tunnel Syndrome

The ulnar nerve is made up of fibers from C6-T1 spinal roots. The nerve lies anterior and inferior to the axillary artery in the 3 o'clock–to–6 o'clock quadrant. Exiting the axilla, the ulnar nerve descends into the upper arm along with the brachial artery. At the middle of the upper arm, the nerve courses medially to pass between the olecranon process and medial epicondyle of the humerus. The nerve then passes between the heads of the flexor carpi ulnaris muscle, continuing downward, moving radially along with the ulnar artery. At a point approximately 1 inch proximal to the crease of the wrist, the ulnar divides into the dorsal and palmar branches. The dorsal branch provides sensation to the ulnar aspect of the dorsum of the hand and the dorsal aspect of the little finger and the ulnar half of the ring finger. The palmar branch provides sensory innervation to the ulnar aspect of the palm of the hand and the palmar aspect of the little finger and the ulnar half of the ring finger. Like the carpal tunnel, the ulnar tunnel is a closed space and is bounded on one side by the pisiform and the other side by the hook of the hamate. The ulnar nerve must pass between the transverse carpal ligament and the volar carpal ligament. In addition to the ulnar nerve, the ulnar tunnel contains the ulnar artery, which may compress the nerve. Unlike the carpal tunnel, the ulnar tunnel does not contain flexor tendon sheaths.

To perform injection of the ulnar tunnel, the patient is placed in a supine position with the arm fully adducted at the patient's side and the elbow slightly flexed with the dorsum of the hand resting on a folded towel. A total of 3 mL of local anesthetic and 40 mg of methylprednisolone are drawn up in a 5-mL sterile syringe. The clinician then has the patient make a fist and at the same time flex his or her wrist to aid in identification of the flexor carpi ulnaris tendon. After preparation of the skin with antiseptic solution, a ⅝-inch, 25-gauge needle is inserted on the radial side of the tendon and just proximal to the crease of the wrist at a 30-degree angle (Fig. 269-1). The needle is slowly advanced until the tip is just beyond the tendon.

Paresthesia in the distribution of the ulnar nerve is often elicited, and the patient should be warned of this. The patient should be told that should paresthesia occur, he or she is to say "There!" as soon as the paresthesia is felt. If paresthesia is elicited, the needle is withdrawn slightly away from the ulnar nerve. Gentle aspiration is then carried out to identify blood. If the aspiration test is negative and no persistent paresthesia into the distribution of the ulnar nerve remains, 3 mL solution is slowly injected, with the patient being monitored closely for signs of local anesthetic toxicity. If no paresthesia is elicited and the needle tip hits bone, the needle is withdrawn out of the periosteum, and, after careful aspiration, 3 mL of solution is slowly injected.

Injection of the ulnar nerve at the wrist to treat ulnar tunnel syndrome is a relatively safe procedure, with the major complications being inadvertent intravascular injection into the ulnar artery and persistent paresthesia secondary to needle trauma to the nerve. Like the carpal tunnel, Guyon's canal is a closed space and care should be taken to inject slowly in order to avoid additional compromise of the nerve. This technique can be performed safely in the presence of anticoagulation by using a 25- or 27-gauge needle, albeit at increased risk of hematoma, if the clinical situation dictates a favorable risk-to-benefit ratio. These complications can be decreased if manual pressure is applied to the area of the block immediately after injection. Application of cold packs for 20-minute periods following the block also decreases the amount of postprocedure pain and bleeding the patient may experience.

SUGGESTED READING

Waldman SD: Ulnar tunnel syndrome. In: Atlas of Pain Management Injection Techniques. Philadelphia, Saunders, 2007.

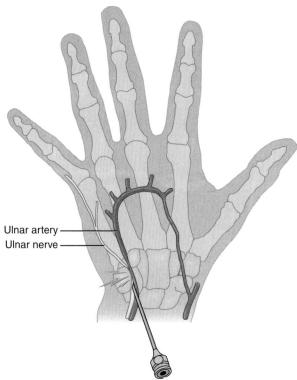

Ulnar artery
Ulnar nerve

FIGURE 269–1 Injection technique for ulnar tunnel syndrome. (From Waldman SD: Atlas of Pain Management Injection Techniques. Philadelphia, Saunders, 2007, p 264.)

CHAPTER 270

Technique for Intra-articular Injection of the Carpometacarpal Joint of the Thumb

The carpometacarpal joint of the thumb is a synovial, saddle-shaped joint that serves as the articulation between the trapezium and the base of the first metacarpal. The joint's primary function is to optimize the pinch function of the hand. The joint allows flexion, extension, abduction, adduction, and a small amount of rotation. The joint is lined with synovium and the resultant synovial space allows intra-articular injection. The entire joint is covered by a relatively weak capsule that surrounds the entire joint and is susceptible to trauma if the joint is subluxed. The carpometacarpal joint may also become inflamed as a result of direct trauma or overuse of the joint.

To perform intra-articular injection of the carpometacarpal joint of the thumb, the patient is placed in a supine position with the arm fully adducted at the patient's side with the hand in neutral position with the ulnar aspect against the table. Traction is then placed on the affected thumb to open the joint. A total of 1.5 mL of local anesthetic and 40 mg of methylprednisolone are drawn up in a 5-mL sterile syringe.

After sterile preparation of skin overlying the carpometacarpal joint of the thumb, the space between the metacarpal and trapezium is identified. The joint can be more easily identified by abducting and adducting the thumb. Using strict aseptic technique, a 1-inch, 25-gauge needle is inserted in the center of the joint through the skin, subcutaneous tissues, and joint capsule into the joint (Fig. 270-1). If bone is encountered, the needle is withdrawn into the subcutaneous tissues and redirected medially. After entering the joint space, the contents of the syringe are gently injected. There should be little resistance to injection. If resistance is encountered, the needle is probably in a tendon and should be advanced slightly into the joint space until the injection proceeds without significant resistance. The needle is then removed, and a sterile pressure dressing and ice pack are placed at the injection site.

Side Effects and Complications

The major complication of intra-articular injection of the carpometacarpal joint of the thumb is infection, which should be exceedingly rare if strict aseptic technique is adhered to. Approximately 25% of patients complain of a transient increase in pain following intra-articular injection of the carpometacarpal joint; the patient should be warned of this.

SUGGESTED READING

Waldman SD: Intra-articular injection of the carpometacarpal joint of the thumb. In: Atlas of Pain Management Injection Techniques, ed. 2. Philadelphia, Saunders, 2007.

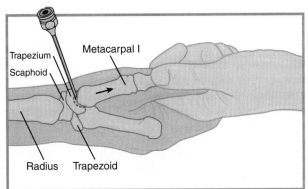

FIGURE 270–1 Intra-articular injection of the carpometacarpal joint of the thumb. (From Waldman SD: Atlas of Pain Management Injection Techniques, ed. 2. Philadelphia, Saunders, 2007, p 224.)

Intra-articular Injection of the Carpometacarpal Joint of the Fingers

The carpometacarpal joints of the fingers are synovial plane joints that serve as the articulation between the carpals and the metacarpals and also allow articulation of the bases of the metacarpal bones with one another. Movement of the joints is limited to a slight gliding motion, with the carpometacarpal joint of the little finger possessing the greatest range of motion. The joint's primary function is to optimize the grip function of the hand. In most patients, there is a common joint space. The joint is strengthened by anterior, posterior, and interosseous ligaments.

To perform intra-articular injection of the carpometacarpal joints of the fingers, the patient is placed in a supine position with the arm fully adducted at the patient's side with the hand in neutral position with the palmar aspect resting on a folded towel. A total of 1.5 mL of local anesthetic and 40 mg of methylprednisolone is drawn up in a 5-mL sterile syringe.

After sterile preparation of skin overlying the affected carpometacarpal joint, the space between the carpal and metacarpal is identified. The joint can be more easily identified by gliding the joint back and forth. Using strict aseptic technique, a 1-inch, 25-gauge needle is inserted in the center of the joint through the skin, subcutaneous tissues, and joint capsule into the joint

(Fig. 271-1). If bone is encountered, the needle is withdrawn into the subcutaneous tissues and redirected medially. After entering the joint space, the contents of the syringe are gently injected. There should be little resistance to injection. If resistance is encountered, the needle is probably in a tendon and should be advanced slightly into the joint space until the injection proceeds without significant resistance. The needle is then removed, and a sterile pressure dressing and ice pack are placed at the injection site.

The major complication of intra-articular injection of the carpometacarpal joints is infection, which should be exceedingly rare if strict aseptic technique is adhered to. Approximately 25% of patients complain of a transient increase in pain following intra-articular injection of the carpometacarpal joint; the patient should be warned of this.

SUGGESTED READING

Waldman SD: Intra-articular injection of the carpometacarpal joint of the fingers. In: Atlas of Pain Management Injection Techniques, ed. 2. Philadelphia, Saunders, 2007.

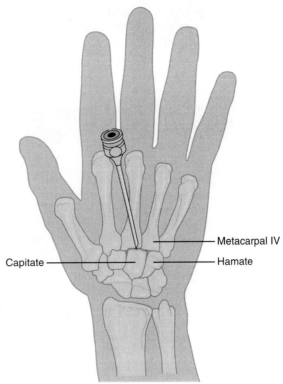

FIGURE 271–1 Intra-articular injection of the carpometacarpal joint of the fingers. (From Waldman SD: Atlas of Pain Management Injection Techniques, ed. 2. Philadelphia, Saunders, 2007, p 227.)

CHAPTER 272

Intra-articular Injection of the Metacarpophalangeal Joints

The metacarpophalangeal joint is a synovial, ellipsoid-shaped joint that serves as the articulation between the base of the proximal phalanges and the head of its respective metacarpal. The joint's primary role is to optimize the gripping function of the hand. The joint allows flexion, extension, abduction, and adduction. The joint is lined with synovium, and the resultant synovial space allows intra-articular injection. The entire joint is covered by a capsule that surrounds the entire joint and is susceptible to trauma if the joint is subluxed. Ligaments help strengthen the joints; the palmar ligaments are particularly strong.

To perform intra-articular injection of the metacarpophalangeal joints, the patient is placed in a supine position with the arm fully adducted at the patient's side with the hand in neutral position with the palmar aspect resting on a folded towel. A total of 1.5 mL of local anesthetic and 40 mg of methylprednisolone is drawn up in a 5-mL sterile syringe.

After sterile preparation of skin overlying the affected metacarpophalangeal joint, the space between the base of the proximal phalanges and the head of the respective metacarpal is identified. The joint can be identified more easily by flexing and extending the joint. Using strict aseptic technique, a 1-inch, 25-gauge needle is inserted in the center of the joint through the skin, subcutaneous tissues, and joint capsule into the joint (Fig. 272-1). If bone is encountered, the needle is withdrawn into the subcutaneous tissues and redirected medially. After entering the joint space, the contents of the syringe are gently injected. There should be little resistance to injection. If resistance is encountered, the needle is probably in a tendon and should be advanced slightly into the joint space until injection proceeds without significant resistance. The needle is then removed, and a sterile pressure dressing and ice pack are placed at the injection site.

The major complication of intra-articular injection of the metacarpophalangeal joints is infection, which should be exceedingly rare if strict aseptic technique is adhered to. Approximately 25% of patients complain of a transient increase in pain after intra-articular injection of the metacarpophalangeal joint; the patient should be warned of this.

SUGGESTED READING

Waldman SD: Intra-articular injection of the metacarpophalangeal joints. In: Atlas of Pain Management Injection Techniques, ed. 2. Philadelphia, Saunders, 2007.

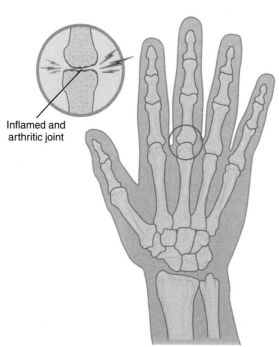

Inflamed and
arthritic joint

FIGURE 272–1 Intra-articular injection of the metacarpophalangeal joints. (From Waldman SD: Atlas of Pain Management Injection Techniques, ed. 2. Philadelphia, Saunders, 2007, p 250.)

Intra-articular Injection of the Interphalangeal Joints

The interphalangeal joints are synovial hinge-shaped joints that serve as the articulation between the phalanges. The interphalangeal joint's primary role is to optimize the gripping function of the hand. The joint allows flexion and extension. The joint is lined with synovium, and the resultant synovial space allows intra-articular injection. The entire joint is covered by a capsule that surrounds the entire joint and is susceptible to trauma if the joint is subluxed. Volar and collateral ligaments help strengthen the joint; the palmar ligaments are particularly strong.

To perform intra-articular injection of the interphalangeal joint, the patient is placed in a supine position with the arm fully adducted at the patient's side with the hand in neutral position with the palmar aspect resting on a folded towel. A total of 1.0 mL of local anesthetic and 40 mg of methylprednisolone is drawn up in a 5-mL sterile syringe.

After sterile preparation of the skin overlying the affected interphalangeal joint, the space between the affected phalanges is identified. The joint can be identified more easily by flexing and extending the joint. Using strict aseptic technique, a 1-inch, 25-gauge needle is inserted in the center of the joint through the skin, subcutaneous tissues, and joint capsule into the joint

(Fig. 273-1). If bone is encountered, the needle is withdrawn into the subcutaneous tissues and redirected medially. After entering the joint space, the contents of the syringe are gently injected. There should be little resistance to injection. If resistance is encountered, the needle is probably in a tendon and should be advanced slightly into the joint space until the injection proceeds without significant resistance. The needle is then removed, and a sterile pressure dressing and ice pack are placed at the injection site.

The major complication of intra-articular injection of the interphalangeal joints is infection, which should be exceedingly rare if strict aseptic technique is adhered to. Approximately 25% of patients complain of a transient increase in pain following intra-articular injection of the interphalangeal joint; the patient should be warned of this.

SUGGESTED READING

Waldman SD: Intra-articular injection of the interphalangeal joints. In: Atlas of Pain Management Injection Techniques, ed. 2. Philadelphia, Saunders, 2007.

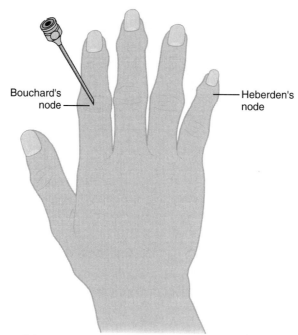

FIGURE 273–1 Intra-articular injection of the interphalangeal joints. (From Waldman SD: Atlas of Pain Management Injection Techniques, ed. 2. Philadelphia, Saunders, 2007, p 253.)

CHAPTER 274

Thoracic Epidural Block

The superior boundary of the epidural space is the fusion of the periosteal and spinal layers of dura at the foramen magnum. The epidural space continues inferiorly to the sacrococcygeal membrane. The thoracic epidural space is bounded anteriorly by the posterior longitudinal ligament and posteriorly by the vertebral laminae and the ligamentum flavum. The vertebral pedicles and intervertebral foramina form the lateral limits of the epidural space. The thoracic epidural space is 3 to 4 mm at the C7-T1 interspace with the cervical spine flexed and approximately 5 mm at the T11-12 interspace. The thoracic epidural space contains fat, veins, arteries, lymphatics, and connective tissue.

When performing thoracic epidural block in the midline, the needle traverses the following structures. After traversing the skin and subcutaneous tissues, the styletted epidural needle impinges on the supraspinous ligament, which runs vertically between the apices of the spinous processes. The supraspinous ligament offers some resistance to the advancing needle. This ligament is dense enough to hold a needle in position even when the needle is released.

The interspinous ligament, which runs obliquely between the spinous processes, is encountered next, offering additional resistance to needle advancement. Because the interspinous ligament is contiguous with the ligamentum flavum, the pain management specialist may perceive a "false" loss of resistance when the needle tip enters the space between the interspinous ligament and the ligamentum flavum. This phenomenon is more pronounced in the thoracic region than in the lumbar region as a result of the less well-defined ligaments.

A significant increase in resistance to needle advancement signals that the needle tip is impinging on the dense ligamentum flavum. Because the ligament is made up almost entirely of elastin fibers, there is a continued increase in resistance as the needle traverses the ligamentum flavum owing to the drag of the ligament on the needle. A sudden loss of resistance occurs as the needle tip enters the epidural space. There should be essentially no resistance to drugs injected into the normal epidural space.

The upper thoracic vertebral interspaces from T1-2 and the lower thoracic vertebral interspaces from T10-12 are functionally equivalent insofar as the technique of epidural block is concerned (Fig. 274-1). The technique for performing epidural block at the level of the upper and the lower thoracic vertebral interspaces is analogous to that for lumbar epidural block. The thoracic vertebral interspaces between T3 and T9 are functionally unique because of the acute downward angle of the spinous processes. Blockade of these middle thoracic interspaces requires use of the paramedian approach to the thoracic epidural space.

Thoracic epidural nerve block may be carried out in the sitting, lateral, or prone position, with the sitting position being favored for simplicity of patient positioning when compared with the lateral position. The prone position should be avoided because it makes patient monitoring more difficult.

Midline Approach

After the patient is placed in an optimal sitting position with the thoracic spine flexed and forehead placed on a padded bedside table, the skin is prepared with an antiseptic solution. For epidural blockade at the upper T1-2 or lower T10-12 interspaces, the operator's middle and index fingers are placed on each side of the spinous processes. The position of the interspace is reconfirmed with palpation using a rocking motion in the superior and inferior planes. The midline of the selected interspace is identified by palpating the spinous processes above and below the interspace using a lateral rocking motion to ensure that the needle entry site is exactly in the midline. One milliliter of local anesthetic is used to infiltrate the skin, subcutaneous tissues, and the supraspinous and interspinous ligaments at the midline.

A 2-inch, 25-gauge or a 3½-inch, 18- or 20-gauge Hustead needle is inserted exactly in the midline in the previously anesthetized area through the supraspinous ligament into the interspinous ligament. Smaller, shorter needles are being used at some centers with equally good results. After attaching a syringe containing either preservative-free saline or the intended injectate of local anesthetic, narcotic, and/or steroid, with constant pressure being applied to the plunger of the syringe with the thumb of the right hand, the needle and syringe are continuously advanced in a slow and deliberate manner with the left hand. The right-handed physician holds the epidural needle firmly at the hub with his or her left thumb and index finger. The left hand is placed firmly against the

patient's neck to ensure against uncontrolled needle movements should the patient unexpectedly move. With constant pressure being applied to the plunger of the syringe with the thumb of the right hand, the needle and syringe are continuously advanced in a slow and deliberate manner with the left hand. As soon as the needle bevel passes through the ligamentum flavum and enters the epidural space, there will be a sudden loss of resistance to injection and the plunger will effortlessly surge forward. The syringe is gently removed from the needle.

An air or saline acceptance test is carried out by injecting 0.5 to 1 mL of air or sterile preservative-free saline with a well-lubricated sterile glass syringe to help confirm that the needle is within the epidural space. The force required for injection should not exceed that necessary to overcome the resistance of the needle. Any significant pain or sudden increase in resistance during injection suggests incorrect needle placement, and one should stop injecting immediately and reassess the position of the needle.

When satisfactory needle position is confirmed, a syringe containing 5 to 7 mL of solution to be injected in the upper thoracic region, or 8 to 10 mL of solution to be injected in the lower thoracic region, is carefully attached to the needle. Gentle aspiration is carried out to identify cerebrospinal fluid or blood. If cerebrospinal fluid is aspirated, the epidural block may be repeated at a different interspace. In this situation, drug dosages should be adjusted accordingly because subarachnoid migration of drugs through the dural rent can occur. If aspiration of blood occurs, the needle should be rotated slightly and the aspiration test repeated. If no blood is present, incremental doses of local anesthetic and other drugs may be administered while monitoring the patient carefully for signs of local anesthetic toxicity.

For diagnostic and prognostic blocks, 1.0% preservative-free lidocaine is a suitable local anesthetic. For therapeutic blocks, 0.25% preservative-free bupivacaine in combination with 80 mg of depot methylprednisolone is injected. Subsequent nerve blocks are carried out in a similar manner, substituting 40 mg of methylprednisolone for the initial 80-mg dose. Daily thoracic epidural nerve blocks with local anesthetic and/or steroid may be required to treat the previously mentioned acute painful conditions. Chronic conditions such as thoracic radiculopathy, tension-type headaches, and diabetic polyneuropathy are treated on an every-other-day to once-a-week basis or as the clinical situation dictates.

If the upper thoracic epidural route is chosen for administration of opioids, 1 mg of preservative-free morphine sulfate formulated for epidural use is a reasonable initial dose in opioid-tolerant patients. For the lower thoracic region, 4 to 5 mg of morphine is an appropriate starting dose. More lipid-soluble opioids such as fentanyl must be delivered by continuous infusion via a thoracic epidural catheter. An epidural catheter may be placed into the thoracic epidural space through a Hustead needle to allow continuous infusions.

Paramedian Approach

Mid-thoracic epidural nerve block using the paramedian approach may be carried out in the sitting, lateral, or prone position, with the sitting position being favored for simplicity of patient positioning when compared with the lateral position. The prone position should be avoided because it makes patient monitoring more difficult.

After the patient is placed in an optimal sitting position with the thoracic spine flexed and forehead placed on a padded bedside table, the skin is prepared with an antiseptic solution. For epidural blockade of the T3-9 interspaces, the operator's middle and index fingers are placed on each side of the spinous processes. The position of the interspace is reconfirmed with palpation using a rocking motion in the superior and inferior planes. The midline of the selected interspace is identified by palpating the spinous processes above and below the interspace using a lateral rocking motion to ensure accurate identification of the midline. At a point approximately ½ inch lateral to the midline at the level of the inferior border of the spinous process, 1 mL of local anesthetic is used to infiltrate the skin, subcutaneous tissues, muscle, and any ligaments encountered (Fig. 274-2).

The 3½-inch, 18- or 20-gauge Hustead needle is inserted perpendicular to the skin into the subcutaneous tissues. The needle is then redirected slightly medial and craniad and advanced approximately ½ inch. The needle stylet is removed, and a well-lubricated 5-mL glass syringe filled with preservative-free sterile saline is attached.

The right-handed physician holds the epidural needle firmly at the hub with his or her left thumb and index finger. The left hand is placed firmly against the patient's neck to ensure against uncontrolled needle movements should the patient unexpectedly move. With constant pressure being applied to the plunger of the syringe with the thumb of the right hand, the needle and syringe are continuously advanced in a slow and deliberate manner with the left hand. As soon as the needle bevel passes through the ligamentum flavum and enters the epidural space, there will be a sudden loss of resistance to injection and the plunger will effortlessly surge forward (Fig. 274-3). If bony contact is made, the needle is withdrawn and redirected in a slightly more medial and cranial trajectory. After the epidural space is identified, the syringe is gently removed from the needle.

An air or saline acceptance test is carried out by injecting 0.5 to 1 mL of air or sterile preservative-free saline with a well-lubricated sterile glass syringe to help confirm that the needle is within the epidural space. The force required for injection should not exceed that necessary to overcome the resistance of the needle. Any significant pain or sudden increase in resistance during injection suggests incorrect needle placement, and one should *stop* injecting immediately and reassess the position of the needle.

When satisfactory needle position is confirmed, a syringe containing 6 to 7 mL of solution to be injected is carefully attached to the needle. Gentle aspiration is carried out to identify cerebrospinal fluid or blood. If cerebrospinal fluid is aspirated, the epidural block may be repeated at a different interspace. In this situation, drug dosages should be adjusted accordingly because subarachnoid migration of drugs through the dural rent can occur. If aspiration of blood occurs, the needle should be rotated slightly and the aspiration test repeated. If no blood is present, incremental doses of local anesthetic and other drugs may be administered while monitoring the patient carefully for signs of local anesthetic toxicity.

For diagnostic and prognostic blocks, 1.0% preservative-free lidocaine is a suitable local anesthetic. For therapeutic blocks, 0.25% preservative-free bupivacaine in combination with 80 mg of depot methylprednisolone is injected. Subsequent nerve blocks are carried out in a similar manner, substituting 40 mg of methylprednisolone for the initial 80-mg dose. Daily thoracic epidural nerve blocks with local anesthetic and/or steroid may be required to treat the previously mentioned acute painful conditions. Chronic conditions such as thoracic radiculopathy, postherpetic neuralgia, and diabetic polyneuropathy are treated on an every-other-day to once-a-week basis or as the clinical situation dictates.

If the mid-thoracic epidural route is chosen for administration of opioids, 3 mg of preservative-free morphine sulfate formulated for epidural use is a reasonable initial dose in opioid-tolerant patients. More lipid soluble opioids such as fentanyl must be delivered by continuous infusion via a thoracic epidural catheter. An epidural catheter may be placed into the thoracic epidural space through a Hustead needle to allow continuous infusions.

Because of the potential for hematogenous spread via Batson's plexus, local infection and sepsis represent absolute contraindications to the thoracic approach to the epidural space. In contradistinction to the caudal approach to the epidural space, anticoagulation and coagulopathy represent absolute contraindications to thoracic epidural nerve block because of the risk of epidural hematoma.

Inadvertent dural puncture occurring during thoracic epidural nerve block should occur less than 0.5% of the time. Failure to recognize inadvertent dural puncture can result in immediate total spinal anesthetic with associated loss of consciousness, hypotension, and apnea.

If epidural doses of opioids are accidentally placed into the subarachnoid space, significant respiratory and central nervous system depression will result. It is also possible to inadvertently place a needle or catheter intended for the epidural space into the subdural space. If subdural placement is unrecognized and epidural doses of local anesthetics are administered, the signs and symptoms are similar to those of massive subarachnoid injection, although the resulting motor and sensory block may be spotty.

The thoracic epidural space is highly vascular. The intravenous placement of the epidural needle occurs in approximately 0.5% to 1% of patients undergoing thoracic epidural anesthesia. This complication is increased in those patients with distended epidural veins, such as the parturient and patients with large intra-abdominal tumor mass. If the misplacement is unrecognized, injection of local anesthetic directly into an epidural vein will result in significant local anesthetic toxicity.

Needle trauma to the epidural veins may result in self-limited bleeding that may cause postprocedure pain. Uncontrolled bleeding into the epidural space may result in compression of the spinal cord with the rapid development of neurologic deficit. Although the incidence of significant neurologic deficit secondary to epidural hematoma after thoracic epidural block is exceedingly rare, this devastating complication should be considered whenever there is rapidly developing neurologic deficit after thoracic epidural nerve block.

Neurologic complications after thoracic nerve block are uncommon if proper technique is used. Direct trauma to the spinal cord and/or nerve roots is usually accompanied by pain. If significant pain occurs during placement of the epidural needle or catheter or during injection, the physician should immediately stop and ascertain the cause of the pain to avoid the possibility of additional neural trauma.

Although uncommon, infection in the epidural space remains an ever-present possibility, especially in the immunocompromised AIDS or cancer patient. If epidural abscess occurs, emergent surgical drainage to avoid spinal cord compression and irreversible neurologic deficit is usually required. Early detection and treatment of infection are crucial to avoid potentially life-threatening sequelae.

SUGGESTED READINGS

Waldman SD: Thoracic epidural block: Midline approach. In: Atlas of Interventional Pain Management, ed 2. Philadelphia, Saunders, 2004.

Waldman SD: Thoracic epidural block: Paramedian approach. In: Atlas of Interventional Pain Management, ed 2. Philadelphia, Saunders, 2004.

Waldman SD: Thoracic epidural block: Transforaminal approach. In: Atlas of Interventional Pain Management, ed 2. Philadelphia, Saunders, 2004.

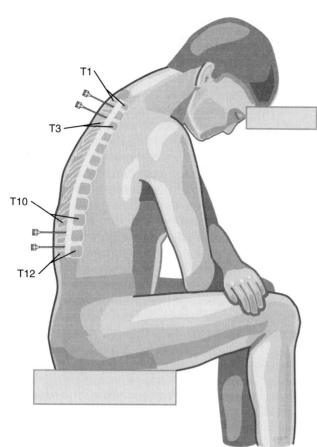

FIGURE 274–1 The upper thoracic vertebral interspaces from T1-2 and the lower thoracic vertebral interspaces from T10-12 are functionally equivalent insofar as the technique of epidural block is concerned. (From Waldman SD: Atlas of Interventional Pain Management, ed 2. Philadelphia, Saunders, 2004, p 213.)

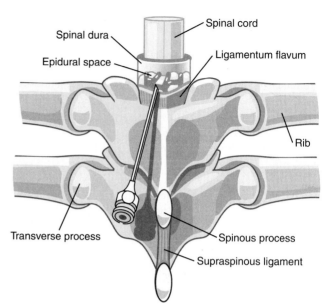

FIGURE 274–2 Thoracic epidural block: paramedian approach. (From Waldman SD: Atlas of Interventional Pain Management, ed 2. Philadelphia, Saunders, 2004, p 219.)

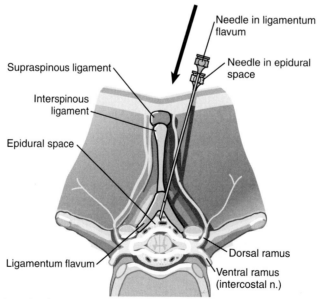

FIGURE 274–3 Correct needle position for the paramedian approach. (From Waldman SD: Atlas of Interventional Pain Management, ed 2. Philadelphia, Saunders, 2004, p 220.)

Thoracic Paravertebral Block

The thoracic paravertebral nerves exit their respective intervertebral foramina just beneath the transverse process of the vertebra. After exiting the intervertebral foramen, the thoracic paravertebral nerve gives off a recurrent branch that loops back through the foramen to provide innervation to the spinal ligaments, meninges, and its respective vertebra. The thoracic paravertebral nerve also interfaces with the thoracic sympathetic chain via the myelinated preganglionic fibers of the white rami communicantes as well as the unmyelinated postganglionic fibers of the gray rami communicantes. After providing these intercommunications with the thoracic sympathetic nervous system as well as the recurrent branch, the thoracic paravertebral nerve divides into a posterior and an anterior primary division. The posterior division courses posteriorly and, along with its branches, provides innervation to the facet joints and the muscles and skin of the back. The larger, anterior division courses laterally to pass into the subcostal groove beneath the rib to become the respective intercostal nerves. The 12th thoracic nerve courses beneath the 12th rib and is called the subcostal nerve. The intercostal and subcostal nerves provide the innervation to the skin, muscles, ribs, and the parietal pleura and parietal peritoneum. Because blockade of the thoracic paravertebral nerve is performed at the point at which the nerve is beginning to give off its various branches, it is possible to block the anterior division and the posterior division as well as the recurrent and sympathetic components of each respective thoracic paravertebral nerve.

To perform thoracic paravertebral block, the patient is placed in the prone position with a pillow under the lower chest to slightly flex the thoracic spine. The spinous process of the vertebra just above the nerve to be blocked is palpated. At a point just below and 1½ inches lateral to the spinous process, the skin is prepared with antiseptic solution. A 22-gauge, 3½-inch needle is attached to a 12-mL syringe and is advanced perpendicular to the skin aiming for the middle of the transverse process. The needle should impinge on bone after being advanced approximately 1½ inches. After bony contact is

made, the needle is withdrawn into the subcutaneous tissues and redirected inferiorly and "walked off" the inferior margin of the transverse process (Fig. 275-1). As soon as bony contact is lost, the needle is slowly advanced approximately ¾ inch deeper until paresthesia in the distribution of the thoracic paravertebral nerve to be blocked is elicited. Once the paresthesia has been elicited and careful aspiration reveals no blood or cerebrospinal fluid, 5 mL of 1.0% preservative-free lidocaine is injected. If there is an inflammatory component to the pain, the local anesthetic is combined with 80 mg of methylprednisolone and is injected in incremental doses. Subsequent daily nerve blocks are carried out in a similar manner, substituting 40 mg of methylprednisolone for the initial 80-mg dose. Because of overlapping innervation of the posterior elements from the medial branch of the posterior division from adjacent vertebrae, the paravertebral nerves above and below the nerve suspected of subserving the painful condition will have to be blocked.

The proximity to the spinal cord and exiting nerve roots makes it imperative that this procedure be carried out only by those well versed in the regional anatomy and experienced in performing interventional pain management techniques. Given the proximity of the pleural space, pneumothorax after thoracic paravertebral nerve block is a distinct possibility. Needle placement too medial may result in epidural, subdural, or subarachnoid injections or trauma to the spinal cord and exiting nerve roots. Placing the needle too deep between the transverse processes may result in trauma to the exiting thoracic nerve roots. Although uncommon, infection remains an ever-present possibility, especially in the immunocompromised cancer patient. Early detection of infection is crucial to avoid potentially life-threatening sequelae.

SUGGESTED READING

Waldman SD: Thoracic paravertebral block. In: Atlas of Interventional Pain Management, ed 2. Philadelphia, Saunders, 2004.

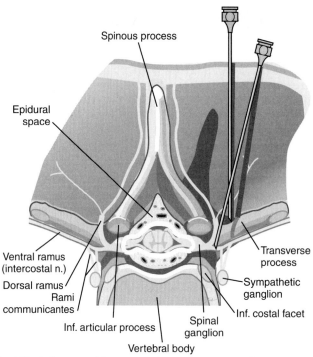

FIGURE 275–1 Thoracic paravertebral block. (From Waldman SD: Atlas of Interventional Pain Management, ed 2. Philadelphia, Saunders, 2004, p 229.)

CHAPTER 276

Thoracic Facet Block

The thoracic facet joints are formed by the articulations of the superior and inferior articular facets of adjacent vertebrae. The thoracic facet joints are true joints in that they are lined with synovium and possess a true joint capsule. This capsule is richly innervated and supports the notion of the facet joint as a pain generator. The thoracic facet joint is susceptible to arthritic changes and trauma secondary to acceleration-deceleration injuries. Such damage to the joint results in pain secondary to synovial joint inflammation and adhesions.

Each facet joint receives innervation from two spinal levels. Each joint receives fibers from the dorsal ramus at the same level as the vertebra as well as fibers from the dorsal ramus of the vertebra above. This fact has clinical import in that it provides an explanation for the ill-defined nature of facet-mediated pain and explains why the dorsal nerve from the vertebra above the offending

level must often also be blocked to provide complete pain relief.

At each level, the dorsal ramus provides a medial branch that exits the intertransverse space crossing over the top of the transverse process at the point where the transverse process joins the vertebra. The nerve then travels inferiorly and medially across the posterior surface of the transverse process to innervate the facet joint. In a manner analogous to lumbar facet block, the medial branch is blocked at the point at which the nerve curves around the top of the transverse process. It should be noted that in the mid-thoracic region, the medial branch of the dorsal ramus may travel superior to the point at which the transverse process joins the vertebra. This probably does not have any clinical significance unless radiofrequency lesioning or cryoneurolysis of the nerve is being considered. In this case, the needle or cryoprobe may have to be placed superior to the junction of the transverse process and vertebra.

Medial Branch Technique

Thoracic facet block using the medial branch technique is the preferred route of treating thoracic facet syndrome. It may be done either blind or under fluoroscopic guidance. The patient is placed in a prone position. Pillows are placed under the chest to allow the thoracic spine to be moderately flexed without discomfort to the patient. The forehead is allowed to rest on a folded blanket.

BLIND TECHNIQUE

If a blind technique is used, the spinous process at the level to be blocked is identified by palpation. A point slightly inferior and 5 cm lateral to the spinous process is then identified as the site of needle insertion. After preparation of the skin with antiseptic solution, a skin wheal of local anesthetic is raised at the site of needle insertion. Then 3 mL of preservative-free local anesthetic is drawn up in a 5-mL sterile syringe. When treating pain thought to be secondary to an inflammatory process, a total of 80 mg of depot steroid is added to the local anesthetic with the first block and 40 mg of depot steroid is added with subsequent blocks.

An 18-gauge, 1-inch needle is inserted through the skin and into the subcutaneous tissue at the previously identified insertion site to serve as an introducer. The introducer needle is then repositioned with a slightly superior and medial trajectory, pointing directly toward the superior portion of the junction of the transverse process and the vertebra at the level to be blocked. A 25-gauge, 3½-inch styletted spinal needle is then inserted through the 18-gauge introducer and directed toward this junction of the transverse process and the vertebra. After bony contact is made, the depth of the contact is noted and the spinal needle is withdrawn. The introducer needle is then repositioned aiming toward the most superior and medial aspect of the junction of the transverse process with the vertebra. The 25-gauge spinal needle is then readvanced until it impinges on the lateralmost aspect of the border of the articular pillar (Fig. 276-1). Should the spinal needle "walk off" the top of the transverse process, it is withdrawn and redirected slightly medially and inferiorly and carefully advanced to the depth of the previous bony contact.

After the needle is felt to be in satisfactory position, the stylet is removed from the 25-gauge spinal needle and the hub is observed for blood or cerebrospinal fluid (CSF). If neither is present, gentle aspiration of the needle is carried out. If the aspiration test is negative, 1.5 mL of solution is injected through the spinal needle.

FLUOROSCOPIC TECHNIQUE

If fluoroscopy is used, the beam is rotated in a sagittal plane from anterior to posterior position, which allows identification and visualization of the junction of the transverse process and vertebra at the level to be blocked. After preparation of the skin with antiseptic solution, a skin wheal of local anesthetic is raised at a point slightly inferior and approximately 5 cm off the midline. An 18-gauge, 1-inch needle is inserted at the insertion site to serve as an introducer. The fluoroscopy beam is aimed directly through the introducer needle, which will appear as a small point on the fluoroscopy screen. The introducer needle is then repositioned under fluoroscopic guidance until this small point is visualized pointing directly toward the most superior and medial point at which the transverse process joins the vertebra.

A total of 5 mL of contrast medium suitable for intrathecal use is drawn up in a sterile 12-mL syringe. Then, 3 mL of preservative-free local anesthetic is drawn up in a separate 5-mL sterile syringe. When treating pain thought to be secondary to an inflammatory process, a total of 80 mg of depot steroid is added to the local anesthetic with the first block and 40 mg of depot steroid is added with subsequent blocks.

A 25-gauge, 3½-inch styletted spinal needle is then inserted through the 18-gauge introducer and directed toward the most superior and medial point at which the transverse process joins the vertebra. After bony contact is made, the spinal needle is withdrawn and the introducer needle is redirected to allow the spinal needle to impinge on the most superior and medial point at which the transverse process joins the vertebra. This procedure is repeated until the tip of the 25-gauge spinal needle rests against the most superior and medial point at which the transverse process joins the vertebra.

After confirmation of needle placement by biplanar fluoroscopy, the stylet is removed from the 25-gauge spinal needle, and the hub is observed for blood or CSF. If neither is present, gentle aspiration of the needle is carried out. If the aspiration test is negative, 1 mL of contrast medium is slowly injected under fluoroscopy to reconfirm needle placement. After correct needle placement is confirmed, 1.5 mL of local anesthetic with or without steroid is injected through the spinal needle.

Intra-articular Technique

Thoracic facet block using the intra-articular technique may be performed either blind or under fluoroscopic guidance. The patient is placed in a prone position. Pillows are placed under the chest to allow the thoracic spine to be moderately flexed without discomfort to the patient. The forehead is allowed to rest on a folded blanket.

BLIND TECHNIQUE

If a blind technique is used, the spinous process at the level to be blocked is identified by palpation. A point two spinal levels lower and 2.5 cm lateral to the spinous process is then identified as the site of needle insertion. Then 3 mL of preservative-free local anesthetic is drawn up in a 5-mL sterile syringe. After preparation of the skin with antiseptic solution, a skin wheal of local anesthetic is raised at the site of needle insertion. When treating pain thought to be secondary to an inflammatory process, a total of 80 mg of depot steroid is added to the local anesthetic with the first block and 40 mg of depot steroid is added with subsequent blocks.

An 18-gauge, 1-inch needle is inserted through the skin and into the subcutaneous tissue at the previously identified insertion site to serve as an introducer. The introducer needle is then repositioned with a superior and ventral trajectory, pointing directly toward the inferior margin of the facet joint at the level to be blocked. The angle of the needle from the skin is approximately 25 degrees. A 25-gauge, 3½-inch styletted spinal needle is then inserted through the 18-gauge introducer and directed toward the articular pillar just below the joint to be blocked. Care must be taken to be sure the trajectory of the needle does not drift either laterally or medially. Medial drift can allow the needle to enter the epidural, subdural, or subarachnoid space and to traumatize the dorsal root or spinal cord. Lateral drift can allow the needle to pass beyond the lateral border of the articular pillar and traumatize the exiting nerve roots.

After bony contact is made, the depth of the contact is noted and the spinal needle is withdrawn. The introducer needle is then redirected slightly more superiorly. The spinal needle is then advanced through the introducer needle until it impinges on the bone of the articular pillar. This maneuver is repeated until the spinal needle slides into the facet joint (Fig. 276-2). A pop is often felt as the needle slides into the joint cavity.

After the needle is felt to be in satisfactory position, the stylet is removed from the 25-gauge spinal needle and the hub is observed for blood or CSF. If neither is present, gentle aspiration of the needle is carried out. If the aspiration test is negative, 1 mL of solution is injected slowly through the spinal needle. Rapid or forceful injection may rupture the joint capsule and exacerbate the patient's pain.

FLUOROSCOPIC TECHNIQUE

If fluoroscopy is used, the beam is rotated in a sagittal plane from anterior to posterior position, which allows identification and visualization of the articular pillars of the respective vertebrae and the adjacent facet joints. After preparation of the skin with antiseptic solution, a skin wheal of local anesthetic is raised at the site of needle insertion. An 18-gauge, 1-inch needle is inserted at the insertion site to serve as an introducer. The fluoroscopy beam is aimed directly through the introducer needle, which will appear as a small point on the fluoroscopy screen. The introducer needle is then repositioned under fluoroscopic guidance until this small point is visualized pointing directly toward the inferior aspect of the facet joint to be blocked.

A total of 5 mL of contrast medium suitable for intrathecal use is drawn up in a sterile 12-mL syringe. Then, 2 mL of preservative-free local anesthetic is drawn up in a separate 5-mL sterile syringe. When treating pain thought to be secondary to an inflammatory process, a total of 80 mg of depot steroid is added to the local anesthetic with the first block and 40 mg of depot steroid is added with subsequent blocks.

A 25-gauge, 3½-inch styletted spinal needle is then inserted through the 18-gauge introducer and directed toward the articular pillar just below the joint to be blocked. After bony contact is made, the spinal needle is withdrawn and the introducer needle repositioned superiorly, aiming toward the facet joint itself. The 25-gauge spinal needle is then re-advanced through the introducer needle until it enters the target joint.

After confirmation of needle placement by biplanar fluoroscopy, the stylet is removed from the 25-gauge spinal needle, and the hub is observed for blood or CSF. If neither is present, gentle aspiration of the needle is carried out. If the aspiration test is negative, 1 mL of contrast medium is slowly injected under fluoroscopy to reconfirm needle placement. After correct needle placement is confirmed, 1 mL of local anesthetic with or without steroid is slowly injected through the spinal needle. Rapid or forceful injection may rupture the joint capsule and exacerbate the patient's pain.

The proximity to the spinal cord and exiting nerve roots makes it imperative that this procedure be carried out only by those well versed in the regional anatomy and experienced in performing interventional pain management techniques. Given the proximity of the pleural space, pneumothorax after thoracic facet block is a distinct possibility. Needle placement too medial may result in epidural, subdural, or subarachnoid injections or trauma to the spinal cord and exiting nerve roots. Placing the needle too deep between the transverse processes may result in trauma to nerve roots.

SUGGESTED READINGS

Waldman SD: Thoracic paravertebral block: Medial branch technique. In: Atlas of Interventional Pain Management, ed 2. Philadelphia, Saunders, 2004.

Waldman SD: Thoracic paravertebral block: Intra-articular technique. In: Atlas of Interventional Pain Management, ed 2. Philadelphia, Saunders, 2004.

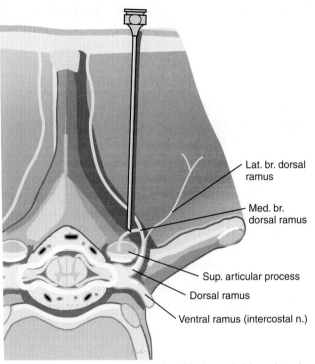

FIGURE 276–1 Thoracic paravertebral block: medial branch technique. (From Waldman SD: Atlas of Interventional Pain Management, ed 2. Philadelphia, Saunders, 2004, p 232.)

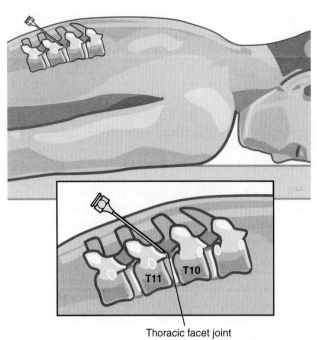

FIGURE 276–2 Thoracic paravertebral block: intra-articular technique. (From Waldman SD: Atlas of Interventional Pain Management, ed 2. Philadelphia, Saunders, 2004, p 236.)

CHAPTER 277

Thoracic Sympathetic Block

The preganglionic fibers of the thoracic sympathetics exit the intervertebral foramen along with the respective thoracic paravertebral nerves. After exiting the intervertebral foramen, the thoracic paravertebral nerve gives off a recurrent branch that loops back through the foramen to provide innervation to the spinal ligaments, meninges, and its respective vertebra. The thoracic paravertebral nerve also interfaces with the thoracic sympathetic chain via the myelinated preganglionic fibers of the white rami communicantes as well as the unmyelinated postganglionic fibers of the gray rami communicantes. At the level of the thoracic sympathetic ganglia, preganglionic and postganglionic fibers synapse. Additionally, some of the postganglionic fibers return to their respective somatic nerves via the gray rami communicantes. These fibers provide sympathetic innervation to the vasculature, sweat glands, and pilomotor muscles of the skin. Other thoracic sympathetic postganglionic fibers travel to the cardiac plexus and course up and down the sympathetic trunk to terminate in distant ganglia.

The first thoracic ganglion is fused with the lower cervical ganglion to help make up the stellate ganglion. As the chain moves caudad, it changes its position with the upper thoracic ganglia just beneath the rib and the lower thoracic ganglia moving more anterior to rest along the posterolateral surface of the vertebral body. The pleural space lies lateral and anterior to the thoracic sympathetic chain. Given the proximity of the thoracic somatic nerves to the thoracic sympathetic chain, the potential exists for both neural pathways to be blocked when performing blockade of the thoracic sympathetic ganglion.

To perform thoracic sympathetic block, the patient is placed in the prone position with a pillow under the lower chest to slightly flex the thoracic spine. The spinous process of the vertebra just above the nerve to be blocked is palpated. At a point just below and 1½ inches lateral to the spinous process, the skin is prepared with antiseptic solution. A 22-gauge, 3½-inch needle is attached to a 12-mL syringe and is advanced perpendicular to the skin aiming for the middle of the transverse process (Fig. 277-1). The needle should impinge on bone after being advanced approximately 1½ inches. After bony contact is made, the needle is withdrawn into the subcutaneous tissues and redirected inferiorly and "walked off" the inferior margin of the transverse process. As soon as bony contact is lost, the needle is slowly advanced approximately 1 inch deeper. Given the proximity of the thoracic sympathetic chain to the somatic nerve, paresthesia in the distribution of the corresponding thoracic paravertebral nerve may be elicited. If this occurs, the needle should be withdrawn and redirected slightly more cephalad, with care being taken to keep the needle close to the vertebral body to avoid pneumothorax. Once the needle is in position and careful aspiration reveals no blood or cerebrospinal fluid, 5 mL of 1.0% preservative-free lidocaine is injected.

The proximity to the spinal cord and exiting nerve roots makes it imperative that this procedure be carried out only by those well versed in the regional anatomy and experienced in performing interventional pain management techniques. Given the proximity of the pleural space, pneumothorax after thoracic sympathetic ganglion block is a distinct possibility. The incidence of pneumothorax will be decreased if care is taken to keep the needle placed medially against the vertebral body. Needle placement too medial may result in epidural, subdural, or subarachnoid injections or trauma to the spinal cord and exiting nerve roots. Although uncommon, infection remains an ever-present possibility, especially in the immunocompromised cancer patient. Early detection of infection is crucial to avoid potentially life-threatening sequelae.

SUGGESTED READING

Waldman SD: Thoracic sympathetic block. In: Atlas of Interventional Pain Management, ed 2. Philadelphia, Saunders, 2004.

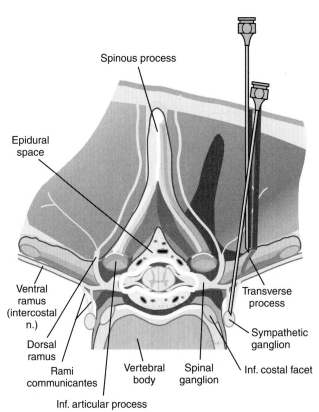

FIGURE 277–1 Thoracic sympathetic block. (From Waldman SD: Atlas of Interventional Pain Management, ed 2. Philadelphia, Saunders, 2004, p 240.)

Intercostal Nerve Block

The intercostal nerves arise from the anterior division of the thoracic paravertebral nerve. A typical intercostal nerve has four major branches. The first branch is the unmyelinated postganglionic fibers of the gray rami communicantes, which interface with the sympathetic chain. The second branch is the posterior cutaneous branch, which innervates the muscles and skin of the paraspinal area. The third branch is the lateral cutaneous division, which arises in the anterior axillary line. The lateral cutaneous division provides the majority of the cutaneous innervation of the chest and abdominal wall. The fourth branch is the anterior cutaneous branch supplying innervation to the midline of the chest and abdominal wall. Occasionally, the terminal branches of a given intercostal nerve may actually cross the midline to provide sensory innervation to the contralateral chest and abdominal wall. The 12th nerve is called the subcostal nerve and is unique in that it gives off a branch to the first lumbar nerve, thus contributing to the lumbar plexus.

To perform intercostal nerve block, the patient is placed in the prone position with the patient's arms hanging loosely off the side of the cart. Alternatively, this block can be done in the sitting or lateral position. The rib to be blocked is identified by palpating its path at the posterior axillary line. The index and middle fingers are then placed on the rib bracketing the site of needle insertion. The skin is then prepared with antiseptic solution. A 22-gauge, 1½-inch needle is attached to a 12-mL syringe and is advanced perpendicular to the skin aiming for the middle of the rib in between the index and middle fingers. The needle should impinge on bone after being advanced approximately ¾ inch. After bony contact is made, the needle is withdrawn into the subcutaneous tissues, and the skin and subcutaneous tissues are retracted with the palpating fingers inferiorly.

This allows the needle to be "walked off" the inferior margin of the rib (Fig. 278-1). As soon as bony contact is lost, the needle is slowly advanced approximately 2 mm deeper. This will place the needle in proximity to the costal grove, which contains the intercostal nerve as well as the intercostal artery and vein. After careful aspiration reveals no blood or air, 3 to 5 mL of 1.0% preservative-free lidocaine is injected. If there is an inflammatory component to the pain, the local anesthetic is combined with 80 mg of methylprednisolone and is injected in incremental doses. Subsequent daily nerve blocks are carried out in a similar manner, substituting 40 mg of methylprednisolone for the initial 80-mg dose. Because of the overlapping innervation of the chest and upper abdominal wall, the intercostal nerves above and below the nerve suspected of subserving the painful condition will have to be blocked.

Given the proximity of the pleural space, pneumothorax after intercostal nerve block is a distinct possibility. The incidence of the complication is less than 1%, but it occurs with greater frequency in patients with chronic obstructive pulmonary disease. Because of the proximity to the intercostal nerve and artery, the pain management specialist should carefully calculate the total milligram dosage of local anesthetic administered because vascular uptake via these vessels is high. Although uncommon, infection remains an ever-present possibility, especially in the immunocompromised cancer patient. Early detection of infection is crucial to avoid potentially life-threatening sequelae.

SUGGESTED READING

Waldman SD: Intercostal nerve block. In: Atlas of Interventional Pain Management, ed 2. Philadelphia, Saunders, 2004.

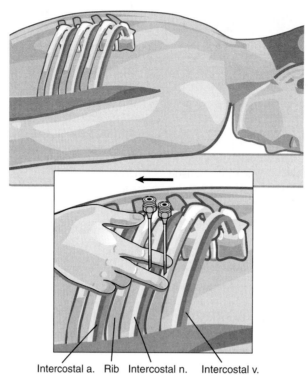

Intercostal a.   Rib   Intercostal n.   Intercostal v.

FIGURE 278–1 Intercostal nerve block. (From Waldman SD: Atlas of Interventional Pain Management, ed 2. Philadelphia, Saunders, 2004, p 243.)

CHAPTER 279

Radiofrequency Lesioning—Intercostal Nerves

The intercostal nerves arise from the anterior division of the thoracic spinal nerve. A typical intercostal nerve has four major branches. The first branch is made up of the unmyelinated postganglionic fibers of the gray rami communicantes, which interface with the sympathetic chain. The second branch is the posterior cutaneous branch, which innervates the muscles and skin of the paraspinal area. The third branch is the lateral cutaneous division, which arises in the anterior axillary line. The lateral cutaneous division provides the majority of the cutaneous innervation of the chest and abdominal wall. The fourth branch is the anterior cutaneous branch supplying innervation to the midline of the chest and abdominal wall. Occasionally, the terminal branches of a given intercostal nerve may actually cross the midline to provide sensory innervation to the contralateral chest and abdominal wall.

The 12th nerve is called the subcostal nerve and is unique in that it gives off a branch to the first lumbar nerve, thus contributing to the lumbar plexus.

To perform radiofrequency lesioning of the intercostal nerves, the patient is placed in the prone position with the patient's arms hanging loosely off the side of the cart. Alternatively, this block can be done in the sitting or lateral position based on the patient's ability to assume the desired position. The rib to be blocked is identified by palpating its path at the posterior axillary line or by fluoroscopy. The index and middle fingers are then placed on the rib bracketing the site of needle insertion. The skin is then prepared with antiseptic solution. A 54-mm, 22-gauge radiofrequency needle with a 4-mm active tip is then advanced, perpendicular to the skin using a slight medial direction to lie as parallel as possible to the nerve, aiming for the middle of the rib in between the index and middle fingers. The needle should impinge on bone after being advanced approximately ¾ inch. After bony contact is made, the needle is withdrawn into the subcutaneous tissues, and the skin and subcutaneous tissues are retracted with the palpating fingers inferiorly. This allows the needle to be "walked off" the inferior margin of the rib (Fig. 279-1). As soon as bony contact is lost, the needle is slowly advanced approximately 2 mm deeper. This will place the needle in proximity to the costal groove, which contains the intercostal nerve as well as the intercostal artery and vein. Trial sensory stimulation is then carried out with 2 V at 50 Hz. If the needle is in proper position, the patient should experience paresthesia in the distribution of the target intercostal nerve. If a proper stimulation pattern is identified, a pulsed radiofrequency lesion is created by heating at 40° C to 45° C for 5 minutes or heating at 49° C to 60° C for 90 seconds. This technique is repeated for each affected nerve root.

Given the proximity of the pleural space, pneumothorax after intercostal nerve block is a distinct possibility. The incidence of the complication is less than 1%, but it occurs with greater frequency in patients with chronic obstructive pulmonary disease. Because of the proximity to the intercostal nerve and artery, the pain management specialist should carefully calculate the total milligram dosage of local anesthetic administered because vascular uptake via these vessels is high. Although uncommon, infection remains an ever-present possibility, especially in the immunocompromised cancer patient. Early detection of infection is crucial to avoid potentially life-threatening sequelae. Even with perfect technique, post-procedure intercostal neuritis can occur, especially with increasing temperatures. In most patients this responds to injection of 40 mg of methylprednisolone and 0.5% preservative-free bupivacaine injected onto the affected nerve. Occasionally, a short course of gabapentin will also be required to manage postprocedure neuritis.

SUGGESTED READING

Waldman SD: Intercostal nerve block: Radiofrequency lesioning. In: Atlas of Interventional Pain Management, ed 2. Philadelphia, Saunders, 2004.

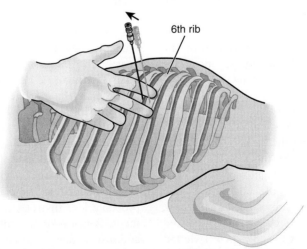

6th rib

FIGURE 279–1 Intercostal nerve block: radiofrequency lesioning. (From Waldman SD: Atlas of Interventional Pain Management, ed 2. Philadelphia, Saunders, 2004, p 247.)

CHAPTER 280

Interpleural Nerve Block

The pleural space extends from the apex to the base of the lung. It also envelopes the anterior and posterior mediastinum. Local anesthetics placed into the interpleural space diffuse out of the interpleural space to block the thoracic somatic and lower cervical and thoracic sympathetic nerves that lie in proximity to the pleural space. Because the density and duration of the block depend on the amount and concentration of local anesthetic in contact with the nerve, it is possible to influence these variables by alterations in the patient's position during and after injection of the interpleural catheter.

The choice of patient position is based on selection of the nerves that are to be blocked. For blockade of the lower cervical and upper thoracic sympathetic chain to treat sympathetically mediated pain, the patient is placed with the affected side up. After injection of the catheter, the patient is placed in the head down position. This position will avoid a dense block of the thoracic somatic nerves. For a dense blockade of the thoracic somatic nerves including the thoracic spinal nerves and corresponding intercostal nerves as well as the thoracic sympathetic chain, the patient is placed in the oblique position with the affected side down and the patient's back propped against a pillow to encourage pooling of the local anesthetic into the interpleural gutter next to the thoracic spine. This will allow the maximum amount of local anesthetic to diffuse onto both the somatic and sympathetic nerves. If the patient cannot lie on the affected side owing to fractured ribs, the interpleural catheter can be placed with the patient in the sitting position or with the affected side up. After injection of the catheter, the patient is then turned to the supine position with the patient tilted away from the affected side to encourage the flow of local anesthetic toward the interpleural gutter next to the thoracic spine.

After the patient is placed in the appropriate position, the eighth rib on the affected side is identified. The path of the rib is then traced posteriorly. At a point approximately 10 cm from the origin of the rib, the skin is marked and then prepared with antiseptic solution (Fig. 280-1A). The index and middle fingers are then placed on the rib bracketing the site of needle insertion. The skin and subcutaneous tissues are then anesthetized with local anesthetic. An 18-gauge, 3½-inch styletted Hustead needle is then placed through the anesthetized area and is advanced perpendicular to the skin, aiming for the middle of the rib in between the index and middle fingers. The needle should impinge on bone after being advanced approximately ½ inch. After bony contact is made, the needle is withdrawn into the subcutaneous tissues, and the skin and subcutaneous tissues are retracted with the palpating fingers superiorly. This allows the needle to be "walked over" the superior margin of the rib, avoiding trauma to the neurovascular bundle that runs beneath the rib (Fig. 280-1B). As soon as bony contact is lost, the stylet is then removed, and the needle is attached to a well-lubricated 5-mL syringe containing air. The needle and syringe are slowly advanced toward the interpleural space. A click will be felt when the parietal pleura is penetrated with the tip of the needle bevel, and at this point the plunger of the syringe will usually advance under its own response to the negative pressure of the interpleural space (Fig. 280-1C). The syringe is removed, and a catheter is advanced 6 to 8 cm into the interpleural space (Figs. 280-1D and 280-2). If no blood or air is identified after careful aspiration, the catheter is taped in place with sterile tape, and the patient is placed in the appropriate position to allow blockade of the desired nerves. From 20 to 30 mL of local anesthetic is then injected in incremental doses, with careful observation for signs of local anesthetic toxicity. If more concentrated, longer-acting local anesthetics such as 0.5% bupivacaine are used, smaller volumes on the order of 10 to 12 mL are given in incremental doses, with the total milligram dosage of drug gradually titrated upward to avoid toxic reactions. Alternatively, continuous infusions of local anesthetic can be administered by pump via the interpleural catheter. If there is an inflammatory component to the pain, the local anesthetic is combined with 80 mg of methylprednisolone and is injected in incremental doses. On subsequent days, 40 mg of methylprednisolone can be added to the local anesthetic.

Given the proximity of the pleural space, pneumothorax after interpleural nerve block is a distinct possibility. The incidence of clinically significant pneumothorax is probably less than 1% after interpleural catheter placement. Because of the proximity to the intercostal vein and artery, the pain management specialist should carefully calculate the total milligram dosage of local anesthetic administered because vascular uptake via these vessels is high. Although uncommon, infection remains an ever-present possibility, especially in the immunocompromised cancer patient. Early detection of infection is crucial to avoid potentially life-threatening sequelae.

SUGGESTED READING

Waldman SD: Interpleural nerve block: Percutaneous technique. In: Atlas of Interventional Pain Management, ed 2. Philadelphia, Saunders, 2004.

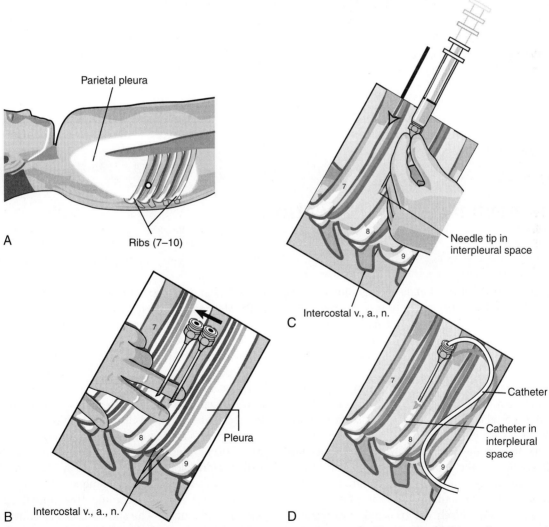

FIGURE 280–1 Interpleural nerve block: percutaneous technique. **A,** Patient positioning. **B,** Identification of anatomic landmarks. **C,** Needle insertion. **D,** Catheter insertion. (From Waldman SD: Atlas of Interventional Pain Management, ed 2. Philadelphia, Saunders, 2004, pp 250-251.)

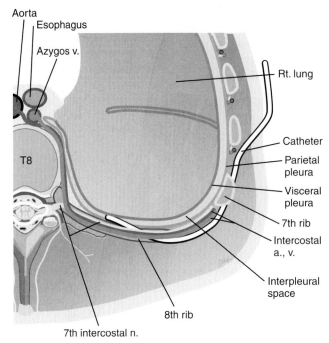

FIGURE 280–2 Interpleural nerve block: clinically relevant anatomy. (From Waldman SD: Atlas of Interventional Pain Management, ed 2. Philadelphia, Saunders, 2004, p 252.)

CHAPTER 281

Sternoclavicular Joint Injection

The sternoclavicular joint is a double gliding joint with an actual synovial cavity. Articulation occurs between the sternal end of the clavicle, the sternal manubrium, and the cartilage of the first rib. The clavicle and sternal manubrium are separated by an articular disc. The joint is reinforced in front and back by the sternoclavicular ligaments. Additional support is provided by the costoclavicular ligament, which runs from the junction of the first rib and its costal cartilage to the inferior surface of the clavicle. The joint is dually innervated by both the supraclavicular nerve and the nerve supplying the subclavius muscle. Posterior to the joint are a number of large arteries and veins, including the left common carotid and brachiocephalic vein and, on the right, the brachiocephalic artery. These vessels are susceptible to needle-induced trauma if the needle is placed too deeply.

The serratus anterior muscle produces forward movement of the clavicle at the sternoclavicular joint, with backward movement at the joint produced by the rhomboid and trapezius muscles. Elevation of the clavicle at the sternoclavicular joint is produced by the sternocleidomastoid, rhomboid, and levator scapulae. Depression of the clavicle at the joint is produced by the pectoralis minor and subclavius muscle.

To perform sternoclavicular joint injection, the patient is placed in the supine position and proper preparation with antiseptic solution of the skin overlying the root of the neck anteriorly as well as the skin overlying the proximal clavicle is carried out. A sterile syringe containing 1.0 mL of 0.25% preservative-free bupivacaine and 40 mg of methylprednisolone is attached to a 1½-inch, 25-gauge needle using strict aseptic technique.

With strict aseptic technique, the sternal end of the clavicle is identified. The sternoclavicular joint should be easily palpable as a slight indentation at the point where the clavicle meets the sternal manubrium. The needle is then carefully advanced through the skin and subcutaneous tissues medially at a 45-degree angle from the skin, through the joint capsule into the joint (Fig. 281-1). If bone is encountered, the needle is withdrawn into the subcutaneous tissues and redirected slightly more medially. After entering the joint space, the contents of the syringe are gently injected. There should be some resistance to injection, because the joint space is small and the joint capsule is dense. If significant resistance is encountered, the needle is probably in a ligament and should be advanced or withdrawn slightly into the joint space until the injection proceeds with only limited resistance. The needle is then removed and a sterile pressure dressing and ice pack are placed at the injection site.

The major complication of this injection technique is pneumothorax if the needle is placed too laterally or deeply and invades the pleural space. Infection, although rare, can occur if strict aseptic technique is not adhered to. The possibility of trauma to the large arteries and veins in proximity to the sternoclavicular joint remains an ever-present possibility as does inadvertent intravascular injection; this complication can be greatly decreased if the clinician pays close attention to accurate needle placement.

SUGGESTED READING

Waldman SD: Injection technique for sternoclavicular joint. Atlas of Pain Management Injection Techniques, ed. 2. Philadelphia, Saunders, 2007.

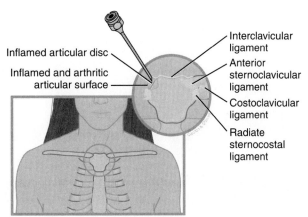

FIGURE 281–1 Injection technique for sternoclavicular joint. (From Waldman SD: Atlas of Pain Management Injection Techniques, ed. 2. Philadelphia, Saunders, 2007, p 285.)

CHAPTER 282

Suprascapular Nerve Block

The suprascapular nerve is formed from fibers originating from the C5 and C6 nerve roots of the brachial plexus, with some contribution of fibers from the C4 root in most patients. The nerve passes inferiorly and posteriorly from the brachial plexus to pass underneath the coracoclavicular ligament through the suprascapular notch. The suprascapular artery and vein accompany the nerve through the suprascapular notch. The suprascapular nerve provides much of the sensory innervation to the shoulder joint and provides innervation to two of the muscles of the rotator cuff, the supraspinatus and infraspinatus.

To perform suprascapular nerve block, the patient is placed in the sitting position with the arms hanging loosely at the patient's side. A total of 10 mL of local anesthetic and 40 mg of methylprednisolone is drawn up in a 20-mL sterile syringe. The spine of the scapula is identified, and the clinician then palpates along the length of the scapular spine laterally to identify the acromion. At the point at which the thicker acromion fuses with the thinner scapular spine, the skin is prepped with antiseptic solution. At this point, the skin and subcutaneous tissues are anesthetized using a 1½-inch needle. After adequate anesthesia is obtained, a 3½-inch, 25-gauge needle is inserted in an inferior trajectory toward the body of the scapula (Fig. 282-1). The needle should make contact with the body of the scapula at a depth of about 1 inch. The needle is then gently walked superiorly and medially until the needle tip "walks off" the scapular body into the suprascapular notch. If the notch is not identified, the same maneuver is repeated, directing the needle superiorly and laterally until the needle tip walks off the scapular body into the

suprascapular notch. Paresthesia is often encountered as the needle tip enters the notch, and the patient should be warned of this. If paresthesia is not elicited after the needle has entered the suprascapular notch, advance the needle an additional ½ inch to place the needle tip beyond the substance of the coracoclavicular ligament. The needle should never be advanced deeper or pneumothorax is likely to occur.

After paresthesia is elicited or the needle has been advanced into the notch as described, gentle aspiration is carried out to identify blood or air. If the aspiration test is negative, the solution is slowly injected, with the patient being monitored closely for signs of local anesthetic toxicity.

The proximity to the suprascapular artery and vein suggests the potential for inadvertent intravascular injection or local anesthetic toxicity from intravascular absorption. The clinician should carefully calculate the total milligram dosage of local anesthetic that may be safely given when performing this injection technique. Because of the proximity of the lung, pneumothorax is a possibility if the needle is advanced too deeply through the suprascapular notch. Although uncommon, infection following this injection can occur if careful attention to sterile technique is not followed.

SUGGESTED READING

Waldman SD: Suprascapular nerve block. In: Atlas of Pain Management Injection Techniques, ed. 2. Philadelphia, Saunders, 2007.

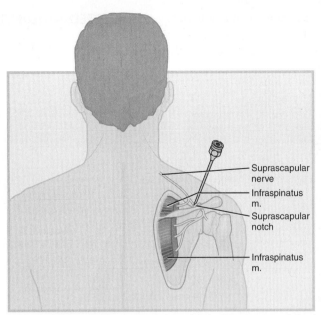

FIGURE 282–1 Suprascapular nerve block. (From Waldman SD: Atlas of Pain Management Injection Techniques, ed. 2. Philadelphia, Saunders, 2007, p 292.)

CHAPTER 283

Costosternal Joint Injection

The cartilage of the true ribs articulates with the sternum via the costosternal joints. The cartilage of the first rib articulates directly with the manubrium of the sternum and is a synarthrodial joint that allows a limited gliding movement. The cartilage of the second through sixth ribs articulates with the body of the sternum via true arthrodial joints. These joints are surrounded by a thin articular capsule. The costosternal joints are strengthened by ligaments but can be subluxed or dislocated by blunt trauma to the anterior chest. Posterior to the costosternal joint are the structures of the mediastinum. These structures are susceptible to needle-induced trauma if the needle is placed too deeply. The pleural space may be entered if the needle is placed too deeply and laterally; pneumothorax may result.

To perform costosternal joint injection, the patient is placed in the supine position and proper preparation with antiseptic solution of the skin overlying the affected costosternal joints is carried out. A sterile syringe containing 1.0 mL of 0.25% preservative-free bupivacaine for each joint to be injected and 40 mg of methylprednisolone is attached to a 1½-inch, 25-gauge needle using strict aseptic technique.

With strict aseptic technique, the costovertebral joints are identified. The costosternal joints should be easily palpable as a slight bulging at the point where the rib attaches to the sternum. The needle is then carefully advanced through the skin and subcutaneous tissues medially with a slight cephalad trajectory into proximity with the joint (Fig. 283-1). If bone is encountered, the needle is withdrawn out of the periosteum. After the needle is in proximity to the joint, 1 mL of solution is gently injected. There should be limited resistance to injection. If significant resistance is encountered, the needle should be withdrawn slightly until the injection proceeds with only limited resistance. This procedure is repeated for each affected joint. The needle is then removed, and a sterile pressure dressing and ice pack are placed at the injection site.

The major complication of this injection technique is pneumothorax if the needle is placed too laterally or deeply and invades the pleural space. Infection, although rare, can occur if strict aseptic technique is not adhered to. The possibility of trauma to the contents of the mediastinum including the esophagus, trachea, and heart remains an ever-present possibility; these complications can be greatly decreased if the clinician pays close attention to accurate needle placement.

SUGGESTED READING

Waldman SD: Costosternal syndrome. In: Atlas of Pain Management Injection Techniques. Philadelphia, Saunders, 2007.

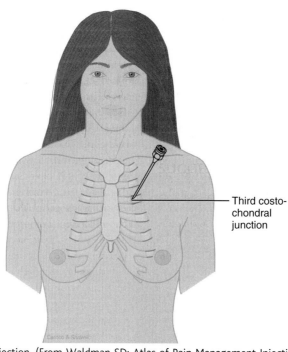

Third costochondral junction

FIGURE 283–1 Costosternal joint injection. (From Waldman SD: Atlas of Pain Management Injection Techniques. Philadelphia, Saunders, 2007, p 302.)

Anterior Cutaneous Nerve Block

The intercostal nerves arise from the anterior division of the thoracic paravertebral nerve. A typical intercostal nerve has four major branches. The first branch is the unmyelinated postganglionic fibers of the gray rami communicantes, which interface with the sympathetic chain. The second branch is the posterior cutaneous branch, which innervates the muscles and skin of the paraspinal area. The third branch is the lateral cutaneous division, which arises in the anterior axillary line and provides the majority of the cutaneous innervation of the chest and abdominal wall. The fourth branch is the anterior cutaneous branch, supplying innervation to the midline of the chest and abdominal wall. The anterior cutaneous branch pierces the fascia of the abdominal wall at the lateral border of the rectus abdominis muscle. The nerve turns sharply in an anterior direction to provide innervation to the anterior wall. The nerve passes through a firm fibrous ring as it pierces the fascia, and it is at this point that the nerve is subject to entrapment. The nerve is accompanied through the fascia by an epigastric artery and vein. Occasionally, the terminal branches of a given intercostal nerve may actually cross the midline to provide sensory innervation to the contralateral chest and abdominal wall. The 12th nerve is called the subcostal nerve and is unique in that it gives off a branch to the first lumbar nerve, thus contributing to the lumbar plexus.

To perform anterior cutaneous nerve block, the patient is placed in the lateral position and proper preparation with antiseptic solution of the skin overlying the affected anterior cutaneous branch of the intercostal nerve is carried out. This usually is at approximately the anterior axillary line. A sterile syringe containing 3.0 mL of 0.25% preservative-free bupivacaine for each nerve to be injected and 40 mg of methylprednisolone is attached to a 1½-inch, 25-gauge needle using strict aseptic technique.

With strict aseptic technique, the rib of the affected intercostal nerve is identified. The lower margin of each affected rib is identified and marked with a sterile marker. The needle is then carefully advanced at the point marked through the skin and subcutaneous tissues until the needle tip impinges on the periosteum of the underlying rib. The needle is then withdrawn back into the subcutaneous tissues and "walked" inferiorly off the inferior rib margin (Fig. 284-1). The needle should be advanced just beyond the inferior rib margin, but no further or pneumothorax or damage to the abdominal viscera could result. After careful aspiration to ensure that the needle tip is not in an intercostal vein or artery, 1 mL of solution is gently injected. There should be limited resistance to injection. If significant resistance is encountered, the needle should be withdrawn slightly until the injection proceeds with only limited resistance. This procedure is repeated for each affected nerve. The needle is then removed, and a sterile pressure dressing and ice pack are placed at the injection site.

The major complication of this injection technique is pneumothorax or damage to the abdominal viscera if the needle is placed too deeply and invades the pleural space or peritoneal cavity. Infection, although rare, can occur if strict aseptic technique is not adhered to. These complications can be greatly decreased if the clinician pays close attention to accurate needle placement. Because this technique blocks the intercostal nerve corresponding to the rib injected, the patient should be warned to expect some transient numbness of the chest and abdominal wall, as well as bulging of the abdomen in the subcostal region due to blockade of the motor innervation to these muscles.

SUGGESTED READING

Waldman SD: Anterior cutaneous nerve entrapment syndrome. In: Atlas of Pain Management Injection Techniques. Philadelphia, Saunders, 2007.

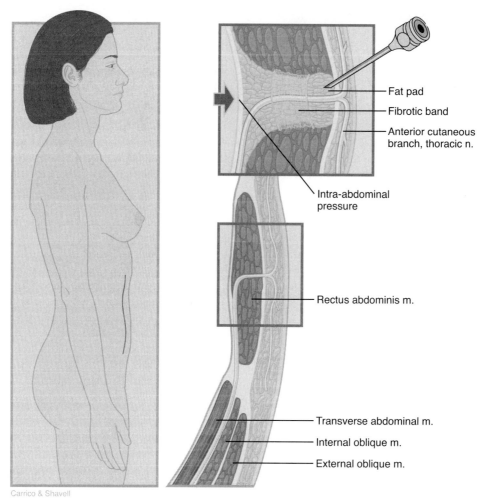

Fat pad

Fibrotic band

Anterior cutaneous
branch, thoracic n.

Intra-abdominal
pressure

Rectus abdominis m.

Transverse abdominal m.

Internal oblique m.

External oblique m.

Carrico & Shavell

FIGURE 284–1 Anterior cutaneous nerve block. (From Waldman SD: Atlas of Pain Management Injection Techniques. Philadelphia, Saunders, 2007, p 327.)

CHAPTER 285

Injection Technique for Lumbar Myofascial Pain Syndrome

The muscles of the back work together as a functional unit to stabilize and allow coordinated movement of the low back and allow one to maintain an upright position. Trauma to an individual muscle can result in dysfunction of the entire functional unit. The rhomboids, latissimus dorsi, iliocostalis quadratus lumborum, multifidus, psoas, and quadratus lumborum muscles are frequent sites of myofascial pain syndrome. The points of origin and attachments of these muscles are particularly susceptible to trauma and the subsequent development of myofascial trigger points (Fig. 285-1). Injection of these trigger points serves as both a diagnostic and therapeutic maneuver.

Careful preparation of the patient prior to trigger point injection helps to optimize results. Trigger point injections are directed at the primary trigger point, rather than in the area of referred pain. It should be explained to the patient that the goal of trigger point injection is to block the trigger of the persistent pain and, it is hoped, to provide long-lasting relief. It is important that the patient understand that with most patients who suffer from myofascial pain syndrome, more than one treatment modality is required to provide optimal pain relief. The use of the prone or lateral position when identifying and marking trigger points as well as when performing the actual trigger point injection helps decrease the incidence of vasovagal reactions. The skin overlying the trigger point to be injected should always be prepared with antiseptic solution prior to injection in order to avoid infection.

After the goals of trigger point injection are explained to the patient and proper preparation of the patient has been carried out, the trigger point to be injected is re-identified by palpation with the sterile gloved finger. A syringe containing 10 mL of 0.25% preservative-free bupivacaine and 40 mg of methylprednisolone to be injected is attached to a 25-gauge needle of a length adequate to reach the trigger point. For the deeper muscles of posture in the low back, a 3½-inch needle is required. A volume of 0.5 to 1.0 mL of solution is then injected into each trigger point. A series of two to five treatment sessions may be required to completely abolish the trigger point; the patient should be informed of this.

The proximity to the spinal cord and exiting nerve roots makes it imperative that this procedure be carried out only by those well versed in the regional anatomy and experienced in performing interventional pain management techniques. Many patients also complain of a transient increase in pain following injection of trigger points. If long needles are used, pneumothorax or damage to the retroperitoneal organs, including the kidneys, may also occur.

SUGGESTED READING

Waldman SD: Lumbar myofascial pain syndrome. In: Atlas of Pain Management Injection Techniques, ed. 2. Philadelphia, Saunders, 2007.

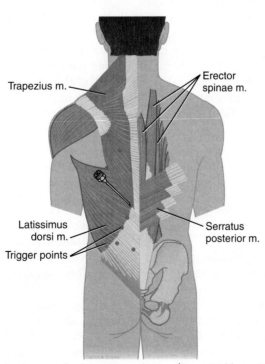

FIGURE 285–1 Injection technique for lumbar myofascial pain syndrome. (From Waldman SD: Atlas of Pain Management Injection Techniques, ed. 2. Philadelphia, Saunders, 2007, p 330.)

CHAPTER 286

Splanchnic Nerve Block

The sympathetic innervation of the abdominal viscera originates in the anterolateral horn of the spinal cord. Preganglionic fibers from T5-12 exit the spinal cord in conjunction with the ventral roots to join the white communicating rami on their way to the sympathetic chain. Rather than synapsing with the sympathetic chain, these preganglionic fibers pass through it to ultimately synapse on the celiac ganglia. The greater, lesser, and least splanchnic nerves provide the major preganglionic contribution to the celiac plexus and transmit the majority of nociceptive information from the viscera. The splanchnic nerves are contained in a narrow compartment made up by the vertebral body and the pleural laterally, the posterior mediastinum ventrally, and the pleural attachment to the vertebra dorsally. This compartment is bounded caudally by the crura of the diaphragm. The volume of this compartment is approximately 10 mL on each side.

The greater splanchnic nerve has its origin from the T5-10 spinal roots. The nerve travels along the thoracic paravertebral border through the crus of the diaphragm into the abdominal cavity, ending on the celiac ganglion of its respective side. The lesser splanchnic nerve arises from the T10-11 roots and passes with the greater nerve to end at the celiac ganglion. The least splanchnic nerve arises from the T11-12 spinal roots and passes through the diaphragm to the celiac ganglion.

Intrapatient anatomic variability of the celiac ganglia is significant, but the following generalizations can be drawn from anatomic studies of the celiac ganglia. The number of ganglia varies from one to five and range in diameter from 0.5 to 4.5 cm. The ganglia lie anterior and anterolateral to the aorta. The ganglia located on the left are uniformly more inferior than their right-sided counterparts by as much as a vertebral level, but both groups of ganglia lie below the level of the celiac artery. The ganglia usually lie approximately at the level of the first lumbar vertebra.

Postganglionic fibers radiate from the celiac ganglia to follow the course of the blood vessels to innervate the abdominal viscera. These organs include much of the distal esophagus, stomach, duodenum, small intestine, ascending and proximal transverse colon, adrenal glands, pancreas, spleen, liver, and biliary system. It is these postganglionic fibers, the fibers arising from the preganglionic splanchnic nerves, and the celiac ganglion that make up the celiac plexus. The celiac plexus is anterior to the crus

of the diaphragm. The plexus extends in front of and around the aorta, with the greatest concentration of fibers anterior to the aorta. The relationship of the celiac plexus to the surrounding structures is as follows: The aorta lies anterior and slightly to the left of the anterior margin of the vertebral body. The inferior vena cava lies to the right, with the kidneys posterolateral to the great vessels. The pancreas lies anterior to the celiac plexus. All of these structures lie within the retroperitoneal space.

Preblock preparation includes the administration of adequate amounts of oral or intravenous fluids to attenuate the hypotension associated with splanchnic nerve block. Evaluation for coagulopathy is indicated if the patient has undergone antiblastic therapy or has a history of significant alcohol abuse. If radiographic contrast is to be used, evaluation of the patient's renal status is also indicated.

The technique for splanchnic nerve block differs little from the classic retrocrural approach to the celiac plexus except that the needles are aimed more cephalad to ultimately rest at the anterolateral margin of the T12 vertebral body. It is imperative that both needles be placed medially against the vertebral body to reduce the incidence of pneumothorax. The patient is placed in the prone position with a pillow placed under the abdomen to flex the thoracolumbar spine. For comfort, the patient's head is turned to the side and the arms are permitted to hang freely off each side of the table. The inferior margins of the 12th ribs are identified and traced to the T12 vertebral body. The spinous process of the L1 vertebral body is then identified and marked with a sterile marker. A point approximately 2 inches just inferior and lateral to each side of the spinous process of L1 is identified. The injection sites are then prepared with antiseptic solution.

The skin, subcutaneous tissues, and musculature are infiltrated with 1.0% lidocaine at the points of needle entry. Then 20-gauge, 13-cm styletted needles are inserted bilaterally through the previously anesthetized area. The needles are initially oriented 45 degrees toward the midline and about 35 degrees cephalad to ensure contact with the T12 vertebral body (Fig. 286-1). Once bony contact is made and the depth noted, the needles are withdrawn to the level of the subcutaneous tissue and redirected slightly less mesiad (about 60 degrees from the midline) so as to "walk off" the lateral surface of the T12 vertebral body. The needles are replaced to the depth at which contact with the vertebral body was first noted. At this point, if no bone is contacted, the left-sided needle is gradually advanced 1.5 cm. The right-sided needle is then advanced slightly farther (i.e., 2 cm past contact with the bone). Ultimately, the tips of the needles should be just anterior to the lateral border of the vertebral body and just behind the aorta and vena cava in the retrocrural space (Fig. 286-2).

The stylets of the needles are removed and the needle hubs inspected for the presence of blood, cerebrospinal fluid, or urine. If radiographic guidance is being used, a small amount of contrast material is injected through each needle, and its spread is observed radiographically. On the fluoroscopic anteroposterior view, contrast is confined to the midline and concentrated near the T12 vertebral body. A smooth posterior contour can be observed that corresponds to the psoas fascia on the lateral view. Alternatively, if computed tomographic guidance is used, contrast should appear lateral to and behind the aorta. The contrast should be observed to be entirely retrocrural. If there is precrural spread, the needles are withdrawn slightly back through the crura of the diaphragm.

If radiographic guidance is not used, a rapid-onset local anesthetic is used in sufficient concentration to produce motor block (e.g., 1.5% lidocaine or 3.0% 2-chloroprocaine) prior to administration of neurolytic agents. If the patient experiences no motor or sensory block in the lumbar dermatomes after an adequate time, additional drugs injected through the needles will probably not reach the somatic nerve roots if given in like volumes.

For diagnostic and prognostic splanchnic nerve block, 7- to 10-mL volume of 1.5% lidocaine or 3.0% 2-chloroprocaine is administered through the needle. For therapeutic block, 7 to 10 mL of 0.5% bupivacaine is administered. Because of the potential for local anesthetic toxicity, all local anesthetics should be administered in incremental doses. A 10-mL volume of absolute alcohol or 6.0% aqueous phenol is used for neurolytic block. After neurolytic solution is injected, each needle should be flushed with sterile saline solution, because there have been anecdotal reports of neurolytic solution being tracked posteriorly with the needles as they are withdrawn.

Because of the proximity to vascular structures, splanchnic nerve block is contraindicated in patients who are receiving anticoagulant therapy or suffer from coagulopathy secondary to antiblastic cancer therapies or liver abnormalities associated with ethanol abuse. Intravascular injection of solutions may result in thrombosis of the nutrient vessels to the spinal cord with secondary paraplegia. Local and/or intra-abdominal infection, as well as sepsis, are absolute contraindications to splanchnic nerve block.

Because blockade of the splanchnic nerve results in increased bowel motility, this technique should be avoided in patients with bowel obstruction. Postblock diarrhea occurs in approximately 50% of patients. Splanchnic nerve block should be deferred in patients who suffer from chronic abdominal pain and who are chemically dependent or exhibit drug-seeking behavior until these issues have been adequately addressed. Alcohol should not be used as a neurolytic agent in patients on disulfiram therapy for alcohol abuse.

The proximity to the spinal cord, exiting nerve roots, pleural space, and viscera makes it imperative that this procedure be performed only by those well versed in the regional anatomy and experienced in interventional pain management techniques. Needle placement that is too medial may result in epidural, subdural, or subarachnoid injections or trauma to the spinal cord and exiting nerve roots. Such incorrect needle placement can result in severe neurologic deficits, including paraplegia. Medial needle placement may also result in intradiscal placement and resultant discitis. Because the needle terminus is retrocrural when the classic two-needle approach to splanchnic nerve block is used, there is an increased incidence of neurologic complications, including neurolysis of the lumbar nerve roots with resultant hip flexor weakness and lower extremity numbness. Techniques that result in precrural needle placement, such as the transcrural and transaortic approaches to splanchnic nerve block, have a lower incidence of this complication and should be considered by the pain management specialist.

Given the proximity of the pleural space, pneumothorax after splanchnic nerve block may occur if the needle is placed too cephalad or anterior. Trauma to the thoracic duct with resultant chylothorax may also occur. If the needles are placed too laterally, trauma to the kidneys and ureters is a distinct possibility.

SUGGESTED READING

Waldman SD: Splanchnic nerve block. In: Atlas of Interventional Pain Management, ed 2. Philadelphia, Saunders, 2004.

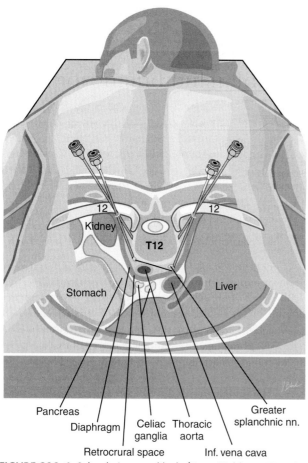

FIGURE 286–1 Splanchnic nerve block. (From Waldman SD: Atlas of Interventional Pain Management, ed 2. Philadelphia, Saunders, 2004, p 262.)

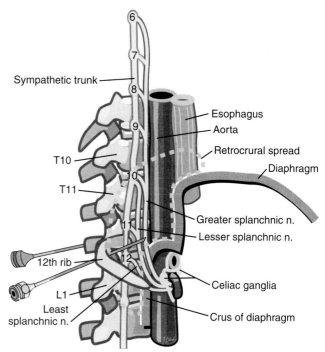

FIGURE 286–2 Correct needle orientation for the splanchnic nerve block. (From Waldman SD: Atlas of Interventional Pain Management, ed 2. Philadelphia, Saunders, 2004, p 263.)

CHAPTER 287

Celiac Plexus Block

The sympathetic innervation of the abdominal viscera originates in the anterolateral horn of the spinal cord. Preganglionic fibers from T5-12 exit the spinal cord in conjunction with the ventral roots to join the white communicating rami on their way to the sympathetic chain. Rather than synapsing with the sympathetic chain, these preganglionic fibers pass through it to ultimately synapse on the celiac ganglia. The greater, lesser, and least splanchnic nerves provide the major preganglionic contribution to the celiac plexus. The greater splanchnic nerve has its origin from the T5-10 spinal roots. The nerve travels along the thoracic paravertebral border through the crus of the diaphragm into the abdominal cavity, ending on the celiac ganglion of its respective side. The lesser splanchnic nerve arises from the T10-11 roots and passes with the greater nerve to end at the celiac ganglion. The least splanchnic nerve arises from the T11-12 spinal roots and passes through the diaphragm to the celiac ganglion.

Interpatient anatomic variability of the celiac ganglia is significant, but the following generalizations can be drawn from anatomic studies of the celiac ganglia: The number of ganglia varies from one to five and range in diameter from 0.5 to 4.5 cm. The ganglia lie anterior and anterolateral to the aorta. The ganglia located on the left are uniformly more inferior than their right-sided counterparts by as much as a vertebral level, but both groups of ganglia lie below the level of the celiac artery. The ganglia usually lie approximately at the level of the first lumbar vertebra.

Postganglionic fibers radiate from the celiac ganglia to follow the course of the blood vessels to innervate the abdominal viscera. These organs include much of the distal esophagus, stomach, duodenum, small intestine, ascending and proximal transverse colon, adrenal glands, pancreas, spleen, liver, and biliary system. It is these postganglionic fibers, the fibers arising from the preganglionic splanchnic nerves, and the celiac ganglion that make up the celiac plexus. The celiac plexus is anterior to the crus of the diaphragm. The plexus extends in front of and around the aorta, with the greatest concentration of fibers anterior to the aorta. The relationship of the celiac plexus to the surrounding structures is as follows: The aorta lies anterior and slightly to the left of the anterior margin of the vertebral body. The inferior vena cava lies to the right, with the kidneys posterolateral to the great vessels. The pancreas lies anterior to the celiac plexus. All of these structures lie within the retroperitoneal space.

Pre–celiac plexus block preparation includes the administration of adequate amounts of oral or intravenous fluids to attenuate the hypotension associated with celiac plexus block. Evaluation for coagulopathy is indicated if the patient has undergone antiblastic therapy or has a history of significant alcohol abuse. If radiographic contrast is to be used, evaluation of the patient's renal status is also indicated.

Two-Needle Retrocrural Technique

The patient is placed in the prone position with a pillow placed under the abdomen to flex the thoracolumbar spine. For comfort, the patient's head is turned to the side and the arms are permitted to hang freely off each side of the table. The inferior margins of the 12th ribs are identified and traced to the T12 vertebral body. The spinous process of the L1 vertebral body is then identified and marked with a sterile marker. A point approximately 2½ inches just inferior and lateral to each side of the transverse process of L1 is identified. The injection sites are then prepared with antiseptic solution.

The skin, subcutaneous tissues, and musculature are infiltrated with 1.0% lidocaine at the points of needle entry. Then 20-gauge, 13-cm styletted needles are inserted bilaterally through the previously anesthetized area. The needles are initially oriented 45 degrees toward the midline and about 15 degrees cephalad to ensure contact with the L1 vertebral body. Once bone is contacted and the depth noted, the needles are withdrawn to the level of the subcutaneous tissue and redirected slightly less mesiad (about 60 degrees from the midline) so as to "walk off" the lateral surface of the L1 vertebral body (Fig. 287-1). The needles are replaced to the depth at which contact with the vertebral body was first noted. At this point, if no bone is contacted, the left-sided needle is gradually advanced 1.5 to 2 cm, or until the pulsation emanating from the aorta and transmitted to the advancing needle is noted. The right-sided needle is then advanced slightly further (i.e., 3 to 4 cm past contact with the bone). Ultimately, the tips of the needles should be just posterior to the aorta on the left and to the anterolateral aspect of the aorta on the right (Fig. 287-2).

The stylets of the needles are removed, and the needle hubs are inspected for the presence of blood, cerebrospinal fluid, or urine. If radiographic guidance is being used, a small amount of contrast material is injected through each needle, and its spread is observed radiographically. On the fluoroscopic anteroposterior view, contrast is confined to the midline and concentrated near the L1 vertebral body (Fig. 287-3). A smooth posterior contour can be observed that corresponds to the psoas fascia on the lateral view (Fig. 287-4). Alternatively, if computed tomographic (CT) guidance is used, contrast should appear lateral to and behind the aorta. If the contrast is entirely retrocrural, the needles should be advanced to the precrural space to avoid any risk of spread of local anesthetic or neurolytic agent posteriorly to the somatic nerve roots.

If radiographic guidance is not used, a rapid-onset local anesthetic is used in sufficient concentration to produce motor block (e.g., 1.5% lidocaine or 3.0% 2-chloroprocaine) prior to administration of neurolytic agents. If the patient experiences no motor or sensory block in the lumbar dermatomes after an adequate time, additional drugs injected through the needles will probably not reach the somatic nerve roots if given in like volumes.

For diagnostic and prognostic block using the retrocrural technique, a 12- to 15-mL volume of 1.0% lidocaine or 3.0% 2-chloroprocaine is administered through each needle. For therapeutic block, 10 to 12 mL of 0.5% bupivacaine is administered through each needle. Because of the potential for local anesthetic toxicity, all local anesthetics should be administered in incremental doses. When treating acute pancreatitis or pain of malignant origin, an 80-mg dose of depot methylprednisolone is advocated for the initial celiac plexus block, with a 40-mg dose given for subsequent blocks.

A 10- to 12-mL volume of absolute alcohol or 6.0% aqueous phenol is injected through each needle for retrocrural neurolytic block. Alternatively, 25 mL of 50% ethyl alcohol can be injected via each needle. After neurolytic solution is injected, each needle should be flushed with sterile saline solution, because there have been anecdotal reports of neurolytic solution being tracked posteriorly with the needles as they are withdrawn.

Single-Needle Periaortic Technique

To perform celiac plexus block using the single-needle periaortic technique, the patient is placed in the prone position with a pillow placed under the abdomen to flex the thoracolumbar spine. For comfort, the patient's head is turned to the side and the arms are permitted to hang freely off each side of the table. The inferior margins of the 12th ribs are identified and traced to the T12 vertebral body. The spinous process of the L1 vertebral body is then identified and marked with a sterile marker. A point approximately 2½ inches just inferior and lateral to the left side of the transverse process of L1 is identified. The injection site is then prepared with antiseptic solution.

The skin, subcutaneous tissues, and musculature are infiltrated with 1.0% lidocaine at the point of needle entry. A 20-gauge, 13-cm styletted needle is inserted bilaterally through the previously anesthetized area. The needle is initially oriented 45 degrees toward the midline and about 15 degrees cephalad to ensure contact with the L1 vertebral body. Once bone is contacted and the depth noted, the needle is withdrawn to the level of the subcutaneous tissue and redirected less mesiad (about 65 degrees from the midline) so as to "walk off" the lateral surface of the L1 vertebral body (Fig. 287-5). The needle is reinserted to the depth at which the vertebral body was first contacted. At this point, if no bone is contacted, the needle is gradually advanced 3 to 4 cm, or until the pulsation emanating from the aorta and transmitted to the advancing needle is noted. If aortic pulsations are noted, the pain specialist may either convert the block into a transaortic celiac plexus technique or note the depth to which the needle has been placed, withdraw the needle into the subcutaneous tissues, and then redirect the needle less mesiad to slide laterally to the aorta. Ultimately, the tip of the needle should be just lateral and anterior to the side of the aorta (Fig. 287-6). This periaortic precrural placement decreases the incidence of inadvertent spread of injected solutions onto the lumbar somatic nerve roots.

The stylet of the needle is removed, and the needle hub is inspected for the presence of blood, cerebrospinal fluid, or urine. If radiographic guidance is being used, a small amount of contrast material is injected through the needle, and its spread is observed radiographically. On the fluoroscopic anteroposterior view, contrast is confined primarily to the left of the midline near the L1 vertebral body. A smooth curvilinear shadow can be observed that corresponds to contrast in the preaortic space on the lateral view. Alternatively, if CT guidance is used, contrast should appear periaortic or, if adenopathy or tumor is present, contrast should be confined to the periaortic space to the left of the aorta. If this limitation of spread of contrast occurs, one should consider redirecting the needle more medially to pass through the aorta to place the needle tip just in front of the aorta. If the contrast is entirely retrocrural, the needle should be advanced to the precrural space to avoid any risk of spread of local anesthetic or neurolytic agent posteriorly to the somatic nerve roots.

If radiographic guidance is not used, a rapid-onset local anesthetic is used in sufficient concentration to produce motor block (e.g., 1.5% lidocaine or 3.0% 2-chloroprocaine) prior to administration of neurolytic agents. If the patient experiences no motor or sensory block in the lumbar dermatomes after an adequate time, additional drugs injected through the needles will probably not reach the somatic nerve roots if given in like volumes.

For diagnostic and prognostic block via the single-needle periaortic technique, 12 to 15 mL of 1.0% lidocaine or 3.0% 2-chloroprocaine is administered through the needle. For therapeutic block, 10 to 12 mL of 0.5% bupivacaine is administered through the needle. Because of the potential for local anesthetic toxicity, all local anesthetics should be administered in incremental doses. When treating acute pancreatitis or pain of malignant origin, 80 mg of depot methylprednisolone is advocated for the initial celiac plexus block, with a 40-mg dose given for subsequent blocks.

A 10- to 12-mL volume of absolute alcohol or 6.0% aqueous phenol is injected through the needle for neurolytic block. Alternatively, 25 mL of 50% ethyl alcohol can be injected via the needle. After neurolytic solution is injected, the needle should be flushed with sterile saline solution, because there have been anecdotal reports of neurolytic solution being tracked posteriorly with the needle as it is withdrawn.

Single-Needle Transaortic Technique

The single-needle transaortic approach to celiac plexus block is analogous to the transaxillary approach to brachial plexus block. Despite concerns about the potential for aortic trauma and subsequent occult retroperitoneal hemorrhage with the transaortic approach to celiac plexus block, it may in fact be safer than the classic two-needle posterior approach. The lower incidence of complications is thought to be due in part to the use of a single fine needle rather than two larger ones. The fact that the aorta is relatively well supported in this region by the diaphragmatic crura and prevertebral fascia also contributes to this technique's relative safety.

FLUOROSCOPICALLY GUIDED TECHNIQUE

The fluoroscopically guided single-needle transaortic approach uses the usual landmarks for the posterior placement of a left-sided 22-gauge, 13-cm styletted needle. Some investigators use a needle entry point 1 to 1.5 cm closer to the midline relative to the classic retrocrural approach combined with a needle trajectory closer to the perpendicular to reduce the incidence of renal trauma. The needle is advanced with the goal of passing just lateral to the anterolateral aspect of the L1 vertebral body. If the L1 vertebral body is encountered, the needle is withdrawn into the subcutaneous tissues and redirected in a manner analogous to the classic retrocrural approach. The styletted needle is gradually advanced until its tip rests in the posterior periaortic space. As the needle impinges on the posterior aortic wall, the operator feels transmitted aortic pulsations via the needle and increased resistance to needle passage.

Passing the needle through the wall of the aorta has been likened to passing a needle through a large rubber band. Free flow of arterial blood when the stylet is removed is evidence that the needle is within the aortic lumen. The stylet is replaced as the needle is advanced until it impinges on the intraluminal anterior wall of the aorta. At this point, the operator again feels an increased resistance to needle advancement. A pop is felt as the needle tip passes through the anterior aortic wall, indicating the needle tip's probable location within the preaortic fatty connective tissue and the substance of the celiac plexus (Figs. 287-7 and 287-8). A saline loss-of-resistance technique, as described later, may help to identify the preaortic space.

Because the needle is sometimes inadvertently advanced beyond the retroperitoneal space into the peritoneal cavity, confirmatory fluoroscopic views of injected contrast medium are advisable, especially during neurolytic blockade. On anteroposterior views, the contrast medium should be confined to the midline, with a tendency toward greater concentration around the anterolateral margins of the aorta. Lateral views should demonstrate a predominantly preaortic orientation extending from around T12-L2, sometimes accompanied by pulsations. Incomplete penetration of the anterior wall is indicated by a narrow longitudinal "line image."

The contrast medium may fail to completely surround the anterior aorta with extensive infiltration of the preaortic region by tumor or in patients who have undergone previous pancreatic surgery or radiation therapy. Experience shows that a lower success rate is to be expected when preaortic spread of contrast medium is poor. In this setting, selective alcohol neurolysis of the splanchnic nerves may provide better pain relief.

For diagnostic and prognostic block via the fluoroscopically guided transaortic technique, 10 to 12 mL of 1.5% lidocaine or 3.0% 2-chloroprocaine is administered through the needle. For therapeutic block, 10 to 12 mL of 0.5% bupivacaine is administered through the needle. Because of the potential for local anesthetic toxicity, all local anesthetics should be administered in incremental doses. For treatment of acute pancreatitis, 80 mg of depot methylprednisolone for the initial block and 40 mg for subsequent blocks is recommended. A 12- to 15-mL volume of absolute alcohol or 6.5% aqueous phenol is used for neurolytic block.

COMPUTED TOMOGRAPHIC–GUIDED TECHNIQUE

The patient is prepared for CT-guided transaortic celiac plexus block in a manner analogous to the earlier-mentioned techniques. After proper positioning on the CT table, a scout film is obtained to identify the T12-L1 interspace (Fig. 287-9). A CT scan is then taken through the interspace. The scan is reviewed for the position of the aorta relative to the vertebral body, the position of intra-abdominal and retroperitoneal organs, and distortion of normal anatomy due to tumor, previous surgery, or adenopathy. The aorta at this level is evaluated for significant aortic aneurysm, mural thrombus, or calcifications that would recommend against a transaortic approach.

The level at which the scan was taken is identified on the patient's skin and marked with a gentian violet marker. The skin is prepared with antiseptic solution. The skin, subcutaneous tissues, and muscle are anesthetized with 1.0% lidocaine at a point approximately 2½ inches from the left of the midline. A 22-gauge, 13-cm styletted needle is placed through the anesthetized area and is advanced until the posterior wall of the aorta is encountered, as evidenced by the transmission of arterial pulsations and an increased resistance to needle advancement. The needle is advanced into the lumen of the aorta. The stylet is removed, and the needle hub is observed for a free flow of arterial blood. A well-lubricated, 5-mL glass syringe filled with preservative free saline is attached to the needle hub. The needle and syringe are then advanced through the anterior wall of the aorta via a loss-of-resistance technique in a manner analogous to the loss-of-resistance technique used to identify the epidural space. The glass syringe is removed, and 3 mL of 1.5% lidocaine in solution is injected through the needle with an equal amount of water-soluble contrast media.

A CT scan at the level of the needle is taken. The scan is reviewed for the placement of the needle and, most important, for the spread of contrast medium. The contrast medium should be seen in the preaortic area and surrounding the aorta (Fig. 287-10). No contrast should be observed in the retrocrural space. After satisfactory needle placement and spread of contrast is confirmed, 12 to 15 mL of absolute alcohol or 6% aqueous phenol is injected through the needle. The needle is flushed with a small amount of sterile saline and then removed. The patient is observed carefully for hemodynamic changes, including hypotension and tachycardia secondary to the resulting profound sympathetic blockade.

Because of the proximity to vascular structures, celiac plexus block is contraindicated in patients who are receiving anticoagulant therapy or suffer from coagulopathy secondary to antiblastic cancer therapies or liver abnormalities associated with ethanol abuse. Intravascular injection of solutions may result in thrombosis of the nutrient vessels to the spinal cord with secondary paraplegia. Local or intra-abdominal infection, as well as sepsis, are absolute contraindications to celiac plexus block.

Because blockade of the celiac plexus results in increased bowel motility, this technique should be avoided in patients with bowel obstruction. Postblock diarrhea occurs in approximately 50% of patients. Celiac plexus block should be deferred in patients who suffer from chronic abdominal pain, who are chemically dependent, or who exhibit drug-seeking behavior until these issues have been adequately addressed. Alcohol should not be used as a neurolytic agent in patients on disulfiram therapy for alcohol abuse.

The proximity to the spinal cord, exiting nerve roots, pleural space, and viscera makes it imperative that this procedure be performed only by those well versed in the regional anatomy and experienced in interventional pain management techniques. Needle placement that is too medial may result in epidural, subdural, or subarachnoid injections or trauma to the spinal cord and exiting nerve roots. Such incorrect needle placement can result in severe neurologic deficits, including paraplegia. Medial needle placement may also result in intradiscal placement and resultant discitis. Because the needle terminus is retrocrural when the classic two-needle approach to splanchnic nerve block is used, there is an increased incidence of neurologic complications, including neurolysis of the lumbar nerve roots with resultant hip flexor weakness and lower extremity numbness. Techniques that result in precrural needle placement, such as the transcrural and transaortic approaches to celiac plexus block, have a lower incidence of this complication and should be considered by the pain management specialist.

Given the proximity of the pleural space, pneumothorax after celiac plexus block may occur if the needle is placed too cephalad. Trauma to the thoracic duct with resultant chylothorax may also occur. If the needles are placed too laterally, trauma to the kidneys and ureters is a distinct possibility.

SUGGESTED READINGS

Waldman SD: Celiac plexus block: Classic two-needle retrocrural technique. In: Atlas of Interventional Pain Management, ed 2. Philadelphia, Saunders, 2004.

Waldman SD: Celiac plexus block: Two-needle transcrural technique. In: Atlas of Interventional Pain Management, ed 2. Philadelphia, Saunders, 2004.

Waldman SD: Celiac plexus block: Single-needle periaortic technique. In: Atlas of Interventional Pain Management, ed 2. Philadelphia, Saunders, 2004.

Waldman SD: Celiac plexus block: Single-needle transaortic technique. In: Atlas of Interventional Pain Management, ed 2. Philadelphia, Saunders, 2004.

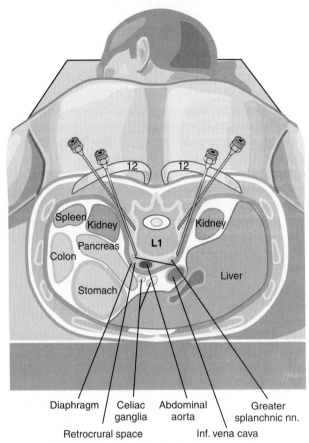

FIGURE 287–1 Celiac plexus block: classic two-needle retrocrural technique. (From Waldman SD: Atlas of Interventional Pain Management, ed 2. Philadelphia, Saunders, 2004, p 267.)

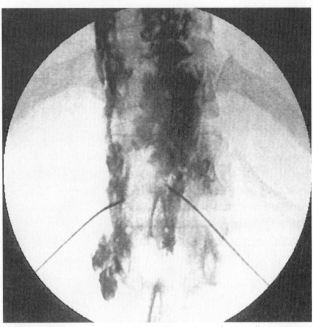

FIGURE 287–3 Fluoroscopic anterior view shows the contrast confined to the midline and concentrated near the L1 vertebral body. (From Waldman SD: Atlas of Interventional Pain Management, ed 2. Philadelphia, Saunders, 2004, p 269.)

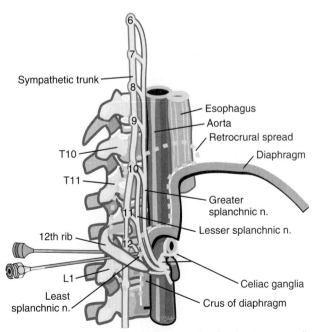

FIGURE 287–2 Correct needle orientation for the classic two-needle retrocrural technique. (From Waldman SD: Atlas of Interventional Pain Management, ed 2. Philadelphia, Saunders, 2004, p 268.)

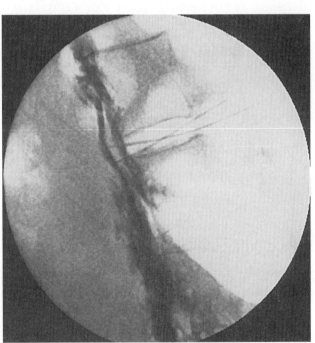

FIGURE 287–4 Lateral view showing a smooth posterior contour that corresponds to the psoas fascia. (From Waldman SD: Atlas of Interventional Pain Management, ed 2. Philadelphia, Saunders, 2004, p 269.)

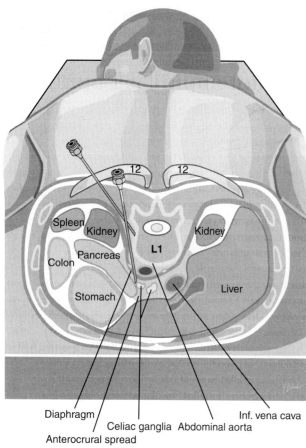

FIGURE 287–5 Celiac plexus block: single-needle periaortic technique. (From Waldman SD: Atlas of Interventional Pain Management, ed 2. Philadelphia, Saunders, 2004, p 279.)

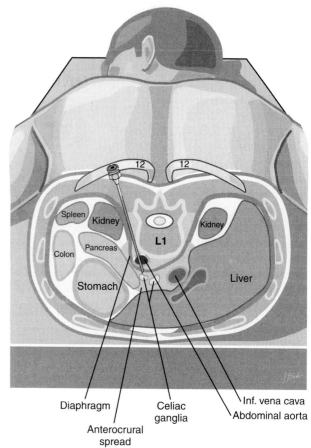

FIGURE 287–7 Celiac plexus block: single-needle transaortic technique. (From Waldman SD: Atlas of Interventional Pain Management, ed 2. Philadelphia, Saunders, 2004, p 286.)

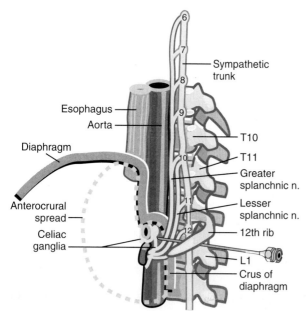

FIGURE 287–6 Correct needle orientation for the single-needle periaortic celiac plexus block. (From Waldman SD: Atlas of Interventional Pain Management, ed 2. Philadelphia, Saunders, 2004, p 280.)

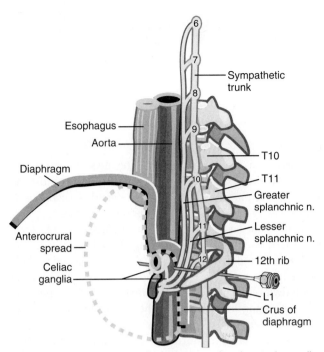

FIGURE 287–8 Correct needle orientation for the single-needle transaortic celiac plexus block. (From Waldman SD: Atlas of Interventional Pain Management, ed 2. Philadelphia, Saunders, 2004, p 287.)

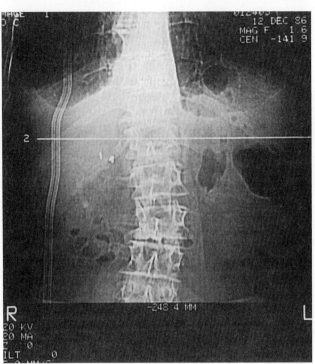

FIGURE 287–9 After proper positioning of the patient on the CT table, a scout film is obtained to identify the T12-L1 interspace, through which a CT scan is then taken. (From Waldman SD: Atlas of Interventional Pain Management, ed 2. Philadelphia, Saunders, 2004, p 288.)

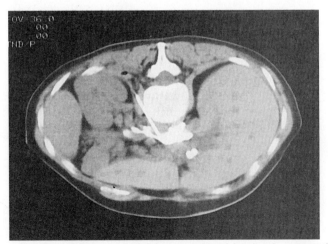

FIGURE 287–10 A CT scan taken at the level of the needle. The scan is reviewed for the placement of the needle and the spread of the contrast medium. The contrast medium should be seen in the preaortic area and surrounding the aorta. (From Waldman SD: Atlas of Interventional Pain Management, ed 2. Philadelphia, Saunders, 2004, p 288.)

CHAPTER **288**

Ilioinguinal Nerve Block

The ilioinguinal nerve is a branch of the L1 nerve root with a contribution from T12 in some patients. The nerve follows a curvilinear course that takes it from its origin of the L1 and occasionally T12 somatic nerves to inside the concavity of the ilium. The ilioinguinal nerve continues anteriorly to perforate the transverse abdominal muscle at the level of the anterior superior iliac spine. The nerve may interconnect with the iliohypogastric nerve as it continues to pass along its course medially and inferiorly, where it accompanies the spermatic cord through the inguinal ring and into the inguinal canal. The distribution of the sensory innervation of the ilioinguinal nerves varies from patient to patient because there may be considerable overlap with the iliohypogastric nerve. In general, the ilioinguinal nerve provides sensory innervation to the upper portion of the skin of the inner thigh and the root of the penis and upper scrotum in men or the mons pubis and lateral labia in women.

To perform ilioinguinal nerve block, the patient is placed in the supine position with a pillow under the knees if extending the legs increases the patient's pain because of traction on the nerve. The anterior superior iliac spine is identified by palpation. A point 2 inches medial and 2 inches inferior to the anterior superior iliac spine is then identified and prepared with antiseptic solution. A 1½-inch, 25-gauge needle is then advanced at an oblique angle toward the pubic symphysis (Fig. 288-1). From 5 to 7 mL of 1.0% preservative-free lidocaine is injected in a fanlike manner as the needle pierces the fascia of the external oblique muscle. Care must be taken not to place the needle too deep and enter the peritoneal cavity and perforate the abdominal viscera.

If the pain has an inflammatory component, the local anesthetic is combined with 80 mg of methylprednisolone and is injected in incremental doses. Subsequent daily nerve blocks are performed similarly, substituting 40 mg of methylprednisolone for the initial 80-mg dose. Because of overlapping innervation of the ilioinguinal and iliohypogastric nerves, it is not unusual to block branches of each nerve when performing ilioinguinal nerve block. After the solution is injected, pressure is applied to the injection site to decrease the incidence of postblock ecchymosis and hematoma formation, which can be dramatic, especially when the patient is receiving anticoagulants.

The main side effect of ilioinguinal nerve block is postblock ecchymosis and hematoma formation. If needle placement is too deep and enters the peritoneal cavity, perforation of the colon may result in intra-abdominal abscess and fistula formation. Early detection of infection is crucial to avoid potentially life-threatening sequelae.

SUGGESTED READING

Waldman SD: Ilioinguinal nerve block. In: Atlas of Interventional Pain Management, ed 2. Philadelphia, Saunders, 2004.

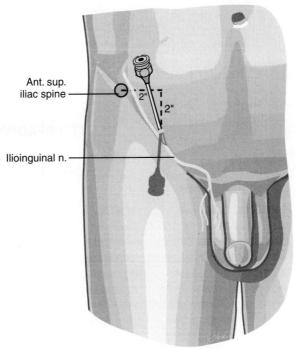

FIGURE 288–1 Ilioinguinal nerve block. (From Waldman SD: Atlas of Interventional Pain Management, ed 2. Philadelphia, Saunders, 2004, p 297.)

CHAPTER 289

Iliohypogastric Nerve Block

The iliohypogastric nerve is a branch of the L1 nerve root with a contribution from T12 in some patients. The nerve follows a curvilinear course that takes it from its origin of the L1 and occasionally T12 somatic nerves to inside the concavity of the ilium. The iliohypogastric nerve continues anteriorly to perforate the transverse abdominal muscle to lie between it and the external oblique muscle. At this point, the iliohypogastric nerve divides into an anterior and a lateral branch. The lateral branch provides cutaneous sensory innervation to the posterolateral gluteal region. The anterior branch pierces the external oblique muscle just beyond the anterior superior iliac spine to provide cutaneous sensory innervation to the abdominal skin above the pubis. The nerve may interconnect with the ilioinguinal nerve along its course, resulting in variation of the distribution of the sensory innervation of the iliohypogastric and ilioinguinal nerves.

To perform iliohypogastric nerve block, the patient is placed in the supine position with a pillow under the knees if extending the legs increases the patient's pain because of traction on the nerve. The anterior superior iliac spine is identified by palpation. A point 1 inch medial and 1 inch inferior to the anterior superior iliac spine is then identified and prepared with antiseptic solution. A 25-gauge, 1½-inch needle is then advanced at an oblique angle toward the pubic symphysis (Fig. 289-1). From 5 to 7 mL of 1.0% preservative-free lidocaine is injected in a fanlike manner as the needle pierces the fascia of the external oblique muscle. Care must be taken not to place the needle too deep and enter the peritoneal cavity and perforate the abdominal viscera.

If the pain has an inflammatory component, the local anesthetic is combined with 80 mg of methylprednisolone and is injected in incremental doses. Subsequent daily nerve blocks are performed similarly, substituting 40 mg of methylprednisolone for the initial 80-mg dose. Because of overlapping innervation of the ilioinguinal and iliohypogastric nerves, it is not unusual to block branches of each nerve when performing iliohypogastric nerve block. After injection of the solution, pressure is applied to the injection site to decrease the incidence of postblock ecchymosis and hematoma formation, which can be dramatic, especially in the patient receiving anticoagulants.

The main side effect of iliohypogastric nerve block is postblock ecchymosis and hematoma formation.

If needle placement is too deep and enters the peritoneal cavity, perforation of the colon may result in intra-abdominal abscess and fistula formation. Early detection of infection is crucial to avoid potentially life-threatening sequelae.

SUGGESTED READING

Waldman SD: Iliohypogastric nerve block. In: Atlas of Interventional Pain Management, ed 2. Philadelphia, Saunders, 2004.

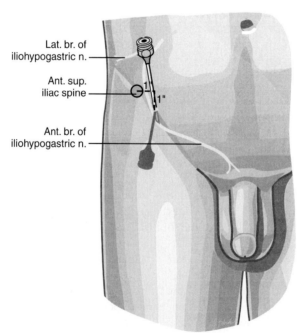

Lat. br. of iliohypogastric n.

Ant. sup. iliac spine

Ant. br. of iliohypogastric n.

FIGURE 289–1 Iliohypogastric nerve block. (From Waldman SD: Atlas of Interventional Pain Management, ed 2. Philadelphia, Saunders, 2004, p 301.)

Genitofemoral Nerve Block

The genitofemoral nerve is a branch of the L1 nerve root with a contribution from T12 in some patients. The nerve follows a curvilinear course that takes it from its origin of the L1 and occasionally T12 and L2 somatic nerves to inside the concavity of the ilium. The genitofemoral nerve descends obliquely in an anterior course through the psoas major muscle to emerge on the abdominal surface opposite L3 or L4. The nerve descends superitoneally behind the ureter and divides into a genital and femoral branch just above the inguinal ligament. In males, the genital branch travels through the inguinal canal passing inside the deep inguinal ring to innervate the cremaster muscle and skin of the scrotum. In females, the genital branch follows the course of the round ligament and provides innervation to the ipsilateral mons pubis and labia majora. In males and females, the femoral branch descends lateral to the external iliac artery to pass behind the inguinal ligament. The nerve enters the femoral sheath lateral to the femoral artery to innervate the skin of the anterior superior femoral triangle.

To block the genital branch of the genitofemoral nerve, the pubic tubercle and the inguinal ligament are identified. A point just lateral to the pubic tubercle just below the inguinal ligament is then identified and prepared with antiseptic solution. A 1½-inch, 25-gauge needle is then advanced through the skin and subcutaneous tissues (Fig. 290-1). Then 5 mL of 1.0% preservative-free lidocaine is injected after careful aspiration. Care must be taken not to place the needle too deep and enter the peritoneal cavity and perforate the abdominal viscera or to inadvertently inject the local anesthetic into the femoral artery.

If the pain has an inflammatory component, the local anesthetic for the blocks described is combined with 80 mg of methylprednisolone and is injected in incremental doses. Subsequent daily nerve blocks are performed similarly, substituting 40 mg of methylprednisolone for the initial 80-mg dose. Because of overlapping innervation of the genitofemoral, ilioinguinal and iliohypogastric nerves, it is not unusual to block branches of each nerve when performing genitofemoral nerve block. After the solution is injected, pressure is applied to the injection site to decrease the incidence of postblock ecchymosis and hematoma formation, which can be dramatic, especially when the patient is receiving anticoagulants.

The main side effect of genitofemoral nerve block is postblock ecchymosis and hematoma formation. If needle placement is too deep and enters the peritoneal cavity, perforation of the colon may result in intra-abdominal abscess and fistula formation. Early detection of infection is crucial to avoid potentially life-threatening sequelae.

SUGGESTED READING

Waldman SD: Genitofemoral nerve block. In: Atlas of Interventional Pain Management, ed 2. Philadelphia, Saunders, 2004.

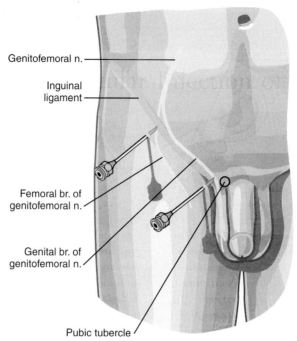

FIGURE 290–1 Genitofemoral nerve block. (From Waldman SD: Atlas of Interventional Pain Management, ed 2. Philadelphia, Saunders, 2004, p 305.)

CHAPTER 291

Lumbar Sympathetic Ganglion Block

The preganglionic fibers of the lumbar sympathetics exit the intervertebral foramina along with the lumbar paravertebral nerves. After exiting the intervertebral foramen, the lumbar paravertebral nerve gives off a recurrent branch that loops back through the foramen to provide innervation to the spinal ligaments, meninges, and its respective vertebra. The upper lumbar paravertebral nerve also interfaces with the lumbar sympathetic chain via the myelinated preganglionic fibers of the white rami communicantes. All five of the lumbar nerves interface with the unmyelinated postganglionic fibers of the gray rami communicantes. At the level of the lumbar sympathetic ganglia, preganglionic and postganglionic fibers synapse. Additionally, some of the postganglionic fibers return to their respective somatic nerves via the gray rami communicantes. Other lumbar sympathetic postganglionic fibers travel to the aortic and hypogastric plexus and course up and down the sympathetic trunk to terminate in distant ganglia.

In many patients, the first and second lumbar ganglia are fused. These ganglia and the remainder of the lumbar chain and ganglia lie at the anterolateral margin of the lumbar vertebral bodies. The peritoneal cavity lies lateral and anterior to the lumbar sympathetic chain. Given the proximity of the lumbar somatic nerves to the lumbar sympathetic chain, the potential exists for both neural pathways to be blocked when performing blockade of the lumbar sympathetic ganglion.

To perform lumbar sympathetic ganglion block, the patient is placed in the prone position with a pillow under the abdomen to gently flex the lumbar spine. The spinous process of the vertebra just above the nerve to be blocked is palpated. At a point just below and 3 inches lateral to the spinous process, the skin is prepared with antiseptic solution. A 22-gauge, 3½-inch needle is attached to a 12-mL syringe and is advanced at a 35- to 45-degree angle to the skin, aiming for the lateral aspect of the vertebral body. The needle should impinge on bone after being advanced approximately 2 inches. If the needle comes into contact with bone at a shallower depth, it has probably impinged on the transverse process. If this occurs, the needle should be directed in a slightly more cephalad trajectory to pass above the transverse process to impinge on the lateral aspect of the vertebral body. After bony contact is made with the vertebral body, the needle is withdrawn into the subcutaneous tissues and redirected at a slightly steeper angle and "walked off" the lateral margin of the vertebral body. As soon as bony contact is lost, the needle is slowly advanced approximately ½ inch deeper (Fig. 291-1). Given the proximity of the lumbar sympathetic chain to the somatic nerve, a paresthesia in the distribution of the corresponding lumbar paravertebral nerve may be elicited. If this occurs, the needle should be withdrawn and redirected slightly more cephalad. The needle is then again slowly advanced until it passes the lateral border of the vertebral body. The needle should ultimately rest at the anterior lateral margin of the vertebral body. If fluoroscopy is used, a small amount of contrast medium may be added to the local anesthetic. The contrast medium should appear just anterior to the vertebral body on the posteroanterior view and just lateral to the vertebral body on the lateral view. If computed tomographic guidance is used, the contrast should be seen surrounding the sympathetic chain anterolateral to the vertebral body (Fig. 291-2). Once the needle is in position and careful aspiration reveals no blood or cerebrospinal fluid, 12 to 15 mL of 1.0% preservative-free lidocaine is injected.

The proximity to the spinal cord and exiting nerve roots makes it imperative that this procedure be carried out only by those well versed in the regional anatomy and experienced in performing interventional pain management techniques. Given the proximity of the peritoneal cavity, damage to the abdominal viscera during lumbar sympathetic ganglion block is a distinct possibility. Proximity to the great vessels makes inadvertent vascular injection a distinct possibility. The incidence of this complication will be decreased if care is taken to place the needle just beyond the anterolateral margin of the vertebral body. Needle placement too medial may result in epidural, subdural, or subarachnoid injections or trauma to the intervertebral disc, spinal cord, and exiting nerve roots. Although uncommon, infection remains an ever-present possibility, especially in the immunocompromised cancer patient. Early detection of infection, including discitis, is crucial to avoid potentially life-threatening sequelae.

SUGGESTED READING

Waldman SD: Lumbar sympathetic ganglion block. In: Atlas of Interventional Pain Management, ed 2. Philadelphia, Saunders, 2004.

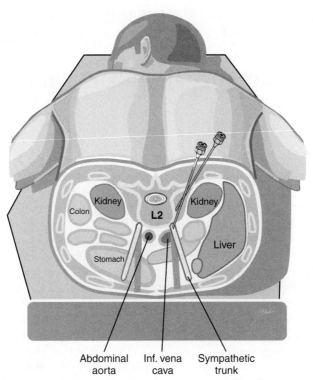

FIGURE 291–1 Lumbar sympathetic ganglion block (From Waldman SD: Atlas of Interventional Pain Management, ed 2. Philadelphia, Saunders, 2004, p 310.)

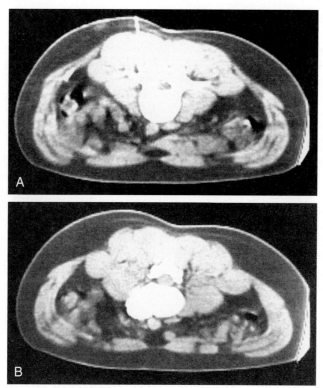

FIGURE 291–2 A, CT-guided needle placement for lumbar sympathetic block. **B,** Proper spread of contrast medium outlining the sympathetic chain. (From Waldman SD: Atlas of Interventional Pain Management, ed 2. Philadelphia, Saunders, 2004, p 312.)

CHAPTER 292

Radiofrequency Lesioning—Lumbar Sympathetic Ganglion

The preganglionic fibers of the lumbar sympathetics exit the intervertebral foramina along with the lumbar paravertebral nerves. After exiting the intervertebral foramen, the lumbar paravertebral nerve gives off a recurrent branch that loops back through the foramen to provide innervation to the spinal ligaments, meninges, and its respective vertebra. The upper lumbar paravertebral nerve also interfaces with the lumbar sympathetic chain via the myelinated preganglionic fibers of the white rami communicantes. All five of the lumbar nerves interface with the unmyelinated postganglionic fibers of the gray rami communicantes. At the level of the lumbar sympathetic ganglia, preganglionic and postganglionic fibers synapse. Additionally, some of the postganglionic fibers return to their respective somatic nerves via the gray rami communicantes. Other lumbar sympathetic

postganglionic fibers travel to the aortic and hypogastric plexus and course up and down the sympathetic trunk to terminate in distant ganglia.

In many patients, the first and second lumbar ganglia are fused. These ganglia and the remainder of the lumbar chain and ganglia lie at the anterolateral margin of the lumbar vertebral bodies. The peritoneal cavity lies lateral and anterior to the lumbar sympathetic chain. Given the proximity of the lumbar somatic nerves to the lumbar sympathetic chain, the potential exists for both neural pathways to be blocked when performing blockade of the lumbar sympathetic ganglion.

The patient is placed in the prone position with a pillow under the abdomen to gently flex the lumbar spine. The spinous process of the vertebra just above the nerve to be blocked is palpated. At a point just below and 3 inches lateral to the spinous process, the skin is prepared with antiseptic solution. A 20-gauge, 150-mm radiofrequency needle with a 10-mm active tip is advanced at a 35- to 45-degree angle to the skin, aiming for the lateral aspect of the L2 vertebral body. The needle should impinge on bone after being advanced approximately 2 inches. If the needle comes into contact with bone at a shallower depth, it has probably impinged on the transverse process. If this occurs, the needle should be directed in a slightly more cephalad trajectory to pass above the transverse process to impinge on the lateral aspect of the vertebral body. After bony contact is made with the vertebral body, the needle is withdrawn into the subcutaneous tissues and redirected at a slightly steeper angle and "walked off" the lateral margin of the vertebral body. As soon as bony contact is lost, the needle is slowly advanced approximately ½ inch deeper (Figs. 292-1 and 292-2). Given the proximity of the lumbar sympathetic chain to the somatic nerve, a paresthesia in the distribution of the corresponding lumbar paravertebral nerve may be elicited. If this occurs, the needle should be withdrawn and redirected slightly more cephalad. The needle is then again slowly advanced until it passes the lateral border of the vertebral body. The needle should ultimately rest at the anterior lateral margin of the vertebral body (Fig. 292-3). A small amount of contrast medium is then injected through the needle. The contrast medium should appear just anterior to the vertebral body on the posteroanterior view and just lateral to the vertebral body on the lateral view. If computed tomographic guidance is used, the contrast can be seen surrounding the sympathetic chain anterolateral to the vertebral body. Once the needle is in position and careful aspiration reveals no blood or cerebrospinal fluid, trial stimulation at 50 Hz at 1 V is carried out. The patient should experience pain localized to the low back. If pain is felt in the groin, the needle is in proximity of the genitofemoral nerve or L1 or L2 nerve roots and must be repositioned. If pain is felt in the lower extremity, the needle is in proximity to the lower lumbar nerve roots and must be repositioned. Motor stimulation should be negative with 3 V at 2 Hz. If stimulation trials are satisfactory, a lesion is created for 60 seconds at 80° C. Based on the patient's clinical response, additional lesions below initial lesions may be required to provide long-lasting pain relief.

The proximity to the spinal cord and exiting nerve roots makes it imperative that this procedure be carried out only by those well versed in the regional anatomy and experienced in performing interventional pain management techniques. Given the proximity of the peritoneal cavity, damage to the abdominal viscera during lumbar sympathetic ganglion radiofrequency lesioning is a distinct possibility. The incidence of this complication will be decreased if care is taken to place the needle just beyond the anterolateral margin vertebral body. Needle placement too medial may result in epidural, subdural, or subarachnoid injections or trauma to the intervertebral disc, spinal cord, and exiting nerve roots. Lesioning with the needle in proximity to the genitofemoral nerve may result in persistent genitofemoral neuritis that can be difficult to treat. Although uncommon, infection remains an ever-present possibility, especially in the immunocompromised cancer patient. Early detection of infection, including discitis, is crucial to avoid potentially life-threatening sequelae.

SUGGESTED READING

Waldman SD: Radiofrequency lesioning—Lumbar sympathetic ganglion. In: Atlas of Interventional Pain Management, ed 2. Philadelphia, Saunders, 2004.

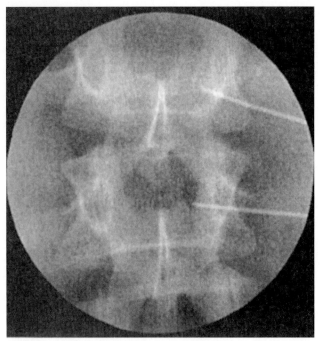

FIGURE 292–1 Posteroanterior radiograph shows the radiofrequency cannula positions during lesioning of the lumbar sympathetic chain. Note that the tips of the radiofrequency cannulas are directly behind the facet joint line. (From Waldman SD: Atlas of Interventional Pain Management, ed 2. Philadelphia, Saunders, 2004, p 315.)

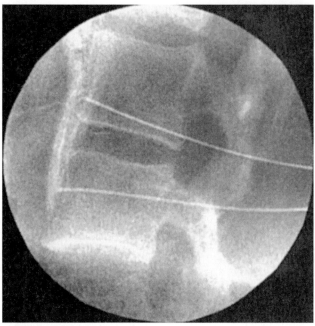

FIGURE 292–2 Lateral radiograph shows the radiofrequency cannula positions at the L2 and L3 levels for lesioning of the lumbar sympathetic chain. (From Waldman SD: Atlas of Interventional Pain Management, ed 2. Philadelphia, Saunders, 2004, p 315.)

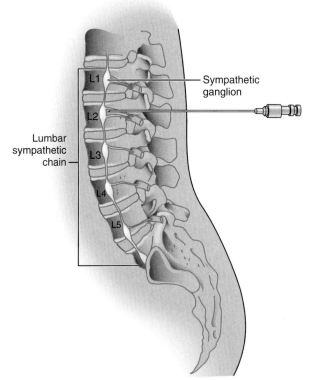

FIGURE 292–3 Correct needle orientation for radiofrequency lesioning of the lumbar sympathetic ganglion. (From Waldman SD: Atlas of Interventional Pain Management, ed 2. Philadelphia, Saunders, 2004, p 316.)

Lumbar Paravertebral Block

The lumbar paravertebral nerves exit their respective intervertebral foramina just beneath the transverse process of the vertebra. After exiting the intervertebral foramen, the lumbar paravertebral nerve gives off a recurrent branch that loops back through the foramen to provide innervation to the spinal ligaments, meninges, and its respective vertebra. The lumbar paravertebral nerve then divides into posterior and anterior primary divisions. The posterior division courses posteriorly and, along with its branches, provides innervation to the facet joints and the muscles and skin of the back. The larger anterior division courses laterally and inferiorly to enter the body of the psoas muscle. Within the muscle, the first four lumbar paravertebral nerves join to form the lumbar plexus. The lumbar plexus also receives a contribution from the 12th thoracic paravertebral nerve. The lumbar plexus provides innervation to the lower abdominal wall, groin, portions of the external genitalia, and portions of the lower extremity.

To perform lumbar paravertebral block, the patient is placed in the prone position with a pillow under the abdomen to slightly flex the lumbar spine. The spinous process of the vertebra at the level to be blocked is palpated. At a point 1½ inches lateral to the spinous process, the skin is prepared with antiseptic solution. A 22-gauge, 3½-inch needle is attached to a 12-mL syringe and is advanced perpendicular to the skin aiming for the middle of the transverse process. The needle should impinge on bone after being advanced approximately 1½ inches. After bony contact is made, the needle is withdrawn into the subcutaneous tissues and redirected inferiorly and walked off the inferior margin of the transverse process. As soon as bony contact is lost, the needle is slowly advanced ½ to ¾ inch deeper until paresthesia in the distribution of the lumbar paravertebral nerve to be blocked is elicited (Fig. 293-1). Once the paresthesia has been elicited and careful aspiration reveals no blood or cerebrospinal fluid, 3 mL of 1.0% preservative-free lidocaine is injected. If there is an inflammatory component to the pain, the local anesthetic is combined with 80 mg of methylprednisolone and is injected in incremental doses. Subsequent daily nerve blocks are carried out in a similar manner, substituting 40 mg of methylprednisolone for the initial 80-mg dose. Because of overlapping innervation of the posterior elements from the medial branch of the posterior division from the vertebra above, the lumbar paravertebral nerves above and below the nerve suspected of subserving the painful condition will have to be blocked.

The proximity of the lumbar paravertebral nerve to the spinal cord and exiting nerve roots makes it imperative that this procedure be carried out only by those well versed in the regional anatomy and experienced in performing interventional pain management techniques. Needle placement too medial may result in epidural, subdural, or subarachnoid injections or trauma to the spinal cord and exiting nerve roots. Placing the needle too deep between the transverse processes may result in trauma to the exiting lumbar nerve roots. Although uncommon, infection remains an ever-present possibility, especially in the immunocompromised cancer patient. Early detection of infection is crucial to avoid potentially life-threatening sequelae.

SUGGESTED READING

Waldman SD: Lumbar paravertebral block. In: Atlas of Interventional Pain Management, ed 2. Philadelphia, Saunders, 2004.

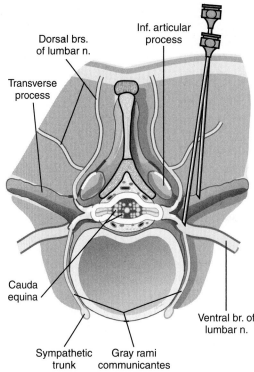

FIGURE 293–1 Lumbar paravertebral block. (From Waldman SD: Atlas of Interventional Pain Management, ed 2. Philadelphia, Saunders, 2004, p 319.)

CHAPTER 294

Lumbar Facet Block

The lumbar facet joints are formed by the articulations of the superior and inferior articular facets of adjacent vertebrae. The lumbar facet joints are true joints in that they are lined with synovium and possess a true joint capsule. This capsule is richly innervated and supports the notion of the facet joint as a pain generator. The lumbar facet joint is susceptible to arthritic changes and trauma secondary to acceleration-deceleration injuries. Such damage to the joint results in pain secondary to synovial joint inflammation and adhesions.

Each facet joint receives innervation from two spinal levels. Each joint receives fibers from the dorsal ramus at the same level as the vertebra as well as fibers from the dorsal ramus of the vertebra above. This fact has clinical importance in that it provides an explanation for the ill-defined nature of facet-mediated pain and explains why

the dorsal nerve from the vertebra above the offending level must often also be blocked to provide complete pain relief.

At each level, the dorsal ramus provides a medial branch that exits the intertransverse space crossing over the top of the transverse process in a groove at the point where the transverse process joins the vertebra. The nerve then travels inferiorly and medially across the posterior surface of the vertebral lamina where it gives off branches to innervate the facet joint. The medial branch is blocked at the point at which the nerve curves around the top of the transverse process.

At the L5 level, it is the dorsal ramus of L5 rather than the medial branch that crosses the sacral ala at the junction of the superior articular process. After crossing the sacral ala, the dorsal ramus then gives off a medial branch that provides innervation for the lumbosacral facet joint. During performance of the lumbar facet block using the medial branch approach, the L5 nerve is blocked at this point rather than at the superomedial junction of the transverse process with the vertebra, as is done when blocking the L1-4 medial branches.

Medial Branch Technique

Lumbar facet block using the medial branch technique is the preferred route of treating lumbar facet syndrome. It may be done either blind or under fluoroscopic guidance.

The patient is placed in a prone position. Pillows are placed under the chest to allow the lumbar spine to be moderately flexed without discomfort to the patient. The forehead is allowed to rest on a folded blanket.

BLIND TECHNIQUE

To block the L1-4 facets using a blind technique, the spinous process at the level to be blocked is identified by palpation. A point slightly inferior and 5 cm lateral to the spinous process is then identified as the site of needle insertion. After preparation of the skin with antiseptic solution, a skin wheal of local anesthetic is raised at the site of needle insertion. Then 3 mL of preservative-free local anesthetic is drawn up in a 5-mL sterile syringe. When treating pain believed to be secondary to an inflammatory process, a total of 80 mg of depot steroid is added to the local anesthetic with the first block, and 40 mg of depot steroid is added with subsequent blocks.

An 18-gauge, 1-inch needle is inserted through the skin and into the subcutaneous tissue at the previously identified insertion site to serve as an introducer. The introducer needle is then repositioned with a slightly superior and medial trajectory, pointing directly toward the superior portion of the junction of the transverse process and the vertebra at the level to be blocked. A 25-gauge, 2- to 3½-inch needle is then inserted through the 18-gauge introducer and directed toward this junction of the transverse process and the vertebra. After bony contact is made, the depth of the contact is noted and the spinal needle is withdrawn. The introducer needle is then repositioned, aiming toward the most superomedial aspect of the junction of the transverse process with the vertebra (Fig. 294-1). The 25-gauge spinal needle is then re-advanced until it impinges on the lateralmost aspect of the border of the articular pillar. Should the spinal needle "walk off" the top of the transverse process, it is withdrawn and redirected slightly medially and inferiorly and carefully advanced to the depth of the previous bony contact.

After the needle is felt to be in a satisfactory position, the stylet is removed from the 25-gauge spinal needle and the hub is observed for blood or cerebrospinal fluid. If neither is present, gentle aspiration of the needle is carried out. If the aspiration test is negative, 1.5 mL of solution is injected through the spinal needle.

For blockade of the dorsal ramus of L5, this same technique is used, but the needle tip is placed more laterally to block the nerve as it passes through the groove between the sacral ala and the superior articular process of the sacrum.

FLUOROSCOPIC TECHNIQUE

If fluoroscopy is used to block the L1-4 facets, the beam is rotated in a sagittal plane from an anterior to posterior position, which allows identification and visualization of the junction of the transverse process and vertebra at the level to be blocked. After preparation of the skin with antiseptic solution, a skin wheal of local anesthetic is raised at a point slightly inferior and approximately 5 cm off the midline. An 18-gauge, 1-inch needle is inserted at the insertion site to serve as an introducer. The fluoroscopy beam is aimed directly through the introducer needle, which will appear as a small point on the fluoroscopy screen. The introducer needle is then repositioned under fluoroscopic guidance until this small point is visualized pointing directly toward the most superomedial point at which the transverse process joins the vertebra.

A total of 5 mL of contrast medium suitable for intrathecal use is drawn up in a sterile 12-mL syringe. Then, 3 mL of preservative-free local anesthetic is drawn up in a separate 5-mL sterile syringe. When treating pain thought to be secondary to an inflammatory process, a total of 80 mg of depot steroid is added to the local anesthetic with the first block, and 40 mg of depot steroid is added with subsequent blocks.

A 25-gauge, 2- to 3½-inch needle is then inserted through the 18-gauge introducer and directed toward the most superomedial point at which the transverse process joins the vertebra. After bony contact is made, the spinal needle is withdrawn and the introducer needle is redirected to allow the spinal needle to impinge on the most superomedial point at which the transverse process joins the vertebra. This procedure is repeated until the tip of the 25-gauge spinal needle rests against the most superior and medial point at which the transverse process joins the vertebra.

After confirmation of needle placement by biplanar fluoroscopy, the hub of the 25-gauge needle is observed for blood or cerebrospinal fluid. If neither is present, gentle aspiration of the needle is carried out. If the aspiration test is negative, 1 mL of contrast medium is slowly injected under fluoroscopy to reconfirm needle placement. After correct needle placement is confirmed, 1.5 mL of local anesthetic with or without steroid is injected through the spinal needle.

To block the L5 facet, the needle tip is placed under fluoroscopic guidance to rest in the groove between the sacral ala and the superior articular process of the sacrum. A foam wedge placed under the pelvis helps rotate the posterior superior iliac crest out of the way.

Intra-articular Approach

Lumbar facet block using the intra-articular technique may be performed either blind or under fluoroscopic guidance. The patient is placed in a prone position. Pillows are placed under the chest to allow the lumbar spine to be moderately flexed without discomfort to the patient. The forehead is allowed to rest on a folded blanket.

BLIND TECHNIQUE

To block the L1-4 facet joints using the blind technique, the spinous process at the level to be blocked is identified by palpation. A point one spinal level lower and 3.5 cm lateral to the spinous process is then identified as the site of needle insertion. Then 3 mL of preservative-free local anesthetic is drawn up in a 5-mL sterile syringe. After preparation of the skin with antiseptic solution, a skin wheal of local anesthetic is raised at the site of needle insertion. When treating pain believed to be secondary to an inflammatory process, a total of 80 mg of depot steroid is added to the local anesthetic with the first block, and 40 mg of depot steroid is added with subsequent blocks.

An 18-gauge, 1-inch needle is inserted through the skin and into the subcutaneous tissue at the previously identified insertion site to serve as an introducer. The introducer needle is then repositioned with a superior and ventral trajectory, pointing directly toward the inferior margin of the facet joint at the level to be blocked. The angle of the needle from the skin is approximately 35 degrees. A 25-gauge, 3½-inch styletted spinal needle is then inserted through the 18-gauge introducer and directed toward the bone just below the joint to be blocked. Care must be taken to be sure the trajectory of the needle does not drift either laterally or medially. Medial drift can allow the needle to enter the epidural, subdural, or subarachnoid space and to traumatize the dorsal root or spinal cord. Lateral drift can allow the needle to pass beyond the lateral border of the vertebra and traumatize the exiting nerve roots.

After bony contact is made, the depth of the contact is noted and the spinal needle is withdrawn. The introducer needle is then redirected slightly more superiorly. The spinal needle is then advanced through the introducer needle until it either enters the facet joint or again impinges on bone. If the needle again impinges on bone, the maneuver is repeated until the spinal needle slides into the facet joint (Fig. 294-2). A "pop" is often felt as the needle slides into the joint cavity.

After the needle is felt to be in satisfactory position, the stylet is removed from the 25-gauge spinal needle and the hub is observed for blood or cerebrospinal fluid. If neither is present, gentle aspiration of the needle is carried out. If the aspiration test is negative, 1 mL of solution is injected slowly through the spinal needle. Rapid or forceful injection may rupture the joint capsule and exacerbate the patient's pain.

To block the lumbosacral (L5) facet joint using the intra-articular technique, the previously discussed technique is used, but it may be necessary to move the needle insertion point slightly more inferior and lateral to avoid the posterior superior iliac crest. Placing a foam wedge under the pelvis to rotate the iliac crest may also help.

FLUOROSCOPIC TECHNIQUE

If fluoroscopy is used to block the L1-4 joints, the beam is rotated in a sagittal plane from an anterior to posterior position, which allows identification and visualization of the articular pillars of the respective vertebrae and the adjacent facet joints. After preparation of the skin with antiseptic solution, a skin wheal of local anesthetic is raised at the site of needle insertion. An 18-gauge, 1-inch needle is inserted at the insertion site to serve as an introducer. The fluoroscopy beam is aimed directly through the introducer needle, which will appear as a small point on the fluoroscopy screen. The introducer needle is then repositioned under fluoroscopic guidance until this small point is visualized pointing directly toward the inferior aspect of the facet joint to be blocked.

A total of 5 mL of contrast medium suitable for intrathecal use is drawn up in a sterile 12-mL syringe. Then, 2 mL of preservative-free local anesthetic is drawn up in a separate 5-mL sterile syringe. When treating pain believed to be secondary to an inflammatory process, a total of 80 mg of depot steroid is added to the local anesthetic with the first block, and 40 mg of depot steroid is added with subsequent blocks.

A 25-gauge, 2- to 3½-inch needle is then inserted through the 18-gauge introducer and directed toward the articular pillar just below the joint to be blocked. After bony contact is made, the spinal needle is withdrawn and the introducer needle repositioned superiorly, aiming toward the facet joint. The 25-gauge spinal needle is then readvanced through the introducer needle until it enters the target joint. To block the lumbosacral (L5) facet joint using the intra-articular technique, the technique discussed earlier is used, but it may be necessary to move the needle insertion point slightly more inferior and lateral to avoid the posterior superior iliac crest. Placing a foam wedge under the pelvis to rotate the iliac crest may also help.

After confirmation of needle placement by biplanar fluoroscopy, the stylet is removed from the 25-gauge spinal needle and the hub is observed for blood or cerebrospinal fluid. If neither is present, gentle aspiration of the needle is carried out. If the aspiration test is negative, 1 mL of contrast medium is slowly injected under fluoroscopy to reconfirm needle placement. After correct needle placement is confirmed, 1 mL of local anesthetic with or without steroid is slowly injected through the spinal needle. Rapid or forceful injection may rupture the joint capsule and exacerbate the patient's pain.

The proximity to the spinal cord and exiting nerve roots makes it imperative that this procedure be carried out only by those well versed in the regional anatomy and experienced in performing interventional pain management techniques. Placing the needle too medially can result in inadvertent subdural, subarachnoid, or epidural injection. Although rare, infection remains an ever-present possibility. Many patients also complain of a transient increase in lumbar pain after injection into the joint.

SUGGESTED READINGS

Waldman SD: Lumbar facet block: Medial branch technique. In: Atlas of Interventional Pain Management, ed 2. Philadelphia, Saunders, 2004.

Waldman SD: Lumbar facet block: Intra-articular technique. In: Atlas of Interventional Pain Management, ed 2. Philadelphia, Saunders, 2004.

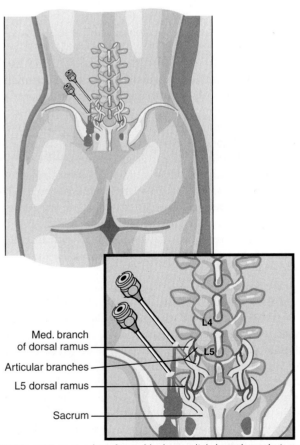

FIGURE 294–1 Lumbar facet block: medial branch technique. (From Waldman SD: Atlas of Interventional Pain Management, ed 2. Philadelphia, Saunders, 2004, p 322.)

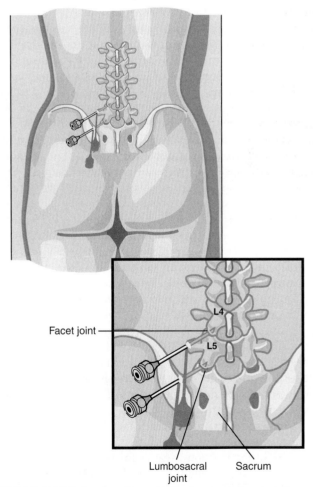

FIGURE 294–2 Lumbar facet block: intra-articular technique. (From Waldman SD: Atlas of Interventional Pain Management, ed 2. Philadelphia, Saunders, 2004, p 335.)

CHAPTER 295

Lumbar Epidural Block

The superior boundary of the epidural space is the fusion of the periosteal and spinal layers of dura at the foramen magnum. The epidural space continues inferiorly to the sacrococcygeal membrane. The lumbar epidural space is bounded anteriorly by the posterior longitudinal ligament and posteriorly by the vertebral laminae and the ligamentum flavum (Fig. 295-1). The vertebral pedicles and intervertebral foramina form the lateral limits of the epidural space. The lumbar epidural space is 5 to 6 mm at the L2-3 interspace with the lumbar spine flexed. The lumbar epidural space contains fat, veins, arteries, lymphatics, and connective tissue (Fig. 295-2).

During performance of lumbar epidural block in the midline, the needle will traverse the following structures (Fig. 295-3). After traversing the skin and subcutaneous tissues, the styletted epidural needle will impinge on the supraspinous ligament, which runs vertically between the apices of the spinous processes. The supraspinous ligament offers some resistance to the advancing needle. This ligament is dense enough to hold a needle in position even when the needle is released.

The interspinous ligament that runs obliquely between the spinous processes is next encountered, offering additional resistance to needle advancement. Because the interspinous ligament is contiguous with the ligamentum flavum, the pain management specialist may perceive a "false" loss of resistance when the needle tip enters the space between the interspinous ligament and the ligamentum flavum.

A significant increase in resistance to needle advancement signals that the needle tip is impinging on the dense ligamentum flavum. Because the ligament is made up almost entirely of elastin fibers, there is a continued increase in resistance as the needle traverses the ligamentum flavum, owing to the drag of the ligament on the needle. A sudden loss of resistance occurs as the needle tip enters the epidural space. There should be essentially no resistance to drugs injected into the normal epidural space.

Lumbar epidural nerve block may be carried out with the patient in a sitting, lateral, or prone position.

The sitting position is easier for both the patient and the pain management specialist. This position enhances the ability to identify the midline and also avoids the problem of rotation of the spine inherent in the use of the lateral position, which may make identification of the epidural space difficult. Some investigators believe that the effects of gravity on local anesthetics is enhanced in the sitting position, improving the ability to block the S1 nerve roots, which can be difficult because of their larger size.

After the patient is placed in optimal position with the lumbar spine flexed and forearms resting on a padded bedside table, the skin is prepared with an antiseptic solution. At the L3-4 interspace, the operator's middle and index fingers are placed on each side of the spinous processes. The position of the interspace is reconfirmed with palpation using a rocking motion in the superior and inferior planes. The midline of the selected interspace is identified by palpating the spinous processes above and below the interspace using a lateral rocking motion to ensure that the needle entry site is exactly in the midline. Then 1 mL of local anesthetic is used to infiltrate the skin, subcutaneous tissues, and supraspinous and interspinous ligament at the midline.

A 25-gauge, 2- to 2½-inch needle or a 3½-inch, 18- or 20-gauge Hustead needle is inserted exactly in the midline in the previously anesthetized area through the supraspinous ligament into the interspinous ligament. Smaller, shorter needles are being used more frequently with equally good results. The needle stylet is removed and a well-lubricated 5-mL glass syringe filled with preservative-free sterile saline is attached. Alternatively, the physician can simply use a 12-mL plastic syringe filled with the intended injectate for the following loss of resistance maneuver. This approach has the advantage of not attaching and removing the glass syringe with the attendant risk of inadvertently moving the needle out of the epidural space.

The right-handed physician holds the epidural needle firmly at the hub with his or her left thumb and index finger. The left hand is placed firmly against the patient's back to ensure against uncontrolled needle movements should the patient unexpectedly move. With constant pressure being applied to the plunger of the syringe with the thumb of the right hand, the needle and syringe are continuously advanced in a slow and deliberate manner with the left hand. As soon as the needle bevel passes through the ligamentum flavum and enters the epidural space, there will be a sudden loss of resistance to injection and the plunger will effortlessly surge forward. The syringe is gently removed from the needle.

An air or saline acceptance test is carried out by injecting 0.5 to 1 mL of air or sterile preservative-free saline with a well-lubricated sterile glass syringe to help confirm that the needle is within the epidural space. The force required for injection should not exceed that necessary to overcome the resistance of the needle. Any significant pain or sudden increases in resistance during injection suggest incorrect needle placement, and one should stop injecting immediately and reassess the position of the needle. A small amount of contrast medium may also be injected through the needle to confirm placement within the epidural space. Most experienced pain management specialists do not require the added step to correctly place the needle into the epidural space.

When satisfactory needle position is confirmed, a syringe containing 10 to 12 mL of solution to be injected is carefully attached to the needle. Gentle aspiration is carried out to identify cerebrospinal fluid or blood. If cerebrospinal fluid is aspirated, the epidural block may be repeated at a different interspace. In this situation, drug dosages should be adjusted accordingly because subarachnoid migration of drugs through the dural rent can occur. If aspiration of blood occurs, the needle should be rotated slightly and the aspiration test repeated. If no blood is present, incremental doses of local anesthetic and other drugs may be administered while monitoring the patient carefully for signs of local anesthetic toxicity.

For diagnostic and prognostic blocks, 1.0% preservative-free lidocaine is a suitable local anesthetic. For therapeutic blocks, 0.25% preservative-free bupivacaine in combination with 80 mg of depot methylprednisolone is injected. Subsequent nerve blocks are carried out in a similar manner substituting 40 mg of methylprednisolone for the initial 80-mg dose. Daily lumbar epidural nerve blocks with local anesthetic and/or steroid may be required to treat the previously mentioned acute painful conditions. Chronic conditions such as lumbar radiculopathy, spinal stenosis, vertebral compression fractures, and diabetic polyneuropathy are treated on an every-other-day to once-a-week basis or as the clinical situation dictates.

If the lumbar epidural route is chosen for administration of opioids, 5 to 7 mg of preservative-free morphine sulfate formulated for epidural use is a reasonable initial dose in opioid-tolerant patients. More lipid-soluble opioids such as fentanyl must be delivered by continuous infusion via a lumbar epidural catheter. An epidural catheter may be placed into the lumbar epidural space through a Hustead needle to allow continuous infusions.

Transforaminal Approach

Lumbar epidural injection using the transforaminal approach is carried out with the patient in the prone position. Although some experienced pain practitioners perform this technique without radiographic guidance, many pain practitioners use fluoroscopy to aid in needle placement to help avoid placing the needle too deeply into the spinal canal and inadvertently injecting into the intrathecal space, subdural, or the spinal cord. Because the procedure is usually done in the prone position, special attention to patient monitoring is mandatory.

With the patient in the prone position on the fluoroscopy table, the end plates of the affected vertebra are aligned. The fluoroscopy beam is then rotated ipsilaterally to align the superior articular process of the vertebra below with the 6-o'clock position of the pedicle above (Fig. 295-4).

The skin is then prepared with an antiseptic solution, and a skin wheal of local anesthetic is placed at a point overlying or just lateral to the tip of the superior articular process of the level below the indicated neural foramen. A 22- or 25-gauge, 3½-inch needle is then placed through the previously anesthetized area and advanced until the tip impinges on bone over the pedicle at a lateral to the 6-o'clock position. Failure to impinge on bone at the point may indicate that the needle has passed into and through the spinal canal and rests within the intrathecal space. Failure to identify this problem can lead to disastrous results.

After this bony landmark is identified, the needle is redirected inferiorly into the targeted spinal nerve canal. An anteroposterior fluoroscopic view is obtained to verify that the needle is not medial to the 6-o'clock position on the pedicle to avoid placement of the needle too deeply into the spinal nerve canal with its attendant risk of entry into the dural sleeve or spinal canal. A lateral view is then used to verify needle position. Special care should be taken when performing left upper lumbar transforaminal blocks to avoid advancing the needle beyond the halfway point of the foramen on lateral view to avoid damage to the segmental artery of Adamkiewicz, which lies in the superior ventral aspect of the foramen with its attendant risk of spinal cord ischemia and paraplegia.

After satisfactory needle position is confirmed, 0.2 to 0.4 mL of contrast medium suitable for subarachnoid use is gently injected under fluoroscopic guidance. The contrast should be seen to flow proximally around the pedicle into the epidural space. Flow distal along the nerve root sheath is usually appreciated. The injection of contrast should be stopped immediately if the patient complains of significant pain on injection. After satisfactory flow of contrast is observed and there is no evidence of subdural, subarachnoid, or intravascular spread of contrast, 6 mg of betamethasone suspension/solution or 20 to 40 mg of methylprednisolone or triamcinolone suspension with 0.5 to 2.0 mL of 2.0% to 4.0% preservative-free lidocaine or 0.5% to 0.75% bupivacaine is slowly injected to a total volume of 1 to 3 mL. Injection of the local anesthetic and/or steroid should be discontinued if the patient complains of any significant pain on injection. Transient mild pressure paresthesia is often noted. After satisfactory injection of the local anesthetic and/or steroid and washout of contrast by the local anesthetic and steroid solution is noted, the needle is removed and pressure is placed on the injection site. The technique may be repeated at additional levels as a diagnostic and/or therapeutic maneuver.

Because of the potential for hematogenous spread via Batson's plexus, local infection and sepsis represent absolute contraindications to the lumbar approach to the epidural space. In contradistinction to the caudal approach to the epidural space, anticoagulation or coagulopathy represent absolute contraindications to lumbar epidural nerve block because of the risk of epidural hematoma.

Inadvertent dural puncture occurring during lumbar epidural nerve block should occur less than 0.5% of the time. Failure to recognize inadvertent dural puncture can result in immediate total spinal anesthetic with associated loss of consciousness, hypotension, and apnea. If epidural doses of opioids are accidentally placed into the subarachnoid space, significant respiratory and central nervous system depression will result. It is also possible to inadvertently place a needle or catheter intended for the epidural space into the subdural space. If subdural placement is unrecognized and epidural doses of local anesthetic are administered, the signs and symptoms are similar to that of massive subarachnoid injection although the resulting motor and sensory block may be spotty.

The lumbar epidural space is highly vascular. The intravenous placement of the epidural needle occurs in 0.5% to 1% of patients undergoing lumbar epidural anesthesia. This complication is increased in those patients with distended epidural veins (i.e., the parturient and patients with large intra-abdominal tumor mass). If the misplacement is unrecognized, injection of local anesthetic directly into an epidural vein will result in significant local anesthetic toxicity.

Needle trauma to the epidural veins may result in self-limited bleeding, which may cause postprocedural pain. Uncontrolled bleeding into the epidural space may result in compression of the spinal cord, with the rapid development of neurologic deficit. Although the incidence of significant neurologic deficit secondary to epidural hematoma after lumbar epidural block is exceedingly rare, this devastating complication should be considered whenever there is rapidly developing neurologic deficit after lumbar epidural nerve block.

Neurologic complications after lumbar nerve block are uncommon if proper technique is used. Direct trauma to the spinal cord and/or nerve roots is usually accompanied by pain. If significant pain occurs during placement of the epidural needle or catheter or during injection, the physician should immediately stop and ascertain the cause of the pain to avoid the possibility of additional neural trauma. The transforaminal approach to lumbar epidural block has a statistically significant increase in the incidence of persistent paresthesias and trauma to neural structures including the spinal cord compared with the midline approach. As mentioned, when using the transforaminal approach, placement of the needle too far into the neural foramina may result in unintentional injection into the spinal cord with resultant paraplegia. Injection into the segmental artery can lead to disastrous morbidity due to spinal cord ischemia.

Although uncommon, infection in the epidural space remains an ever-present possibility, especially in the immunocompromised AIDS or cancer patient. If epidural abscess occurs, emergent surgical drainage to avoid spinal cord compression and irreversible neurologic deficit is usually required. Early detection and treatment of infection are crucial to avoid potentially life-threatening sequelae.

SUGGESTED READINGS

Waldman SD: Lumbar epidural nerve block. In: Atlas of Interventional Pain Management, ed. 2. Philadelphia, Saunders, 2004.

Waldman SD: Lumbar epidural nerve block: Transforaminal approach. In: Atlas of Interventional Pain Management, ed 2. Philadelphia, Saunders, 2004.

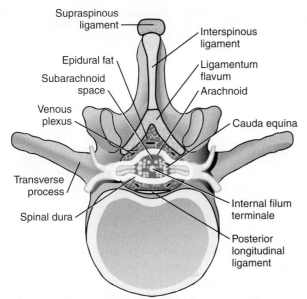

FIGURE 295–1 Anatomy of the lumbar epidural space. (From Waldman SD: Atlas of Interventional Pain Management, ed 2. Philadelphia, Saunders, 2004, p 342.)

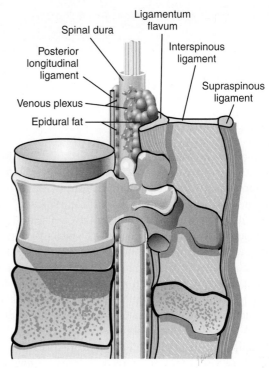

FIGURE 295–2 The contents of the lumbar epidural space. (From Waldman SD: Atlas of Interventional Pain Management, ed 2. Philadelphia, Saunders, 2004, p 343.)

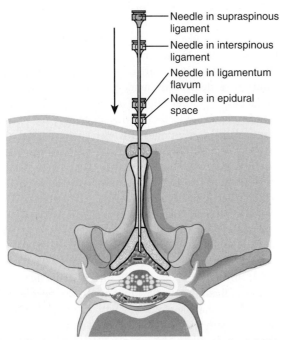

FIGURE 295–3 Needle position for the lumbar epidural block. (From Waldman SD: Atlas of Interventional Pain Management, ed 2. Philadelphia, Saunders, 2004, p 344.)

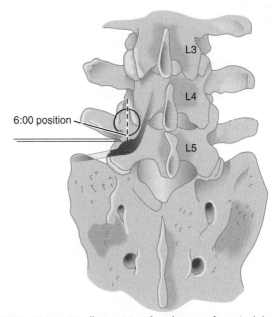

FIGURE 295–4 Needle position for the transforaminal lumbar epidural block. (From Waldman SD: Atlas of Interventional Pain Management, ed 2. Philadelphia, Saunders, 2004, p 353.)

CHAPTER 296

Lumbar Subarachnoid Block

The spinal cord ends at approximately L2 in the majority of adults and at approximately L4 in most infants. Therefore, in most settings, lumbar subarachnoid nerve block should be performed below these levels to avoid the potential for trauma to the spinal cord. The spinal cord is surrounded by three layers of protective connective tissue: the dura, the arachnoid, and the pia mater. The dura is the outermost layer and is composed of tough fibroelastic fibers that form a mechanical barrier to protect the spinal cord. The next layer is the arachnoid. The arachnoid is separated from the dura by only a small potential space, which is filled with serous fluid. The arachnoid is a barrier to the diffusion of substances and effectively serves to limit the spread of drugs administered into the epidural space from diffusing into the spinal fluid. The innermost layer is the pia, a vascular structure that helps provide lateral support to the spinal cord.

To reach the subarachnoid space, a needle placed via the paramedian approach at the L3-4 interspace will pass through the skin, subcutaneous tissues, the inner margin of the interspinous ligament, the ligamentum flavum, the epidural space, dura, the subdural space, and arachnoid. Drugs administered into the subarachnoid space are placed between the arachnoid and pia, although inadvertent subdural injection is possible. Subdural injection of local anesthetic is characterized by a spotty, incomplete block.

Lumbar subarachnoid nerve block via the paramedian approach may be carried out in the sitting, lateral, or prone position. The sitting position is easier for both the patient and the pain management specialist. This position enhances the ability to identify the midline and also avoids the problem of rotation of the spine inherent in the use of the lateral position. Such rotation may make placement of the needle into the subarachnoid space difficult. If the lateral position is chosen, careful attention to patient positioning, including identification of the midline, avoiding rotation of the spine, and maximizing flexion of the lumbar spine, is essential to successfully complete subarachnoid nerve block. The prone position is best used with the patient in the jackknife position to maximize flexion of the lumbar spine. It is occasionally used for administration of hypobaric solutions for midline procedures such as hemorrhoidectomy. Although this position limits the amount of rotation of the spine possible and simplifies midline identification, the inherent dangers of

the prone position, including difficulty in monitoring the patient and problems with airway management, militate against the routine use of the prone position for lumbar subarachnoid nerve block.

After the patient is placed in optimal position with the lumbar spine flexed and without rotation, the iliac crests are identified. The spinous process of L4 is approximately on an imaginary line drawn between the two iliac crests. The skin is then prepared with an antiseptic solution. At the L3-4 interspace, the operator's middle and index fingers are placed on each side of the spinous processes. The position of the interspace is reconfirmed with palpation using a rocking motion in the superior and inferior planes. The midline of the selected interspace is identified by palpating the spinous processes above and below the interspace using a lateral rocking motion. Failure to accurately identify the midline is the number one reason for failed lumbar subarachnoid nerve block. At a point 1 cm lateral and 1 cm below the midline of the L4-5 interspace, local anesthetic is used to infiltrate the skin, subcutaneous tissues, and the edge of interspinous ligament, aiming toward the center of the interspace (Fig. 296-1).

The choice of needle for lumbar subarachnoid block is based in part on the experience of the operator and in part in the desire to decrease the incidence of postdural puncture headache. In general, smaller-gauge needles with points that separate, rather than cut, dural fibers will result in a decreased incidence of postdural puncture headaches, all other things being equal. The use of an introducer needle facilitates the successful use of smaller-gauge needles. A longer 5- or 6-inch needle is often needed to reach the subarachnoid space when using the paramedian approach, especially in larger individuals. The chosen styletted spinal needle is inserted through the previously anesthetized area and advanced with a 10- to 15-degree cephalomedial trajectory. It is advanced through the subcutaneous tissues and supraspinous ligament into the interspinous ligament. The operator will perceive an increase in resistance to needle advancement as the needle passes through the edge of the interspinous ligament and the dense ligamentum flavum. Should the needle impinge on bone, the needle should be withdrawn and readvanced with a slightly more cephalad trajectory. Care must be taken not to allow the needle to cross the midline by directing the needle too laterally or trauma to the spinal cord or exiting nerve roots on the side opposite needle placement may result (Fig. 296-2). The needle will then traverse the epidural space, and the operator will feel a "pop" as the needle pierces the dura. The needle is slowly advanced an additional 1 mm, and the stylet is removed. A free flow of spinal fluid should be observed; or if a smaller spinal needle has been used, cerebrospinal fluid should appear in the hub. If no spinal fluid is observed, the stylet is replaced and the needle is advanced slightly and then rotated 90 degrees. The stylet is again removed, and the hub is again observed for spinal fluid. If no spinal fluid appears, the needle should be removed and the midline re-identified before attempting to repeat the previous technique. After spinal fluid is observed, the needle is fixed in position by the operator placing his or her hand against the patient's back. A drug suitable for subarachnoid administration is chosen, and the addition of glucose to make a hyperbaric solution and/or vasoconstrictors such as epinephrine or phenylephrine to prolong the duration of spinal block is considered. The solution is slowly injected, with the injection immediately being discontinued if the patient reports any pain. The needle is then removed.

Because of the potential for hematogenous spread via Batson's plexus, local infection and sepsis represent absolute contraindications to the paramedian approach to the subarachnoid space. In contradistinction to the caudal approach to the epidural space, anticoagulation or coagulopathy represent absolute contraindications to lumbar subarachnoid nerve block owing to the risk of epidural and subarachnoid hematoma.

Hypotension is a common side effect of lumbar subarachnoid nerve block and is the result of the profound sympathetic blockade attendant with this procedure. Prophylactic intramuscular or intravenous administration of vasopressors and fluid loading may help avoid this potentially serious side effect of lumbar subarachnoid nerve block. If it is ascertained that a patient would not tolerate hypotension because of other serious systemic disease, more peripheral regional anesthetic techniques such as lumbar plexus block may be preferable to lumbar subarachnoid nerve block.

It is also possible to inadvertently place a needle or catheter intended for the subarachnoid space into the subdural space. If subdural placement is unrecognized, the resulting block will be spotty. This problem can be avoided if the operator advances the needle slightly after perceiving the pop of the needle as it pierces the dura.

Neurologic complications after lumbar subarachnoid nerve block are uncommon if proper technique is used. Direct trauma to the spinal cord and/or nerve roots is usually accompanied by pain. If significant pain occurs during placement of the spinal needle or catheter or during injection, the physician should immediately stop and ascertain the cause of the pain to avoid the possibility of additional neural trauma. Delayed neurologic complications due to chemical irritation of the coverings of the spinal cord, nerves, and the spinal cord have been reported. Most severe complications have been attributed to contaminants to the local anesthetic, although the addition of steroids and vasopressors and the use of concentrated hyperbaric solutions have also been implicated.

Although uncommon, infection in the subarachnoid space remains an ever-present possibility, especially in the immunocompromised AIDS or cancer patient. If epidural abscess occurs, emergent surgical drainage to avoid spinal cord compression and irreversible neurologic deficit is usually required. Meningitis occurring after lumbar subarachnoid nerve block may require subarachnoid administration of antibiotics. Early detection and treatment of infection are crucial to avoid potentially life-threatening sequelae.

SUGGESTED READING

Waldman SD: Lumbar subarachnoid block: Paramedian approach. In: Atlas of Interventional Pain Management, ed 2. Philadelphia, Saunders, 2004.

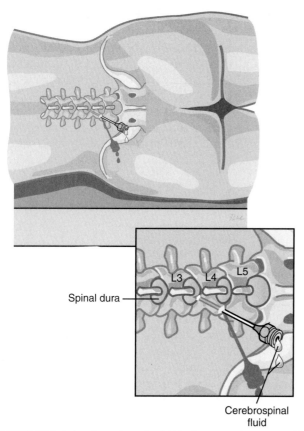

FIGURE 296–1 Lumbar subarachnoid block: paramedian approach. (From Waldman SD: Atlas of Interventional Pain Management, ed 2. Philadelphia, Saunders, 2004, p 371.)

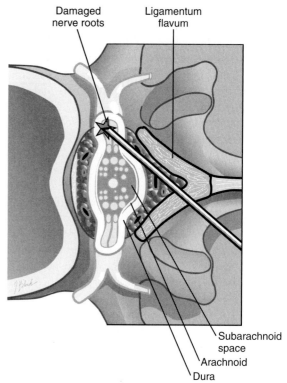

FIGURE 296–2 Needle position for the paramedian lumbar subarachnoid block. (From Waldman SD: Atlas of Interventional Pain Management, ed 2. Philadelphia, Saunders, 2004, p 372.)

CHAPTER 297

Caudal Epidural Nerve Block

The triangular sacrum consists of the five fused sacral vertebrae, which are dorsally convex. The sacrum inserts in a wedgelike manner between the two iliac bones, articulating superiorly with the fifth lumbar vertebra and caudad with the coccyx. On the anterior concave surface, there are four pairs of unsealed anterior sacral foramina that allow passage of the anterior rami of the upper four sacral nerves. The posterior sacral foramina are smaller than their anterior counterparts. Leakage of drugs injected into the sacral canal is effectively prevented by the sacrospinal and multifidus muscles. The vestigial remnants of the inferior articular processes project downward on each side of the sacral hiatus. These bony projections are called the sacral cornua and represent important clinical landmarks when performing caudal epidural nerve block.

Although there are gender- and race-determined differences in the shape of the sacrum, they are of little importance relative to the ultimate ability to successfully perform caudal epidural nerve block on a given patient. The triangular coccyx is made up of three to five rudimental vertebrae. Its superior surface articulates with the inferior articular surface of the sacrum. The tip of the coccyx is an important clinical landmark when performing caudal epidural nerve block.

The sacral hiatus is formed by the incomplete midline fusion of the posterior elements of the lower portion of the S4 and the entire S5 vertebrae. This U-shaped space is covered posteriorly by the sacrococcygeal ligament, which is also an important clinical landmark when performing caudal epidural nerve block. Penetration of the sacrococcygeal ligament provides direct access to the epidural space of the sacral canal.

A continuation of the lumbar spinal canal, the sacral canal continues inferiorly to terminate at the sacral hiatus. The volume of the sacral canal with all of its contents removed averages approximately 34 mL in dried bone specimens. It should be emphasized that much smaller volumes of local anesthetic (i.e., 5 to 10 mL) are used in day-to-day pain management practice. The use of large volumes of local anesthetic, especially in the area of pain management, will result in an unacceptable level of local anesthetic–induced side effects, such as incontinence and urinary retention, and should be avoided.

The sacral canal contains the inferior termination of the dural sac, which ends between S1 and S3 (Fig. 297-1). The five sacral nerve roots and the coccygeal nerve all traverse the canal, as does the terminal filament of the spinal cord, the filum terminale. The anterior and posterior rami of the S1-4 nerve roots exit from their respective anterior and posterior sacral foramina. The S5 roots and coccygeal nerves leave the sacral canal via the sacral hiatus. These nerves provide sensory and motor innervation to their respective dermatomes and myotomes. They also provide partial innervation to several pelvic organs, including the uterus, fallopian tubes, bladder, and prostate.

The sacral canal also contains the epidural venous plexus, which generally ends at S4 but may continue inferiorly. Most of these vessels are concentrated in the anterior portion of the canal. Both the dural sac and epidural vessels are susceptible to trauma by advancing needles or catheters cephalad into the sacral canal. The remainder of the sacral canal is filled with fat, which is subject to an age-related increase in its density. Some investigators believe this change is responsible for the increased incidence of "spotty" caudal epidural nerve blocks in adults.

Caudal epidural nerve block can be performed in either the prone or lateral position. To perform caudal epidural nerve block in the prone position, the patient is placed in the prone position. The patient's head is placed on a pillow and turned away from the pain management physician. The legs and heels are abducted to prevent tightening of the gluteal muscles, which can make identification of the sacral hiatus more difficult.

Preparation of a wide area of skin with antiseptic solution is then carried out so that all of the landmarks can be palpated aseptically. A fenestrated sterile drape is placed to avoid contamination of the palpating finger.

The middle finger of the nondominant hand is placed over the sterile drape into the natal cleft with the fingertip at the tip of the coccyx. This maneuver allows easy confirmation of the sacral midline and is especially important when using the lateral position.

After careful identification of the midline, the area under the proximal interphalangeal joint is located. The middle finger is then moved cephalad to the area that was previously located under the proximal interphalangeal joint. This spot is palpated using a lateral rocking motion to identify the sacral cornua. The sacral hiatus will be found at this level if the pain management physician's glove size is 7½ or 8. If the pain management physician's glove size is smaller, the location of the sacral hiatus will be just superior to the area located below the operator's proximal interphalangeal joint when the fingertip is at the tip of the coccyx. If the pain management physician's glove size is larger, the location of the sacral hiatus will be just inferior to the area located below the proximal interphalangeal joint when the fingertip is at the tip of the coccyx.

Although there is normally significant anatomic variation of the sacrum and sacral hiatus, the spatial relationship between the tip of the coccyx and the location of the sacral hiatus remains amazingly constant.

After locating the sacral hiatus, a 25-gauge, 1½-inch needle is inserted through the anesthetized area at a 45-degree angle into the sacrococcygeal ligament (Fig. 297-2). A 25-gauge, ⅝-inch needle is indicated for pediatric applications. The use of longer needles will increase the incidence of complications, including intravascular injection and inadvertent dural puncture, yet add nothing to the overall success of this technique.

As the sacrococcygeal ligament is penetrated, a "pop" will be felt. If contact with the interior bony wall of the sacral canal occurs, the needle should be withdrawn slightly. This will disengage the needle tip from the periosteum. The needle is then advanced approximately 0.5 cm into the canal. This is to ensure that the entire needle bevel is beyond the sacrococcygeal ligament to avoid injection into the ligament.

An air acceptance test is performed by the injection of 1 mL of air through the needle. There should be no bulging or crepitus of the tissues overlying the sacrum. The force required for injection should not exceed that necessary to overcome the resistance of the needle. If there is initial resistance to injection, the needle should be rotated 180 degrees in case the needle is correctly placed in the canal but the needle bevel is occluded by the internal wall of the sacral canal. Any significant pain or sudden increases in resistance during injection suggest incorrect needle placement, and the pain management physician should stop injecting immediately and reassess the position of the needle.

When the needle is satisfactorily positioned, a syringe containing 5 to 10 mL of 1.0% preservative-free lidocaine is attached to the needle. A larger volume of local anesthetic, on the order of 20 to 30 mL, is used if surgical anesthesia is required. When treating pain believed to be secondary to an inflammatory process, a total of 80 mg of depot steroid is added to the local anesthetic with the first block and 40 mg of depot steroid is added with subsequent blocks.

Gentle aspiration is carried out to identify cerebrospinal fluid or blood. Although rare, inadvertent dural puncture can occur, and careful observation for spinal fluid must be carried out. Aspiration of blood occurs more commonly. This can be due either to damage to veins during insertion of the needle into the caudal canal or, less commonly, to intravenous placement of the needle. Should the aspiration test be positive for either spinal fluid or blood, the needle is repositioned and the aspiration test repeated. If the test is negative, subsequent injections of 0.5-mL increments of local anesthetic are undertaken. Careful observation for signs of local anesthetic toxicity or subarachnoid spread of local anesthetic during the injection and after the procedure is indicated. Clinical experience has led to the use of smaller volumes of local anesthetic without sacrificing the clinical efficacy of caudal steroid epidural blocks. The use of smaller volumes of local anesthetic has markedly decreased the number of local anesthetic-related side effects.

Daily caudal epidural nerve blocks with local anesthetic and/or steroid may be required to treat the previously mentioned acute painful conditions. Chronic conditions such as lumbar radiculopathy and diabetic polyneuropathy are treated on an every-other-day to once-a-week basis or as the clinical situation dictates. Our extensive clinical experience with caudal steroid epidural blocks suggests that using this technique on an every-other-day basis improves the outcome compared with once-a-week nerve blocks and should be considered when treating radiculopathy and other conditions amenable to treatment with caudal steroid epidural nerve blocks.

If selective neurolytic block of an individual sacral nerve is desired, incremental 0.1-mL injections of 6.5% phenol in glycerin or alcohol to a total volume of 1 mL may be used after first confirming the level of pain relief and potential side effects with local anesthetic blocks. If the caudal epidural route is chosen for administration of opioids, 4 to 5 mg of morphine sulfate formulated for epidural use is a reasonable initial dose. More lipid-soluble opioids such as fentanyl must be delivered by continuous infusion via a caudal catheter.

It is possible to insert the needle incorrectly when performing caudal epidural nerve block. The needle may be placed outside the sacral canal, resulting in the injection of air and/or drugs into the subcutaneous tissues. Palpation of crepitus and bulging of tissues overlying the sacrum during injection indicate this needle malposition. An increased resistance to injection accompanied by pain is also noted. A second possible needle misplacement is when the needle tip is placed into the periosteum of the sacral canal. This needle misplacement is suggested by considerable pain on injection, a very high resistance to injection, and the inability to inject more than a few milliliters of drug. A third possibility of needle malposition is partial placement of the needle bevel in the sacrococcygeal ligament. Again, there is significant resistance to injection, as well as significant pain as the drugs are injected into the ligament. A fourth possible needle malposition is to force the point of the needle into the marrow cavity of the sacral vertebra, resulting in very high blood levels of local anesthetic. This needle malposition is detected by the initial easy acceptance of a few milliliters of local anesthetic, followed by a rapid increase in resistance to injection as the noncompliant bony cavity fills with local anesthetic. Significant local anesthetic toxicity can occur as a result of this complication. The fifth and most serious needle malposition occurs when the needle is inserted through the sacrum or lateral to the coccyx into the pelvic cavity beyond. This can result in the needle entering both the rectum and birth canal, resulting in contamination of the needle. The repositioning of the contaminated needle into the sacral canal will carry with it the danger of infection.

The caudal epidural space is highly vascular; therefore, the possibility of intravascular uptake of local anesthetic is significant with this technique. Careful aspiration and incremental dosing of local anesthetic is important to allow early detection of local anesthetic toxicity. Careful observation of the patient during and after the procedure is mandatory. Use of smaller volumes of local anesthetic (i.e., the 5 to 10 mL recommended for therapeutic blocks) will help avoid this complication, as will the use of shorter, smaller-gauge needles. The incidence of significant neurologic deficit secondary to epidural hematoma after caudal block is exceedingly rare.

Neurologic complications after caudal nerve block are rare. Usually these complications are associated with a preexisting neurologic lesion or with surgical or obstetric trauma rather than from the caudal block itself. The application of local anesthetic and opioids to the sacral nerve roots results in an increased incidence of urinary retention. This side effect occurs more commonly in elderly males and multiparous females and after inguinal and perineal surgery. Again, the use of smaller doses of local anesthetic will help avoid these bothersome complications without affecting the efficacy of caudal steroid epidural nerve blocks when treating painful conditions.

Although uncommon, infection remains an ever-present possibility, especially in the immunocompromised AIDS or cancer patient. Early detection of infection is crucial to avoid potentially life-threatening sequelae.

SUGGESTED READING

Waldman SD: Caudal epidural nerve block. In: Atlas of Interventional Pain Management, ed 2. Philadelphia, Saunders, 2004.

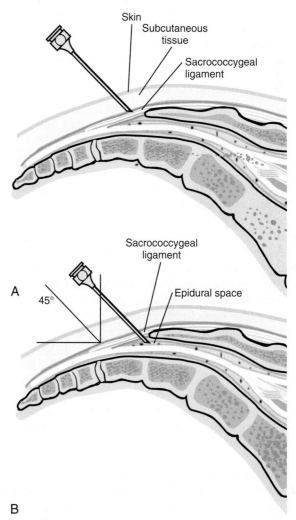

FIGURE 297–2 Caudal epidural nerve block. (From Waldman SD: Atlas of Interventional Pain Management, ed 2. Philadelphia, Saunders, 2004, p 388.)

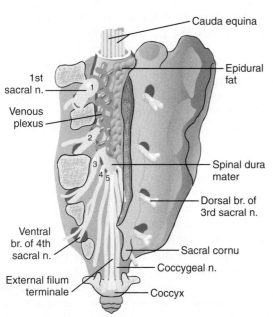

FIGURE 297–1 The sacral canal. (From Waldman SD: Atlas of Interventional Pain Management, ed 2. Philadelphia, Saunders, 2004, p 382.)

CHAPTER 298

Lysis of Epidural Adhesions: Racz Technique

Lysis of epidural adhesions has been used to treat a variety of painful conditions. It is postulated that the common denominator in each of these pain syndromes is the compromise of spinal nerve roots as they traverse and exit the epidural space by adhesions and scarring. It is thought that these adhesions and scar tissue not only restrict the free movement of the nerve roots as they emerge from the spinal cord and travel through the intervertebral foramina but also result in dysfunction of epidural venous blood and lymph flow. This dysfunction results in additional nerve root edema, which further compromises the affected nerves. Inflammation may also play a part in the genesis of pain as these nerves are repeatedly traumatized each time the nerve is stretched against the adhesions and scar tissue.

Diagnostic categories thought to be amenable to treatment with lysis of epidural adhesions using the Racz technique include failed back surgery with associated perineural fibrosis, herniated disc, traumatic and nontraumatic vertebral body compression fracture, metastatic carcinoma to the spine and epidural space, multilevel degenerative arthritis, facet joint pain, epidural scarring following infection, and other pain syndromes of the spine that have their basis in epidural scarring that have failed to respond to more conservative treatments.

To perform lysis of epidural adhesions using the Racz technique, intravenous access is obtained for administration of intravenous sedation during the injection of solutions via the catheter. Sedation during injection may be necessary because of pain produced by the distraction of the nerve roots as the solution lyses the perineural adhesions. After venous access is obtained, the patient is placed in the prone position with legs moderately abducted and heels inverted to relax the gluteus medius muscles and facilitate identification of the sacral hiatus.

Preparation of a wide area of skin with antiseptic solution is then carried out so that all the landmarks can be palpated aseptically. A fenestrated sterile drape is placed to avoid contamination of the palpating finger. The middle finger of the nondominant hand is placed over the sterile drape into the natal cleft with the fingertip at the tip of the coccyx. This maneuver allows easy confirmation of the sacral midline and is especially important when using the lateral position.

After careful identification of the midline, the area under the proximal interphalangeal joint is located. The middle finger is then moved cephalad to the area that was previously located under the proximal interphalangeal joint. This spot is palpated using a lateral rocking motion to identify the sacral cornua. The sacral hiatus is found at this level if the pain management physician's glove size is 7½ or 8. If the pain management physician's glove size is smaller, the location of the sacral hiatus will be just superior to the area located below the operator's proximal interphalangeal joint when the fingertip is at the tip of the coccyx. If the pain management physician's glove size is larger, the location of the sacral hiatus will be just inferior to the area located below the proximal interphalangeal joint when the fingertip is at the tip of the coccyx. Although there is normally significant anatomic variation of the sacrum and sacral hiatus, the spatial relationship between the tip of the coccyx and the location of the sacral hiatus remains amazingly constant.

After locating the sacral hiatus, a point 1 inch lateral and ½ inch below the sacral hiatus is identified, and the skin and subcutaneous tissues down to the sacrococcygeal ligament are infiltrated with local anesthetic. This lateral needle placement facilitates direction of the catheter toward the affected nerve roots. A 16-gauge, 3½-inch styletted needle suitable for catheter placement is inserted through the anesthetized area at a 45-degree angle toward the sacral hiatus. As the sacrococcygeal ligament is penetrated, a "pop" will be felt. If contact with the interior bony wall of the sacral canal occurs, the needle should be withdrawn slightly. This will disengage the needle tip from the periosteum. The needle is then advanced to approximately the level of the S2 foramen (Fig. 298-1).

An air acceptance test is performed by the injection of 1 mL of air through the needle. There should be no bulging or crepitus of the tissues overlying the sacrum. The force required for injection should not exceed that necessary to overcome the resistance of the needle. If there is initial resistance to injection, the needle should be rotated slightly in case the needle is correctly placed in the canal but the needle bevel is occluded by the internal wall of the sacral canal. Any significant pain or sudden increase in resistance during injection suggests incorrect needle placement, and the pain management physician should stop injecting immediately and reassess the position of the needle. Needle position should be confirmed by fluoroscopy on both anteroposterior and lateral views.

After negative aspiration for blood and cerebrospinal fluid (CSF), 10 mL of a water-soluble contrast medium such as iohexol or metrizamide is slowly injected under fluoroscopy. The pain specialist should check closely for any evidence of contrast medium in the epidural venous plexus, which would suggest intravenous placement of the needle, or subdural or subarachnoid placement, which appears as a more concentrated centrally located density. As the epidural space fills with contrast material, a Christmas tree shape will appear as the contrast medium surrounds the perineural structures. Defects in this classic Christmas tree appearance are indicative of epidural perineural adhesions.

After confirming proper needle placement and ensuring that no blood or CSF can be aspirated from the needle, 12 to 14 mL of 0.25% preservative-free bupivacaine and 40 mg of triamcinolone acetate are slowly injected through the epidural needle while observing the fluoroscope screen. The local anesthetic will force the contrast medium around the adhesions, further identifying affected nerve roots.

After the area of adhesions is identified on epiduralgram, the bevel of the epidural needle is turned toward the ventrolateral aspect of the caudal canal of the affected side. This facilitates passage of the catheter toward the affected nerves and decreases the chance of catheter breakage or shearing (Fig. 298-2). The use of a wire spiral catheter such as the Racz Tun-L-Kath epidural catheter will further decrease the incidence of this complication.

The catheter is then passed through the needle into the area of adhesions. Multiple attempts may be required to obtain placement of the catheter into the adhesions. The Racz needle allows for the catheter to be withdrawn and repositioned and is preferred over the standard Crawford epidural needle.

After the catheter is placed within the area of adhesions, the catheter is aspirated for blood or CSF. If the aspiration test is negative, an additional 7 to 10 mL of contrast medium is slowly injected through the catheter. This additional contrast medium should be seen spreading into the area of the adhesion. If the contrast material is observed to flow in satisfactory position, an additional 10 mL of 0.25% bupivacaine and 40 mg of triamcinolone are injected through the catheter to further lyse the remaining adhesions. Some investigators also recommend the addition of hyaluronidase to facilitate the spread of solutions injected. Approximately 3% of the population may experience some degree of allergic reaction to this drug, and this fact may limit its use.

Thirty minutes after the second injection of bupivacaine, after negative aspiration, 10 mL of 10% saline is injected in small increments over 20 to 30 minutes. The hyperosmolar properties of the hypertonic saline further shrink the nerve root and help treat the perineural edema caused by the venous obstruction secondary to the adhesions. The injection of 10% saline into the epidural space is quite painful, and intravenous sedation may be required if the saline spreads beyond the area previously anesthetized by the 0.25% bupivacaine. This pain is transient in nature and is generally gone within 10 minutes. After the final injection of 10% saline, the catheter is carefully secured and a sterile dressing is placed. Intravenous cephalosporin antibiotics are recommended by Dr. Racz to prevent bacterial colonization of the catheter while it is in place.

This injection procedure of bupivacaine followed by 10% saline is repeated for 3 days. Epiduralgrams are repeated only if there is a question of catheter migration, as the contrast medium can be irritating to the nerve roots and is quite expensive. The catheter is removed after the last injection. The patient is instructed to keep the area clean and dry and to call at the first sign of elevated temperature or infection.

Complications directly related to epidural lysis of adhesions are generally self-limited, although occasionally, even in the best of hands, severe complications can occur. Self-limited complications include pain at the injection site, transient back pain, ecchymosis and hematoma formation over the sacral hiatus, and unintended subdural or subarachnoid injection of local anesthetic. Severe complications of epidural lysis of adhesions include unintended subdural or subarachnoid injection of hypertonic saline, persistent sensory deficit in the lumbar and sacral dermatomes, paraparesis or paraplegia, persistent bowel and/or bladder dysfunction, sexual dysfunction, and infection. Although uncommon, unrecognized infection in the epidural space can result in paraplegia and death. Clinically, the signs and symptoms of epidural abscess present as a high fever, spine pain, and progressive neurologic deficit. If epidural abscess is suspected, blood and urine cultures should be taken, antibiotics started, and emergent magnetic resonance imaging of the spine obtained to allow identification and drainage of any abscess formation prior to irreversible neurologic deficit.

SUGGESTED READING

Waldman SD: Lysis of epidural adhesions: Racz technique. In: Atlas of Interventional Pain Management, ed 2. Philadelphia, Saunders, 2004.

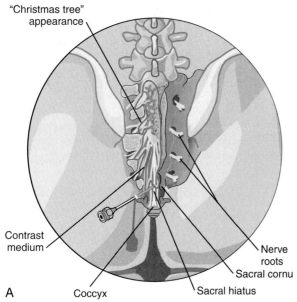

FIGURE 298–1 "Christmas tree" appearance of the contrast spread. (From Waldman SD: Atlas of Interventional Pain Management, ed 2. Philadelphia, Saunders, 2004, p 402.)

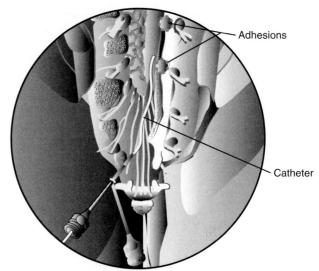

FIGURE 298–2 Lysis of epidural adhesions. (From Waldman SD: Atlas of Interventional Pain Management, ed 2. Philadelphia, Saunders, 2004, p 403.)

CHAPTER 299

Sacral Nerve Block

The convex dorsal surface of the sacrum has an irregular surface secondary to the fusing of the elements of the sacral vertebrae. Dorsally, there is a midline crest called the median sacral crest. Eight posterior sacral foramina allow the passage of four pairs of the primary posterior divisions of the sacral nerve roots. The posterior sacral foramina are smaller than their anterior counterparts. Leakage of drugs injected onto the sacral nerves through the posterior neural foramina is effectively prevented by the sacrospinal and multifidus muscles. The fifth sacral nerves exit the sacral canal via the sacral hiatus. The sacral nerves provide sensory innervation to the anorectal region and motor innervation to the external anal sphincter and levator ani muscles. The second through fourth sacral nerves provide the majority of visceral innervation to the bladder and urethra as well as the external genitalia.

Sacral nerve block via the transsacral approach is carried out in either the prone or the lateral position. Each position has its own advantages and disadvantages. The prone position is easier for the pain management

physician, but its use may be limited because of the patient's inability to rest comfortably on his or her abdomen or because of the presence of ostomy appliances such as colostomy and ileostomy bags. Furthermore, easy access to the airway is limited should problems occur while the patient is prone. The lateral position allows better access to the airway but is technically a more demanding approach. As with the caudal block, identification of the sacral hiatus is crucial to successfully perform sacral nerve block.

Before the procedure is begun, 18 mL of 1.0% preservative-free lidocaine is drawn into a sterile 20-mL syringe. When treating pain believed to be secondary to an inflammatory process, a total of 80 mg of depot steroid is added to the local anesthetic with the first block, and 40 mg of depot steroid is added with subsequent blocks.

The patient is placed in the prone position. Preparation of a wide area of skin with antiseptic solution is then carried out so that all of the landmarks can be palpated aseptically. A fenestrated sterile drape is placed to avoid contamination of the palpating finger. The middle finger of the non-dominant hand is placed over the sterile drape into the natal cleft with the fingertip at the tip of the coccyx. This maneuver allows easy confirmation of the sacral midline and is especially important when using the lateral position.

After careful identification of the midline, the area under the proximal interphalangeal joint is located. The middle finger is then moved cephalad to the area that was previously located under the proximal interphalangeal joint. This spot is palpated using a lateral rocking motion to identify the sacral cornua. The sacral hiatus will be found at this level if the pain management physician's glove size is 7½ or 8. If the pain management physician's glove size is smaller, the location of the sacral hiatus will be just superior to the area located below the operator's proximal interphalangeal joint when the fingertip is at the tip of the coccyx. If the pain management physician's glove size is larger, the location of the sacral hiatus will be just inferior to the area located below the proximal interphalangeal joint when the fingertip is at the tip of the coccyx.

Although there is normally significant anatomic variation of the sacrum and sacral hiatus, the spatial relationship between the tip of the coccyx and the location of the sacral hiatus remains amazingly constant.

The S5 sacral nerves can be blocked as they exit the sacral foramen. The sacral cornu are identified, and at a point just medial to their inferior border, a 25-gauge, 1½-inch needle is advanced just deep to the cornu and 2 to 3 mL of solution is injected (Fig. 299-1).

To block the S4 sacral nerves, after locating the sacral hiatus, a point ½ inch superior and ½ inch lateral to the sacral cornu is identified. A 25-gauge, 1½-inch needle is inserted at this point and is advanced slowly perpendicular to the skin into the S4 posterior foramen. If bony contact is made, the needle is withdrawn into the subcutaneous tissues and readvanced in a slightly more superior and lateral trajectory. This maneuver is repeated until the needle is walked off the posterior sacrum into the S4 foramen. The needle is advanced ½ inch into the foramen (see Fig. 299-1). A paresthesia may be elicited, and the patient should be warned of such. Careful aspiration for blood and cerebrospinal fluid is carried out. If the aspiration test is negative, 2 to 3 mL of the solution is injected.

The S3 foramen is then identified approximately ½ inch superior and ½ inch lateral to the S4 foramen. Again, the needle is placed and the injection carried out as with the technique described for S4 nerve block. This maneuver is repeated for the S2 nerve, the foramen of which is ½ inch superior and ½ inch lateral to the S3 foramen. The maneuver is again repeated in an analogous manner for the S1 nerve, the foramen of which is ½ inch superior and ½ inch lateral to the S2 foramen.

If selective neurolytic block of an individual sacral nerve is desired, incremental 0.1-mL injections of 6.5% phenol in glycerin or alcohol to a total volume of 1 mL may be used after first confirming the level of pain relief and potential side effects with local anesthetic blocks. Because of the potential for spread of drugs injected via the transsacral approach onto other sacral nerves, incremental dosing is crucial to avoid accidentally applying neurolytic solution to the wrong sacral nerve. Radiofrequency lesioning or cryoneurolysis can help avoid this problem.

Sacral nerve block is a simple and safe procedure so long as there is an understanding of the potential for spread of solutions injected onto nerves for which the drugs were not intended. This fact is especially important when using neurolytic solutions.

This anatomic region is highly vascular; therefore, the possibility of intravascular uptake of local anesthetic is significant with this technique when multiple sacral nerves are blocked. Careful aspiration and incremental dosing of local anesthetic is important to allow early detection of local anesthetic toxicity. Careful observation of the patient during and after the procedure is mandatory.

The epidural venous plexus generally ends at S4 but may descend the entire length of the canal in some patients. Needle trauma to this plexus may result in bleeding, thus causing postprocedural pain. Subperiosteal injection of drugs may also result in bleeding and is associated with significant pain both during and after injection. Both of these complications, as well as the incidence of ecchymosis at the injection site, can be reduced by the use of short, small-gauge needles. The incidence of significant neurologic deficit secondary to hematoma after sacral block is exceedingly rare.

Although uncommon, infection remains an ever-present possibility, especially in the immunocompromised AIDS or cancer patient. Early detection of infection is crucial to avoid potentially life-threatening sequelae.

The application of local anesthetic to the sacral nerve roots results in an increased incidence of urinary bladder dysfunction. This side effect of sacral nerve block is seen more commonly in elderly males and multiparous females and after inguinal and perineal surgery. Overflow incontinence or dribbling may occur in this patient population if they are unable to void or bladder catheterization is not used. It is advisable that all patients undergoing sacral nerve block void before discharge from the pain center.

SUGGESTED READING

Waldman SD: Sacral nerve block. In: Atlas of Interventional Pain Management, ed 2. Philadelphia, Saunders, 2004.

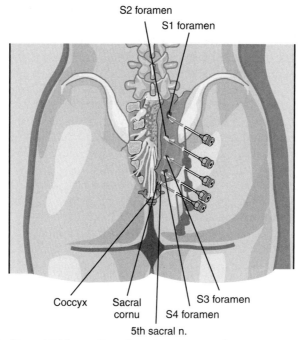

FIGURE 299–1 Sacral nerve block. (From Waldman SD: Atlas of Interventional Pain Management, ed 2. Philadelphia, Saunders, 2004, p 409.)

CHAPTER 300

Hypogastric Plexus Block

In the context of neural blockade, the hypogastric plexus can simply be thought of as a continuation of the lumbar sympathetic chain that can be blocked in a manner analogous to lumbar sympathetic nerve block. The preganglionic fibers of the hypogastric plexus find their origin primarily in the lower thoracic and upper lumbar region of the spinal cord. These preganglionic fibers interface with the lumbar sympathetic chain via the white communicantes. Postganglionic fibers exit the lumbar sympathetic chain and, together with fibers from the parasympathetic sacral ganglion, make up the superior hypogastric plexus. The superior hypogastric plexus lies in front of L4 as a coalescence of fibers. As these fibers descend, at a level of L5, they begin to divide into the hypogastric nerves following in close proximity the iliac vessels. As the hypogastric nerves continue their lateral and inferior course, they are accessible for neural blockade as they pass in front of the L5-S1 interspace. The hypogastric nerves pass downward from this point, following

the concave curve of the sacrum and passing on each side of the rectum to form the inferior hypogastric plexus. These nerves continue their downward course along each side of the bladder to provide innervation to the pelvic viscera and vasculature.

Single-Needle Blind Technique

The patient is placed in the prone position with a pillow placed under the lower abdomen to gently flex the lumbar spine and maximize the space between the transverse process of L5 and the sacral alae. The L4-5 interspace is located by identifying the iliac crests and finding the interspace at that level. The skin at this level is prepared with antiseptic solution. A point 6 cm from the midline at this level is identified, and the skin and subcutaneous tissues are anesthetized with 1.0% lidocaine. A 20-gauge, 13-cm needle is then inserted through the previously anesthetized area and directed approximately 30 degrees caudad and 30 degrees mesiad toward the anterolateral portion of the L5-S1 interspace. If the transverse process of L5 is encountered, the needle is withdrawn and redirected slightly more caudad. If the vertebral body of L5 is encountered, the needle is withdrawn and redirected slightly more lateral until, in a manner analogous to lumbar sympathetic block, the needle is "walked off" the anterolateral aspect of the vertebral body.

A 5-mL glass syringe filled with preservative-free saline is then attached to the needle. The needle is then slowly advanced into the prevertebral space while maintaining constant pressure on the plunger of the syringe in a manner analogous to the loss-of-resistance technique used for identification of the epidural space. A "pop" and loss of resistance will be felt as the needle pierces the anterior fascia of the psoas muscle and enters the prevertebral space (Fig. 300-1). After careful aspiration for blood, cerebrospinal fluid, and urine, 10 mL of 1.0% preservative-free lidocaine is slowly injected in incremental doses while observing the patient closely for signs of local anesthetic toxicity. If there is believed to be an inflammatory component to the pain, the local anesthetic is combined with 80 mg of methylprednisolone and is injected in incremental doses. Subsequent daily nerve blocks are carried out in a similar manner, substituting 40 mg of methylprednisolone for the initial 80-mg dose. The needle is then removed, and an ice pack is placed on the injection site to decrease postblock bleeding and pain.

Single-Needle Computed Tomography–Guided Technique

The patient is placed in the prone position on the computed tomography (CT) gantry with a pillow placed under the lower abdomen to gently flex the lumbar spine and maximize the space between the transverse process of L5 and the sacral alae. A CT scout film of the lumbar spine is taken, and the L4-5 interspace is identified. The skin overlying the L4-5 interspace is prepared with antiseptic solution, and sterile drapes are placed. At a point approximately 6 cm from midline, the skin and subcutaneous tissues are anesthetized with 1% lidocaine using a 25-gauge, 3.8-cm needle. A 20-gauge, 13-cm needle is then inserted through the previously anesthetized area and directed approximately 30 degrees caudad and 30 degrees mesiad toward the anterolateral portion of the L5-S1 interspace. If the transverse process of L5 is encountered, the needle is withdrawn and redirected slightly more caudad. If the vertebral body of L5 is encountered, the needle is withdrawn and redirected slightly more lateral and "walked off" the anterolateral aspect of the vertebral body in a manner analogous to lumbar sympathetic block. A 5-mL glass syringe filled with preservative-free saline

is then attached to the needle. The needle is then slowly advanced into the prevertebral space while maintaining constant pressure on the plunger of the syringe. A "pop" and loss of resistance will be felt as the needle pierces the anterior fascia of the psoas muscle. After careful aspiration, 2 to 3 mL of water-soluble contrast medium is injected through the needle and a CT scan is taken to confirm current retroperitoneal needle placement. Because of contralateral spread of the contrast medium in the prevertebral space, it is often unnecessary to place a second needle as is advocated by some pain specialists. A total volume of 10 mL of 1.0% preservative-free lidocaine is then injected in divided doses after careful aspiration for blood, cerebrospinal fluid, and urine. If adequate pain relief is obtained, incremental doses of absolute alcohol or 6.5% aqueous phenol may be injected in a similar manner after it is ascertained that the patient is experiencing no untoward bowel or bladder effects from blockade of the hypogastric plexus.

Two-Needle Blind Technique

The patient is placed in the prone position with a pillow placed under the lower abdomen to gently flex the lumbar spine and maximize the space between the transverse process of L5 and the sacral alae. The L4-5 interspace is located by identifying the iliac crests and finding the interspace at that level. The skin at this level is prepared with antiseptic solution. A point 6 cm from the midline at this level is identified, and the skin and subcutaneous tissues are anesthetized with 1.0% lidocaine. A 20-gauge, 13-cm needle is then inserted through the previously anesthetized area and directed approximately 30 degrees caudad and 30 degrees mesiad toward the anterolateral portion of the L5-S1 interspace. If the transverse process of L5 is encountered, the needle is withdrawn and redirected slightly more caudad. If the vertebral body of L5 is encountered, the needle is withdrawn and redirected slightly more lateral until, in a manner analogous to lumbar sympathetic block, the needle is walked off the anterolateral aspect of the vertebral body.

A 5-mL glass syringe filled with preservative-free saline is then attached to the needle. The needle is then slowly advanced into the prevertebral space while maintaining constant pressure on the plunger of the syringe in a manner analogous to the loss-of-resistance technique used for identification of the epidural space. A "pop" and loss of resistance will be felt as the needle pierces the anterior fascia of the psoas muscle and enters the prevertebral space. A contralateral needle is then inserted in a similar manner using the trajectory and depth of the first needle as a guide (Fig. 300-2). After careful aspiration for blood, cerebrospinal fluid, and urine, 5 mL of 1.0% preservative-free lidocaine is slowly injected in incremental doses while observing the patient closely for signs of local anesthetic toxicity. If there is believed to be an inflammatory component to the pain, the local anesthetic is combined with 80 mg of methylprednisolone and is injected in incremental doses. Subsequent daily nerve blocks are carried out in a similar manner, substituting 40 mg of methylprednisolone for the initial 80-mg dose. Each needle is then removed, and an ice pack is placed on the injection site to decrease postblock bleeding and pain.

Two-Needle Computed Tomography– Guided Technique

The patient is placed in the prone position on the CT gantry with a pillow placed under the lower abdomen to gently flex the lumbar spine and maximize the space between the transverse process of L5 and the sacral alae. A CT scout film of the lumbar spine is taken, and the L4-5 interspace is identified. The skin overlying the L4-5 interspace is prepared with antiseptic solution, and sterile drapes are placed. At a point approximately 6 cm from midline, the skin and subcutaneous tissues are anesthetized with 1% lidocaine using a 25-gauge, 3.8-cm needle. A 20-gauge, 13-cm needle is then inserted through the previously anesthetized area and directed approximately 30 degrees caudad and 30 degrees mesiad toward the anterolateral portion of the L5-S1 interspace. If the transverse process of L5 is encountered, the needle is withdrawn and redirected slightly more caudad. If the vertebral body of L5 is encountered, the needle is withdrawn and redirected slightly more lateral and walked off the anterolateral aspect of the vertebral body in a manner analogous to lumbar sympathetic block. A 5-mL glass syringe filled with preservative-free saline is then attached to the needle. The needle is then slowly advanced into the prevertebral space while maintaining constant pressure on the plunger of the syringe. A "pop" and loss of resistance will be felt as the needle pierces the anterior fascia of the psoas muscle. After careful aspiration, 2 to 3 mL of water-soluble contrast medium is injected through the needle and a CT scan is taken to confirm current retroperitoneal needle placement. If no contralateral spread of the

contrast medium in the prevertebral space is observed, a contralateral needle is inserted in a similar manner using the trajectory and depth of the first needle as a guide. A total volume of 5 mL of 1.0% preservative-free lidocaine is then injected in divided doses after careful aspiration for blood, cerebrospinal fluid, and urine. If adequate pain relief is obtained, incremental doses of absolute alcohol or 6.5% aqueous phenol may be injected in a similar manner after it is ascertained that the patient is experiencing no untoward bowel or bladder effects from blockade of the hypogastric plexus. Each needle is then removed, and an ice pack is placed on the injection site to decrease postblock bleeding and pain.

The proximity of the hypogastric nerves to the iliac vessels means that the potential for bleeding or inadvertent intravascular injection remains a distinct possibility. The relationship of the cauda equina and exiting nerve roots makes it imperative that this procedure be carried out only by those well versed in the regional anatomy and experienced in performing lumbar sympathetic nerve block. Given the proximity of the pelvic cavity, damage to the pelvic viscera including the ureters during hypogastric plexus block is a distinct possibility. The incidence of this complication will be decreased if care is taken to place the needle just beyond the anterolateral margin of the L5-S1 interspace. Needle placement too medial may result in epidural, subdural, or subarachnoid injections or trauma to the intervertebral disc, spinal cord, and exiting nerve roots. Although uncommon, infection remains an ever-present possibility, especially in the immunocompromised cancer patient. Early detection of infection, including discitis, is crucial to avoid potentially life-threatening sequelae.

SUGGESTED READINGS

Waldman SD: Hypogastric plexus block: Single-needle technique. In: Atlas of Interventional Pain Management, ed 2. Philadelphia, Saunders, 2004.

Waldman SD: Hypogastric plexus block: Classic two-needle technique. In: Atlas of Interventional Pain Management, ed 2. Philadelphia, Saunders, 2004.

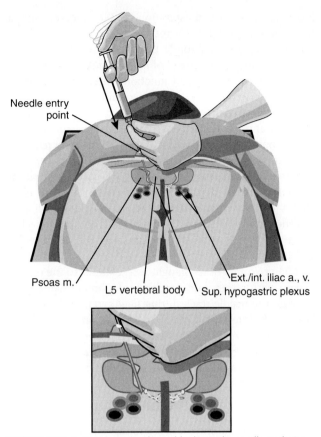

FIGURE 300–1 Hypogastric plexus block: single-needle technique. (From Waldman SD: Atlas of Interventional Pain Management, ed 2. Philadelphia, Saunders, 2004, p 413.)

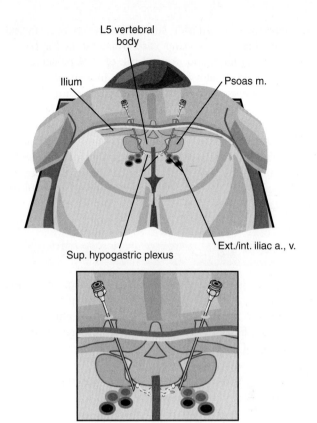

FIGURE 300–2 Hypogastric plexus block: classic two-needle technique. (From Waldman SD: Atlas of Interventional Pain Management, ed 2. Philadelphia, Saunders, 2004, p 417.)

Ganglion of Walther (Impar) Block

In the context of neural blockade, the ganglion of Walther can simply be thought of as the terminal coalescence of the sympathetic chain. The ganglion of Walther lies in front of the sacrococcygeal junction and is amenable to blockade at this level. The ganglion receives fibers from the lumbar and sacral portions of the sympathetic and parasympathetic nervous system and provides sympathetic innervation to portions of the pelvic viscera and genitalia.

Blind Technique

The patient is placed in the jackknife position to facilitate access to the inferior margin of the gluteal cleft.

The midline is identified, and the skin just below the tip of the coccyx that overlies the anococcygeal ligament is prepared with antiseptic solution. The skin and subcutaneous tissues at this point are anesthetized with 1.0% lidocaine. A 3½-inch spinal needle is then bent at a point 1 inch from its hub to a 30-degree angle to allow placement of the needle tip in proximity to the anterior aspect of the sacrococcygeal junction. The needle may be bent again at a point 2 inches from the hub to accommodate those patients with an exaggerated coccygeal curve to allow placement of the needle tip to rest against the sacrococcygeal junction.

The bent needle is then placed through the previously anesthetized area and is advanced until the needle tip impinges on the anterior surface of the sacrococcygeal junction (Fig. 301-1). After careful aspiration for blood, cerebrospinal fluid, and urine, 3 mL of 1.0% preservative-free lidocaine is slowly injected in incremental doses. If there is believed to be an inflammatory component to the pain, the local anesthetic is combined with 80 mg of methylprednisolone and is injected in incremental doses. Subsequent daily nerve blocks are carried out in a similar manner, substituting 40 mg of methylprednisolone for the initial 80-mg dose. The needle is then removed, and an ice pack is placed on the injection site to decrease postblock bleeding and pain.

Computed Tomography–Guided Technique

The patient is placed in the prone position on the computed tomography (CT) gantry with a pillow placed under the pelvis to facilitate access to the inferior gluteal cleft. A CT scout film is taken, and the sacrococcygeal junction and the tip of the coccyx are identified. The midline is also identified, and the skin just below the tip of the coccyx that overlies the anococcygeal ligament is prepared with antiseptic solution. The skin and subcutaneous tissues at this point are anesthetized with 1.0% lidocaine. A 3½-inch spinal needle is then bent at a point 1 inch from its hub to a 30-degree angle to allow placement of the needle tip in proximity to the anterior aspect of the sacrococcygeal junction. The needle may be bent again at a point 2 inches from the hub to accommodate patients with an exaggerated coccygeal curve to allow the needle tip to rest against the anterior sacrococcygeal junction.

The needle is then placed through the previously anesthetized area and is advanced until the needle tip impinges on the anterior surface of the sacrococcygeal junction. After careful aspiration for blood, cerebrospinal fluid, and urine, 2 to 3 mL of water-soluble contrast medium is injected through the needle and a CT scan is taken to confirm the spread of contrast medium just anterior to the sacrococcygeal junction. After correct needle placement is confirmed, a total volume of 3 mL of 1.0% preservative-free lidocaine is injected in divided doses after careful aspiration for blood, cerebrospinal fluid, and urine. If adequate pain relief is obtained, incremental doses of absolute alcohol or 6.5% aqueous phenol may be injected in a similar manner after it is ascertained that the patient is experiencing no untoward bowel or bladder effects from local anesthetic blockade of the ganglion of Walther. The needle is then removed, and an ice pack is placed on the injection site to decrease postblock bleeding and pain.

The proximity of the ganglion of Walther to the rectum makes perforation and tracking of contaminants back through the needle track during needle removal a distinct possibility. Infection and fistula formation, especially in those patients who are immunocompromised or have received radiation therapy to the perineum, can represent a devastating and potentially life-threatening complication to this block. The relationship of the cauda equina and exiting sacral nerve roots makes it imperative that this procedure be carried out only by those well versed in the regional anatomy and experienced in performing interventional pain management techniques.

SUGGESTED READING

Waldman SD: Ganglion of Walther (Impar) block. In: Atlas of Interventional Pain Management, ed 2. Philadelphia, Saunders, 2004.

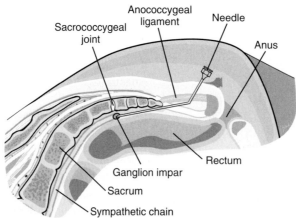

FIGURE 301–1 Ganglion of Walther (Impar) block. (From Waldman SD: Atlas of Interventional Pain Management, ed 2. Philadelphia, Saunders, 2004, p 421.)

Pudendal Nerve Block

The pudendal nerve is made up of fibers from the S2, S3, and S4 nerves. The nerve passes inferiorly between the piriformis and coccygeal muscles. Along with the pudendal vessels, the pudendal nerve leaves the pelvis via the greater sciatic foramen. It then passes around the medial portion of the ischial spine to reenter the pelvis through the lesser sciatic foramen. The pudendal nerve is amenable to blockade at this point via the transvaginal approach. The nerve then divides into three terminal branches: (1) the inferior rectal nerve, which provides innervation to the anal sphincter and perianal region; (2) the perineal nerve, which supplies the posterior two thirds of the scrotum or labia majora and muscles of the urogenital triangle; and (3) the dorsal nerve of the penis or clitoris, which supplies sensory innervation to the dorsum of the penis or clitoris.

The Transvaginal Approach

To perform pudendal nerve block using the transvaginal approach, the patient is placed in the lithotomy position. The index and middle fingers of the pain specialist's nondominant hand are inserted into the vagina to bracket the ischial spine. The needle guide is inserted between the fingers, and its tip is placed against the vaginal mucosa just in front of the ischial spine. A 20-gauge, 6-inch needle is then placed through the guide and is advanced through the sacrospinous ligament just beyond the ischial spine (Fig. 302-1). A loss of resistance will be felt as the needle passes beyond the ligament. After negative aspiration for blood, 10 mL of 1.0% preservative-free lidocaine is injected. An additional 3 to 4 mL of local anesthetic may be injected as the needle is withdrawn into the vagina to ensure blockade of the inferior rectal nerve.

The Transperineal Approach

The patient is placed in the lithotomy position. The ischial tuberosity is identified by palpation, and an area 1 inch lateral and 1 inch posterior to the tuberosity is then prepared with antiseptic solution. A skin wheal is raised at this point with local anesthetic. The index finger of the pain specialist's nondominant hand is inserted into the rectum to identify the ischial spine. A 6-inch needle is then placed through the previously anesthetized area and directed toward the ischial spine. The finger placed in the rectum will help guide the needle just beyond the ischial spine (Fig. 302-2). After careful aspiration for blood is negative, 10 mL of 1.0% lidocaine is injected. An additional 3 to 4 mL of local anesthetic may be injected as the needle is withdrawn to ensure blockade of the inferior rectal nerve.

The proximity of the pudendal nerve to the pudendal artery and vein makes the potential for intravascular injection a distinct possibility. Despite proximity to the rectum, infection with the transvaginal approach to pudendal nerve block does not appear to be a problem, although, theoretically, infection and fistula formation, especially in those patients who are immunocompromised or have received radiation therapy to the perineum, could represent a devastating and potentially life-threatening complication to this block.

SUGGESTED READINGS

Waldman SD: Pudendal nerve block: Transvaginal approach. In: Atlas of Interventional Pain Management, ed 2. Philadelphia, Saunders, 2004.

Waldman SD: Pudendal nerve block: Transperineal approach. In: Atlas of Interventional Pain Management, ed 2. Philadelphia, Saunders, 2004.

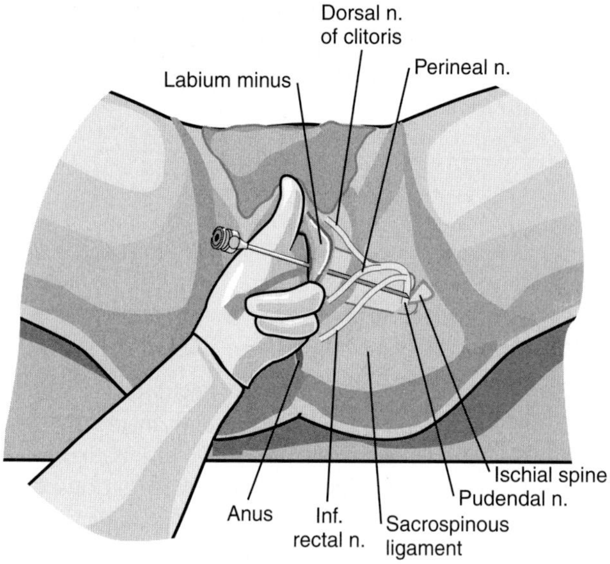

FIGURE 302–1 Pudendal nerve block: transvaginal approach. (From Waldman SD: Atlas of Interventional Pain Management, ed 2. Philadelphia, Saunders, 2004, p 425.)

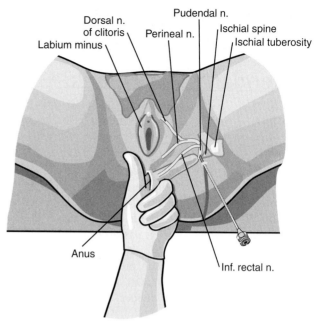

FIGURE 302–2 Pudendal nerve block: transperineal approach. (From Waldman SD: Atlas of Interventional Pain Management, ed 2. Philadelphia, Saunders, 2004, p 428.)

CHAPTER 303

Sacroiliac Joint Injection

The sacroiliac joint is formed by the articular surfaces of the sacrum and iliac bones. These articular surfaces have corresponding elevations and depressions, which give the joints their irregular appearance on radiographs. The strength of the sacroiliac joint comes primarily from the posterior and interosseous ligaments rather than the bony articulations. The sacroiliac joints bear the weight of the trunk and are thus subject to the development of strain and arthritis. As the joint ages, the intra-articular space narrows making intra-articular injection more challenging. The ligaments and the sacroiliac joint itself receive their innervation from L3 to S3 nerve roots, with L4 and L5 providing the greatest contribution to the innervation of the joint. This diverse innervation may help explain the ill-defined nature of sacroiliac pain. The sacroiliac joint has a very limited range of motion and that motion is induced by changes in the forces placed on the joint by shifts in posture and joint loading.

To perform injection of the sacroiliac joint, the patient is placed in the supine position and proper preparation with antiseptic solution of the skin overlying the affected sacroiliac joint space is carried out. A sterile syringe containing 4.0 mL of 0.25% preservative-free bupivacaine and 40 mg of methylprednisolone is attached to a 3½-inch, 25-gauge needle using strict aseptic technique. With strict aseptic technique, the posterior superior spine of the ilium is identified. At this point, the needle is then carefully advanced through the skin and subcutaneous tissues at a 45-degree angle toward the affected sacroiliac joint (Fig. 303-1). If bone is encountered, the needle is withdrawn into the subcutaneous tissues and redirected superiorly and slightly more lateral. After entering the joint space, the contents of the syringe are gently injected. There should be little resistance to injection. If resistance is encountered, the needle is probably in a ligament and should be advanced slightly into the joint space until the injection proceeds without significant resistance. The needle is then removed, and a sterile pressure dressing and ice pack are placed at the injection site.

The major complication of intra-articular injection of the sacroiliac is infection. This complication should be exceedingly rare if strict aseptic technique is adhered to. Approximately 25% of patients will complain of a transient increase in pain following intra-articular injection of the sacroiliac joint and should be warned of such. Care must be taken to avoid injection too laterally or the needle may traumatize the sciatic nerve.

SUGGESTED READING

Waldman SD: Sacroiliac joint block. In: Atlas of Interventional Pain Management, ed 2. Philadelphia, Saunders, 2004.

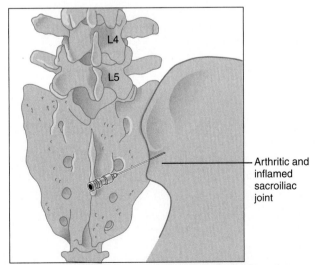

FIGURE 303–1 Sacroiliac joint block. (From Waldman SD: Atlas of Interventional Pain Management, ed 2. Philadelphia, Saunders, 2004, p 432.)

CHAPTER 304

Intra-articular Injection of the Hip Joint

The rounded head of the femur articulates with the cup-shaped acetabulum of the hip. The articular surface is covered with hyaline cartilage, which is susceptible to arthritis. The rim of the acetabulum is composed of a fibrocartilaginous layer called the acetabular labrum, which is susceptible to trauma should the femur be subluxed or dislocated. The joint is surrounded by a capsule that allows the wide range of motion of the hip joint. The joint capsule is lined with a synovial membrane that attaches to the articular cartilage. This membrane gives rise to synovial tendon sheaths and bursae that are subject to inflammation. The hip joint is innervated by the femoral, obturator, and sciatic nerves. The major ligaments of the hip joint include the iliofemoral, pubofemoral, ischiofemoral, and transverse acetabular, which provide strength to the hip joint. The muscles of the hip and their attaching tendons are susceptible to trauma and to wear and tear from overuse and misuse.

The goals of this injection technique are explained to the patient. The patient is placed in the supine position, and proper preparation with antiseptic solution of the skin overlying the hip, subacromial region, and joint space is carried out. A sterile syringe containing 4.0 mL of 0.25% preservative-free bupivacaine and 40 mg of methylprednisolone is attached to a 2-inch, 25-gauge needle using strict aseptic technique. With strict aseptic technique, the femoral artery is identified. At a point approximately 2 inches lateral to the femoral artery just below the inguinal ligament, the hip joint space is identified. The needle is then carefully advanced through the skin and subcutaneous tissues through the joint capsule into the joint (Fig. 304-1). If bone is encountered, the needle is withdrawn into the subcutaneous tissues and redirected superiorly and slightly more medial. After entering the joint space, the contents of the syringe are gently injected. There should be little resistance to injection. If resistance is encountered, the needle is probably in a ligament or tendon and should be advanced slightly into the joint space until the injection proceeds without significant resistance. The needle is then removed, and a sterile pressure dressing and ice pack are placed at the injection site.

The major complication of intra-articular injection of the hip is infection, which should be exceedingly rare if strict aseptic technique is adhered to. Approximately 25% of patients complain of a transient increase in pain following intra-articular injection of the hip joint; the patient should be warned of this.

SUGGESTED READING

Waldman SD: Intra-articular injection of the hip joint. In: Atlas of Pain Management Injection Techniques. Philadelphia, Saunders, 2007.

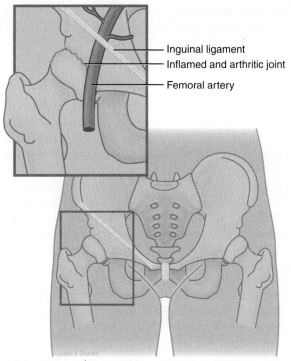

— Inguinal ligament
— Inflamed and arthritic joint
— Femoral artery

FIGURE 304–1 Intra-articular injection of the hip joint. (From Waldman SD: Atlas of Pain Management Injection Techniques. Philadelphia, Saunders, 2007, p 339.)

CHAPTER 305

Injection Technique for Ischial Bursitis

The ischial bursa is vulnerable to injury from both acute trauma and repeated microtrauma. Acute injuries frequently take the form of direct trauma to the bursa from direct falls onto the buttocks and from overuse, such as prolonged riding of horses or bicycles. Running on uneven or soft surfaces such as sand also may cause ischial bursitis. If the inflammation of the ischial bursa becomes chronic, calcification of the bursa may occur.

The patient suffering from ischial bursitis frequently complains of pain at the base of the buttock with resisted extension off the lower extremity. The pain is localized to the area over the ischial tuberosity with referred pain noted into the hamstring muscle, which also may develop coexistent tendinitis. Often, the patient is unable to sleep on the affected hip and may complain of a sharp "catching" sensation when extending and flexing the hip, especially on first awakening. Physical examination may

reveal point tenderness over the ischial tuberosity. Passive straight leg raising and active resisted extension of the affected lower extremity reproduces the pain. Sudden release of resistance during this maneuver markedly increases the pain.

Plain radiographs or magnetic resonance imaging of the hip may reveal calcification of the bursa and associated structures consistent with chronic inflammation. Magnetic resonance imaging is also indicated if disruption of the hamstring musculotendinous unit is suspected. The injection technique described here serves as both a diagnostic and therapeutic maneuver and also treats hamstring tendinitis.

The ischial bursa lies between the gluteus maximus muscle and the ischial tuberosity. The action of the gluteus maximus muscle includes the flexion of trunk on thigh when maintaining a sitting position while riding a horse. This action can irritate the ischial bursa, as can repeated pressure against the bursa that forces it against the ischial tuberosity. The hamstring muscles find a common origin at the ischial tuberosity and can be irritated from overuse or misuse. The action of the hamstrings includes flexion of the lower extremity at the knee. Running on soft or uneven surfaces can cause a tendinitis at the origin of the hamstring muscles.

The goals of this injection technique are explained to the patient. The patient is placed in the lateral position with the affected side up and the affected leg flexed at the knee. Proper preparation with antiseptic solution of the skin overlying the ischial tuberosity is then carried out. A syringe containing 4.0 mL of 0.25% preservative-free bupivacaine and 40 mg of methylprednisolone is attached to a 1½-inch, 25-gauge needle. The ischial tuberosity is then identified with a sterilely gloved finger. Prior to needle placement, the patient should be advised to say "There!" as soon as paresthesia is felt in the lower extremity, indicating that the needle has impinged on the sciatic nerve. Should paresthesia occur, the needle should be immediately withdrawn and repositioned more medially.

The needle is then carefully advanced at that point through the skin, subcutaneous tissues, muscle, and tendon until it impinges on the bone of the ischial tuberosity (Fig. 305-1). Care must be taken to keep the needle in the midline and not to advance it laterally or it could impinge on the sciatic nerve. After careful aspiration and if no paresthesia is present, the contents of the syringe are then gently injected into the bursa.

The proximity to the sciatic nerve makes it imperative that this procedure be carried out only by those well versed in the regional anatomy and experienced in performing injection techniques. Many patients also complain of a transient increase in pain following injection of the bursa and tendons mentioned. Although rare, infection after injection of the ischial bursa remains an ever-present possibility.

SUGGESTED READING

Waldman SD: Injection technique for ischial bursitis. In: Atlas of Pain Management Injection Techniques, ed. 2. Philadelphia, Saunders, 2007.

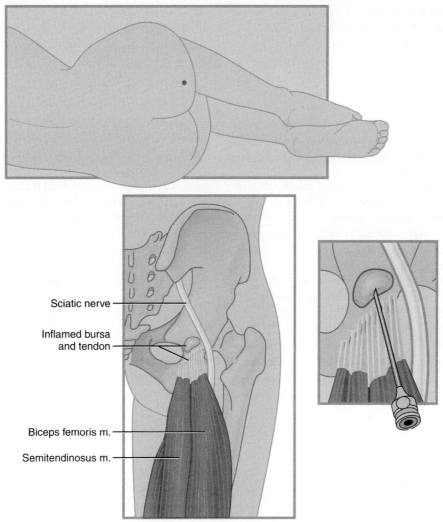

FIGURE 305–1 Injection technique for ischial bursitis pain. (From Waldman SD: Atlas of Pain Management Injection Techniques, ed. 2. Philadelphia, Saunders, 2007, p 347.)

CHAPTER 306

Injection Technique for Gluteal Bursitis

The gluteal bursae are vulnerable to injury from both acute trauma and repeated microtrauma. Acute injuries frequently take the form of direct trauma to the bursa from falls directly onto the buttocks or repeated intramuscular injections, as well as from overuse such as running for long distances, especially on soft or uneven surfaces.

If the inflammation of the gluteal bursae becomes chronic, calcification of the bursae may occur.

The patient who suffers from gluteal bursitis frequently complains of pain at the upper outer quadrant of the buttock and with resisted abduction and extension of the lower extremity. The pain is localized to the area over the upper outer quadrant of the buttock, with referred pain noted into the sciatic notch. Often, the patient is unable to sleep on the affected hip and may complain of a sharp "catching" sensation when extending and abducting the hip, especially on first awakening. Physical examination may reveal point tenderness in the upper outer quadrant of the buttocks. Passive flexion and adduction reproduces the pain, as does active resisted extension and abduction of the affected lower extremity. Sudden release of resistance during this maneuver markedly increases the pain.

Plain radiographs of the hip may reveal calcification of the bursa and associated structures consistent with chronic inflammation. Magnetic resonance imaging scan is indicated if occult mass or tumor of the hip is suspected. The injection technique described here serves as both a diagnostic and therapeutic maneuver.

There is significant intrapatient variability in the size, number, and location of the gluteal bursae. The gluteal bursae lie between the gluteal maximus, medius, and minimus muscles, as well as between these muscles and the underlying bone. The action of the gluteus maximus muscle includes the flexion of trunk on thigh when maintaining a sitting position while riding a horse. This action can irritate the gluteal bursae, as can repeated trauma from repetitive activity, including running.

To perform injection of the gluteal bursa, the patient is placed in the lateral position with the affected side up and the affected leg flexed at the knee. Proper preparation with antiseptic solution of the skin overlying the upper outer quadrant of the buttocks is then carried out. A syringe containing 4.0 mL of 0.25% preservative-free bupivacaine and 40 mg of methylprednisolone is attached to a 3½-inch, 25-gauge needle. The point of maximal tenderness within the upper outer quadrant of the buttocks is then identified with a sterile gloved finger. Prior to needle placement, the patient should be advised to say "There!" immediately if paresthesia into the lower extremity is felt, indicating that the needle has impinged on the sciatic nerve. Should paresthesia occur, the needle should be immediately withdrawn and repositioned more medially. The needle is then carefully advanced perpendicular to the skin at the previously identified point until it impinges on the wing of the ilium (Fig. 306-1). Care must be taken to keep the needle medial and not to advance it laterally or it could impinge on the sciatic nerve. After careful aspiration and if no paresthesia is present, the contents of the syringe are then gently injected into the bursa. There should be minimal resistance to injection.

The proximity to the sciatic nerve makes it imperative that this procedure be carried out only by those well versed in the regional anatomy and experienced in performing injection techniques. Many patients also complain of a transient increase in pain after injection of the bursae.

SUGGESTED READING

Waldman SD: Injection technique for gluteal bursitis. In: Atlas of Pain Management Injection Techniques. Philadelphia, Saunders, 2007.

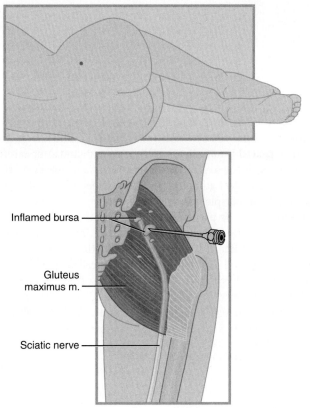

FIGURE 306–1 Injection technique for gluteal bursitis pain. (From Waldman SD: Atlas of Pain Management Injection Techniques. Philadelphia, Saunders, 2007, p 351.)

CHAPTER 307

Injection Technique for Psoas Bursitis

The psoas bursa is vulnerable to injury from both acute trauma and repeated microtrauma. Acute injuries frequently take the form of direct trauma to the bursa from seat belt injuries as well as from overuse injuries requiring repeated hip flexion, such as javelin throwing and ballet. If the inflammation of the psoas bursa becomes chronic, calcification of the bursa may occur.

The patient suffering from psoas bursitis will frequently complain of pain in the groin. The pain is localized to the area just below the crease of the groin anteriorly with referred pain noted into the hip joint. Often, the patient will be unable to sleep on the affected hip and may complain of a sharp "catching" sensation with range of motion of the hip.

Physical examination may reveal point tenderness in the upper thigh just below the crease of the groin. Passive flexion, adduction, and abduction, as well as active resisted flexion and adduction of the affected lower extremity, reproduce the pain. Sudden release of resistance during this maneuver will markedly increase the pain.

Plain radiographs of the hip may reveal calcification of the bursa and associated structures consistent with chronic inflammation. Magnetic resonance imaging is indicated if occult mass or tumor of the hip or groin is suspected. The injection technique described here will serve as both a diagnostic and therapeutic maneuver.

The psoas bursa lies between the psoas tendon and the anterior aspect of the femoral neck. The bursa lies deep to the femoral artery, vein, and nerve. The psoas muscle arises from the transverse processes, vertebral bodies, and intervertebral discs of the T12-L5 vertebrae and inserts into the lesser trochanter of the femur. The psoas muscle flexes the thigh on the trunk or, if the thigh is fixed, flexes the trunk on the thigh as when moving from a supine to sitting position. This action can irritate the psoas bursa as can repeated trauma from repetitive activity including running up stairs or overuse of exercise equipment for lower extremity strengthening. The psoas muscle is innervated by the lumbar plexus.

To perform injection of the psoas bursa, the patient is placed in the supine position, and the pulsation of the femoral artery at the midpoint of the inguinal ligament is identified. At a point 2½ inches down and 2½ inches lateral to these femoral arterial pulsations lies the entry point of the needle. This point should be at the medial edge of the sartorius muscle. Proper preparation with antiseptic solution of the skin overlying this point is then carried out. A syringe containing the 9.0 mL of 0.25% preservative-free bupivacaine and 40 mg of methylprednisolone is attached to a 3½-inch, 25-gauge needle.

Prior to needle placement, the patient should be advised to say "There!" immediately if he or she feels paresthesia into the lower extremity, indicating that the needle has impinged on the femoral nerve. Should paresthesia occur, the needle should be immediately withdrawn and repositioned more laterally. The needle is then carefully advanced through the previously identified point at a 45-degree angle medially and cephalad to allow the needle to safely pass beneath the femoral artery, vein, and nerve. The needle is advanced very slowly to avoid trauma to the femoral nerve until it hits the bone of the femoral neck (Fig. 307-1). The needle is then withdrawn back out of the periosteum and after careful aspiration for blood, and if no paresthesia is present, the contents of the syringe are gently injected into the bursa. There should be minimal resistance to injection.

The proximity to the femoral artery, vein, and nerve makes it imperative that this procedure be carried out only by those well versed in the regional anatomy and experienced in performing injection techniques to avoid trauma to these important structures. Many patients will also complain of a transient increase in pain after injection of the bursa. Although rare, infection following injection of the psoas bursa remains an ever-present possibility.

SUGGESTED READING

Waldman SD: Injection technique for psoas bursitis. In: Atlas of Pain Management Injection Techniques. Philadelphia, Saunders, 2007.

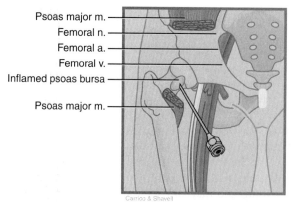

FIGURE 307–1 Injection technique for psoas bursitis pain. (From Waldman SD: Atlas of Pain Management Injection Techniques. Philadelphia, Saunders, 2007, p 357.)

Injection Technique for Iliopectineal Bursitis

The iliopectineal bursa is vulnerable to injury from both acute trauma and repeated microtrauma. Acute injuries frequently take the form of direct trauma to the bursa via hip injuries, as well as from overuse injuries. If the inflammation of the iliopectineal bursa becomes chronic, calcification of the bursa may occur.

The patient who suffers from iliopectineal bursitis frequently complains of pain in the anterior hip and groin. The pain is localized to the area just below the crease of the groin anteriorly, with referred pain noted into the hip joint and anterior pelvis. Often, the patient is unable to sleep on the affected hip and may complain of a sharp "catching" sensation with range of motion of the hip. Iliopectinate bursitis often coexists with arthritis of the hip joint.

Physical examination may reveal point tenderness in the upper thigh just below the crease of the groin. Passive flexion, adduction, and abduction, as well as active resisted flexion and adduction of the affected lower extremity, reproduce the pain. Sudden release of resistance during this maneuver markedly increases the pain.

Plain radiographs of the hip may reveal calcification of the bursa and associated structures consistent with chronic inflammation. Magnetic resonance imaging is indicated if occult mass or tumor of the hip or groin is suspected. The injection technique described here serves as both a diagnostic and therapeutic maneuver.

The iliopectineal bursa lies between the psoas and iliacus muscles and the iliopectineal eminence. The iliopectineal eminence is the point at which the ilium and the pubis bone merge. The psoas and iliacus muscles join at the lateral side of the psoas, and the combined fibers are referred to as the iliopsoas muscle. Like the psoas, the iliacus flexes the thigh on the trunk or, if the thigh is fixed, flexes the trunk on the thigh, as when moving from a supine to sitting position. This action can irritate the iliopectineal bursa, as can repeated trauma from repetitive activity including sit-ups or overuse of exercise equipment for lower extremity strengthening. The iliacus muscle is innervated by the femoral nerve.

To perform injection of the iliopectineal bursa, the patient is placed in the supine position, and the pulsation of the femoral artery at the midpoint of the inguinal ligament is identified. At a point 2½ inches down and 3½ inches lateral to these femoral arterial pulsations lies the entry point of the needle. This point should be at the lateral edge of the sartorius muscle. Proper preparation with antiseptic solution of the skin overlying this point is then carried out. A syringe containing 9.0 mL of 0.25% preservative-free bupivacaine and 40 mg of methylprednisolone is attached to a 3½-inch, 25-gauge needle.

Prior to needle placement, the patient should be advised to say "There!" as soon as paresthesia into the lower extremity is felt, indicating that the needle has impinged on the femoral nerve. Should paresthesia occur, the needle should be immediately withdrawn and repositioned more laterally. The needle is then carefully advanced through the previously identified point at a 45-degree angle cephalad to allow the needle to safely pass beneath the femoral artery, vein, and nerve. The needle is advanced very slowly to avoid trauma to the femoral nerve until it hits the bone at the point where the ilium and pubis bones merge (Fig. 308-1). The needle is then withdrawn back out of the periosteum and, after careful aspiration for blood and if no paresthesia is present, the contents of the syringe are then gently injected into the bursa. There should be minimal resistance to injection.

The proximity to the femoral artery, vein, and nerve makes it imperative that this procedure be carried out only by those well versed in the regional anatomy and experienced in performing injection techniques. Many patients also complain of a transient increase in pain after injection of the bursa.

SUGGESTED READING

Waldman SD: Iliopectineal bursitis. In: Atlas of Pain Management Injection Techniques, ed. 2. Philadelphia, Saunders, 2007.

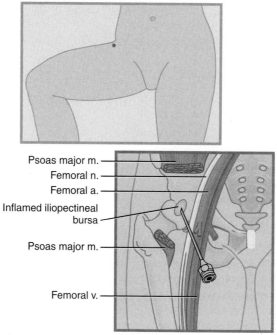

Psoas major m.
Femoral n.
Femoral a.
Inflamed iliopectineal bursa
Psoas major m.
Femoral v.

FIGURE 308–1 Injection technique for iliopectinate bursitis pain. (From Waldman SD: Atlas of Pain Management Injection Techniques, ed. 2. Philadelphia, Saunders, 2007, p 359.)

CHAPTER 309

Injection Technique for Trochanteric Bursitis

The trochanteric bursa is vulnerable to injury from both acute trauma and repeated microtrauma. Acute injuries frequently take the form of direct trauma to the bursa via falls directly onto the greater trochanter or previous hip surgery, as well as from overuse injuries, including running on soft or uneven surfaces. If the inflammation of the trochanteric bursa becomes chronic, calcification of the bursa may occur.

The patient who suffers from trochanteric bursitis frequently complains of pain in the lateral hip that can radiate down the leg, mimicking sciatica. The pain is localized to the area over the trochanter. Often, the patient is unable to sleep on the affected hip and may complain of a sharp "catching" sensation with range of motion of the hip, especially on first rising. The patient may note that walking upstairs is increasingly more difficult. Trochanteric bursitis often coexists with arthritis of the hip joint, back and sacroiliac joint disease, and gait disturbance.

Physical examination may reveal point tenderness in the lateral thigh just over the greater trochanter. Passive adduction and abduction, as well as active resisted abduction of the affected lower extremity, reproduce the pain. Sudden release of resistance during this maneuver markedly increases the pain. There should be no sensory deficit in the distribution of the lateral femoral cutaneous nerve, as is seen with meralgia paresthetica, which often is confused with trochanteric bursitis

Plain radiographs and magnetic resonance imaging (MRI) of the hip may reveal calcification of the bursa and associated structures consistent with chronic inflammation. MRI is indicated if occult mass or tumor of the hip or groin is suspected. Electromyography helps distinguish trochanteric bursitis from meralgia paresthetica and sciatica. The injection technique described here serves as both a diagnostic and therapeutic maneuver.

The trochanteric bursa lies between the greater trochanter and the tendon of the gluteus medius and the iliotibial tract. The gluteus medius muscle has its origin from the outer surface of the ilium, and its fibers pass downward and laterally to attach on the lateral surface of the greater trochanter. The gluteus medius locks the pelvis in place when walking and running. This action can irritate the trochanteric bursa, as can repeated trauma from repetitive activity, including jogging on soft or uneven surfaces or overuse of exercise equipment for lower extremity strengthening. The gluteus medius muscle is innervated by the superior gluteal nerve.

To perform injection of the trochanteric bursa, the goals of this injection technique are explained to the patient and the patient is placed in the lateral decubitus position with the affected side up. The midpoint of the greater trochanter is identified. Proper preparation with antiseptic solution of the skin overlying this point is then carried out. A syringe containing 2.0 mL of 0.25% preservative-free bupivacaine and 40 mg of methylprednisolone is attached to a 3½-inch, 25-gauge needle.

Prior to needle placement, the patient should be advised to say "There!" as soon as paresthesia into the lower extremity is felt, indicating that the needle has impinged on the sciatic nerve. Should paresthesia occur, the needle should be immediately withdrawn and repositioned more laterally. The needle is then carefully advanced through the previously identified point at a right angle to the skin directly toward the center of the greater trochanter. The needle is advanced very slowly to avoid trauma to the sciatic nerve until it hits the bone (Fig. 309-1). The needle is then withdrawn back out of the periosteum and, after careful aspiration for blood and if no paresthesia is present, the contents of the syringe are then gently injected into the bursa. There should be minimal resistance to injection.

The proximity to the sciatic nerve makes it imperative that this procedure be carried out only by those well versed in the regional anatomy and experienced in performing injection techniques. Many patients also complain of a transient increase in pain after injection of the bursa. Infection, although rare, can occur, and careful attention to sterile technique is mandatory.

SUGGESTED READING

Waldman SD: Injection technique for trochanteric bursitis. In: Atlas of Pain Management Injection Techniques. Philadelphia, Saunders, 2007.

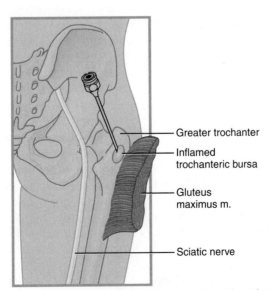

FIGURE 309–1 Injection technique for trochanteric bursitis. (From Waldman SD: Atlas of Pain Management Injection Techniques. Philadelphia, Saunders, 2007, p 365.)

CHAPTER 310

Injection Technique for Meralgia Paresthetica

Meralgia paresthetica is caused by compression of the lateral femoral cutaneous nerve by the inguinal ligament as it passes through or under the inguinal ligament. This entrapment neuropathy presents as pain, numbness, and dysesthesias in the distribution of the lateral femoral cutaneous nerve. These symptoms often begin as a burning pain in the lateral thigh with associated cutaneous sensitivity. Patients who suffer from meralgia paresthetica note that sitting, squatting, or wearing wide belts that compress the lateral femoral cutaneous nerve cause the symptoms of meralgia paresthetica to worsen. Although traumatic lesions to the lateral femoral cutaneous nerve have been implicated in the onset of meralgia paresthetica, in most patients, no obvious antecedent trauma can be identified.

Physical findings include tenderness over the lateral femoral cutaneous nerve at the origin of the inguinal ligament at the anterior superior iliac spine. A positive Tinel's sign may be present over the lateral femoral cutaneous nerve as it passes beneath the inguinal ligament. Careful sensory examination of the lateral thigh reveals a sensory deficit in the distribution of the lateral femoral cutaneous nerve. No motor deficit should be present. Sitting or the wearing of tight waistbands or wide belts that compress the lateral femoral cutaneous nerve may exacerbate the symptoms of meralgia paresthetica.

Meralgia paresthetica often is misdiagnosed as lumbar radiculopathy, trochanteric bursitis, or attributed to primary hip pathology. Radiographs of the hip and electromyography help distinguish meralgia paresthetica from radiculopathy or pain emanating from the hip. Most patients who suffer from a lumbar radiculopathy have back pain associated with reflex, motor, and sensory changes and lower extremity pain, whereas patients with meralgia paresthetica have no back pain and no motor or reflex changes. The sensory changes of meralgia paresthetica are limited to the distribution of the lateral femoral cutaneous nerve and should not extend below the knee. It should be remembered that lumbar radiculopathy and lateral femoral cutaneous nerve entrapment may coexist as the so-called "double crush" syndrome. Occasionally, diabetic femoral neuropathy may produce anterior thigh pain, which may confuse the diagnosis.

Electromyography helps distinguish lumbar radiculopathy and diabetic femoral neuropathy from meralgia paresthetica. Plain radiographs of the back, hip, and pelvis are indicated in all patients who present with meralgia paresthetica in order to rule out occult bony pathology. Based on the patient's clinical presentation, additional testing may be indicated, including complete blood count, uric acid, sedimentation rate, and antinuclear antibody testing. Magnetic resonance imaging of the spine is indicated if herniated disc, spinal stenosis, or a space-occupying lesion is suspected. The injection technique described below serves as both a diagnostic and therapeutic maneuver.

The lateral femoral cutaneous nerve is formed from the posterior divisions of the L2 and L3 nerves. The nerve leaves the psoas muscle and courses laterally and inferiorly to pass just beneath the ilioinguinal nerve at the level of the anterior superior iliac spine. The nerve passes under the inguinal ligament and then travels beneath the fascia lata, where it divides into an anterior and posterior branch. The anterior branch provides limited cutaneous sensory innervation over the anterolateral thigh. The posterior branch provides cutaneous sensory innervation to the lateral thigh from just above the greater trochanter to the knee.

To perform injection for meralgia paresthetica, the patient is placed in the supine position with a pillow under the knees if lying with the legs extended increases the patient's pain due to traction on the nerve. The anterior superior iliac spine is identified by palpation. A point 1 inch medial to the anterior superior iliac spine and just inferior to the inguinal ligament is then identified and prepped with antiseptic solution A 1½-inch, 25-gauge needle is then advanced perpendicular to the skin slowly until the needle is felt to "pop" through the fascia (Fig. 310-1). Paresthesia is often elicited. After careful aspiration, 5 to 7 mL of 1.0% preservative-free lidocaine and 40 mg of methylprednisolone are injected in a fanlike pattern as the needle pierces the fascia of the external oblique muscle. Care must be taken not to place the needle too deep and enter the peritoneal cavity and perforate the abdominal viscera. After injection of the solution, pressure is applied to the injection site to decrease the incidence of postblock ecchymosis and hematoma formation, which can be quite dramatic, especially in the anticoagulated patient.

The main side effect of lateral femoral cutaneous nerve block is postblock ecchymosis and hematoma. If needle placement is too deep and enters the peritoneal cavity, perforation of the colon may result in the formation of intra-abdominal abscess and fistula. Early detection of infection is crucial in order to avoid potentially life-threatening sequelae. If the needle is placed too medial, blockade of the femoral nerve may occur and make ambulation difficult.

SUGGESTED READING

Waldman SD: Injection technique for meralgia paresthetica. In: Atlas of Pain Management Injection Techniques. Philadelphia, Saunders, 2007.

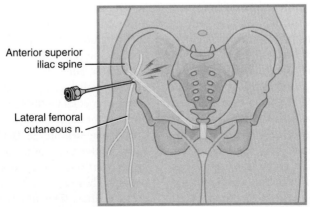

FIGURE 310–1 Injection technique for meralgia paresthetica. (From Waldman SD: Atlas of Pain Management Injection Techniques. Philadelphia, Saunders, 2007, p 359.)

CHAPTER 311

Injection Technique for Piriformis Syndrome

Piriformis syndrome is caused by compression of the sciatic nerve by the piriformis muscle as it passes through the sciatic notch. This entrapment neuropathy manifests as pain, numbness, paresthesias, and associated weakness in the distribution of the sciatic nerve. These symptoms often begin as severe pain in the buttocks that radiates into the lower extremity and foot. Patients who suffer from piriformis syndrome may develop altered gait, which in turn may result in the development of coexistent sacroiliac, back, and hip pain, further confusing the clinical picture. If untreated, progressive motor deficit of the gluteal muscles and lower extremity can result. The onset of symptoms of piriformis syndrome is usually after direct trauma to the sacroiliac and gluteal region and occasionally as a result of repetitive hip and lower extremity motions or repeated pressure on the piriformis muscle and underlying sciatic nerve. Rarely, occult tumors in this anatomic area can also compress the sciatic nerve as it passes through the sciatic notch and produce symptoms identical to piriformis syndrome.

Physical findings include tenderness over the sciatic notch. A positive Tinel's sign over the sciatic nerve as it passes beneath the piriformis muscle often is present. A positive straight-leg raising test is suggestive of sciatic nerve entrapment that may be due to piriformis syndrome. Palpation of the piriformis muscle reveals tenderness and a swollen, indurated muscle belly. Lifting or bending at the waist and hips increases the pain symptomatology in most patients who suffer from piriformis syndrome. Weakness of affected gluteal muscles and the lower extremity and, ultimately, muscle wasting often are seen in advanced untreated piriformis syndrome.

Piriformis syndrome is often misdiagnosed as lumbar radiculopathy or is attributed to primary hip pathology. Radiographs of the hip and electromyography help distinguish piriformis syndrome from radiculopathy of pain emanating from the hip. Most patients who suffer from a lumbar radiculopathy have back pain associated with reflex, motor, and sensory changes that are associated with neck pain, whereas patients with piriformis syndrome have only secondary back pain and no reflex changes. The motor and sensory changes of piriformis syndrome are limited to the distribution of the sciatic nerve below the sciatic notch. It should be remembered that lumbar radiculopathy and sciatic nerve entrapment may coexist as the so-called "double crush" syndrome.

Electromyography helps distinguish lumbar radiculopathy from piriformis syndrome. Plain radiographs of the back, hip, and pelvis are indicated in all patients who present with piriformis syndrome in order to rule out occult bony pathology. Based on the patient's clinical presentation, additional testing may be indicated, including complete blood count, uric acid, erythrocyte sedimentation rate, and antinuclear antibody testing. Magnetic resonance imaging scan of the back is indicated if a herniated disc, spinal stenosis, or space-occupying lesion is suspected. The injection technique described here serves as both a diagnostic and therapeutic maneuver.

The piriformis muscle has its origin from the anterior sacrum. It passes laterally through the greater sciatic foramen to insert on the upper border of the greater trochanter of the femur. The piriformis muscle's primary function is to externally rotate the femur at the hip joint. The piriformis muscle is innervated by the sacral plexus. With internal rotation of the femur, the tendinous insertion and belly of the muscle can compress the sciatic nerve and, if this persists, cause entrapment of the sciatic nerve.

The sciatic nerve provides innervation to the distal lower extremity and foot with the exception of the medial aspect of the calf and foot, which are subserved by the saphenous nerve. The largest nerve in the body, the sciatic nerve, is derived from the L4, L5, and the S1-3 nerve roots. The roots fuse together in front of the anterior surface of the lateral sacrum on the anterior surface of the piriform muscle. The nerve travels inferiorly and leaves the pelvis just below the piriform muscle via the sciatic notch. Just beneath the nerve at this point is the obturator internus muscle. The sciatic nerve lies anterior to the gluteus maximus muscle; at this muscle's lower border, the sciatic nerve lies halfway between the greater trochanter and the ischial tuberosity. The sciatic nerve courses downward past the lesser trochanter to lie posterior and medial to the femur. In the mid-thigh, the nerve gives off branches to the hamstring muscles and the adductor magnus muscle. In most patients, the nerve divides to form the tibial and common peroneal nerves in the upper portion of the popliteal fossa, although in some patients these nerves can remain separate through their entire course. The tibial nerve continues downward to provide innervation to the distal lower extremity, whereas the common peroneal nerve travels laterally to innervate a portion of the knee joint and, via its lateral cutaneous branch, provide sensory innervation to the back and lateral side of the upper calf.

To perform injection for piriformis syndrome, the patient is placed in the Sims' position with the upper leg flexed. The greater trochanter and the ischial tuberosity on the involved side is identified by palpation. Midway between these two bony landmarks lies the sciatic nerve (Fig. 311-1). This midpoint is then identified and prepped with antiseptic solution. A 3½-inch, 25-gauge needle is then advanced perpendicular to the skin very slowly until paresthesia is elicited. The patient should be warned to expect paresthesia and should be told to say "There!" as soon as the paresthesia is felt. Paresthesia usually is elicited at a depth of 2½ to 3 inches. If the needle is felt to impinge on the bone of the sciatic notch, the needle is withdrawn and redirected laterally and slightly superiorly until paresthesia is elicited. Once paresthesia in the distribution of the sciatic nerve is elicited, the needle is withdrawn 1 mm, and the patient is observed to be sure that he or she is not experiencing any persistent paresthesia. If no persistent paresthesia is present and after careful aspiration, 8 mL of 1.0% preservative-free lidocaine and 40 mg of methylprednisolone are slowly injected. Care must be taken not to advance the needle into the substance of the nerve during the injection and to thereby inject solution intraneurally. After injection of the solution, pressure is applied to the injection site to decrease the incidence of postblock ecchymosis and hematoma formation.

The main side effect of this injection technique is postblock ecchymosis and hematoma. As mentioned, pressure should be maintained on the injection site post block to avoid ecchymosis and hematoma formation. Because a paresthesia is elicited with this technique, the potential for needle-induced trauma to the sciatic nerve remains a possibility. By advancing the needle slowly and withdrawing the needle slightly away from the nerve, needle-induced trauma to the sciatic nerve can be avoided.

SUGGESTED READING

Waldman SD: Injection technique for piriformis syndrome. In: Atlas of Pain Management Injection Techniques, ed. 2. Philadelphia, Saunders, 2007.

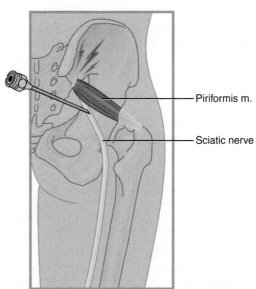

Piriformis m.

Sciatic nerve

FIGURE 311–1 Injection technique for piriformis syndrome. (From Waldman SD: Atlas of Pain Management Injection Techniques, ed. 2. Philadelphia, Saunders, 2007, p 399.)

CHAPTER 312

Lumbar Plexus Block

The lumbar plexus lies within the substance of the psoas muscle. The plexus is made up of the ventral roots of the first four lumbar nerves, and in some patients, a contribution from the 12th thoracic nerve. The nerves lie in front of the transverse processes of their respective vertebrae; as they course inferolaterally, they divide into a number of peripheral nerves. The ilioinguinal and iliohypogastric nerves are branches of the L1 nerves with an occasional contribution of fibers from T12. The genitofemoral nerve is made up of fibers from L1 and L2. The lateral femoral cutaneous nerve is derived from fibers of L2 and L3. The obturator nerve receives fibers from L2 to L4, and the femoral nerve is made up of fibers from L2 to L4. The pain management specialist should be aware of the considerable interpatient variability in terms of the actual spinal nerves that provide fibers to make up these peripheral branches. This variability means that differential neural blockade on an anatomic basis must be interpreted with caution.

The Winnie 3-In-1 Technique

The rationale behind lumbar plexus block using the Winnie 3-in-1 technique is to block the three principal nerves that comprise the lumbar plexus as they lie enclosed by the fascial plane between the quadratus lumborum, the iliacus muscle, and the psoas major muscle. Solutions injected in this fascial plane flow cranially to bathe the lateral femoral cutaneous nerve, the femoral nerve, and the obturator nerve as they pass below the inguinal ligament.

To perform lumbar plexus block using the Winnie 3-in-1 technique, the patient is placed in the supine position. The inguinal ligament and the femoral artery on the side to be blocked are identified. At a point just lateral to the femoral artery and just below the inguinal ligament, the skin is prepared with antiseptic solution. A 22-gauge, 1½-inch needle is slowly advanced in a slightly caudad direction until a paresthesia in the distribution of the femoral nerve is elicited (Fig. 312-1). The patient should be warned of such and instructed to say "There!" immediately on perceiving the paresthesia. If there is no persistent paresthesia in the distribution of the femoral nerve and careful aspiration reveals no blood or cerebrospinal fluid, 25 to 30 mL of 1.0% preservative-free lidocaine is slowly

injected in incremental doses, with care taken to observe the patient for signs of local anesthetic toxicity. Pressure should be applied below the needle to force the solution to flow cranially along the fascial plane rather than distally into the leg. If the pain has an inflammatory component, the local anesthetic is combined with 80 mg of methylprednisolone and is injected in incremental doses. Subsequent daily nerve blocks are carried out in a similar manner, substituting 40 mg of methylprednisolone for the initial 80-mg dose. As mentioned earlier, an intravenous catheter can be placed into the fascial sheath to allow continuous infusion of local anesthetic.

The Psoas Technique

To perform lumbar plexus block utilizing the psoas technique, the patient is placed in the lateral or sitting position with the lumbar spine flexed. If the lateral position is chosen, the side to be blocked should be up. The superior iliac crest is identified, and the spinous process is palpated in a direct line medially with the crest. This is the spinous process of the L4 vertebra in the vast majority of patients. Counting down one level, the L5 spinous process is then identified (Fig. 312-2). At a point 1½ inches lateral to the L5 spinous process, the skin is prepared with antiseptic solution. A 22-gauge, 13-cm styletted needle is advanced perpendicular to the skin, aiming for the middle of the transverse process. The needle should impinge on bone after being advanced approximately 1½ inches (Fig. 312-3). After bone is contacted, the needle is withdrawn into the subcutaneous tissues and redirected superiorly and "walked off" the superior margin of the transverse process. As soon as bony contact is lost, the stylet is removed and a 5-mL, well-lubricated syringe filled with sterile preservative-free saline is attached. The syringe and needle are slowly advanced in a manner analogous to the loss-of-resistance technique used for identification of the epidural space, with constant pressure being placed on the plunger of the syringe (Fig. 312-4). At a depth of 2 to 2½ inches, a loss of resistance is encountered as the needle exits the quadratus lumborum muscle and enters the psoas compartment (Fig. 312-5).

If careful aspiration reveals no blood or cerebrospinal fluid, 25 to 30 mL of 1.0% preservative-free lidocaine is slowly injected in incremental doses, with care taken to observe the patient for signs of local anesthetic toxicity. If the pain has an inflammatory component, the local anesthetic is combined with 80 mg of methylprednisolone and is injected in incremental doses. Subsequent daily nerve blocks are carried out in a similar manner, substituting 40 mg of methylprednisolone for the initial 80-mg dose.

The proximity to the femoral artery and vein makes the possibility of local anesthetic toxicity real when performing lumbar plexus block using the Winnie 3-in-1 approach. Persistent paresthesia secondary to trauma to the femoral nerve has rarely been reported after this technique. Although uncommon, infection remains an ever-present possibility, especially in the immunocompromised cancer patient. Early detection of infection is crucial to avoid potentially life-threatening sequelae. Postblock groin and back pain, as well as ecchymosis and hematoma of the groin, occur often enough that the patient should be warned of such prior to beginning lumbar plexus block using the Winnie 3-in-1 technique.

The proximity to the spinal cord and exiting nerve roots makes it imperative that lumbar plexus block using the psoas technique be performed only by those well versed in the regional anatomy and experienced in interventional pain management techniques. Needle placement that is too medial may result in epidural, subdural, or subarachnoid injections or trauma to the spinal cord and exiting nerve roots. Placing the needle too deep between the transverse processes may result in trauma to the exiting lumbar nerve roots. Although uncommon, infection remains an ever-present possibility, especially in the immunocompromised cancer patient. Early detection of infection is crucial to avoid potentially life-threatening sequelae. Postblock back pain from trauma to the paraspinous musculature is not uncommon after lumbar plexus block using the psoas compartment technique.

SUGGESTED READINGS

Waldman SD. Lumbar plexus nerve block: The Winnie 3-in-1 technique. In: Atlas of Interventional Pain Management, ed 2. Philadelphia, Saunders, 2004.

Waldman SD. Lumbar plexus nerve block: Psoas compartment technique. In: Atlas of Interventional Pain Management, ed 2. Philadelphia, Saunders, 2004.

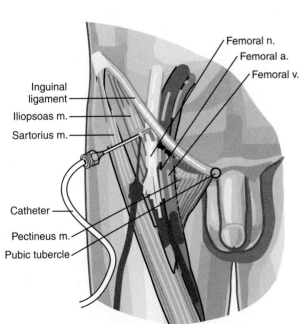

FIGURE 312–1 Lumbar plexus nerve block: The Winnie 3-in-1 technique. (From Waldman SD: Atlas of Interventional Pain Management, ed 2. Philadelphia, Saunders, 2004, p 442.)

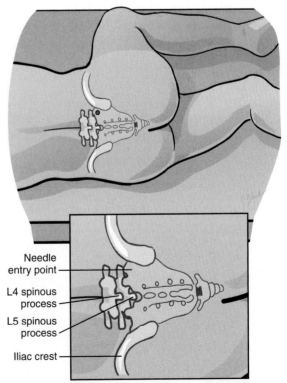

FIGURE 312–2 Needle entry point for the psoas compartment technique. (From Waldman SD: Atlas of Interventional Pain Management, ed 2. Philadelphia, Saunders, 2004, p 445.)

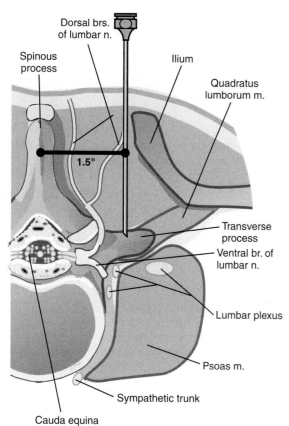

FIGURE 312–3 Correct needle positioning for the psoas compartment technique. (From Waldman SD: Atlas of Interventional Pain Management, ed 2. Philadelphia, Saunders, 2004, p 446.)

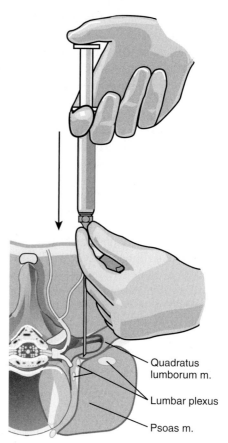

FIGURE 312–4 Injection technique for the psoas compartment approach. (From Waldman SD: Atlas of Interventional Pain Management, ed 2. Philadelphia, Saunders, 2004, p 447.)

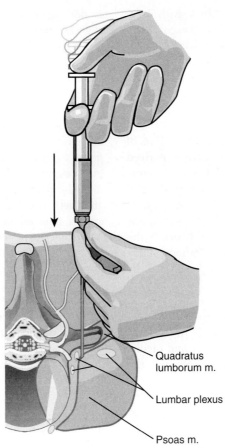

FIGURE 312–5 Loss of resistance technique in the psoas compartment approach. (From Waldman SD: Atlas of Interventional Pain Management, ed 2. Philadelphia, Saunders, 2004, p 448.)

Quadratus lumborum m.

Lumbar plexus

Psoas m.

CHAPTER 313

Femoral Nerve Block

Femoral nerve block is useful in the evaluation and management of lower extremity pain thought to be subserved by the femoral nerve. The technique is also useful to provide surgical anesthesia for the lower extremity when combined with lateral femoral cutaneous, sciatic, and obturator nerve block or lumbar plexus block. It is used for this indication primarily in patients who would not tolerate the sympathetic changes induced by spinal or epidural anesthesia and who need lower extremity surgery. Femoral nerve block with local anesthetic can be used diagnostically during differential neural blockade on an anatomic basis in the evaluation of lower extremity pain.

If destruction of the femoral nerve is being considered, this technique is useful as a prognostic indicator of the degree of motor and sensory impairment that the patient may experience. Femoral nerve block with local anesthetic may be used to palliate acute pain emergencies, including femoral neck and shaft fractures, and for postoperative pain relief while waiting for pharmacologic methods to become effective. Femoral nerve block with local anesthetic and steroid is occasionally used in the treatment of persistent lower extremity pain when the pain is thought to be secondary to inflammation or when entrapment of the femoral nerve as it passes under the inguinal ligament is suspected. Femoral nerve block with local anesthetic and steroid is also indicated in the palliation of pain and motor dysfunction associated with diabetic femoral neuropathy. Destruction of the femoral nerve is occasionally used in the palliation of persistent lower extremity pain secondary to invasive tumor that is mediated by the femoral nerve and has not responded to more conservative measures.

The femoral nerve innervates the anterior portion of the thigh and medial calf. The femoral nerve is derived from the posterior branches of the L2, L3, and L4 nerve roots. The roots fuse together in the psoas muscle and descend laterally between the psoas and iliacus muscles to enter the iliac fossa. The femoral nerve gives off motor fibers to the iliac muscle and then passes beneath the inguinal ligament to enter the thigh. The femoral nerve is just lateral to the femoral artery as it passes beneath the inguinal ligament and is enclosed with the femoral artery and vein within the femoral sheath. The nerve gives off motor fibers to the sartorius, quadriceps femoris, and pectineus muscles. It also provides sensory fibers to the knee joint as well as the skin overlying the anterior and medial thigh. The nerve is easily blocked as it passes through the femoral triangle.

The patient is placed in the supine position with the leg in neutral position. The femoral artery is identified just below the inguinal ligament by palpation. A point just lateral to the pulsations of the femoral artery and just inferior to the inguinal ligament is then identified and prepared with antiseptic solution. A 25-gauge, 1½-inch needle is then advanced at this point slowly with a cephalad trajectory until paresthesia in the distribution of the femoral nerve is elicited (Fig. 313-1). The patient should be warned to expect such and should be told to say "There!" immediately on perceiving the paresthesia. Paresthesia usually is elicited at a depth of ½ to ¾ inch. If paresthesia

is not elicited, the needle is withdrawn and redirected slightly more medially until paresthesia is obtained. Once paresthesia in the distribution of the femoral nerve is elicited, the needle is withdrawn 1 mm, and the patient is observed to be sure he or she is not experiencing any persistent paresthesia. If no persistent paresthesia is present and after careful aspiration, 15 to 18 mL of 1.0% preservative-free lidocaine is slowly injected. Care must be taken not to advance the needle into the substance of the nerve during the injection and inject solution intraneurally.

If the pain has an inflammatory component, the local anesthetic is combined with 80 mg of methylprednisolone and is injected in incremental doses. Subsequent daily nerve blocks are performed in a similar manner, substituting 40 mg of methylprednisolone for the initial 80-mg dose. After injection of the solution, pressure is applied to the injection site to decrease the incidence of postblock ecchymosis and hematoma formation.

The main side effect of femoral nerve block is postblock ecchymosis and hematoma. As mentioned earlier, pressure should be maintained on the injection site post block to avoid ecchymosis and hematoma formation. Because paresthesia is elicited with this technique, needle-induced trauma to the femoral nerve remains a possibility. By advancing the needle slowly and then withdrawing the needle slightly away from the nerve, needle-induced trauma to the femoral nerve can be avoided. Although uncommon, infection following femoral nerve injection can occur.

SUGGESTED READING

Waldman SD: Femoral nerve block. In: Atlas of Interventional Pain Management, ed 2. Philadelphia, Saunders, 2004.

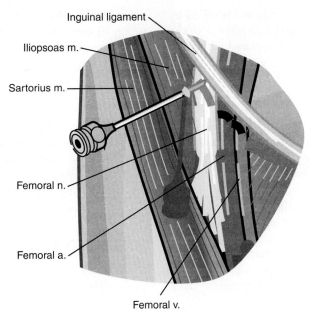

FIGURE 313–1 Femoral nerve block. (From Waldman SD: Atlas of Interventional Pain Management, ed 2. Philadelphia, Saunders, 2004, p 453.)

CHAPTER 314

Obturator Nerve Block

Obturator nerve block is useful in the evaluation and management of hip pain and spasm of the hip adductors thought to be subserved by the obturator nerve. The technique is also useful to provide surgical anesthesia for the lower extremity when combined with lateral femoral cutaneous, femoral, and sciatic nerve block. Obturator nerve block with local anesthetic can be used as a diagnostic tool during differential neural blockade on an anatomic basis in the evaluation of hip pain. If destruction of the obturator nerve is being considered, this technique is useful as a prognostic indicator of the degree of motor and sensory impairment that the patient may experience. Obturator nerve block with local anesthetic may be used to palliate acute pain emergencies, including postoperative pain relief, while waiting for pharmacologic methods to become effective. Obturator nerve block with local anesthetic is also useful in the management of hip adductor spasm, which may make perineal care or urinary catheterization difficult. This technique is also useful to aid in physical therapy following hip surgery. Obturator nerve block with local anesthetic and steroid is also useful in the treatment of persistent hip pain when the pain is thought to be secondary to inflammation or entrapment of the obturator nerve. Destruction of the obturator nerve is occasionally indicated for the palliation of persistent hip pain after trauma to the hip that is mediated by the obturator nerve.

The obturator nerve provides the majority of innervation to the hip joint. It is derived from the posterior divisions of the L2, L3, and L4 nerves. The nerve leaves the medial border psoas muscle and courses inferiorly to pass the pelvis, where it joins the obturator vessels to travel via the obturator canal to enter the thigh. The nerve then divides into an anterior and posterior branch. The anterior branch supplies an articular branch to provide sensory innervation to the hip joint, motor branches to the superficial hip adductors, and a cutaneous branch to the medial aspect of the distal thigh. The posterior branch provides motor innervation to the deep hip adductors and an articular branch to the posterior knee joint.

To perform obturator nerve block, the patient is placed in the supine position with the legs slightly abducted.

The pubic tubercle on the involved side is identified by palpation. A point 1 inch lateral and 1 inch inferior to the pubic tubercle is then identified and prepared with antiseptic solution. A 22-gauge, 3-inch needle is then slowly advanced perpendicular to the skin until the needle is felt to impinge on the superior pubic ramus (Fig. 314-1). The depth of bony contact is noted, and the needle is withdrawn and redirected laterally and slightly inferiorly (Fig. 314-2). The needle is advanced approximately ¾ to 1 inch deeper to place the needle tip in the obturator canal. Paresthesia in the distribution of the obturator nerve may be elicited. After careful aspiration, 10 to 15 mL of 1.0% preservative-free lidocaine is injected. Care must be taken not to place the needle in the obturator artery or vein.

If the pain has an inflammatory component, the local anesthetic is combined with 80 mg of methylprednisolone and is injected in incremental doses. Subsequent daily nerve blocks are carried out in a similar manner, substituting 40 mg of methylprednisolone for the initial 80-mg dose. After injection of the solution, pressure is applied to the injection site to decrease the incidence of postblock ecchymosis and hematoma formation.

The main side effect of obturator nerve block is postblock ecchymosis and hematoma. Because of proximity to the obturator artery and vein, intravascular injection remains an ever-present possibility. As mentioned, pressure should be maintained on the injection site post block to avoid ecchymosis and hematoma formation. Although uncommon, infection following obturator nerve block remains an ever-present possibility.

SUGGESTED READING

Waldman SD: Obturator nerve block. In: Atlas of Interventional Pain Management, ed 2. Philadelphia, Saunders, 2004.

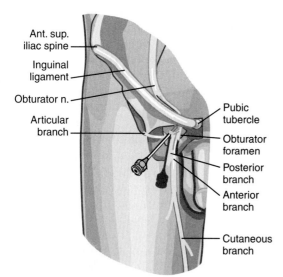

FIGURE 314–1 Obturator nerve anatomy. (From Waldman SD: Atlas of Interventional Pain Management, ed 2. Philadelphia, Saunders, 2004, p 461.)

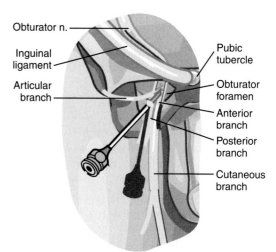

FIGURE 314–2 Obturator nerve block. (From Waldman SD: Atlas of Interventional Pain Management, ed 2. Philadelphia, Saunders, 2004, p 462.)

Sciatic Nerve Block

Sciatic nerve block is useful in the evaluation and management of distal lower extremity pain thought to be subserved by the sciatic nerve. The technique is also useful to provide surgical anesthesia for the distal lower extremity when combined with lateral femoral cutaneous, femoral, and obturator nerve block or lumbar plexus block. It is used for this indication primarily with patients who would not tolerate the sympathetic changes induced by spinal or epidural anesthesia who need distal extremity amputations or débridement. Sciatic nerve block with local anesthetic can be used diagnostically during differential neural blockade on an anatomic basis in the evaluation of distal lower extremity pain. If destruction of the sciatic nerve is being considered, this technique is useful as a prognostic indicator of the degree of motor and sensory impairment that the patient may experience. Sciatic nerve block with local anesthetic may be used to palliate acute pain emergencies, including distal lower extremity fractures and for postoperative pain relief, while waiting for pharmacologic methods to become effective. Sciatic nerve block with local anesthetic and steroid is occasionally used in the treatment of persistent distal lower extremity pain when the pain is thought to be secondary to inflammation or when entrapment of the sciatic nerve at the level of the lesser trochanter is suspected. Destruction of the sciatic nerve is occasionally indicated for the palliation of persistent distal lower extremity pain secondary to invasive tumor that is mediated by the sciatic nerve and has not responded to more conservative measures.

The sciatic nerve innervates the distal lower extremity and foot with the exception of the medial aspect of the calf and foot, which are subserved by the saphenous nerve. The largest nerve in the body, the sciatic nerve is derived from the L4, L5, and the S1-3 nerve roots. The roots fuse together in front of the anterior surface of the lateral sacrum on the anterior surface of the piriform muscle. The nerve travels inferiorly and leaves the pelvis just below the piriform muscle via the sciatic notch. The sciatic nerve lies anterior to the gluteus maximus muscle and, at this muscle's lower border, lies halfway between the greater trochanter and the ischial tuberosity. The sciatic nerve courses downward past the lesser trochanter to lie posterior and medial to the femur. In the mid-thigh, the nerve gives off branches to the hamstring muscles and the adductor magnus muscle. In most patients, the nerve divides to form the tibial and common peroneal nerves in the upper portion of the popliteal fossa, although these nerves sometimes remain separate through their entire course. The tibial nerve continues downward to provide innervation to the distal lower extremity, whereas the common peroneal nerve travels laterally to innervate a portion of the knee joint and, via its lateral cutaneous branch, provides sensory innervation to the back and lateral side of the upper calf.

The Anterior Approach

Sciatic nerve block via the anterior approach is used for patients who cannot assume the Sims' or lithotomy position because of lower extremity trauma. To perform sciatic nerve block using the anterior approach, the patient is placed in the supine position with the leg in neutral position. The greater trochanter and the crease of the groin on the involved side are identified by palpation. An imaginary line is then drawn parallel to the crease of the groin that runs from the greater trochanter to the center of the thigh. This center point is then identified and prepared with antiseptic solution. A 25-gauge, 3½-inch needle is then slowly advanced perpendicular to the skin until it impinges on the femur. The needle is then "walked" slightly superiorly and medially until it walks off the top of the lesser trochanter (Fig. 315-1). A paresthesia in the distribution of the sciatic nerve will be elicited; if a nerve stimulator is used, dorsiflexion and plantar flexion of the foot will be noted. The patient should be warned to expect paresthesia and should be told to say "There!" immediately on perceiving the paresthesia. Paresthesia is usually elicited at a depth 1 inch beyond initial bony contact. Once paresthesia is elicited in the distribution of the sciatic nerve, the needle is withdrawn 1 mm, and the patient is observed to rule out any persistent paresthesia. If no persistent paresthesia is present and after careful aspiration, 15 to 18 mL of 1.0% preservative-free lidocaine is slowly injected. Care must be taken not to advance the needle into the substance of the nerve during the injection and inject solution intraneurally.

If the pain has an inflammatory component, the local anesthetic is combined with 80 mg of methylprednisolone and is injected in incremental doses. Subsequent daily nerve blocks are carried out in a similar manner, substituting 40 mg of methylprednisolone for the initial

80-mg dose. After injection of the solution, pressure is applied to the injection site to decrease the incidence of postblock ecchymosis and hematoma formation.

The Posterior Approach

To perform sciatic nerve block using the posterior approach, the patient is placed in the Sims' position with the upper leg flexed. The greater trochanter and the ischial tuberosity on the involved side are identified by palpation. The sciatic nerve lies midway between these two bony landmarks (Fig. 315-2). This midpoint is then identified and prepared with antiseptic solution. A 25-gauge, 3½-inch needle is then slowly advanced perpendicular to the skin until paresthesia is elicited; if a nerve stimulator is used, dorsiflexion and plantar flexion of the foot are noted. The patient should be warned to expect paresthesia and should be told to say "There!" immediately on perceiving the paresthesia. Paresthesia is usually elicited at a depth of 2½ to 3 inches. If the needle is felt to impinge on the bone of the sciatic notch, the needle is withdrawn and redirected laterally and slightly superiorly until paresthesia is elicited. Once paresthesia is elicited in the distribution of the sciatic nerve, the needle is withdrawn 1 mm, and the patient is observed to rule out any persistent paresthesia. If no persistent paresthesia is present and after careful aspiration, 15 to 18 mL of 1.0% preservative-free lidocaine is slowly injected. Care must

be taken not to advance the needle into the substance of the nerve during the injection and inject solution intraneurally.

If the pain has an inflammatory component, the local anesthetic is combined with 80 mg of methylprednisolone and is injected in incremental doses. Subsequent daily nerve blocks are carried out in a similar manner, substituting 40 mg of methylprednisolone for the initial 80-mg dose. After injection of the solution, pressure is applied to the injection site to decrease the incidence of postblock ecchymosis and hematoma formation.

The main side effect of sciatic nerve block using the anterior approach is postblock ecchymosis and hematoma. As mentioned, pressure should be maintained on the injection site post block to avoid ecchymosis and hematoma formation. Because this technique elicits paresthesia, needle-induced trauma to the sciatic nerve remains possible. By advancing the needle slowly and withdrawing the needle slightly away from the nerve, one can avoid needle-induced trauma to the sciatic nerve.

SUGGESTED READINGS

Waldman SD: Sciatic nerve block: Anterior approach. In: Atlas of Interventional Pain Management, ed 2. Philadelphia, Saunders, 2004.

Waldman SD: Sciatic nerve block: Posterior approach. In: Atlas of Interventional Pain Management, ed 2. Philadelphia, Saunders, 2004.

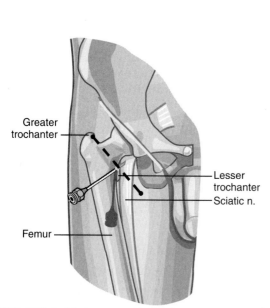

FIGURE 315–1 Sciatic nerve block: anterior approach. (From Waldman SD: Atlas of Interventional Pain Management, ed 2. Philadelphia, Saunders, 2004, p 467.)

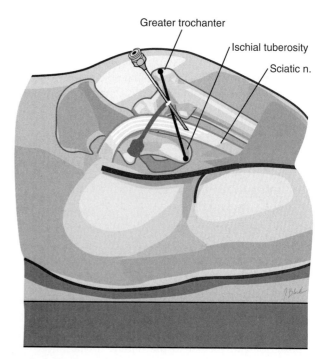

FIGURE 315–2 Sciatic nerve block: posterior approach. (From Waldman SD: Atlas of Interventional Pain Management, ed 2. Philadelphia, Saunders, 2004, p 47ø.)

Tibial Nerve Block at the Knee

Tibial nerve block at the knee is useful in the evaluation and management of foot and ankle pain thought to be subserved by the tibial nerve. The technique is also useful to provide surgical anesthesia for the distal lower extremity when combined with common peroneal and saphenous nerve block or lumbar plexus block. It is used for this indication primarily in patients who would not tolerate the sympathetic changes induced by spinal or epidural anesthesia and who need distal lower extremity surgery, such as débridement or distal amputation. Tibial nerve block at the knee with local anesthetic can be used as a diagnostic tool during differential neural blockade on an anatomic basis in the evaluation of lower extremity pain. If destruction of the tibial nerve is being considered, this technique is useful as a prognostic indicator of the degree of motor and sensory impairment that the patient may experience. Tibial nerve block at the knee with local anesthetic may be used to palliate acute pain emergencies, including ankle and foot fractures and postoperative pain relief, when combined with the blocks mentioned while waiting for pharmacologic methods to become effective. Tibial nerve block at the knee with local anesthetic and steroid is occasionally used in the treatment of persistent ankle and foot pain when the pain is thought to be secondary to inflammation or when entrapment of the tibial nerve at the popliteal fossa is suspected. Tibial nerve block at the knee with local anesthetic and steroid is also indicated in the palliation of pain and motor dysfunction associated with diabetic neuropathy. Destruction of the tibial nerve block at the knee is occasionally used in the palliation of persistent lower extremity pain secondary to invasive tumor that is mediated by the tibial nerve and has not responded to more conservative measures.

The tibial nerve is one of the two major continuations of the sciatic nerve, the other being the common peroneal nerve. The tibial nerve provides sensory innervation to the posterior portion of the calf, the heel, and the medial plantar surface. The tibial nerve splits from the sciatic nerve at the superior margin of the popliteal fossa and descends in a slightly medial course through the popliteal fossa. The tibial nerve block at the knee lies just beneath the popliteal fascia and is readily accessible for neural blockade. The tibial nerve continues its downward course, running between the two heads of the gastrocnemius muscle, passing deep to the soleus muscle. The nerve

courses medially between the Achilles tendon and the medial malleolus, where it divides into the medial and lateral plantar nerves, providing sensory innervation to the heel and medial plantar surface. The tibial nerve is occasionally subject to compression at this point and is known as posterior tarsal tunnel syndrome.

To perform tibial nerve block at the knee, the patient is placed in the prone position with the leg slightly flexed. The skin crease of the knee and margins of the semitendinosus and biceps femoris muscles in the upper popliteal fossa are palpated. The margins of these muscles can be more easily identified by having the patient flex his or her leg under resistance. An imaginary triangle is envisioned with the apex being the convergence of these two muscles and the base being the skin crease of the knee (Fig. 316-1). At a point in the center of this imaginary apex, the skin is prepared with antiseptic solution. A 25-gauge, 1½-inch needle is then slowly advanced perpendicular to the skin through this point toward the tibial nerve until paresthesia is elicited in the distribution of the tibial nerve. The patient should be warned to expect paresthesia and should be told to say "There!" immediately on perceiving the paresthesia. Paresthesia is usually elicited at a depth of ½ to ¾ inch. If paresthesia is not elicited, the needle is withdrawn and redirected slightly more medially until paresthesia is obtained. Once paresthesia is elicited in the distribution of the tibial nerve, the needle is withdrawn 1 mm and the patient is observed to rule out any persistent paresthesia. If no persistent paresthesia is present and after careful aspiration, 8 mL of 1.0% preservative-free lidocaine is slowly injected. Care must be taken not to advance the needle into the substance of the nerve during the injection and inject solution intraneurally. Given the proximity to the common peroneal nerve, this nerve may also be blocked when performing tibial nerve block at the knee.

If the pain has an inflammatory component, the local anesthetic is combined with 80 mg of methylprednisolone and is injected in incremental doses. Subsequent daily nerve blocks are carried out in a similar manner, substituting 40 mg of methylprednisolone for the initial 80-mg dose. After injection of the solution, pressure is applied to the injection site to decrease the incidence of postblock ecchymosis and hematoma formation.

The main side effect of tibial nerve block at the knee is postblock ecchymosis and hematoma. As mentioned earlier, pressure should be maintained on the injection site post block to avoid ecchymosis and hematoma formation. Because this technique elicits paresthesia, needle-induced trauma to the tibial nerve remains possible. By advancing the needle slowly and withdrawing the needle slightly away from the nerve prior to injection, one can avoid needle-induced trauma to the tibial nerve.

SUGGESTED READING

Waldman SD: Tibial nerve block at the knee. In: Atlas of Interventional Pain Management, ed 2. Philadelphia, Saunders, 2004.

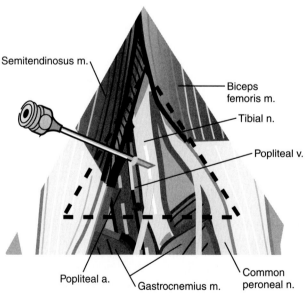

FIGURE 316–1 Tibial nerve block at the knee. (From Waldman SD: Atlas of Interventional Pain Management, ed 2. Philadelphia, Saunders, 2004, p 482.)

Tibial Nerve Block at the Ankle

Tibial nerve block at the ankle is useful in the evaluation and management of foot and ankle pain thought to be subserved by the tibial nerve. The technique is also useful to provide surgical anesthesia for the ankle and foot when combined with common peroneal and saphenous nerve block or lumbar plexus block. It is used for this indication primarily in patients who would not tolerate the sympathetic changes induced by spinal or epidural anesthesia and who need distal lower extremity surgery, such as débridement or distal amputation. Tibial nerve block at the ankle with local anesthetic can be used as a diagnostic tool during differential neural blockade on an anatomic basis in the evaluation of lower extremity pain. If destruction of the tibial nerve is being considered, this technique is useful as a prognostic indicator of the degree of motor and sensory impairment. Tibial nerve block at the ankle with local anesthetic may be used to palliate acute pain emergencies, including ankle and foot fractures and for postoperative pain relief, when combined with the blocks mentioned while waiting for pharmacologic methods to become effective. Tibial nerve block at the ankle with local anesthetic and steroid is occasionally used in the treatment of persistent ankle and foot pain when the pain is thought to be secondary to inflammation or when entrapment of the tibial nerve at the posterior tarsal tunnel is suspected. Tibial nerve block at the ankle with local anesthetic and steroid is also indicated in the palliation of pain and motor dysfunction associated with diabetic neuropathy. Destruction of the tibial nerve block at the ankle is occasionally used in the palliation of persistent lower extremity pain secondary to invasive tumor that is mediated by the distal tibial nerve and has not responded to more conservative measures.

The tibial nerve is one of the two major continuations of the sciatic nerve, the other being the common peroneal nerve. The tibial nerve provides sensory innervation to the posterior portion of the calf, the heel, and the medial plantar surface. The tibial nerve splits from the sciatic nerve at the superior margin of the popliteal fossa and descends in a slightly medial course through the popliteal fossa. The tibial nerve block at the ankle lies just beneath the popliteal fascia and is readily accessible for neural blockade. The tibial nerve continues its downward course, running between the two heads of the gastrocnemius muscle, passing deep to the soleus muscle. The nerve courses medially between the Achilles tendon and the medial malleolus, where it divides into the medial and lateral plantar nerves, providing sensory innervation to the heel and medial plantar surface. The tibial nerve is subject to compression at this point, which is known as posterior tarsal tunnel syndrome.

The patient is placed in the lateral position with the affected leg in the dependent position and slightly flexed. The posterior tibial artery at this level is then palpated. The area between the medial malleolus and the Achilles tendon is identified and prepared with antiseptic solutions. A 25-gauge, 1½-inch needle is inserted at this level and directed anteriorly toward the pulsations of the posterior tibial artery. If the arterial pulsations cannot be identified, the needle is directed toward the posterior, superior border of the medial malleolus. The needle is then advanced slowly toward the tibial nerve, which lies in the posterior groove of the medial malleolus, until paresthesia is elicited in the distribution of the tibial nerve (Fig. 317-1). The patient should be warned to expect paresthesia and should be told to say "There!" immediately on perceiving the paresthesia. Paresthesia is usually elicited after the needle is advanced ½ to ¾ inch. If paresthesia is not elicited, the needle is withdrawn and redirected slightly more cephalad until paresthesia is obtained. Once paresthesia is elicited in the distribution of the tibial nerve, the needle is withdrawn 1 mm and the patient is observed to rule out any persistent paresthesia. If no persistent paresthesia is present and after careful aspiration, 6 mL of 1.0% preservative-free lidocaine is slowly injected. Care must be taken not to advance the needle into the substance of the nerve during the injection and inject solution intraneurally.

If the pain has an inflammatory component, the local anesthetic is combined with 80 mg of methylprednisolone and is injected in incremental doses. Subsequent daily nerve blocks are carried out in a similar manner, substituting 40 mg of methylprednisolone for the initial 80-mg dose. After injection of the solution, pressure is applied to the injection site to decrease the incidence of postblock ecchymosis and hematoma formation.

The main side effect of tibial nerve block at the ankle is postblock ecchymosis and hematoma. As mentioned earlier, pressure should be maintained on the injection site post block to avoid ecchymosis and hematoma formation. Because this technique elicits paresthesia, needle-induced trauma to the tibial nerve remains possible. By advancing the needle slowly and withdrawing the needle slightly away from the nerve prior to injection, one can avoid needle-induced trauma to the tibial nerve. This technique can safely be performed in the presence of anticoagulation by using a 25- or 27-gauge needle, albeit at increased risk of hematoma, if the clinical situation dictates a favorable risk-to-benefit ratio.

SUGGESTED READING

Waldman SD: Tibial nerve block at the ankle. In: Atlas of Interventional Pain Management, ed 2. Philadelphia, Saunders, 2004.

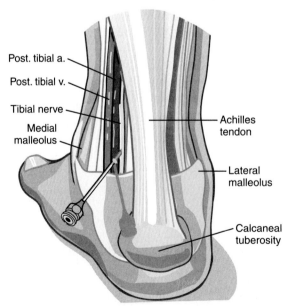

FIGURE 317–1 Tibial nerve block at the ankle. (From Waldman SD: Atlas of Interventional Pain Management, ed 2. Philadelphia, Saunders, 2004, p 486.)

Saphenous Nerve Block at the Knee

Saphenous nerve block at the knee is useful in the evaluation and management of distal lower extremity pain thought to be subserved by the saphenous nerve. The technique is also useful to provide surgical anesthesia for the distal lower extremity when combined with tibial and common peroneal nerve block or lumbar plexus block. It is used for this indication primarily in patients who would not tolerate the sympathetic changes induced by spinal or epidural anesthesia and who need distal lower extremity surgery, such as débridement or distal amputation. Saphenous nerve block at the knee with local anesthetic can be used diagnostically during differential neural blockade on an anatomic basis in the evaluation of lower extremity pain. If destruction of the saphenous nerve is being considered, this technique is useful as a prognostic indicator of the degree of motor and sensory impairment that the patient may experience. Saphenous nerve block at the knee with local anesthetic may be used to palliate acute pain emergencies, including distal lower extremity fractures and for postoperative pain relief, when combined with the previously mentioned blocks while waiting for pharmacologic methods to become effective. Saphenous nerve block at the knee with local anesthetic and steroid is occasionally used in the treatment of persistent distal lower extremity pain when the pain is thought to be secondary to inflammation or when entrapment of the saphenous nerve as it passes through Hunter's canal is suspected. Saphenous nerve block at the knee with local anesthetic and steroid is also indicated in the palliation of pain and motor dysfunction associated with diabetic neuropathy. Destruction of the saphenous nerve is occasionally used in the palliation of persistent lower extremity pain secondary to invasive tumor that is mediated by the saphenous nerve and has not responded to more conservative measures.

The saphenous nerve is the largest sensory branch of the femoral nerve. The saphenous nerve provides sensory innervation to the medial malleolus, the medial calf, and a portion of the medial arch of the foot. The saphenous nerve is derived primarily from the fibers of the L3 and L4 nerve roots. The nerve travels along with the femoral artery through Hunter's canal and moves superficially as it approaches the knee. It passes over the medial condyle of the femur, splitting into terminal sensory branches. The saphenous nerve is subject to trauma or compression anywhere along its course. The nerve is frequently traumatized during vein harvest procedures for coronary artery bypass grafting procedures. The saphenous nerve is also subject to compression as it passes over the medial condyle of the femur.

To perform saphenous nerve block at the knee, the patient is placed in the lateral position with the leg slightly flexed. The medial condyle of the femur is palpated. A point just in front of the posterior edge of the medial condyle is then identified and prepared with antiseptic solution. A 25-gauge, ½-inch needle is then slowly advanced through this point toward the medial condyle of the femur until paresthesia is elicited in the distribution of the saphenous nerve (Fig. 318-1). The patient should be warned to expect paresthesia and should be told to say "There!" immediately on perceiving the paresthesia. Paresthesia usually is elicited at a depth of ¼ to ½ inch. If paresthesia is not elicited, the needle is withdrawn and redirected slightly more anteriorly until paresthesia is obtained. Once paresthesia is elicited in the distribution of the saphenous nerve, the needle is withdrawn 1 mm, and the patient is observed to rule out any persistent paresthesia. If no persistent paresthesia is present and after careful aspiration, 5 mL of 1.0% preservative-free lidocaine is slowly injected. Care must be taken not to advance the needle into the substance of the nerve during the injection and inject solution intraneurally.

If the pain has an inflammatory component, the local anesthetic is combined with 80 mg of methylprednisolone and is injected in incremental doses. Subsequent daily nerve blocks are carried out in a similar manner, substituting 40 mg of methylprednisolone for the initial 80-mg dose. After injection of the solution, pressure is applied to the injection site to decrease the incidence of postblock ecchymosis and hematoma formation.

The main side effect of saphenous nerve block at the knee is postblock ecchymosis and hematoma, because the nerve is close to the greater saphenous artery. As mentioned, pressure should be maintained on the injection site post block to avoid ecchymosis and hematoma formation. Because this technique elicits a paresthesia, needle-induced trauma to the saphenous nerve remains possible. By advancing the needle slowly and withdrawing the needle slightly away from the nerve prior to injection, one can avoid needle-induced trauma to the saphenous nerve.

SUGGESTED READING

Waldman SD: Saphenous nerve block at the knee. In: Atlas of Interventional Pain Management, ed 2. Philadelphia, Saunders, 2004.

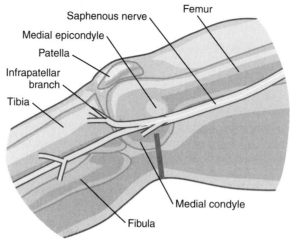

FIGURE 318–1 Saphenous nerve block at the knee. (From Waldman SD: Atlas of Interventional Pain Management, ed 2. Philadelphia, Saunders, 2004, p 490.)

CHAPTER 319

Common Peroneal Nerve Block at the Knee

Common peroneal nerve block is useful in the evaluation and management of distal lower extremity pain thought to be subserved by the common peroneal nerve. The technique is also useful to provide surgical anesthesia for the distal lower extremity when combined with tibial and saphenous nerve block or lumbar plexus block. It is used for this indication primarily in patients who would not tolerate the sympathetic changes induced by spinal or epidural anesthesia who need distal lower extremity surgery, such as débridement or distal amputation. Common peroneal nerve block with local anesthetic can be used as a diagnostic tool when performing differential neural blockade on an anatomic basis in the evaluation of lower extremity pain. If destruction of the common peroneal nerve is being considered, this technique is useful as a prognostic indicator of the degree of motor and sensory impairment that the patient may experience. Common peroneal nerve block with local anesthetic may be used to palliate acute pain emergencies, including distal lower extremity fractures and postoperative pain relief, when combined with the previously mentioned blocks while waiting for pharmacologic methods to become effective. Common peroneal nerve block with local anesthetic and steroid is occasionally used in the treatment of persistent distal lower extremity pain when the pain is thought to be

secondary to inflammation or when entrapment of the common peroneal nerve as it passes the head of the fibula is suspected. Common peroneal nerve block with local anesthetic and steroid is also indicated in the palliation of pain and motor dysfunction associated with diabetic neuropathy. Destruction of the common peroneal nerve is occasionally used in the palliation of persistent lower extremity pain secondary to invasive tumor that is mediated by the common peroneal nerve and has not responded to more conservative measures.

The common peroneal nerve is one of the two major continuations of the sciatic nerve, the other being the tibial nerve. The common peroneal nerve provides sensory innervation to the inferior portion of the knee joint and the posterior and lateral skin of the upper calf. The common peroneal nerve is derived from the posterior branches of the L4, L5, and S1-2 nerve roots. The nerve splits from the sciatic nerve at the superior margin of the popliteal fossa and descends laterally behind the head of the fibula. The common peroneal nerve is subject to compression at this point by such circumstances as improperly applied casts and tourniquets. The nerve is also subject to compression as it continues its lateral course, winding around the fibula through the fibular tunnel, which is made up of the posterior border of the tendinous insertion of the peroneus longus muscle and the fibula itself. Just distal to the fibular tunnel the nerve divides into its two terminal branches, the superficial and the deep peroneal nerves. Each of these branches is subject to trauma and may be blocked individually as a diagnostic and therapeutic maneuver.

To perform common peroneal nerve block at the knee, the patient is placed in the lateral position with the leg slightly flexed. The head of the fibula and the junction of fibular head and neck are palpated. A point just below the fibular head is then identified and prepared with antiseptic solution. A 25-gauge, ½-inch needle is then slowly advanced through this point toward the neck of the fibula until a paresthesia is elicited in the distribution of the common peroneal nerve (Fig. 319-1). The patient should be warned to expect a paresthesia and should be told to say "There!" immediately on perceiving the paresthesia. Paresthesia is usually elicited at a depth of ¼ to ½ inch. If paresthesia is not elicited, the needle is withdrawn and redirected slightly more posteriorly until a paresthesia is obtained. Once paresthesia is elicited in the distribution of the common peroneal nerve, the needle is withdrawn 1 mm, and the patient is observed to rule out any persistent paresthesia. If no persistent paresthesia is present and after careful aspiration, 5 mL of 1.0% preservative-free lidocaine is slowly injected. Care must be taken not to advance the needle into the substance of the nerve during the injection and inject solution intraneurally.

If the pain has an inflammatory component, the local anesthetic is combined with 80 mg of methylprednisolone and is injected in incremental doses. Subsequent daily nerve blocks are carried out in a similar manner, substituting 40 mg of methylprednisolone for the initial 80-mg dose. After injection of the solution, pressure is applied to the injection site to decrease the incidence of postblock ecchymosis and hematoma formation.

The main side effect of common peroneal nerve block is postblock ecchymosis and hematoma. As mentioned, pressure should be maintained on the injection site post block to avoid ecchymosis and hematoma formation. Because this technique elicits paresthesia, needle-induced trauma to the common peroneal nerve remains possible. By advancing the needle slowly and withdrawing the needle slightly away from the nerve prior to injection, one can avoid needle-induced trauma to the common peroneal nerve.

SUGGESTED READING

Waldman SD: Common peroneal nerve block at the knee. In: Atlas of Interventional Pain Management, ed 2. Philadelphia, Saunders, 2004.

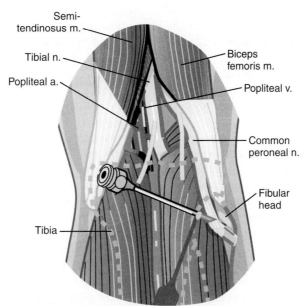

FIGURE 319–1 Common peroneal nerve block at the knee. (From Waldman SD: Atlas of Interventional Pain Management, ed 2. Philadelphia, Saunders, 2004, p 499.)

CHAPTER 320

Deep Peroneal Nerve Block at the Ankle

Deep peroneal nerve block is useful in the evaluation and management of foot pain thought to be subserved by the deep peroneal nerve. The technique is also useful to provide surgical anesthesia for the foot when combined with tibial and saphenous nerve block or lumbar plexus block. It is used for this indication primarily in patients who would not tolerate the sympathetic changes induced by spinal or epidural anesthesia who need foot surgery such as débridement or toe or forefoot amputation. Deep peroneal nerve block with local anesthetic can be used as a diagnostic tool when performing differential neural blockade on an anatomic basis in the evaluation of distal lower extremity pain. If destruction of the deep peroneal nerve is being considered, this technique is useful as a prognostic indicator of the degree of motor and sensory impairment that the patient may experience. Deep peroneal nerve block with local anesthetic may be used to palliate acute pain emergencies, including foot fractures and postoperative pain relief, when combined with the previously mentioned blocks while waiting for pharmacologic methods to become effective. Deep peroneal nerve block with local anesthetic and steroid is occasionally used in the treatment of persistent foot pain when the pain is thought to be secondary to inflammation or when entrapment of the deep peroneal nerve as it passes through the anterior tarsal tunnel is suspected. Deep peroneal nerve block with local anesthetic and steroid is also indicated in the palliation of pain and motor dysfunction associated with diabetic neuropathy. Destruction of the deep peroneal nerve is occasionally used in the palliation of persistent foot pain secondary to invasive tumor that is mediated by the deep peroneal nerve and has not responded to more conservative measures.

The common peroneal nerve is one of the two major continuations of the sciatic nerve, the other being the tibial nerve. The common peroneal nerve provides sensory innervation to the inferior portion of the knee joint and the posterior and lateral skin of the upper calf. The common peroneal nerve is derived from the posterior branches of the L4, L5, and S1-2 nerve roots. The nerve splits from the sciatic nerve at the superior margin of the popliteal fossa and descends laterally behind the head of the fibula. The common peroneal nerve is subject to compression at this point by such circumstances as improperly applied casts and tourniquets. The nerve is also subject to compression as it continues its lateral course, winding around the fibula through the fibular tunnel, which is made up of the posterior border of the tendinous insertion of the peroneus longus muscle and the fibula itself. Just distal to the fibular tunnel, the nerve divides into its two terminal branches, the superficial and the deep peroneal nerves. Each of these branches are subject to trauma and may be blocked individually as a diagnostic and therapeutic maneuver.

The deep branch continues down the leg in conjunction with the tibial artery and vein to provide sensory innervation to the web space of the first and second toes and adjacent dorsum of the foot. Although this distribution of sensory fibers is small, this area is often the site of Morton's neuroma surgery and thus is important to the regional anesthesiologist. The deep peroneal nerve provides motor innervation to all of the toe extensors and the anterior tibialis muscles. The deep peroneal nerve passes beneath the dense superficial fascia of the ankle, where it is subject to an entrapment syndrome known as the anterior tarsal tunnel syndrome.

To perform deep peroneal nerve block at the ankle, the patient is placed in the supine position with the leg extended. The extensor hallucis longus tendon is identified by having the patient extend his or her big toe against resistance. A point just medial to the tendon at the skin crease of the ankle is identified and prepared with antiseptic solution. A 25-gauge, 1½-inch needle is then slowly advanced through this point toward the tibia until a paresthesia is elicited into the web space between the first and second toe (Fig. 320-1). The patient should be warned to expect a paresthesia and should be told to say "There!" immediately on perceiving the paresthesia. Paresthesia is usually elicited at a depth of ¼ to ½ inch. If a paresthesia is not elicited, the needle is withdrawn and redirected slightly more posteriorly until paresthesia is obtained. Once paresthesia is elicited in the distribution of the deep peroneal nerve, the needle is withdrawn 1 mm, and the patient is observed to rule out any persistent paresthesia. If no persistent paresthesia is present and after careful aspiration, 6 to 8 mL of 1.0% preservative-free lidocaine is slowly injected. Care must be taken not to advance the needle into the substance of the nerve during the injection and inject solution intraneurally.

If the pain has an inflammatory component, the local anesthetic is combined with 80 mg of methylprednisolone and is injected in incremental doses. Subsequent daily nerve blocks are carried out in a similar manner, substituting 40 mg of methylprednisolone for the initial 80-mg dose. After injection of the solution, pressure is applied to the injection site to decrease the incidence of postblock ecchymosis and hematoma formation.

The main side effect of deep peroneal nerve block is postblock ecchymosis and hematoma. As mentioned earlier, pressure should be maintained on the injection site post block to avoid ecchymosis and hematoma formation. Because this technique elicits a paresthesia, needle-induced trauma to the deep peroneal nerve remains possible.

By advancing the needle slowly and withdrawing the needle slightly away from the nerve prior to injection, one can avoid needle-induced trauma to the deep peroneal nerve.

SUGGESTED READING

Waldman SD: Deep peroneal nerve block at the ankle. In: Atlas of Interventional Pain Management, ed 2. Philadelphia, Saunders, 2004.

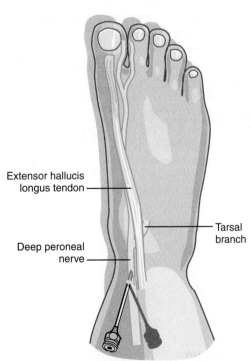

FIGURE 320–1 Deep peroneal nerve block at the ankle. (From Waldman SD: Atlas of Interventional Pain Management, ed 2. Philadelphia, Saunders, 2004, p 502.)

CHAPTER 321

Superficial Peroneal Nerve Block at the Ankle

The common peroneal nerve is one of the two major continuations of the sciatic nerve, the other being the tibial nerve. The common peroneal nerve provides sensory innervation to the inferior portion of the knee joint and the posterior and lateral skin of the upper calf. The common peroneal nerve is derived from the posterior branches of the L4, L5, and S1-2 nerve roots. The nerve splits from the sciatic nerve at the superior margin of the popliteal fossa and descends laterally behind the head of the fibula. The common peroneal nerve is subject to compression at this point by such circumstances as improperly applied casts and tourniquets. The nerve is also subject to compression as it continues its lateral course, winding around the fibula through the fibular tunnel, which is made up of the posterior border of the tendinous insertion of the peroneus longus muscle and the fibula itself. Just distal to the fibular tunnel, the nerve divides into its two terminal branches, the superficial and the deep peroneal nerves. Each of these branches is subject to trauma and may be blocked individually as a diagnostic and therapeutic maneuver.

The superficial branch continues down the leg in conjunction with the extensor digitorum longus muscle. The nerve divides into terminal branches at a point just above the ankle. These fibers of these terminal branches provide sensory innervation to most of the dorsum of the foot except for the area adjacent to the web space of the first and second toes, which is supplied by the deep peroneal nerve. The superficial peroneal nerve also provides sensory innervation to the toes except for the area between the first and second toe, which is supplied by the deep peroneal nerve.

To perform superficial nerve block at the ankle, the patient is placed in the supine position with the leg extended. One identifies the extensor hallucis longus tendon by having the patient extend his or her big toe against resistance. A point just medial to the tendon at the skin crease of the ankle is identified and prepared with antiseptic solution. A 25-gauge, 1½-inch needle is then slowly advanced through this point; during injection, the needle is advanced subcutaneously toward the lateral malleolus (Fig. 321-1). A total of 7 to 8 mL of 1.0% preservative-free lidocaine should be injected to ensure that all the terminal branches of the superficial peroneal nerve are blocked.

If the pain has an inflammatory component, the local anesthetic is combined with 80 mg of methylprednisolone and is injected in incremental doses. Subsequent daily nerve blocks are carried out in a similar manner, substituting 40 mg of methylprednisolone for the initial 80-mg dose. After injection of the solution, pressure is applied to the injection site to decrease the incidence of postblock ecchymosis and hematoma formation.

The main side effect of superficial peroneal nerve block is postblock ecchymosis and hematoma. As mentioned, pressure should be maintained on the injection site post block to avoid ecchymosis and hematoma formation. Because of proximity to the deep peroneal nerve, this nerve frequently is blocked during superficial peroneal nerve block.

SUGGESTED READING

Waldman SD: Superficial peroneal nerve block at the ankle. In: Atlas of Interventional Pain Management, ed 2. Philadelphia, Saunders, 2004.

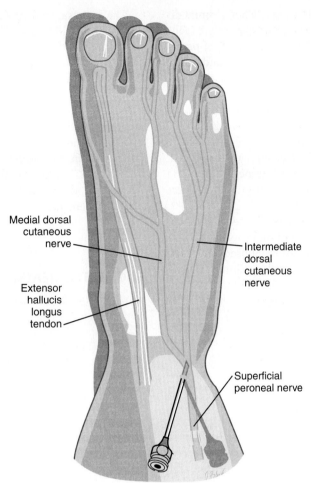

FIGURE 321–1 Superficial peroneal nerve block at the ankle. (From Waldman SD: Atlas of Interventional Pain Management, ed 2. Philadelphia, Saunders, 2004, p 508.)

Medial dorsal cutaneous nerve

Extensor hallucis longus tendon

Intermediate dorsal cutaneous nerve

Superficial peroneal nerve

CHAPTER 322

Sural Nerve Block at the Ankle

The sural nerve is a branch of the posterior tibial nerve. The sural nerve passes from the posterior calf around the lateral malleolus to provide sensor innervation of the posterior lateral aspect of the calf and the lateral surface of the foot and fifth toe and the plantar surface of the heel. The sural nerve is subject to compression at the ankle and is known as *boot syndrome* because it is associated with compression of the nerve by boots that are too tight.

To perform sural nerve block at the ankle, the patient is placed in the lateral position with the affected leg in the superior position and slightly flexed. The posterior groove behind the lateral malleolus is identified by palpation. The area between the lateral malleolus and the Achilles tendon is identified and prepared with antiseptic solutions. A 25-gauge, 1½-inch needle is inserted at this level and directed anteriorly toward the lateral malleolus. The needle is then advanced slowly toward the sural nerve, which lies in the posterior groove of the lateral malleolus, until paresthesia is elicited in the distribution of the sural nerve (Fig. 322-1). The patient should be warned to expect a paresthesia and should be told to say "There!" immediately on perceiving the paresthesia. Paresthesia is usually elicited after the needle is advanced ½ to ¾ inch. If paresthesia is not elicited, the needle is withdrawn and redirected slightly more cephalad until paresthesia is obtained. Once paresthesia is elicited in the distribution of the sural nerve, the needle is withdrawn 1 mm, and the patient is observed to rule out any persistent paresthesia. If no persistent paresthesia is present and after careful aspiration, 6 mL of 1.0% preservative-free lidocaine is slowly injected. Care must be taken not to advance the needle into the substance of the nerve during the injection and to inject solution intraneurally.

If the pain has an inflammatory component, the local anesthetic is combined with 80 mg of methylprednisolone and is injected in incremental doses. Subsequent daily nerve blocks are carried out in a similar manner, substituting 40 mg of methylprednisolone for the initial 80-mg dose. After injection of the solution, pressure is applied to the injection site to decrease the incidence of postblock ecchymosis and hematoma formation.

The main side effect of sural nerve block at the ankle is postblock ecchymosis and hematoma. As mentioned, pressure should be maintained on the injection site post block to avoid ecchymosis and hematoma formation. Because this technique elicits paresthesia, needle-induced trauma to the sural nerve remains possible. By advancing the needle slowly and withdrawing the needle slightly away from the nerve, one can avoid needle-induced trauma to the sural nerve. This technique can be safely performed in the presence of anticoagulation by using a 25- or 27-gauge needle, albeit at increased risk of hematoma, if the clinical situation dictates a favorable risk-to-benefit ratio.

SUGGESTED READING

Waldman SD: Sural nerve block at the ankle. In: Atlas of Interventional Pain Management, ed 2. Philadelphia, Saunders, 2004.

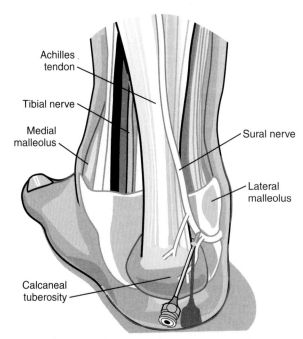

FIGURE 322–1 Sural nerve block at the ankle. (From Waldman SD: Atlas of Interventional Pain Management, ed 2. Philadelphia, Saunders, 2004, p 512.)

CHAPTER **323**

Metatarsal and Digital Nerve Block at the Ankle

Metatarsal and digital nerve block is used primarily in two clinical situations: (1) to provide surgical anesthesia in the distribution of the digital nerves for laceration, tendon, and fracture repair and (2) to provide postoperative pain relief after joint replacement or major surgical procedures on the foot.

In a manner analogous to that of the digital nerves of the hand, the digital nerves of the foot travel through the intrametatarsal space to innervate each toe. The plantar digital nerves, which are derived from the posterior tibial nerve, provide sensory innervation to the major portion of the plantar surface. The dorsal aspect of the foot is innervated by terminal branches of the deep and superficial peroneal nerves. The overlap in the sensory innervation of these nerves may be considerable.

To perform metatarsal and digital nerve block, the patient is placed in a supine position with a pillow placed under the knee to slightly flex the leg. A total of 3 mL per digit of non–epinephrine-containing local anesthetic is drawn up in a 12-mL sterile syringe.

Metatarsal Nerve Block

After preparation of the skin with antiseptic solution, at a point proximal to the metatarsal head, a 25-gauge, 1½-inch needle is inserted just adjacent to the metatarsal bone to be blocked (Fig. 323-1). While the clinician is slowly injecting, the needle is advanced from the dorsal surface of the foot toward the plantar surface. The plantar digital nerve is situated on the dorsal side of the flexor retinaculum—thus, the needle has to be advanced almost to the plantar surface of the foot in order to produce satisfactory anesthesia. The needle is removed, and pressure is placed on the injection site to avoid hematoma formation.

Digital Nerve Block

After preparation of the skin with antiseptic solution, at a point at the base of the toe, a 25-gauge, 1½-inch needle is inserted just adjacent to the bone of the digit to be blocked (Fig. 323-2). While slowly injecting, the needle is advanced from the dorsal surface of the foot toward the plantar surface. The needle is removed, and pressure is placed on the injection site to avoid hematoma formation.

Because of the confined nature of the soft tissue surrounding the metatarsals and digits, the potential for mechanical compression of the blood supply after injection of solution must be considered. The pain specialist must avoid rapidly injecting large volumes of solution into these confined spaces, or vascular insufficiency and gangrene may occur. Furthermore, epinephrine-containing solutions must always be avoided to avoid ischemia and possible gangrene.

This technique can be safely performed in the presence of anticoagulation by using a 25- or 27-gauge needle, albeit at increased risk of hematoma, if the clinical situation dictates a favorable risk-to-benefit ratio. These complications can be decreased if manual pressure is applied to the area of the block immediately after injection. Application of cold packs for 10-minute periods after the block also decreases the amount of postprocedure pain and bleeding. Although uncommon, infection remains an ever present possibility following blockade of the metatarsal and digital nerves.

SUGGESTED READING

Waldman SD: Metatarsal and digital nerve block at the ankle. In: Atlas of Interventional Pain Management, ed 2. Philadelphia, Saunders, 2004.

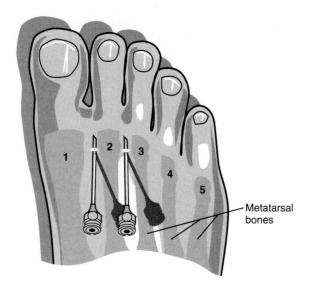

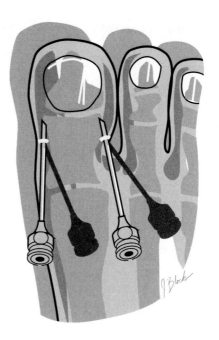

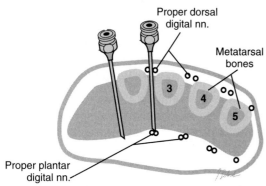

FIGURE 323–1 Metatarsal nerve block at the ankle. (From Waldman SD: Atlas of Interventional Pain Management, ed 2. Philadelphia, Saunders, 2004, p 514.)

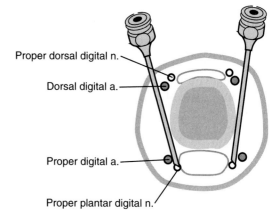

FIGURE 323–2 Digital nerve block at the ankle. (From Waldman SD: Atlas of Interventional Pain Management, ed 2. Philadelphia, Saunders, 2004, p 515.)

CHAPTER 324

Intra-articular Injection of the Knee

The rounded condyles of the femur articulate with the condyles of the tibia below and the patella anteriorly. The articular surface is covered with hyaline cartilage, which is susceptible to arthritis. The joint is surrounded laterally and posteriorly by a capsule that provides support for the joint. The capsule is absent anteriorly, and in its place is the suprapatellar and infrapatellar bursa. Laterally and medially, the joint is strengthened by the tendons of the vastus lateralis and medius muscles. Posteriorly, the joint is strengthened by the oblique popliteal ligament. Also adding to the strength of the joint is a variety of extracapsular ligaments, including the medial and lateral collateral ligaments and the ligamentum patellae anteriorly and the oblique popliteal ligament posteriorly. Within the joint capsule there is also a variety of ligaments that add to the strength of the joint, including the anterior and posterior cruciate ligaments.

The joint capsule is lined with a synovial membrane that attaches to the articular cartilage and gives rise to a number of bursa, including the suprapatellar and infrapatellar bursae. The knee joint is innervated by the femoral, obturator, common peroneal, and tibial nerves. In addition to arthritis, the knee joint is susceptible to the development of tendinitis, bursitis, and disruption of the ligaments, cartilage, and tendons.

To perform intra-articular injection of the knee, the patient is placed in the supine position with a rolled blanket underneath the knee to gently flex the joint. The skin overlying the medial joint is prepped with antiseptic solution. A sterile syringe containing 5.0 mL of 0.25% preservative-free bupivacaine and 40 mg of methylprednisolone is attached to a 1½-inch, 25-gauge needle using strict aseptic technique. With strict aseptic technique, the joint space is identified. The clinician places his or her thumb on the lateral margin of the patella and pushes it medially. At a point at the middle of the medial edge of the patella, the needle is inserted between the patella and femoral condyles. The needle is then carefully advanced through the skin and subcutaneous tissues through the joint capsule into the joint (Fig. 324-1). If bone is encountered, the needle is withdrawn into the subcutaneous tissues and redirected superiorly. After entering the joint space, the contents of the syringe are gently injected. There should be little resistance to injection. If resistance is encountered, the needle is probably in a ligament or tendon and should be advanced slightly into the joint space until the injection proceeds without significant resistance. The needle is then removed, and a sterile pressure dressing and ice pack are placed at the injection site.

The major complication of intra-articular injection of the knee is infection, which should be exceedingly rare if strict aseptic technique is adhered to. Approximately 25% of patients complain of a transient increase in pain after intra-articular injection of the knee joint; the patient should be warned of this.

SUGGESTED READING

Waldman SD: Intra-articular injection of the knee joint. In: Atlas of Pain Management Injection Techniques, ed 2. Philadelphia, Saunders, 2007.

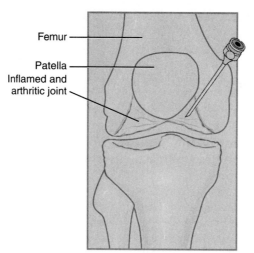

Femur

Patella
Inflamed and
arthritic joint

FIGURE 324–1 Intra-articular injection of the knee. (From Waldman SD: Atlas of Pain Management Injection Techniques, ed 2. Philadelphia, Saunders, 2007, p 420.)

CHAPTER 325

Injection Technique for Suprapatellar Bursitis

The suprapatellar bursa is vulnerable to injury from both acute trauma and repeated microtrauma. Acute injuries frequently take the form of direct trauma to the bursa via falls directly onto the knee or from patellar fractures, as well as from overuse injuries, including running on soft or uneven surfaces, or from jobs that require crawling on the knees such as carpet laying. If the inflammation of the suprapatellar bursa becomes chronic, calcification of the bursa may occur.

The patient who suffers from suprapatellar bursitis frequently complains of pain in the anterior knee above the patella that can radiate superiorly into the distal anterior thigh. Often, the patient is unable to kneel or walk down stairs. The patient also may complain of a sharp "catching" sensation with range of motion of the knee, especially on first rising. Suprapatellar bursitis often coexists with arthritis and tendinitis of the knee joint, and these other pathologic processes may confuse the clinical picture.

Physical examination may reveal point tenderness in the anterior knee just above the patella. Passive flexion as well as active resisted extension of the knee reproduces the pain. Sudden release of resistance during this maneuver markedly increases the pain. There may be swelling in the suprapatellar region with a "boggy" feeling to palpation. Occasionally, the suprapatellar bursa may become infected with systemic symptoms, including fever and malaise, as well as local symptoms, including rubor, color, and dolor being present.

Plain radiographs of the knee may reveal calcification of the bursa and associated structures, including the quadriceps tendon, consistent with chronic inflammation. Magnetic resonance imaging is indicated if internal derangement, occult mass, or tumor of the knee is suspected. Electromyography helps distinguish suprapatellar bursitis from femoral neuropathy, lumbar radiculopathy, and plexopathy. The following injection technique serves as a diagnostic and therapeutic maneuver.

The suprapatellar bursa extends superiorly from beneath the patella under the quadriceps femoris muscle and its tendon. The bursa is held in place by a small portion of the vastus intermedius muscle, called the articularis genus muscle. Both the quadriceps tendon and the suprapatellar bursa are subject to the development of inflammation caused by overuse, misuse, or direct trauma. The quadriceps tendon is made up of fibers from the four muscles that comprise the quadriceps muscle: the vastus lateralis, the vastus intermedius, the vastus medialis, and the rectus femoris. These muscles are the primary extensors of the lower extremity at the knee. The tendons of these muscles converge and unite to form a single, exceedingly strong tendon. The patella functions as a sesamoid bone within the quadriceps tendon, with fibers of the tendon expanding around the patella and forming the medial and lateral patella retinacula, which help strengthen the knee joint. These fibers are called expansions and are subject to strain; the tendon proper is subject to the development of tendinitis. The suprapatellar, infrapatellar, and prepatellar bursae also may concurrently become inflamed with dysfunction of the quadriceps tendon.

To perform injection of the suprapatellar bursa, the patient is placed in the supine position with a rolled blanket underneath the knee to gently flex the joint. The skin overlying the medial aspect of the knee joint is prepped with antiseptic solution. A sterile syringe containing 2.0 mL of 0.25% preservative-free bupivacaine and 40 mg of methylprednisolone is attached to a 1½-inch, 25-gauge needle using strict aseptic technique. With strict aseptic technique, the superior margin of the medial patella is identified. Just above this point, the needle is inserted horizontally to slide just beneath the quadriceps tendon

(Fig. 325-1). If the needle strikes the femur, it is then withdrawn slightly and redirected in a more anterior trajectory. When the needle is in position just below the quadriceps tendon, the contents of the syringe are then gently injected. There should be little resistance to injection. If resistance is encountered, the needle is probably in a ligament or tendon and should be advanced or withdrawn slightly until the injection proceeds without significant resistance. The needle is then removed, and a sterile pressure dressing and ice pack are placed at the injection site.

The major complication of this injection technique is infection, which should be exceedingly rare if strict aseptic technique is adhered to. Approximately 25% of patients complain of a transient increase in pain after injection of the suprapatellar bursa of the knee; the patient should be warned of this.

SUGGESTED READING

Waldman SD: Injection technique for suprapatellar bursitis. In: Atlas of Pain Management Injection Techniques, ed 2. Philadelphia, Saunders, 2007.

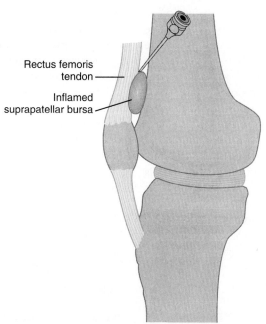

Rectus femoris tendon

Inflamed suprapatellar bursa

FIGURE 325–1 Injection technique for suprapatellar bursitis. (From Waldman SD: Atlas of Pain Management Injection Techniques, ed 2. Philadelphia, Saunders, 2007, p 452.)

CHAPTER 326

Prepatellar Bursitis

The prepatellar bursa is vulnerable to injury from both acute trauma and repeated microtrauma. Acute injuries frequently take the form of direct trauma to the bursa via falls directly onto the knee or from patellar fractures, as well as from overuse injuries, including running on soft or uneven surfaces. Prepatellar bursitis also may result from jobs that require crawling or kneeling such as carpet laying or scrubbing floors; the other name for prepatellar bursitis is "housemaid's knee." If the inflammation of the prepatellar bursa becomes chronic, calcification of the bursa may occur.

The patient who suffers from prepatellar bursitis frequently complains of pain and swelling in the anterior knee over the patella that can radiate superiorly and inferiorly into the area surrounding the knee. Often, the patient is unable to kneel or walk down stairs. The patient also may complain of a sharp "catching" sensation with range of motion of the knee, especially on first rising. Prepatellar bursitis often coexists with arthritis and tendinitis of the knee joint and these other pathologic processes may confuse the clinical picture.

Physical examination may reveal point tenderness in the anterior knee just above the patella. Swelling and fluid accumulation surrounding the patella often is present. Passive flexion as well as active resisted extension of the knee reproduces the pain. Sudden release of resistance during this maneuver markedly increases the pain. The prepatellar bursa may become infected with systemic symptoms, including fever and malaise, as well as local symptoms including rubor, color, and dolor.

Plain radiographs of the knee may reveal calcification of the bursa and associated structures, including the quadriceps tendon, consistent with chronic inflammation. Magnetic resonance imaging is indicated if bursitis, internal derangement, occult mass, or tumor of the knee is suspected. Electromyography helps distinguish prepatellar bursitis from femoral neuropathy, lumbar radiculopathy, and plexopathy. The following injection technique serves as a diagnostic and therapeutic maneuver.

The prepatellar bursa lies between the subcutaneous tissues and the patella. The bursa is held in place by ligamentum patellae. Both the quadriceps tendon and the prepatellar bursa are subject to the development of inflammation caused by overuse, misuse, or direct trauma. The quadriceps tendon is made up of fibers from the four muscles that comprise the quadriceps muscle: the vastus lateralis, the vastus intermedius, the vastus medialis, and the rectus femoris. These muscles are the primary extensors of the lower extremity at the knee. The tendons of these muscles converge and unite to form a single, exceedingly strong tendon. The patella functions as a sesamoid bone within the quadriceps tendon, with fibers of the tendon expanding around the patella and forming the medial and lateral patella retinacula, which help strengthen the knee joint. These fibers are called expansions and are subject to strain; the tendon proper is subject to the development of tendinitis. The prepatellar, infrapatellar, and prepatellar bursa also may concurrently become inflamed with dysfunction of the quadriceps tendon.

To perform injection of the prepatellar bursa, the patient is placed in the supine position with a rolled blanket underneath the knee to gently flex the joint. The skin overlying the patella is prepared with antiseptic solution. A sterile syringe containing 2.0 mL of 0.25% preservative-free bupivacaine and 40 mg of methylprednisolone is attached to a 1½-inch, 25-gauge needle using strict aseptic technique. With strict aseptic technique, the center of the medial patella is identified. Just above this point, the needle is inserted horizontally to slide subcutaneously into the prepatellar bursa (Fig. 326-1). If the needle strikes the patella, it is then withdrawn slightly and redirected in a more anterior trajectory. When the needle is in position in proximity to the prepatellar bursa, the contents of the syringe are then gently injected. There should be little resistance to injection. If resistance is encountered, the needle is probably in a ligament or tendon and should be advanced or withdrawn slightly until the injection proceeds without significant resistance. The needle is then removed, and a sterile pressure dressing and ice pack are placed at the injection site.

The major complication of this injection technique is infection, which should be exceedingly rare if strict aseptic technique is adhered to. Approximately 25% of patients complain of a transient increase in pain after injection of the prepatellar bursa of the knee; the patient should be warned of this.

SUGGESTED READING

Waldman SD: Injection technique for prepatellar bursitis. In: Atlas of Pain Management Injection Techniques, ed. 2. Philadelphia, Saunders, 2007.

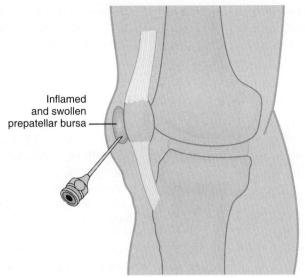

FIGURE 326–1 Injection technique for prepatellar bursitis. (From Waldman SD: Atlas of Pain Management Injection Techniques, ed. 2. Philadelphia, Saunders, 2007, p 455.)

CHAPTER 327

Injection Technique for Superficial Infrapatellar Bursitis

Both infrapatellar bursae are vulnerable to injury from both acute trauma and repeated microtrauma. Acute injuries frequently take the form of direct trauma to the bursae via falls directly onto the knee or from patellar fractures, as well as from overuse injuries, including long-distance running. Infrapatellar bursitis also may result from jobs that require crawling or kneeling, such as carpet laying or scrubbing floors. If the inflammation of the infrapatellar bursae becomes chronic, calcification of the bursae may occur.

The patient suffering from infrapatellar bursitis frequently complains of pain and swelling in the anterior knee below the patella that can radiate inferiorly into the area surrounding the knee. Often, the patient is unable to kneel or walk down stairs. The patient also may complain of a sharp "catching" sensation with range of motion of the knee, especially on first rising. Infrapatellar bursitis often coexists with arthritis and tendinitis of the knee joint, and these other pathologic processes may confuse the clinical picture.

Physical examination may reveal point tenderness in the anterior knee just below the patella. Swelling and fluid accumulation that surrounds the lower patella is often present. Passive flexion as well as active resisted extension of the knee reproduces the pain. Sudden release of resistance during this maneuver markedly increases the pain. The superficial infrapatellar bursa may become infected, with systemic symptoms, including fever and malaise, as well as local symptoms including rubor, color, and dolor being present.

Plain radiographs of the knee may reveal calcification of the bursa and associated structures, including the quadriceps tendon, consistent with chronic inflammation. Magnetic resonance imaging is indicated if bursitis, internal derangement, occult mass, or tumor of the knee is suspected. Electromyography helps distinguish infrapatellar bursitis from neuropathy, lumbar radiculopathy, and plexopathy. The following injection technique serves as a diagnostic and therapeutic maneuver.

The superficial infrapatellar bursa lies between the subcutaneous tissues and the ligamentum patellae. The bursa is held in place by ligamentum patellae. Both the ligamentum patellae as well as the superficial infrapatellar bursa are subject to the development of inflammation caused by overuse, misuse, or direct trauma. The ligamentum patellae attach above to the lower patella and below to the tibia.

The fibers that make up the ligamentum patellae are continuations of the tendon of the quadriceps femoris muscle. The quadriceps tendon is made up of fibers from the four muscles that comprise the quadriceps muscle: the vastus lateralis, the vastus intermedius, the vastus medialis, and the rectus femoris. These muscles are the primary extensors of the lower extremity at the knee. The tendons of these muscles converge and unite to form a single, exceedingly strong tendon. The patella functions as a sesamoid bone within the quadriceps tendon, with fibers of the tendon expanding around the patella, thereby forming the medial and lateral patella retinacula, which help strengthen the knee joint. These fibers are called expansions and are subject to strain; the tendon proper is subject to the development of tendinitis.

To perform injection of the superficial infrapatellar bursa, the patient is placed in the supine position with a rolled blanket underneath the knee to gently flex the joint. The skin overlying the patella is prepped with antiseptic solution. A sterile syringe containing 2.0 mL of 0.25% preservative-free bupivacaine and 40 mg of methylprednisolone is attached to a 1½-inch, 25-gauge needle using strict aseptic technique. With strict aseptic technique, the center of the lower pole of the patella is identified. Just below this point, the needle is inserted at a 45-degree angle to slide subcutaneously into the superficial infrapatellar bursa (Fig. 327-1). If the needle strikes the patella, it is then withdrawn slightly and redirected in a more inferior trajectory. When the needle is in position in proximity to the superficial infrapatellar bursa, the contents of the syringe are then gently injected. There should be little resistance to injection. If resistance is encountered, the needle is probably in a ligament or tendon and should be advanced or withdrawn slightly until the injection proceeds without significant resistance. The needle is then removed, and a sterile pressure dressing and ice pack are placed at the injection site.

The major complication of this injection technique is infection, which should be exceedingly rare if strict aseptic technique is adhered to. Approximately 25% of patients complain of a transient increase in pain after injection of the superficial infrapatellar bursa of the knee; the patient should be warned of this.

SUGGESTED READING

Waldman SD: Injection technique for superficial infrapatellar bursitis. In: Atlas of Pain Management Injection Techniques, ed. 2. Philadelphia, Saunders, 2007.

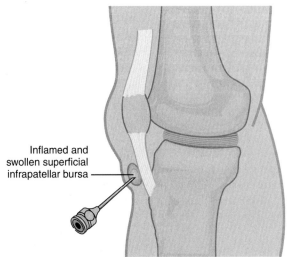

Inflamed and swollen superficial infrapatellar bursa

FIGURE 327–1 Injection technique for superficial infrapatellar bursitis. (From Waldman SD: Atlas of Pain Management Injection Techniques, ed. 2. Philadelphia, Saunders, 2007, p 463.)

Injection Technique for Deep Infrapatellar Bursitis

The infrapatellar bursa is vulnerable to injury from both acute trauma and repeated microtrauma. Acute injuries frequently take the form of direct trauma to the bursae via falls directly onto the knee or from patellar fractures, as well as from overuse injuries, including long-distance running. Infrapatellar bursitis also may result from jobs that require crawling or kneeling, such as carpet laying or scrubbing floors. If the inflammation of the infrapatellar bursae becomes chronic, calcification of the bursae may occur.

The patient who suffers from deep infrapatellar bursitis frequently complains of pain and swelling in the anterior knee below the patella that can radiate inferiorly into the area surrounding the knee. Often, the patient is unable to kneel or walk down stairs. The patient also may complain of a sharp "catching" sensation with range of motion of the knee, especially on first rising. Infrapatellar bursitis often coexists with arthritis and tendinitis of the knee joint, and these other pathologic processes may confuse the clinical picture.

Physical examination may reveal point tenderness in the anterior knee just below the patella. Swelling fluid accumulation that surrounds the lower patella is often present. Passive flexion as well as active resisted extension of the knee reproduces the pain. Sudden release of resistance during this maneuver markedly increases the pain. The deep infrapatellar bursa is not as susceptible to infection as the superficial infrapatellar bursa.

Plain radiographs of the knee may reveal calcification of the bursa and associated structures, including the quadriceps tendon, consistent with chronic inflammation. Magnetic resonance imaging is indicated if bursitis, internal derangement, occult mass, or tumor of the knee is suspected. Electromyography helps distinguish infrapatellar bursitis from neuropathy, lumbar radiculopathy, and plexopathy. The following injection technique serves as a diagnostic and therapeutic maneuver.

The deep infrapatellar bursa lies between the ligamentum patellae and the tibia. The bursa is held in place by ligamentum patellae. Both the ligamentum patellae as well as the deep infrapatellar bursa are subject to the development of inflammation following overuse, misuse, or direct trauma. The ligamentum patellae attaches above to the lower patella and below to the tibia. These fibers that make up the ligamentum patellae are continuations of the tendon of the quadriceps femoris muscle. The quadriceps tendon is made up of fibers from the four muscles that comprise the quadriceps muscle: the vastus lateralis, the vastus intermedius, the vastus medialis, and the rectus femoris. These muscles are the primary extensors of the lower extremity at the knee. The tendons of these muscles converge and unite to form a single, exceedingly strong tendon. The patella functions as a sesamoid bone within the quadriceps tendon, with fibers of the tendon expanding around the patella and thereby forming the medial and lateral patella retinacula, which help strengthen the knee joint. These fibers are called expansions and are subject to strain; the tendon proper is subject to the development of tendinitis.

To perform injection of the deep infrapatellar bursa, the patient is placed in the supine position with a rolled blanket underneath the knee to gently flex the joint. The skin overlying the medial portion of the lower margin of the patella is prepped with antiseptic solution. A sterile syringe containing 2.0 mL of 0.25% preservative-free bupivacaine and 40 mg of methylprednisolone is attached to a 1½-inch, 25-gauge needle using strict aseptic technique. With strict aseptic technique, the medial lower margin of the patella is identified. Just below this point, the needle is inserted at a right angle to the patella to slide beneath the ligamentum patellar into the deep infrapatellar bursa (Fig. 328-1). If the needle strikes the patella, it is then withdrawn slightly and redirected in a more inferior trajectory. When the needle is in position in proximity to the deep infrapatellar bursa, the contents of the syringe are then gently injected. There should be little resistance to injection. If resistance is encountered, the needle is probably in a ligament or tendon and should be advanced or withdrawn slightly until the injection proceeds without significant resistance. The needle is then removed, and a sterile pressure dressing and ice pack are placed at the injection site.

The major complication of this injection technique is infection, which should be exceedingly rare if strict aseptic technique is adhered to. Approximately 25% of patients complain of a transient increase in pain after injection of the deep infrapatellar bursa of the knee; the patient should be warned of this.

SUGGESTED READING

Waldman SD: Injection technique for deep infrapatellar bursitis. In: Atlas of Pain Management Injection Techniques, ed. 2. Philadelphia, Saunders, 2007.

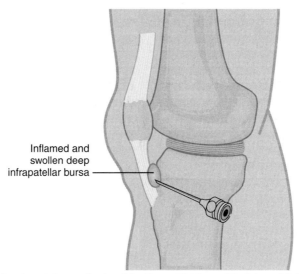

Inflamed and
swollen deep
infrapatellar bursa

FIGURE 328–1 Injection technique for deep infrapatellar bursitis. (From Waldman SD: Atlas of Pain Management Injection Techniques, ed. 2. Philadelphia, Saunders, 2007, p 463.)

CHAPTER 329

Intra-articular Injection of the Ankle Joint

The ankle is a hinge-type articulation between the distal tibia, the two malleoli, and the talus. The articular surface is covered with hyaline cartilage, which is susceptible to arthritis. The joint is surrounded by a dense capsule, which helps strengthen the ankle. The joint capsule is lined with a synovial membrane that attaches to the articular cartilage. The ankle joint is innervated by the deep peroneal and tibial nerves. The major ligaments of the ankle joint include the deltoid, anterior talofibular, calcaneofibular, and posterior talofibular ligaments, which provide the majority of strength to the ankle joint. The muscles of the ankle and their attaching tendons are susceptible to trauma and to wear and tear from overuse and misuse.

To perform intra-articular injection of the ankle joint, the patient is placed in the supine position and proper preparation with antiseptic solution of the skin overlying the ankle joint is carried out. A sterile syringe containing 2.0 mL of 0.25% preservative-free bupivacaine and 40 mg of methylprednisolone is attached to a 1½-inch, 25-gauge needle using strict aseptic technique. With strict aseptic technique, with the foot in neutral position, the junction of the tibia and fibula just above the talus is identified. At this point, a triangular indentation that indicates the joint space is easily palpable. The needle is then carefully advanced through the skin and subcutaneous tissues, through the joint capsule, and into the joint (Fig. 329-1). If bone is encountered, the needle is withdrawn into the subcutaneous tissues and redirected superiorly and slightly more medial. After entering the joint space, the contents of the syringe are gently injected. There should be little resistance to injection. If resistance is encountered, the needle is probably in a ligament or tendon and should be advanced slightly into the joint space until the injection proceeds without significant resistance. The needle is then removed, and a sterile pressure dressing and ice pack are placed at the injection site.

The major complication of intra-articular injection of the ankle is infection, which should be exceedingly rare if strict aseptic technique is adhered to. Approximately 25% of patients complain of a transient increase in pain after intra-articular injection of the ankle joint; the patient should be warned of this.

SUGGESTED READING

Waldman SD: Injection technique for intra-articular injection of the ankle joint. In: Atlas of Pain Management Injection Techniques, ed. 2. Philadelphia, Saunders, 2007.

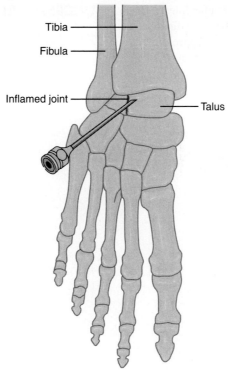

FIGURE 329–1 Intra-articular injection of the ankle joint. (From Waldman SD: Atlas of Pain Management Injection Techniques, ed. 2. Philadelphia, Saunders, 2007, p 463.)

CHAPTER **330**

Intra-articular Injection of the Toe Joints

Each toe joint has its own capsule. The articular surface of these joints is covered with hyaline cartilage, which is susceptible to arthritis. The toe joint capsules are lined with a synovial membrane that attaches to the articular cartilage. The deep transverse ligaments connect the joints of the five toes and provide the majority of strength to the toe joints. The muscles of the toe joint and their attaching tendons are susceptible to trauma and to wear and tear from overuse and misuse.

To perform intra-articular injection of the toe, the patient is placed in the supine position and proper preparation with antiseptic solution of the skin overlying the affected toe joint is carried out. A sterile syringe containing 1.5 mL of 0.25% preservative-free bupivacaine and 40 mg of methylprednisolone is attached to a $\frac{5}{8}$-inch, 25-gauge needle using strict aseptic technique.

With strict aseptic technique, the affected toe is distracted to open the joint space. The joint space is then identified. At this point, the needle is carefully advanced perpendicular to the joint space just next to the extensor tendons, through the skin and subcutaneous tissues, through the joint capsule, and into the joint (Fig. 330-1). If bone is encountered, the needle is withdrawn into the subcutaneous tissues and redirected superiorly. After entering the joint space, the contents of the syringe are gently injected. There should be little resistance to injection. If resistance is encountered, the needle is probably in a ligament or tendon and should be advanced slightly into the joint space until the injection proceeds without significant resistance. The needle is then removed, and a sterile pressure dressing and ice pack are placed at the injection site.

The major complication of intra-articular injection of the toe joint is infection, which should be exceedingly rare if strict aseptic technique is adhered to. Approximately 25% of patients complain of a transient increase in pain after intra-articular injection of the toe joint; the patient should be warned of this.

SUGGESTED READING

Waldman SD: Injection technique for intra-articular injection of the toe joints. In: Atlas of Pain Management Injection Techniques, ed. 2. Philadelphia, Saunders, 2007.

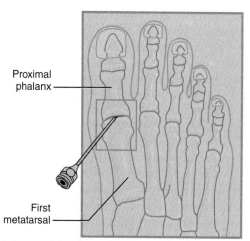

Proximal phalanx

First metatarsal

FIGURE 330–1 Intra-articular injection of the toe joint. (From Waldman SD: Atlas of Pain Management Injection Techniques, ed. 2. Philadelphia, Saunders, 2007, p 509.)

Lumbar Subarachnoid Neurolytic Block

Lumbar subarachnoid neurolytic block is used primarily in patients suffering from pain of malignant origin that is localized to one to three spinal segments and that has failed to respond to other conservative therapy. Because of the potential for serious complications, this technique is rarely used for patients suffering from chronic benign pain, but it may be considered after a careful analysis of the risk-to-benefit ratio in carefully selected patients. Because this technique is most successful when treating pain that is subserved by a limited number of spinal nerves, lumbar subarachnoid neurolytic block has found its greatest utility in the treatment of pain involving lower extremity and lower back pain, such as the pain of tumors invading the lumbar plexus or metastatic prostate or colon malignancy. Given the unique ability of this technique to allow destruction of the sensory component of the spinal root while theoretically sparing the motor component, this technique should probably be considered earlier in the course of a patient's disease than is currently being done. As with neurolytic celiac plexus block, the technique has a highly favorable cost-to-benefit ratio compared with chronic administration of spinal opioids.

The Bell-Magendie law states that the motor fibers exit the ventral aspect of the spinal cord and the sensory fibers exit the dorsal aspect of the spinal cord. This separation of motor and sensory fibers allows for selective destruction of the sensory fibers without concomitant destruction of the motor fibers at the same level. In contradistinction to the cervical region, the lumbar nerve roots leave the spinal cord at levels much higher than they exit the vertebral column. Hence, because the neurolytic solution must be placed on the dorsal root as it leaves the spinal cord, the pain specialist must ascertain the level at which the nerve actually leaves the spinal cord and perform the block at that level rather than at the point at which the spinal nerve root leaves the bony vertebral column.

By placing the patient in a position with the dorsal roots uppermost, a hypobaric neurolytic solution such as alcohol can be floated onto the sensory fibers thought to be responsible for subserving the patient's pain while at the same time avoiding placing solution on the dependent motor fibers. By placing the patient in a position with the dorsal nerve roots being bottommost, a hyperbaric neurolytic solution can be dripped onto the dependent sensory fibers thought to be subserving the patient's pain

while at the same time avoiding the solution's floating onto the uppermost motor fibers.

It should be noted that the deep tissues such as bone may receive their innervation from a different spinal level than the skin overlying it. For this reason, if the patient's pain is thought to be primarily due to bony involvement from metastatic disease, it will be necessary to consult a sclerotome chart to determine which spinal nerve root actually provides innervation to the affected area. Failure to consult a sclerotome chart and simply relying on the dermatomal distribution of the pain may thus result in block of the wrong spinal segment.

In the lumbar region, the spinal cord is surrounded by three layers of protective connective tissue: the dura, the arachnoid, and the pia mater. The dura is the outermost layer and is composed of tough fibroelastic fibers that form a mechanical barrier to protect the spinal cord. The next layer is the arachnoid, which is separated from the dura by only a small potential space that is filled with serous fluid. The arachnoid is a barrier to the diffusion of substances and effectively serves to limit the spread of drugs administered into the epidural space from diffusing into the spinal fluid. The innermost layer is the pia, a vascular structure that helps provide lateral support to the spinal cord. Drugs administered into the subarachnoid space are placed between the arachnoid and pia, although inadvertent subdural injection is possible. Subdural injection of local anesthetic is characterized by a spotty, incomplete block.

The spinal cord ends at L2 in most adults, but given the fact that lumbar subarachnoid neurolytic block must be carried out at the level at which the dorsal sensory fibers actually leave the spinal cord, the potential for needle-induced trauma to the spinal cord itself remains an ever-present possibility.

Hypobaric Neurolytic Solution Technique

Lumbar subarachnoid neurolytic block is usually carried out in the lateral position, although the sitting or semirecumbent position can be used if the patient is unable to lie on his or her side because of bony metastatic disease or because of respiratory insufficiency that makes lying with the head down difficult. The prone position is occasionally used when bilateral neurolytic block of a lumbar segment is desired. Although this position limits the amount of rotation of the spine possible and simplifies midline identification, the inherent dangers of the prone position, including difficulty in monitoring the patient and problems with airway management, militate against the routine use of the prone position for lumbar subarachnoid neurolytic block. As with all other regional anesthesia techniques, proper position is crucial to allow successful completion of the block and to avoid complications. Regardless of the position chosen, careful attention to patient positioning, including identification of the midline, avoiding rotation of the spine, and ensuring flexion of the lumbar spine, is essential to successfully complete lumbar subarachnoid neurolytic block.

After the patient is placed in the lateral position with the affected side uppermost, the head is placed on a pillow, with the lumbar spine flexed and without rotation. The patient is rolled forward toward the abdomen approximately 45 degrees, with the chest and abdomen bolstered on pillows to allow the patient to comfortably remain in this position for the 30 or 40 minutes required to complete the procedure and allow the block to set up. The spinous process at the level at which the nerve thought to be subserving the patient's pain exits the spinal cord is then identified (Fig. 331-1). If bone or deep structures are thought to be the source of the patient's pain, a sclerotome chart is also consulted to determine the spinal nerve that most likely provides sensory innervation to the affected area (Fig. 331-2).

The skin overlying the spinal segment thought to subserve the pain, as well as the skin overlying several levels above and below the selected segment, is then prepared with an antiseptic solution. The spinous process of the selected segment is then identified, and the operator's middle and index fingers are placed on each side of the spinous processes. The position of the interspace is reconfirmed with palpation using a rocking motion in the superior and inferior planes. The midline of this interspace is then identified by palpating the spinous processes above and below the interspace using a lateral rocking motion. Failure to accurately identify the midline is the number one reason for failed lumbar subarachnoid neurolytic block.

At a point in the midline of the chosen interspace, local anesthetic is used to infiltrate the skin, subcutaneous tissues, the supraspinous ligament, and the interspinous ligament down to the ligamentum flavum. A 22-gauge, 3½-inch spinal needle with the stylet in place is then inserted exactly in the midline through the previously anesthetized area. The stylet is removed, and a well-lubricated, 5-mL glass syringe filled with preservative-free saline is attached to the spinal needle. While maintaining constant pressure on the plunger of the syringe, the nondominant hand advances the needle and syringe as a unit, with care being taken to keep the needle fixed against the patient so that any sudden movement by the patient will not allow the needle to advance into the spinal cord. The epidural space is then identified using a loss-of-resistance technique.

After the epidural space has been identified, and if there is no blood or cerebrospinal fluid (CSF) identified in the needle hub, the stylet is replaced and the needle is carefully advanced through the dura and arachnoid into the subarachnoid space (Fig. 331-3). Care must be taken not to advance the needle in an uncontrolled manner because trauma to the spinal cord with subsequent syrinx formation could occur.

The stylet is removed, and a free flow of CSF is identified. A tuberculin syringe containing 1 mL of absolute alcohol is then attached to the needle. Sequential incremental injections of 0.1 mL of absolute alcohol are then administered (Fig. 331-4). The patient should be forewarned that a strong burning sensation will occur for a few seconds following injection and that he or she will be asked where the burning is felt. The patient's perception of the location of the burning will allow the pain specialist to determine whether the burning is at, above, or below the site of the patient's original pain complaint and allow repositioning of the needle accordingly. This verbal feedback is crucial to the overall success of lumbar subarachnoid neurolytic block. For this reason, no local anesthetic should be administered through the spinal needle and no preblock intravenous sedation given in an effort to decrease the amount of procedure-related pain.

If, after injection of alcohol, the burning sensation corresponds to the location of the source of the patient's pain, up to 0.8 mL of absolute alcohol is injected in 0.1-mL incremental doses, with time being given between each dose to ascertain each dose's effects and side effects. If the burning sensation is above or below the site of the patient's pain, the needle is removed and replaced accordingly, and the process is repeated. It is not unusual for several nerves to be blocked in order to provide complete pain relief. This can be done at separate settings in order for the patient to experience the effects of the absolute alcohol on his or her pain and functional ability. After the injection process is completed, the needle is flushed with 0.1 mL of sterile preservative-free saline and the needle is removed. The patient is left in the operative position with the dorsal roots uppermost for an additional 15 minutes. The patient is then returned to the supine position.

Hyperbaric Neurolytic Solution Technique

Phenol (6.5%) in glycerin is the most common neurolytic agent used for hyperbaric lumbar subarachnoid neurolytic block. The block is carried out in a manner identical to the hypobaric technique described earlier, except for patient positioning. In order for hyperbaric solutions to block the dorsal sensory fibers without concomitant blockade of the corresponding ventral motor fibers, the patient must be positioned with the affected side down and the patient turned 45 degrees toward his or her back (Fig. 331-5). Pillows or a foam wedge is placed behind the patient's back to allow him or her to rest comfortably in this position for 30 to 40 minutes. As with the hypobaric technique, the pain specialist injects 0.1-mL increments of the neurolytic solution, with time between injections allowed to ascertain the effects and side effects of each increment (Fig. 331-6). The major limitation with the use of hyperbaric solutions is the fact that the patient must lie with the affected side down, making the procedure more painful than using hypobaric solutions, which allow the patient to lie on the nonaffected side.

Most complications associated with lumbar subarachnoid neurolytic block can be greatly decreased if careful attention is paid to the technical details and in particular the positioning of the patient. Motor and sensory deficits after lumbar subarachnoid neurolytic block can occur even with the best technique. The patient and the patient's family should be forewarned about the potential for the complications to ensure a clear understanding of the risk-to-benefit ratio of the proposed procedure. Bowel or bladder dysfunction occurs with greater frequency after lumbar subarachnoid neurolytic block compared with cervical and upper thoracic subarachnoid neurolytic procedures. Postblock dysesthesias can also occur after seemingly successful neurolytic procedures. Generally, the dysesthesias are thought to represent incomplete destruction of the fibers subserving the pain, and consideration should be given to repeat neurolysis if dysesthesias persist.

Because of the potential for hematogenous spread via Batson's plexus, local infection and sepsis represent absolute contraindications to the subarachnoid nerve block. In contradistinction to the caudal approach to the epidural space, anticoagulation and coagulopathy represent absolute contraindications to lumbar subarachnoid neurolytic block because of the risk of epidural and subarachnoid hematoma.

Hypotension is a common side effect of lumbar subarachnoid neurolytic block and is the result of the profound sympathetic blockade attendant with this procedure. Prophylactic intramuscular or intravenous administration of vasopressors and fluid loading may help avoid this potentially serious side effect of lumbar subarachnoid neurolytic block. If it is ascertained that a patient would not tolerate hypotension because of other serious systemic disease, more peripheral regional anesthetic techniques, such as lumbar plexus neurolysis, may be preferable to lumbar subarachnoid neurolytic block.

It is also possible to inadvertently place a needle or catheter intended for the subarachnoid space into the subdural space. If subdural placement is unrecognized, the resulting block will be spotty and the neurolytic solution may spread onto nerves that were not intended to be blocked. This problem can be avoided if the operator advances the needle slightly after perceiving the "pop" of the needle as it pierces the dura.

Neurologic complications due to needle-induced trauma after lumbar subarachnoid neurolytic block are uncommon if proper technique is used. Direct trauma to the spinal cord and/or nerve roots is usually accompanied by pain. If significant pain occurs during placement of the spinal needle, the physician should immediately stop and ascertain the cause of the pain to avoid the possibility of additional neural trauma. Delayed neurologic complications due to chemical irritation of the coverings of the spinal cord, nerves, and the spinal cord itself have been reported. This problem is usually self-limited, although it must be distinguished from meningitis of infectious etiology.

Although uncommon, infection in the subarachnoid space remains an ever-present possibility, especially in the immunocompromised AIDS or cancer patient. If epidural abscess occurs, emergent surgical drainage to avoid spinal cord compression and irreversible neurologic deficit is usually required. Meningitis after lumbar subarachnoid neurolytic block may require subarachnoid administration of antibiotics. Early detection and treatment of infection are crucial to avoid potentially life-threatening sequelae.

SUGGESTED READING

Waldman SD: Lumbar subarachnoid neurolytic block. In: Atlas of Interventional Pain Management, ed 2. Philadelphia, Saunders, 2004.

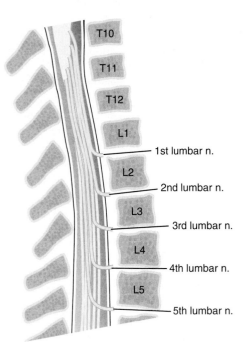

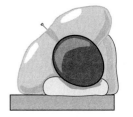

FIGURE 331–1 Anatomy of the lumbar nerve roots. (From Waldman SD: Atlas of Interventional Pain Management, ed 2. Philadelphia, Saunders, 2004, p 527.)

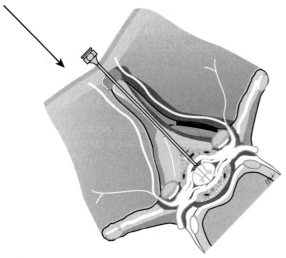

FIGURE 331–3 Patient and needle position for the hypobaric technique. (From Waldman SD: Atlas of Interventional Pain Management, ed 2. Philadelphia, Saunders, 2004, p 529.)

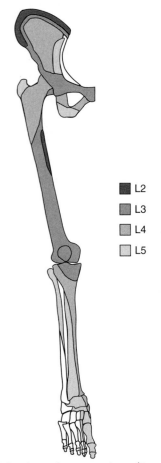

■ L2
■ L3
■ L4
■ L5

FIGURE 331–2 Lumbar sclerotome chart. (From Waldman SD: Atlas of Interventional Pain Management, ed 2. Philadelphia, Saunders, 2004, p 527.)

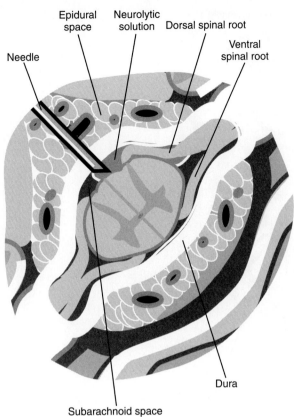

FIGURE 331–4 Postinjection technique. (From Waldman SD: Atlas of Interventional Pain Management, ed 2. Philadelphia, Saunders, 2004, p 530.)

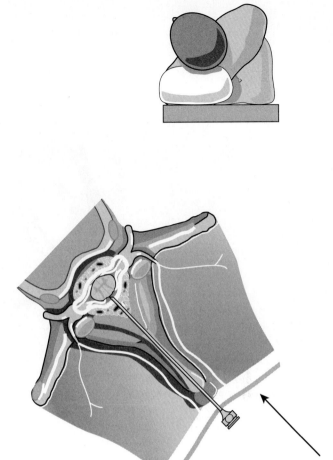

FIGURE 331–5 Patient and needle position for the hyperbaric technique. (From Waldman SD: Atlas of Interventional Pain Management, ed 2. Philadelphia, Saunders, 2004, p 531.)

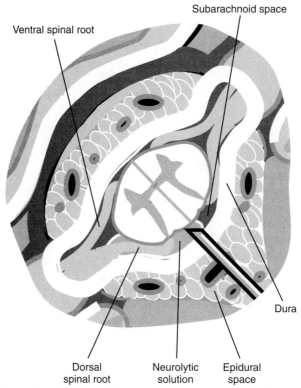

FIGURE 331–6 Postinjection technique. (From Waldman SD: Atlas of Interventional Pain Management, ed 2. Philadelphia, Saunders, 2004, p 531.)

CHAPTER 332

Lumbar Discography

Lumbar discography is indicated as a diagnostic maneuver in a carefully selected subset of patients suffering from back and lumbar radicular pain. Patients who may benefit from discography include (1) those patients with persistent back and/or lumbar radicular pain in whom traditional diagnostic modalities such as magnetic resonance imaging (MRI), computed tomographic (CT) scanning, and electromyography have failed to delineate a cause of the pain; (2) those patients in whom equivocal findings such as bulging lumbar discs are identified on traditional diagnostic modalities, to determine whether such abnormalities are in fact responsible for the pain; (3) those patients who are to undergo lumbar fusion, where discography may help identify which levels need to be fused; (4) those patients who have previously undergone fusion of the lumbar spine, where discography may

help identify whether levels above and below the fusion are responsible for persistent pain; and (5) those patients in whom recurrent disc herniation cannot be separated from scar tissue with traditional imaging techniques. In each of these selected patient populations, the pain management specialist must correlate the data obtained from the injection itself, the provocation of pain on injection, the radiographic appearance of the discogram obtained, and in selected patients, the relief of pain after the disc is injected with local anesthetic. A failure to carefully correlate all of this diagnostic information in the context of the patient's clinical presentation will lead the pain management specialist to erroneously interpret the results of discography and adversely influence clinical decision making.

From a functional anatomic viewpoint, lumbar discs must be thought of as distinct from cervical discs insofar as a source of pain is concerned. Radicular symptomatology solely from disc herniation is much more common in the lumbar region compared with the cervical and thoracic regions. The reason for this is twofold: (1) In order for the lumbar disc to impinge on the lumbar nerve roots, it must herniate posteriorly and laterally. The lumbar nerve roots are not protected from impingement from lumbar disc herniation by the bony wall of the facet joints as are the cervical nerve roots. (2) The posterior longitudinal ligament in the lumbar region is only a single layer, which is thinner and less well developed in its lateral aspects. It is in this lateral region in which lumbar disc herniation with impingement on exiting nerve roots is most likely to occur.

The nuclear material in the lumbar disc is placed more posterior than its cervical counterpart. The gelatinous nucleus pulposus of the lumbar disc is surrounded by a dense, laminated fibroelastic network of fibers known as the annulus. The annular fibers are arranged in concentric layers that run obliquely from adjacent vertebrae. It is this annular layer that receives sensory innervation from a variety of sources. Posteriorly, the annulus receives fibers from the sinuvertebral nerves, which also provide sensory innervation to the posterior elements, including portions of the facet joints. Laterally, fibers from the exiting spinal nerve roots provide sensory innervation, with the anterior portion of the disc receiving fibers from the sympathetic chain. Whether part or all of these fibers play a role in discogenic pain is a subject of controversy among pain specialists.

The lumbar nerve roots leave the spinal cord and travel laterally through the intervertebral foramina. If the posterior lumbar disc herniates laterally, it can impinge on the lumbar root as it travels through the intervertebral foramen, producing classic radicular symptoms. If the lumbar disc herniates posteromedially, it may impinge on the spinal cord itself, producing myelopathy that may include lower extremity as well as bowel and bladder symptoms. Severe compression of the lumbar spinal cord may result in cauda equina syndrome, paraparesis, or, rarely, paraplegia.

To perform lumbar discography, the patient is placed in the prone position with a pillow under the abdomen to slightly flex the lumbar spine as if for a lumbar sympathetic block. The relative positions of the lung, ribs, aorta, vena cava, kidneys, nerve roots, and spinal cord must be considered and these structures can best be visualized with CT (Fig. 332-1). The spinous process of the vertebra just above the disc to be evaluated is palpated. At a point just below and 1½ inches lateral to the spinous process, the skin is prepared with antiseptic solution and the skin and subcutaneous tissues are infiltrated with local anesthetic.

A 22-gauge, 13-cm styletted needle is advanced through the skin under fluoroscopic or CT guidance, with the target being the middle of the disc to be imaged. Given the proximity of the somatic nerve roots, paresthesia in the distribution of the corresponding lumbar paravertebral nerve may be elicited. If this occurs, the needle should be withdrawn and redirected slightly more cephalad. The needle is again readvanced in incremental steps under fluoroscopic or CT guidance, with care being taken to keep the needle trajectory medial to avoid pneumothorax.

The needle is then advanced in incremental steps into the central nucleus. Sequential scanning is indicated to avoid advancing the needle completely through the disc and into the lower limits of the spinal cord or cauda equina. The pain management specialist must also take care not to allow the needle to track too laterally into the lower pleural or retroperitoneal space. Water-soluble contrast medium suitable for intrathecal use is then slowly injected through the needle into the disc in a volume of 0.2 to 0.6 mL.

The resistance to injection should be noted, with an intact disc exhibiting firm resistance at these volumes. Simultaneously, the patient's pain response during injection is noted. The location of the patient's pain and its quality and similarity to the patient's ongoing clinical symptoms are evaluated. The use of a verbal analogue scale may be useful to help the patient quantify the amount of pain experienced compared with that during the injection of adjacent discs.

The nucleogram of a normal lumbar disc appears as a globular mass with occasional posterolateral clefts that occur as part of the normal aging process of the disc (Fig. 332-2). In the damaged disc, the contrast material may flow into tears of the inner annulus, producing a characteristic transverse pattern (Fig. 332-3). If the tears in the annulus extend to the outer layer, a radial pattern is produced (Fig. 332-4). Contrast material may also flow between the layers of annulus, producing a circumferential pattern (Fig. 332-5). Complete disruption of the annulus allows the contrast material to flow into the epidural space or into the cartilaginous end plate of the vertebra itself. Although the greater the damage to the annulus, the greater the likelihood that the disc being evaluated is the source of the patient's pain, the pain management specialist must evaluate all of the information obtained during the discography procedure and place this information into the context of the patient's pain symptomatology.

After evaluation of the nucleogram, a decision must be made whether to proceed with discography of adjacent discs or to inject local anesthetic into the disc currently being imaged. Analgesic discography is useful in those patients whose clinical pain pattern is reproduced or provoked during the injection of contrast medium. If the pain that was provoked during the injection of contrast medium is relieved by a subsequent injection of local anesthetic into the disc, an inference can be drawn that the disc is the likely source of the patient's pain. It must be remembered that if there is disruption of the annulus, the injected local anesthetic may spread into the epidural space and anesthetize somatic and sympathetic nerves that may subserve discs at an adjacent level. If this occurs, erroneous information may be obtained if discography is then performed on adjacent discs.

After injection procedures are completed, the patient is observed for 30 minutes prior to discharge. The patient should be warned to expect minor postprocedure discomfort, including some soreness of the paraspinous musculature. Ice packs placed on the injection site for 20-minute time periods will help decrease these untoward effects. The patient should be instructed to call immediately if any fever or other systemic symptoms occur that might suggest infection.

Complications directly related to discography are generally self-limited, although occasionally, even with the best technique, severe complications can occur. The most common severe complication after discography is infection of the disc, which is commonly referred to as discitis. Because of the limited blood supply of the disc, such infections can be extremely hard to eradicate. Discitis usually manifests as an increase in spine pain several days to a week after discography. Acutely, there will be no change in the patient's neurologic examination as a result of disc infection.

Epidural abscess, which can rarely occur after discography, generally manifests within 24 to 48 hours.

Clinically, the signs and symptoms of epidural abscess are high fever, spine pain, and progressive neurologic deficit. If either discitis or epidural abscess is suspected, blood and urine cultures should be taken, antibiotics started, and emergent MRI of the spine obtained to allow identification and drainage of any abscess formation, to prevent irreversible neurologic deficit.

In addition to infectious complications, pneumothorax may occur after lumbar discography. This complication should rarely occur if CT guidance is used during needle placement. Small pneumothorax after lumbar discography can often be treated conservatively, and tube thoracostomy can be avoided. Trauma to retroperitoneal structures, including the kidney, may also occur if CT guidance is not used to avoid and localize these structures.

Direct trauma to the nerve roots and the spinal cord can occur if the needle is allowed to traverse the entire disc or is placed too laterally. These complications should rarely occur if incremental CT scans are taken while advancing the needle. Such needle-induced trauma to the lower lumbar spinal cord and cauda equina can result in deficits, including cauda equina syndrome and paraplegia.

SUGGESTED READING

Waldman SD: Lumbar discography. In: Atlas of Interventional Pain Management, ed 2. Philadelphia, Saunders, 2004.

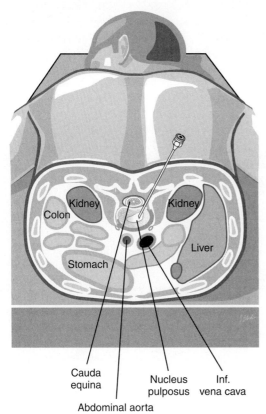

FIGURE 332–1 Technique for lumbar discography. (From Waldman SD: Atlas of Interventional Pain Management, ed 2. Philadelphia, Saunders, 2004, p 563.)

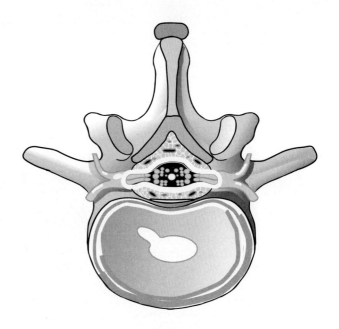

Transverse

FIGURE 332–3 Transverse lumbar disc. (From Waldman SD: Atlas of Interventional Pain Management, ed 2. Philadelphia, Saunders, 2004, p 565.)

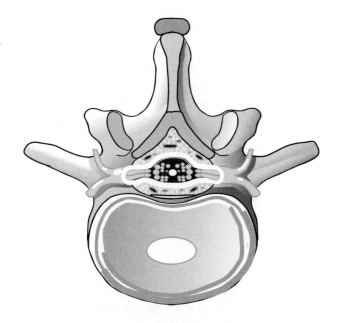

Normal

FIGURE 332–2 Normal lumbar disc. (From Waldman SD: Atlas of Interventional Pain Management, ed 2. Philadelphia, Saunders, 2004, p 565.)

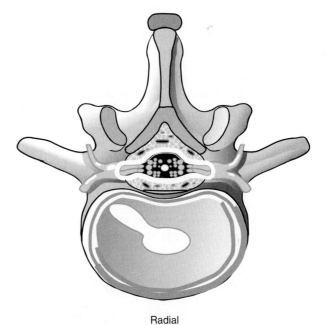

Radial

FIGURE 332–4 Radial lumbar disc. (From Waldman SD: Atlas of Interventional Pain Management, ed 2. Philadelphia, Saunders, 2004, p 566.)

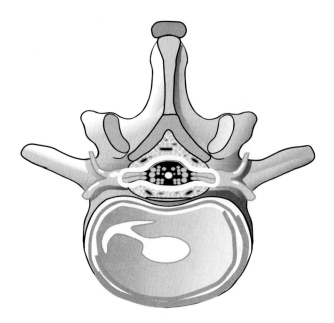

Circumferential

FIGURE 332–5 Circumferential lumbar disc. (From Waldman SD: Atlas of Interventional Pain Management, ed 2. Philadelphia, Saunders, 2004, p 566.)

CHAPTER 333

Vertebroplasty

Vertebroplasty is indicated for those patients suffering from weakening of the vertebral body due to a number of pathologic processes. Idiopathic osteoporosis is by far the most frequent indication for percutaneous vertebroplasty. Other indications include drug-induced osteoporosis, tumor of the vertebral body, hemangioma, and traumatic vertebral crush fractures. It should be noted that percutaneous vertebroplasty is indicated for stabilization of weakened vertebra whether or not pain is present. The best results can be expected when (1) there is limited compression of the vertebral body, (2) the fracture is less than 12 months old, or (3) the lesion is greater than 12 months old and the radionuclide bone scan is still "hot," indicating continued active disease. Percutaneous vertebroplasty is used most commonly in the mid and lower thoracic and lumbar spine.

The vertebral column consists of 24 vertebrae and two fused bones, the sacrum and the coccyx. Its function is to support the body and bear its weight. Its S-shape helps impart strength and adds flexibility. The vertebrae

articulate with each other by means of the facet joints, which are true synovial joints, and the intervertebral discs. These discs act as shock absorbers and help distribute any vertical forces placed on the spine horizontally. Although each area of the spine has minor anatomic differences that allow it to better perform its functions, the typical vertebra has many structural features in common. The body or centrum of the vertebra bears the majority of the weight, which is placed in the vertebral column. The lamina is the arch that encloses the posterior portion of the spinal canal.

The spinous process projects posteriorly and serves as an attachment point for the muscles of the back. The vertebral foramina allow passage of the spinal nerve roots from the spinal canal. The articular facet joints allow flexion, extension, and a limited amount of rotation between each spinal segment.

To perform percutaneous vertebroplasty, the patient is placed in the prone position on the fluoroscopy table, and the vertebra to be treated is identified with anteroposterior and lateral views. The skin overlying the affected vertebra is marked and then prepped with antiseptic solution and draped in a sterile manner. The skin and subcutaneous tissues are then anesthetized with local anesthetic. A 22-gauge, 3½-inch needle is then directed under fluoroscopic guidance against the pedicle of the affected vertebra, and the deep tissues and periosteum of the pedicle are generously infiltrated with local anesthetic. An 11-gauge trocar is used for the lower thoracic and lumbar vertebra, and a 13-gauge trocar is used for the smaller midthoracic vertebra. The trocar is advanced through the previously anesthetized area under fluoroscopic guidance in a trajectory that will allow the tip to make contact with the center of the upper outer third of the pedicle of the affected vertebra.

The trocar is embedded into the pedicle using firm pressure and a back-and-forth twisting motion. Care must be taken in severely osteoporotic patients not to fracture the pedicle by overzealous advancement of the trocar. After the tip of the trocar is firmly embedded in the pedicle, the trocar is advanced toward the affected vertebral body under anteroposterior and lateral fluoroscopic guidance. The trocar is advanced until the tip rests in the anterior third of the vertebral body, which bears the most of the weight (Fig. 333-1)

A long spinal needle is then used to fill the trocar with sterile saline to avoid injecting air into the epidural veins during the injection of contrast medium. Nonionic iodinated contrast medium is then injected slowly through the trocar under continuous fluoroscopic observation. The contrast should initially fill the vertebral body and will appear as a fine reticular blush pattern before flowing into the epidural and paravertebral veins. If the vertebra is fractured, contrast will be seen to leak out of the defect. Contrast injection will also allow the operator to determine whether the end plates and posterior wall of the vertebral body are intact. If the trocar is seen to be in the lumen of a large vertebral body vein, it should be advanced a few millimeters to avoid injection of the polymethylmethacrylate (PMMA) cement into the vein. Too much contrast injection should be avoided because it can obscure the subsequent injection of the PMMA.

After venography and vertebral body contrast injection is completed, the trocar is infused with sterile saline. The PMMA is then mixed according to the manufacturer's directions. Most PMMA contains sterile barium sulfate as an opacifying agent. If there was significant vascular uptake of contrast, the PMMA should be mixed to a more viscous consistency. If the contrast was injected with great difficulty due to dense bone and little vascular uptake was seen, the PMMA should be mixed to a less viscous consistency. The PMMA is then injected under fluoroscopic observation. If significant venous filling is seen, the operator should wait 1 or 2 minutes to allow the injected PMMA to harden and occlude the veins before resuming injection. If the PMMA extrudes through an incompetent end plate into the intervertebral disc, the same strategy is employed. If the injection becomes difficult, the trocar is withdrawn a few millimeters and the injection is slowly resumed. This technique is continued until the vertebral body is well filled. It is often necessary to place a second trocar into the vertebral body via the contralateral pedicle to obtain complete filling of the vertebra. The PMMA will harden in a few minutes. Sitting is allowed after a sedative or anesthetic has worn off, and patients are allowed to stand on the day following the procedure.

If careful attention is paid to the procedure, complications following percutaneous vertebroplasty are uncommon. The risks of significant intravascular or epidural injection are greatly decreased if fluoroscopic guidance is used during the injection process. Unintentional injection of the PMMA into the spinal canal can result in devastating neurologic complications and should rarely occur if careful attention to technique is used. Severe back pain following percutaneous vertebroplasty can be the result of a new vertebral fracture of a different vertebra or of fracture of the pedicle during the procedure. Encroachment on the intervertebral foramina by PMMA may cause new radicular symptoms that may ultimately require surgical decompression. Infection, although rare, remains a possibility, especially in the immunocompromised patient, such as a patient on long-term steroids or suffering from cancer.

SUGGESTED READING

Waldman SD: Percutaneous vertebroplasty. In: Atlas of Interventional Pain Management, ed 2. Philadelphia, Saunders, 2004.

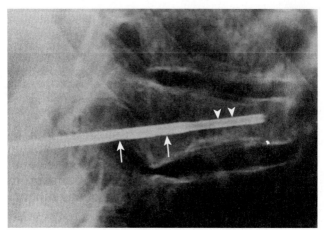

FIGURE 333–1 Trocar in proper position for injection of PMMA. (From Depriester C, et al: Percutaneous vertebroplasty: Indications, techniques, and complications. In Connors JJ, Wojak JC [eds]: Interventional Neuroradiology: Strategies and Practical Techniques. Philadelphia, Saunders, 1999, p 355.)

CHAPTER 334

Spinal Cord Stimulation

A trial of spinal cord stimulation is indicated in patients suffering from the following painful conditions that have failed to respond to more conservative therapy: (1) reflex sympathetic dystrophy, (2) causalgia, (3) ischemic pain secondary to peripheral vascular insufficiency, (4) radiculopathies, (5) failed back syndrome, (6) arachnoiditis, (7) postherpetic neuralgia, (8) phantom limb pain, and possibly (9) intractable angina. Because spinal cord stimulation is a reversible technique for pain relief, it should be considered prior to neurodestructive procedures in most patients.

Patients thought to be candidates for a trial of spinal cord stimulation should be psychologically stable and should have exhausted all traditional less invasive treatment modalities. Furthermore, the patient should not exhibit drug misuse, overuse, and/or continued drug-seeking behaviors. The family and patient must demonstrate a clear understanding of the pros and cons of spinal cord stimulation and accept the potential for hardware revisions and electronic reprogramming to obtain optimal pain relief.

Spinal cord stimulator electrodes can be placed into the epidural space either percutaneously or via a small laminotomy. The superior boundary of the epidural space is the fusion of the periosteal and spinal layers of dura at the foramen magnum. The epidural space continues inferiorly to the sacrococcygeal membrane. The epidural space is bounded anteriorly by the posterior longitudinal ligament and posteriorly by the vertebral laminae and the ligamentum flavum. The vertebral pedicles and intervertebral foramina form the lateral limits of the epidural space. The cervical epidural space is 3 to 4 mm at the C7-T1 interspace with the cervical spine flexed. The lumbar epidural space is 5 to 6 mm at the L2-L3 interspace with the lumbar spine flexed. The epidural space contains fat, veins, arteries, lymphatics, and connective tissue. Spinal cord stimulator electrodes can be placed anywhere along the epidural space from the cervical to the caudal region.

Spinal cord stimulator electrode placement may be carried out with the patient in the sitting, lateral, or prone position. Selection of position is based on the patient's ability to maintain the chosen position for the 30 to 45 minutes needed to place the electrode into the epidural space, position it, and then tunnel the electrode subcutaneously. Because placement of a spinal cord stimulator electrode requires patient feedback, choosing the most comfortable position is important to minimize the need for adjunctive intravenous narcotics or sedation.

After aseptic preparation of the skin to include the midline and electrode exit site, a Tuohy needle is placed into the epidural space at the level of desired electrode placement. The spinal cord–stimulating electrode is then advanced through the Tuohy needle into the epidural space. Spinal cord stimulator electrodes have a tendency to drag against the internal needle wall, and this may result in damage to the electrode insulation. This can be avoided by wetting both the needle and electrode with saline prior to attempting to advance the electrode through the needle.

After the electrode enters the epidural space, it is gently advanced under fluoroscopic guidance to a midline position overlying the spinal segments to be stimulated (Fig. 334-1). A small incision is then made with a No. 15 scalpel extending cranially and caudally approximately 0.5 cm with the epidural needle still in place to avoid inadvertent damage to the electrode. Care must be taken to completely dissect all tissue away from the needle to allow the electrode to fall freely into the incision as the tunneling tool is advanced. The needle is then carefully withdrawn back along the electrode and removed. The electrode is now attached to the pulse generator via a sterile screening cable. Trial stimulation is carried out with the patient describing the type and location of stimulation as well as the effect of the stimulation on the patient's ongoing pain. Ideally, the patient should report perception of the stimulation pattern superimposed on the painful area. It should be noted that more than one electrode is occasionally required to adequately relieve the patient's pain.

After satisfactory electrode position is obtained, the electrode is disconnected from the screening cable, and a sterile extension set is then tunneled subcutaneously to the flank using a malleable tunneling device. The malleable tunneling device is then shaped to match the contour of the flank. The skin of the midline incision is now lifted with thumb forceps, and the tunneling device is introduced subcutaneously and guided laterally. When the tip of the tunneling device has reached the exit point laterally, it is turned away from the patient; this forces the tip against the skin. The scalpel is then used to cut down onto the tip. The tunneling device is then advanced through the incision, bringing the extension set with it. This approach allows for a straight electrode path and decreases the incidence of electrode failure secondary to subcutaneous electrode kinking and subsequent breakage. The distal end of the electrode is then connected to the proximal portion of the extension set in the midline incision. Gentle traction is then placed on the distal end of the extension set to pull any excess portion of the extension set and electrode into the midline wound to allow the incision to be closed. The extension set is then connected to the pulse generator, and repeat trial stimulation is carried out to verify that the patient still perceives an acceptable stimulation pattern. If an acceptable pattern of stimulation is obtained, the midline incision is then closed with interrupted sutures, and sterile dressings are placed. A 48-hour period of trial stimulation is then carried out with careful quantification of the patient's functional ability and pain relief. If satisfactory results of the period of trial stimulation are obtained, it is reasonable to proceed with stage II permanent implantation of a pulse generator or radiofrequency coupling device.

In patients in whom a 48- to 72-hour stage I trial of spinal cord stimulation has been considered successful, it is reasonable to proceed with a stage II permanent implantation of the pulse generator. Prior to proceeding with permanent implantation of a pulse generator, the pain management specialist should carefully review the results of the trial stimulation period, looking not only at the reported pain relief, but functional levels, the need for additional pain medication, or other indications of psychological factors that might make permanent implantation inadvisable.

There are two basic types of spinal cord stimulation systems: (1) a totally implantable electrode and pulse generator system, and (2) a totally implantable electrode and receiver antenna that is used with an external pulse generator. Each type of system has advantages and disadvantages, and thus the ultimate choice of system should be based on matching these factors to the needs of the specific patient.

Spinal cord pulse generator placement may be carried out with the patient in the lateral position. Because patient cooperation is not required for this technique, intravenous sedation may be given if required for the patient to remain in the lateral position for the 30 to 45 minutes needed to disconnect the electrode from the extension set, remove the old extension set, replace it with a new one, and reconnect it to the pulse generator.

After aseptic preparation of the skin to include the midline incision, pulse generator pocket site, and the electrode exit site, the sutures are removed from the midline incision. The connection between the spinal cord stimulator electrode and the extension set is then identified. With care being taken not to dislodge the spinal cord stimulation, the connection is carefully removed from the midline incision. The Silastic cuff is removed, and the set screws are loosened to allow the extension set and electrode to be disconnected. After the electrode is disconnected from the extension set, the extension set is removed from the subcutaneous tunnel. Depending on the type of system implanted, this is accomplished by cutting the connector off the extension set and withdrawing the extension set out of the subcutaneous tunnel and discarding it, or cutting the distal end of the extension set off at the skin line of the exit site and pulling the proximal segment of the extension set back through the subcutaneous tunnel into the midline incision and then discarding it. Either approach can result in contamination of the operative site.

After the extension set is removed, an incision in the anterior subcostal region is made just large enough to accommodate the pulse generator or receiver antenna. A subcutaneous pocket is then created using small, curved blunt-tipped scissors. The pocket must be commodious enough to accommodate the pulse generator or receiver antenna, or the edge of these devices will erode through the skin. However, the pocket must not be made too large or the devices could turn over on themselves, making subsequent programming or stimulation impossible. After the pocket is created, adequate hemostasis must be obtained, or hematoma formation and infection are a distinct possibility. After adequate hemostasis has been obtained, a malleable tunneling device is then passed from the pocket incision back to exit in the reopened midline incision. A new sterile implantable extension set is then attached to the distal end of the tunneling device. The tunneling device is then drawn back out of the midline incision, bringing the extension set with it. The proximal end of the extension set is then attached to the epidural stimulating electrode, and the distal end of the extension set is attached to the pulse generator or receiver antenna. Silastic cuffs should be placed and sutured over these connections if required by the type of stimulator system. Excess electrode or extension set connector is carefully placed in the midline incision (Fig. 334-2). The pulse generator is then activated or the receiver antenna stimulated to verify that the system is working. After this is ascertained, the midline and pulse generator/receiver antenna pocket incisions are closed with two layers of interrupted sutures, which can be removed in 10 to 14 days.

Because of the potential for hematogenous spread via Batson's plexus, local infection and sepsis represent absolute contraindications to the placement of spinal cord stimulator electrodes into the epidural space. Anticoagulation and coagulopathy represent absolute contraindications to placement of epidural spinal cord stimulator electrodes because of the risk of epidural hematoma.

Inadvertent dural puncture occurring during identification of the epidural space should occur less than 0.5% of the time. Failure to recognize inadvertent dural puncture can result in placement of the stimulating electrode into the subdural or subarachnoid space.

Needle- or electrode-induced trauma to the epidural veins may result in self-limited bleeding, which may cause postprocedural pain. Uncontrolled bleeding into the epidural space may result in compression of the spinal cord with the rapid development of neurologic deficit. Although the incidence of significant neurologic deficit secondary to epidural hematoma after placement of epidural spinal cord stimulator electrodes is exceedingly rare, this devastating complication should be considered whenever there is rapidly developing neurologic deficit after placement of epidural spinal cord stimulator electrodes.

Neurologic complications after placement of epidural spinal cord stimulator electrodes are uncommon if proper technique is used. Direct trauma to the spinal cord and/or nerve roots is usually accompanied by pain. If significant pain occurs during placement of the epidural needle or electrode placement, the physician should immediately stop and ascertain the cause of the pain to avoid the possibility of additional neural trauma.

Although uncommon, infection in the epidural space remains an ever-present possibility, especially in the immunocompromised AIDS or cancer patient. If epidural abscess occurs, emergent surgical drainage to avoid spinal cord compression and irreversible neurologic deficit is usually required. Early detection and treatment of infection are crucial to avoid potentially life-threatening sequelae.

Although hardware failure occurs with a greatly decreased frequency compared with the early days of spinal cord stimulation, unfortunately, problems still occur. Damage to the insulation of the stimulating electrode during placement can be avoided if the electrode is wetted with sterile saline prior to advancing it through the epidural needle. The electrode should never be withdrawn against the tip of the epidural needle, because damage to the insulation or shearing of the electrode can occur. Care must be taken to carefully tighten all set screws when connecting the electrode to the extension set or to the pulse generator so they do not subsequently loosen and disrupt electrical contact. Although each spinal cord stimulation system is different, most require that a Silastic cuff be securely placed and sutured over all electrical connections to avoid body fluids from shorting out the connection. The pain management specialist should consult the package insert prior to implantation of a spinal cord stimulation system.

SUGGESTED READINGS

Waldman SD: Spinal cord stimulation: Stage I trial stimulation. In: Atlas of Interventional Pain Management, ed 2. Philadelphia, Saunders, 2004.

Waldman SD: Spinal cord stimulation: Stage II pulse generator implantation. Atlas of Interventional Pain Management, ed 2. Philadelphia, Saunders, 2004.

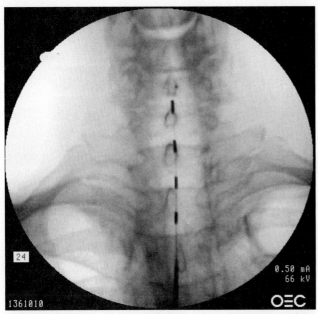

FIGURE 334–1 Spinal cord stimulator electrodes can be placed anywhere along the epidural space from the cervical to the caudal region. (From Waldman SD: Atlas of Interventional Pain Management, ed 2. Philadelphia, Saunders, 2004, p 593.)

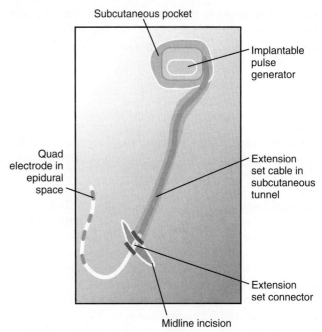

FIGURE 334–2 Spinal cord stimulation: stage II pulse generator implantation. (From Waldman SD: Atlas of Interventional Pain Management, ed 2. Philadelphia, Saunders, 2004, p 600.)

CHAPTER 335

Totally Implantable Infusion Pumps

Implantation of a totally implantable infusion pump is indicated for the infusion of drugs into the epidural or more commonly the subarachnoid space in the following clinical situations: (1) for the administration of epidural drugs for the palliation of pain in cancer patients with a life expectancy of months to years; (2) in carefully selected patients who suffer from chronic benign pain who have experienced palliation of their pain with trial doses of spinal opioids and who have failed to respond to other more conservative treatments; and (3) in those patients suffering from spasticity who have experienced decreased spasms after trial doses of subarachnoid administration of baclofen.

Advantages of totally implantable infusion pumps include the lower incidence of infections relative to tunneled epidural catheters and reservoirs/ports. Furthermore, once the infusion pump is implanted, there is a lower incidence of delivery system failure compared with tunneled catheters. Disadvantages of totally implantable infusion pumps include the fact that implantation, subsequent refill, and pump removal are more technically demanding relative to tunneled catheters and reservoirs/pumps. Additionally, the cost of a totally implantable infusion pump is significantly greater than that of tunneled catheters or reservoirs/ports, although the lower overall cost of drugs, supplies, and medical bills during the time the pump is used may offset the higher initial cost of the pump.

Placement of totally implantable infusion pumps may be carried out with the patient in the sitting, lateral, or prone position. Selection of position is based on the patient's ability to maintain the chosen position for the 25 to 30 minutes needed to place the catheter and pump. Because most infusion pumps are placed on an outpatient basis, choosing the most comfortable position is important to minimize the need for adjunctive intravenous narcotics or sedation. Because each specific type of pump may require additional steps during the implantation process, the pain management specialist should consult the package insert prior to beginning the implantation procedure.

After aseptic preparation of the skin to include the site of tunneling and infusion pump implantation site, a 17-gauge Tuohy needle is placed into the epidural or subarachnoid space at the level of desired catheter placement. The Silastic one-piece catheter is then advanced through the Tuohy needle into the epidural space (Fig. 335-1). Silastic catheters have a tendency to drag against the internal needle wall and fold back onto themselves. This can be avoided by wetting both the needle and catheter with saline prior to attempting to advance the catheter through the needle.

After the catheter enters the epidural or subarachnoid space, it is gently advanced an additional 3 to 4 cm. A small incision is made with a No. 15 scalpel extending cranially and caudally approximately 0.5 cm with the Tuohy needle still in place to avoid inadvertent damage to the catheter. Care must be taken to completely dissect all tissue away from the needle to allow the catheter to fall freely into the incision as the tunneling tool is advanced. If a subarachnoid catheter terminus is planned, a purse-string suture is placed around the needle prior to removal to help decrease the incidence of hygroma formation as a result of cerebrospinal fluid (CSF) tracking back along the catheter into the pump pocket. The needle is then carefully withdrawn back along the catheter until the tip is outside the skin. The catheter wire stylet is withdrawn, and the Tuohy needle is removed from the catheter. The injection port is then attached to the distal end of the catheter, and, after aspiration, a small amount of preservative-free sterile saline is injected to ensure catheter integrity. If the catheter is placed in the epidural space, 5 to 6 mL of 1.5% lidocaine is injected into the epidural space via the catheter to provide dense segmental sensory block for the subcutaneous tunneling. This approach avoids the need for painful subcutaneous infiltration at the tunneling site. If the catheter is placed into the subarachnoid space, infiltration of a local anesthetic containing epinephrine along the tunneling path is recommended.

The malleable tunneling device is then shaped to match the contour of the flank. The skin is now lifted with thumb forceps, and the tunneling device is introduced subcutaneously and guided laterally. When the tip of the tunneling device has reached the exit point laterally in the right upper quadrant of the abdomen, it is turned away from the patient; this forces the tip against the skin. The scalpel is then used to cut down onto the tip. The tunneling device is then advanced through the incision. This approach allows for a straight catheter path and decreases the incidence of catheter failure secondary to

subcutaneous catheter kinking. An incision large enough to accommodate subcutaneous placement of the pump is then extended from each side of the tunneling tool. The injection port is removed from the distal end of the catheter, and the catheter is then threaded onto the stud on the proximal end of the tunneling device. The tunneling device is then withdrawn through the second incision, bringing the catheter with it through the subcutaneous tunnel (Fig. 335-2).

With care being taken not to injure the catheter, a subcutaneous pocket is created using small, curved blunt-tipped scissors. The pocket must be commodious enough to accommodate the infusion pump, or the edge of the pump will erode through the skin. However, the pocket must not be made too large, or the infusion pump can turn over on itself, making subsequent refill impossible. After the pocket is created, adequate hemostasis must be obtained, or hematoma formation and infection are a distinct possibility. After adequate hemostasis has been obtained, excess distal catheter length is removed, and the infusion pump is attached to the distal end of the catheter. The infusion pump is secured to the catheter by the means of interrupted nonabsorbable sutures placed over the Silastic boot. The pump is then placed into the pocket, with care being taken not to twist or kink the catheter (Fig. 335-3). The wound is then closed with a double layer of interrupted sutures, which may be removed in 10 to 14 days.

Because of the potential for hematogenous spread via Batson's plexus, local infection and sepsis represent absolute contraindications to the placement of catheters into the epidural space. Anticoagulation and coagulopathy represent absolute contraindications to placement of epidural catheters because of the risk of epidural hematoma.

Inadvertent dural puncture occurring during identification of the epidural space should occur less than 0.5% of the time. Failure to recognize inadvertent dural puncture can result in immediate total spinal anesthetic with associated loss of consciousness, hypotension, and apnea. If epidural doses of opioids are accidentally placed into the subarachnoid space, significant respiratory and central nervous system depression will result. It is also possible to inadvertently place a needle or catheter intended for the epidural space into the subdural space. If subdural placement is unrecognized and epidural doses of local anesthetic are administered, the signs and symptoms are similar to those of massive subarachnoid injection, although the resulting motor and sensory block may be spotty.

The epidural space is highly vascular. The intravenous placement of the epidural needle or catheter occurs in approximately 0.5% to 1% of patients undergoing placement of epidural catheters. This complication is increased in those patients with distended epidural veins, such as the parturient and patients with large intra-abdominal tumor mass. If the misplacement is unrecognized, injection of local anesthetic directly into an epidural vein will result in significant local anesthetic toxicity.

Needle trauma to the epidural veins may result in self-limited bleeding, which may cause postprocedural pain. Uncontrolled bleeding into the epidural space may result in compression of the spinal cord with the rapid development of neurologic deficit. Although the incidence of significant neurologic deficit secondary to epidural hematoma after placement of epidural catheters is exceedingly rare, this devastating complication should be considered whenever there is rapidly developing neurologic deficit after placement of epidural catheters.

Neurologic complications after placement of epidural or subarachnoid catheters are uncommon if proper technique is used. Direct trauma to the spinal cord and/or nerve roots is usually accompanied by pain. If significant pain occurs during placement of the epidural or subarachnoid needle or catheter or during injection, the physician should immediately stop and ascertain the cause of the pain to avoid the possibility of additional neural trauma.

Although uncommon, infection in the epidural space or meningitis remains an ever-present possibility, especially in the immunocompromised AIDS or cancer patient. If epidural abscess occurs, emergent surgical drainage to avoid spinal cord compression and irreversible neurologic deficit is usually required. Early detection and treatment of infection are crucial to avoid potentially life-threatening sequelae. Infections of the infusion pump pocket can usually be managed with systemic and topical antibiotics and, occasionally, incision and drainage. The patient must be observed closely for spread of infection proximally down the subcutaneous tunnel into the epidural space. If this occurs, the entire delivery system should be removed immediately.

If a subarachnoid catheter terminus is planned, CSF tracking back along the catheter to the pump pocket with hygroma formation is a possibility. Such hygroma formation makes pump refill more difficult and increases the chance of infection. Hygroma formation can be avoided by placement of a purse-string suture around the needle at the time the catheter is placed and placing a pressure dressing over the pump pocket after the implantation procedure. Although rare, a cutaneous/subarachnoid fistula can occur if CSF leakage continues.

Surprisingly, the major complications related to totally implantable infusion pumps are related to pump refill rather than to the implantation technique itself. When refilling a pump with a side port that provides direct access to the subarachnoid or epidural space, scrupulous attention to technique must be followed to avoid placing a lethal bolus of opioid or baclofen directly into the subarachnoid or epidural space.

SUGGESTED READING

Waldman SD: Implantation of totally implantable infusion pumps. In: Atlas of Interventional Pain Management, ed 2. Philadelphia, Saunders, 2004.

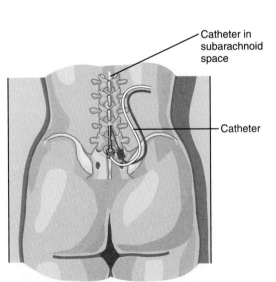

FIGURE 335–1 Needle placement and catheter advancement. (From Waldman SD: Atlas of Interventional Pain Management, ed 2. Philadelphia, Saunders, 2004, p 614.)

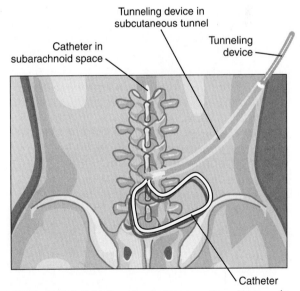

FIGURE 335–2 Withdrawal of the tunneling device. (From Waldman SD: Atlas of Interventional Pain Management, ed 2. Philadelphia, Saunders, 2004, p 614.)

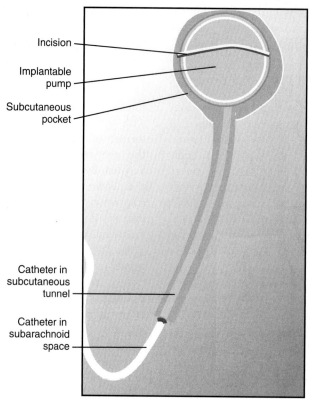

Incision

Implantable
pump

Subcutaneous
pocket

Catheter in
subcutaneous
tunnel

Catheter in
subarachnoid
space

FIGURE 335–3 Placement of the pump. (From Waldman SD: Atlas of Interventional Pain Management, ed 2. Philadelphia, Saunders, 2004, p 615.)

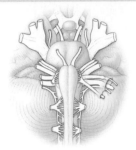

SECTION 6

Physical and Behavioral Modalities

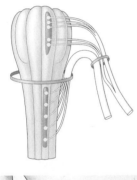

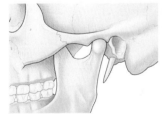

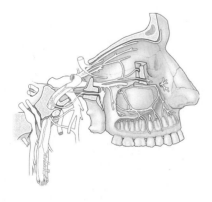

CHAPTER 336

The Physiologic Effects of Therapeutic Heat

The mechanisms by which heat exerts its analgesic effect extend beyond the simple effects of heat locally on the target tissue. Locally, heat elicits the following physiologic responses: (1) increased blood flow, (2) decreased muscle spasm, (3) increased extensibility of connective tissue, (4) decreased joint stiffness, (5) reduction of edema, and, most important, (6) analgesia (Table 336-1). Because the sensation of temperature and pain are both carried to the higher centers via the same neural pathways, it is not unreasonable to imagine that heat exerts a modulating effect at the spinal and supraspinal levels. In addition, the feeling of well-being associated with therapeutic heat most likely causes the release of endorphins and other neurotransmitters, further modifying the pain response. It should be noted that although the beneficial nature of therapeutic heat cannot be denied, this treatment modality is not without side effects. The relative contraindications to the use of therapeutic heat are summarized in Table 336-2. Although these precautions are not absolute, special care should be taken should a decision be made to use therapeutic heat in these clinical settings.

Choosing a Therapeutic Heat Modality

The clinician who is considering the use of therapeutic heat as an adjunct in the treatment of his or her patient's pain has a variety of heating modalities from which to choose (Table 336-3). Although the indications for the use of therapeutic heat apply to all therapeutic heating modalities discussed in this chapter, each modality has its own distinct advantages and disadvantages, which not only can influence the success or failure of this therapeutic intervention but also can determine the incidence of side effects and complications if the wrong modality is

TABLE 336–1 Physiologic Effects of Therapeutic Heat

- Increased blood flow
- Decreased muscle spasm
- Increased extensibility of connective tissue
- Decreased joint stiffness
- Reduction of edema
- Analgesia

TABLE 336–2 Relative Contraindications to Therapeutic Heat

- Lack of or reduced sensation
- Demyelinating diseases
- Acute inflammation
- Bleeding disorders
- Hemorrhage
- Malignancy
- Inability to communicate or respond to pain
- Atrophic skin
- Ischemia
- Scar tissue

chosen or is used in the incorrect clinical situation (Table 336-4). As a practical consideration, the failure to match the modality to the patient will usually result in a less-than-optimal outcome.

When matching the modality to the patient, it is essential to understand the underlying physics of each therapeutic heat modality. Each heat modality accomplishes the delivery of heat to the target tissue by a specific physical mechanism of heat transfer. For sake of organization, these mechanisms can be divided into the categories of conduction, convection, and conversion. Whereas conduction and convection provide primarily superficial heating, conversion has the

TABLE 336–3 Therapeutic Heat Modalities

- Superficial heat modalities
  - Modalities that rely on conduction
  Hydrocollator packs
  Circulating water heating pads
  Chemical heating pads
  Reusable microwavable heating pads
  Paraffin baths
  - Modalities that rely on convection
  Hydrotherapy
  Fluidotherapy
- Deep heat modalities
  - Modalities that rely on conversion
  Ultrasound
  Short wave diathermy
  Microwave diathermy

TABLE 336–4 Indications for the Use of Therapeutic Heat Modalities

- Pain
- Muscle spasm
- Bursitis
- Tenosynovitis
- Collagen vascular diseases
- Contracture
- Fibromyalgia
- Induction of hyperemia
- Hematoma resolution
- Superficial thrombophlebitis
- Reflex sympathetic dystrophy

ability to heat deep tissues. Therefore, the first question when choosing a therapeutic heat modality is whether the superficial or deep heat is the desired goal.

The next step in matching the modality to the patient is understanding which modalities transfer heat by which mechanism (see Table 336-3). The most commonly used heat modality in clinical practice, hot packs, transfers superficial heat by conduction, as do heating pads, circulating water heating pads, chemical heating packs, reusable microwave heating pads, and paraffin baths. Hydrotherapy and fluidotherapy deliver superficial heat to the target tissue by convection. The deep heating modalities of ultrasound, radiant heat, short wave diathermy, and microwave diathermy deliver heat to the target tissues by conversion. By understanding how each heat modality delivers heat, the clinician can then use the unique characteristics of heat modality to best meet the patient's needs. Specific heat modalities are discussed next.

Superficial Heating Modalities

MODALITIES THAT DELIVER HEAT BY CONDUCTION

Hydrocollator Packs

As mentioned, the mechanism by which the various types of hot packs deliver heat to the target tissue is by

TABLE 336–5 Indications for Therapeutic Ultrasound

- Tendinitis
- Bursitis
- Nonacutely inflamed arthritis
- Frozen joints
- Contractures
- Degenerative arthritis
- Fractures
- Plantar fasciitis

conduction. The amount of heat delivered by conduction is directly proportional to the following variables: (1) the area of heat delivery, (2) the length of time the heat is delivered, (3) the temperature gradient between the hot pack and the target tissue, and (4) the thermal conductivity of the surfaces. The amount of heat delivered by conduction is inversely proportional to the thickness of the layers of materials and tissue that the heat must be conducted through. By altering any of these variables, the amount of heat delivered to the target tissue can be increased or decreased as the clinical situation and patient comfort dictates.

Hydrocollator packs are flexible packs which contain a silicate gel product that are heated in a water bath to approximately 170° F. The large surface area and flexible nature make this modality ideally suited for treating low back and dorsal spine pain. Smaller hydrocollator packs are useful in the treatment of neck pain. The packs do not absorb significant amounts of water, but their surface is wet, thus increasing conduction. A terry cloth towel is placed between the patient and the hydrocollator pack with the thickness of towels being the easiest way to control the dosimetry and to allow titration of the temperature to patient comfort. The packs maintain a therapeutic temperature for approximately 20 to 30 minutes to allow for superficial heating of large surface areas. To avoid burning the patient, care must be taken to allow excess water to drain from the pack prior to use. The hydrocollator pack should always be placed on rather than under the patient for easy removal should the patient complain the pad is too hot.

Circulating Water Heating Pads (K-Pads)

Like the hydrocollator pack, the circulating water heating pad is ideally suited for treating low back and dorsal spine pain. More flexible than hydrocollator packs, the circulating water heating pad can also be used on shoulders and extremities. The circulating water pad is thermostatically controlled so that the water temperature remains constant allowing for superficial heating of relative large surface areas. This confers two additional benefits to this heat delivery device: (1) unlike hydrocollator packs, hot water bottles, and microwave heating pads, which cool over time, the circulating water heating pad can deliver a constant temperature to the target tissue over time; and (2) the thermostatically controlled circulation system greatly decreases the risk of thermal injuries associated with traditional electric pads. Despite the increased safety of circulating water pads relative to electric heating pads, because they do not cool spontaneously, their use should be closely monitored and carefully timed.

Chemical Heating Packs

Chemical heating packs are readily available in most pharmacies. They consist of a flexible outer layer that contains internally segregated chemicals that, when mixed together by squeezing or kneading the package, cause an exothermic reaction that releases heat capable of producing superficial heating of the affected body part. Other chemical heating pads produce heat by oxidation when the chemical heating pack is exposed to air. Most chemical heating packs that rely on oxidation contain iron powder, activated charcoal, sodium chloride, and water. Although inexpensive and convenient to use, the chemical heating packs produce varying degrees of heat and may cause burns. Furthermore, the chemicals contained in the packs can cause chemical irritation to the skin if the outer package integrity is compromised. Chemical heating packs have the advantage of being portable and not requiring electricity or external heating.

Reusable Microwavable Heating Pads

The widespread use of microwave ovens has spawned a variety of new reusable heating pad products that are designed to be quickly heated in the microwave oven. These products consist of an outer bag that may be made of cloth or plastic with a sealed inner bag containing gel or grains including rice, corn, or wheat and deliver their heat via conduction to provide superficial heating of the affected tissues. Some products add aromatic substances to provide the added theoretical benefit of aromatherapy. Although convenient and easy to use, these products have some serious drawbacks. First, as with microwave popcorn, variations in the heating abilities of microwave ovens can cause overheating or underheating. Additionally, there is no simple way to verify the actual temperature of the product, and owing to the nature of microwave ovens, there may be significant inconsistencies of surface temperatures, with "hot spots" resulting in serious burns. Like hydrocollator packs and other heat delivery modalities that do not deliver a constant source of heat, cooling can be inconsistent.

Paraffin Baths

Used primarily for the treatment of hand abnormalities associated with rheumatoid arthritis, degenerative arthritis, and the other collagen vascular diseases such as scleroderma, paraffin baths are a useful form of conduction-type heat therapy capable of providing superficial heating of the affected tissues. Paraffin baths are reasonably safe as long as the temperature of the liquid paraffin is checked prior to extremity immersion or application. The paraffin is generally mixed with mineral oil in 7 parts paraffin to 1 part mineral oil and placed in a thermostatically controlled heater. The affected body part is then dipped into the paraffin bath and then removed to allow the paraffin to solidify. This procedure is repeated up to 10 times. The affected body parts are then placed under an insulating sheet for approximately 20 minutes, and then the paraffin is stripped off and returned to the thermostatically controlled heater to remelt and to be used again. This technique is usually not undertaken if there are acutely inflamed joints, but only after anti-inflammatory drugs have began to treat the acute inflammation.

MODALITIES THAT DELIVER HEAT BY CONVECTION

Hydrotherapy

Water is an ideal medium to deliver heat to affected tissues due to its high specific heat. Hydrotherapy utilizes this physical property to advantage by using the agitation of whirlpool to constantly move the layer of heated water that has cooled after contact with the skin and replacing it with water heated to the correct temperature. In addition to the superficial heat delivery properties of hydrotherapy, immersion of the affected body part or entire body in the case of Hubbard tank therapy allows the high specific gravity of water to partially eliminate the effect of gravity adding another potentially therapeutic sensation to the analgesic milieu. The massaging effect of water can also help reduce muscle spasm as well as provide gentle débridement of wounds. For treatment of single limbs, immersion in waters with temperatures of 115° F is generally well tolerated if careful monitoring is carried out. Temperatures above 102° F should be avoided when using total body immersion to avoid overheating. In general, total body immersion should be avoided in patients with multiple sclerosis to avoid the triggering of neurologic deficits that may become permanent.

Fluidotherapy

Fluidotherapy utilizes convection as its mechanism of heat transfer. In contrast to hydrotherapy, which relies on the high specific heat of water delivered at lower temperatures, fluidotherapy relies on the substances with a low affinity for heat, such as glass beads, pulverized corn cobs, etc., and high heat temperatures of 116° F. The result is a dry semifluid mixture that is heated by thermostatically controlled hot air. The patient is able to immerse the affected hand, foot, or portion of an extremity into the mixture. As the affected body part is heated, sweating enhances heat transfer, producing superficial heating. This treatment modality is useful in the treatment of reflex sympathetic dystrophy in that the medium used, such as glass beads, provides gentle tactile desensitization.

Deep Heating Modalities

MODALITIES THAT DELIVER HEAT BY CONVERSION

The heat delivery modalities discussed earlier have in common their ability to produce superficial heating of affected tissues. When heating of the deep tissues is desired, the clinician has several modalities at his or her disposal. These include three modalities in common clinical use: (1) ultrasound, (2) short wave diathermy, and (3) microwave diathermy. These modalities have in common their ability to safely heat deep tissues via the physical property of conversion of physical energy into heat when properly used.

Variables affecting the amount of heat ultimately delivered to deep tissues for each of these modalities include (1) the pattern of relative heating, (2) the specific heat of the tissue being heated, and (3) the physiologic factors affecting the tissues being heated. Each is discussed individually. Relative heating is the relative amount of energy that is converted into heat at any point in the tissue being heated. For sake of consistency, common reference points for the pattern of relative heating include the subcutaneous fat–muscle interface, the muscle–bone interface, and others. The pattern of relative heating is different for each of the deep heat modalities currently in common clinical use.

The specific heat of the tissue also influences how deep heat is distributed through affected tissues. Each type of tissue being heated has its own specific heat. As each of these tissues is heated, the thermal conductivity of the tissue changes as the relative temperatures of each type of tissue reaches equilibrium thus affecting the heat exchange between warmer and cooler tissues.

The physiologic changes induced by deep heating also influence the heat distribution of these deep heating modalities. It does so by modifying the physiologic factors that existed before the deep heat was applied. For example, under normal conditions, the skin temperature is generally lower than that of the deeper muscle tissues. The application of a deep heating modality will further raise the core temperature of the muscle being heating, thus increasing the temperature gradient between skin and deep muscle. However, as the deep heat is applied to muscle, an increase in blood flow to the heated muscle occurs. The incoming blood is cooler than the heated muscle, so the blood with its relatively high specific heat acts as a cooling agent, carrying off excess heat and thus cooling the muscle. The interplay of these and other physiologic factors ultimately affects the pattern of temperature distribution.

Ultrasound

Ultrasound utilizes sound waves to deliver energy to affected tissue. These sound waves occur at a frequency well above the upper level of human hearing (which occurs at approximately 20,000 Hz) and are produced by the use of a piezoelectric crystal that converts electrical energy into sound waves. These sound waves produce both thermal and nonthermal therapeutic effects on tissue, and manipulation of the physical properties of these effects can tailor the therapeutic response delivered, such as high temperature destruction of malignant liver tumors, phonophoresis (the forcing of steroids and anti-inflammatory drugs into tissues with sound), lithotripsy, and, of course, deep heating of tissues.

Although an extensive discussion of the physics involved in the therapeutic use of ultrasound is beyond the purpose of this chapter, a few general comments are useful for the clinician to understand how the modalities are used to produce deep heat for the treatment of pain and the other conditions listed in Table 336-4. For the purposes of our discussion, it is sufficient to note that the two major variables at play that determine the propagation of ultrasonic energy are (1) the absorption characteristics of the tissues being exposed to the sound waves and (2) the reflection of these sound waves as they impinge on tissue interfaces (e.g., muscle, bone). It is these two variables that give ultrasound the unique characteristic of being able to heat deep tissues such as joints with little heating of overlying skin and subcutaneous tissues.

Each variable can dramatically affect the amount of sound energy that is converted to heat. For example, bone absorbs almost 10 times more energy than skeletal muscle and almost 20 times more than of subcutaneous fat, which means that much more of the ultrasonic energy is converted into heat at the bone interface relative to the muscle or subcutaneous fat interface. Likewise, reflection of the ultrasonic energy occurs primarily at the bone interface with very little reflection occurring at the subcutaneous fat or muscle interface. This means that most of the sound energy delivered is able to penetrate the subcutaneous tissues and muscle with the reflected sound waves producing much of their heating effect at the muscle bone interface. This physical property of reflection can produce extremely high temperatures if ultrasound is accidentally used in patients with metal prosthetics and large metal surgical clips, as reflection from these artificial interfaces can produce an intense increase in reflected ultrasonic energy that can cause disastrous deep thermal injury. Thus, the admonition that ultrasound is contraindicated over metal implants should be heeded.

In order for sound waves to be effectively delivered to the intended tissues, coupling between the skin overlying the tissue and the ultrasound wand must be accomplished. This is done by introducing a medium called a coupling agent. Gel and degassed water are commonly used coupling agents. Ultrasound is usually delivered by slowly moving the ultrasound wand, which has been liberally covered with coupling agent, over the affected area for 5 to 10 minutes. For body parts with irregular surfaces such as the ankle, ultrasound can be delivered indirectly by immersing the affected body part in degassed water and placing the ultrasound wand in close proximity to the skin without actually touching it and then slowly moving over the affected areas. This technique is known as *indirect ultrasound* and will require higher energy levels to offset the absorption of sound waves by the water in order to achieve similar deep heating effects compared with direct ultrasound.

Indications for ultrasound are summarized in Table 336-5. Tendinitis and bursitis generally respond well to treatment with ultrasound, as does degenerative arthritis. Although the use of ultrasound is generally avoided when a joint is acutely inflamed, it can be beneficial as the joint inflammation is resolving after intra-articular injection of steroids and/or the implementation of anti-inflammatory drugs. Ultrasound can be used in concert to enhance the effects of active and passive range of motion and stretching of joints that have lost normal range of motion as well as in the treatment of plantar fasciitis.

Short Wave Diathermy

Short wave diathermy utilizes electromagnetic radio waves to convert energy to deep heat. As with ultrasound, short wave diathermy is thought to exert its therapeutic effects by both thermal and nonthermal mechanisms. The primary nonthermal mechanism associated with the use of therapeutic short wave diathermy occurs via vibration induction of tissue molecules when exposed to radio waves. By changing the characteristics of the shortwave applicator, the clinician can target the specific type of tissue he or she wants to heat. By using an inductive applicator that generates a magnetically induced eddy of radio wave currents in the tissues, selective heating of water-rich tissues such as muscle can be obtained. By using a capacity coupled applicator that generates heat via generation of an electrical field, selective heating of water poor tissues such as subcutaneous fat and adjacent soft tissues can be accomplished. With either type of short wave diathermy, metal must be avoided, so the patient must remove all jewelry and treatment must be carried out on a nonconductive treatment table, such as one made of wood. Furthermore, implanted pacemakers, spinal cord stimulators, surgical implants, and copper-containing IUDs should never be exposed to short wave diathermy, to avoid excessive heating and thermal injury. Indications for short wave diathermy mirror those listed for ultrasound, although the ability to heat subcutaneous fat and adjacent soft tissues not reached by superficial heat modalities and less well heated by ultrasound may lead the clinician to choose short wave diathermy to treat painful conditions and other pathologic processes that are thought to find their nidus in more superficial tissues.

Microwave Diathermy

Microwave diathermy utilizes electromagnetic radio waves with frequencies of 915 and 2456 MHz. Based on the physical properties of these waves and the corresponding dimensions of the microwave antennae, microwave diathermy has two unique properties that can be used to clinical advantage. The first is that microwaves are selectively absorbed in tissues with high water content such as muscle. This makes microwave diathermy ideally suited to treat pathologic processes that occur in the muscles and adjacent fat. The second is that microwaves are more easily focused than the short waves used in short wave diathermy, decreasing energy leaking and thus making heating more efficient and circumscribed.

Microwave diathermy also has several unique side effects of which the clinician must be aware. First, microwaves can cause cataract formation, so protective eyewear must be worn whenever microwave diathermy is used. Second, in addition to the precautions and contraindications to the use of short wave diathermy listed earlier, microwave diathermy has a selective affinity to heat water, so this technique should not be used in patients with edema, blisters, or hyperhidrosis because the sweat beads may become heated and cause burns to the skin.

SUGGESTED READING

Waldman SD, Waldman KA, Waldman HJ: Therapeutic heat and cold in the management of pain. In Waldman SD (ed): Pain Management. Philadelphia, Saunders, 2007.

CHAPTER 337

Therapeutic Cold

The application of therapeutic cold exerts both local and remote physiologic effects. Locally, the application of therapeutic cold causes vasoconstriction, which is ultimately followed by a reflex vasodilatation after the vascular smooth muscles are paralyzed from the cold. Therapeutic cold also decreases the metabolic activity of the treated part as well as decreasing muscle tone. As cooling progresses, spasticity will also be decreased. Because cooling slows nerve conduction, analgesia will occur. Indications for the use of therapeutic cold are summarized in Table 337-1.

Choosing a Therapeutic Cold Modality

As with the choice of heat modalities, matching the therapeutic cold modality to the patient is paramount to the success or failure of this treatment modality as well as to help minimize the side effects and complications associated with its use. The major determinants in the choice of therapeutic cold modalities are based primarily on two categories: (1) the body part being treated and (2) whether the modality will be administered by a qualified health care professional. As with therapeutic heat, improper use of therapeutic cold modalities can cause serious complications (Table 337-2).

Therapeutic Cold Modalities

ICE PACKS AND SLUSHES

The high specific heat capacities of ice packs and slushes allow rapid cooling of affected areas. Ice packs can be simply made by placing melting ice and cold water in a "zip-lock" plastic bag. By using crushed ice and more cold

TABLE 337–1 Indications for Therapeutic Cold

- Pain
- Muscle spasm
- Acute musculoskeletal injury
- Bursitis
- Tendinitis
- Adjunct to muscle reeducation

TABLE 337–2 Precautions and Contraindications When Using Therapeutic Cold

- Lack of or reduced sensation
- Ischemia
- Raynaud's phenomenon
- Cold intolerance

water, a slush pack can be made. Commercially available plastic packs that are often covered with a soft fabric that contain gel and may be stored in the refrigerator/freezer until use are also a convenient way of delivering therapeutic cold. The flexible nature of both of these therapeutic cold modalities allows them to be used over joints or to cool larger areas such as the low back. The rate of cooling of the skin is rapid and the rate of the cooling of deeper tissues is largely a function of the thickness of fat interposed between skin and muscle. When used for periods of 20 minutes or less, they are generally safe. The use of a towel between the ice pack or slush and the affected body part will increase tolerance and compliance and decrease the incidence of thermal injury. For home use, a package of frozen peas or corn can serve as an effective and inexpensive ice pack for many painful conditions.

ICED WHIRLPOOLS

Used primarily for athletic injuries, the iced whirlpool can rapidly cool an injured extremity by constantly moving water away that is warmed by contact with the patient's skin and replacing it with colder water. Many patients find that the temperatures required to adequately cool muscle are too uncomfortable to tolerate for the time it takes to achieve the intended therapeutic effect. However, some patients find the iced whirlpool more beneficial than similar heated whirlpool treatments.

ICE RUBS

Useful for applying therapeutic cold to larger surface areas such as the low back, ice rubs using water frozen in a plastic or Styrofoam cup can rapidly achieve therapeutic temperatures with cutaneous anesthesia being achieved within 8 to 10 minutes. Additionally, the rubbing action can produce a relaxing effect and aids in tactile desensitization. In healthy patients, ice rubs for periods of 20 minutes or less are generally safe.

EVAPORATIVE COOLING SPRAYS

Useful in the treatment of trigger points associated with fibromyalgia and as an adjunct to stretching, the application of evaporative cooling sprays can be quite effective. In the past, ethyl chloride spray was the agent of choice; however, the flammability and potential toxicity of the agent have led to the use of the chlorofluoromethane compounds. Although effective, these compounds have been criticized as having a negative effect on the environment. With the use of evaporative sprays, the trigger point or affected muscle is identified and the agent is aimed at the target area from a distance of approximately 1 meter and applied for approximately 10 seconds. Prolonged cooling of a single point with the evaporative agents can result in thermal injury.

CHEMICAL ICE PACKS

There are a large number of disposable ice packs available for home use and for clinical applications. Chemical ice packs are made of a flexible outer layer with a two-compartment inner layer. One inner compartment contains water and the other contains ammonium nitrate, which, when combined by squeezing or kneading the package, creates cooling via an endothermic reaction. These products have the advantage of requiring no refrigeration, being easily moldable to joints given their flexibility, and being relatively inexpensive. As with chemical heat packs, the temperature of chemical ice packs is poorly controlled and thermal injuries or inadequate or uneven cooling may occur. Exposure of the skin to the chemicals contained in the pack may cause chemical irritation.

Contrast Baths

A combination of therapeutic heat and cold, contrast baths are useful in the treatment of reflex sympathetic dystrophy and other sympathetically maintained pain syndromes as well as rheumatoid arthritis. Its efficacy is thought to be due to desensitization of nerves by alternating exposure of the affected extremity to heat and cold. Contrast baths consist of a hot and cold bath with temperatures of 110° F and 60° F, respectively. Therapeutic contrast baths begin with the soaking of the affected extremity in the warm bath for 10 minutes. The extremity is then rapidly transferred to the cold bath for a period of 3 minutes followed by rapid transfer back to the warm bath for 5 minutes. The cycle is repeated four times. For patients with extreme allodynia, less extreme temperatures may be required during initiation of therapy. Contrast baths should be combined with tactile desensitization techniques if optimal results are to be obtained.

SUGGESTED READING

Waldman SD, Waldman KA, Waldman HJ: Therapeutic heat and cold in the management of pain. In Waldman SD (ed): Pain Management. Philadelphia, Saunders, 2007.

CHAPTER 338

Transcutaneous Electrical Nerve Stimulation

Long before the gate control theory of Melzack and Wall, the use of sensory stimulation as a way to relieve pain had gained widespread acceptance. The modalities of heat and cold, massage, burning, scarification, moxibustion, cupping, and the like were the mainstays of nonpharmacologic pain relief. There are reports from ancient Egypt of the use of electric catfish applied to the area of pain as one means of pain control. One must wonder, given that these electric fish could produce a discharge of up to 400 V, whether the patient experienced a miraculous cure just to avoid another treatment.

It was the explanation by Melzack and Wall of how a stimulus could theoretically provide pain relief by modulating or closing a presynaptic gate that allows transmission of pain impulses to the higher centers that finally gave a scientific basis for the use of what heretofore had been highly accepted but largely discounted techniques. It was this impetus that led to renewed interest in the use of electricity as a "counterirritant" or stimulus that could close the gate on pain. The early work by Shealy in dorsal column stimulation spurred a search for less invasive ways to deliver electricity to nerves. One of the results was transcutaneous electrical nerve stimulation (TENS), which was used initially as a noninvasive screening tool to determine whether a patient would experience pain relief with implantation of a dorsal column stimulator. The ease of use and noninvasive nature of TENS made it an instant success. It was these same attributes that led to its overuse and, to a certain extent, to its mediocre reputation as a pain-relieving modality. This chapter discusses the scientific rationale behind TENS and provides the clinician with a practical guide to its use.

Scientific Basis of TENS

As mentioned, the gate control theory was, in essence, the first unified theory of pain. Earlier theories were largely based on the Cartesian view of peripheral nociception carried to the central nervous system and could not explain how a peripheral stimulus for counterirritative techniques (e.g., acupuncture, moxibustion, electric shock) could produce pain relief. The gate control theory changed everything. For the first time, scientists, psychologists, and physicians were presented with an elegantly simple explanation of how pain could be produced or blocked in the periphery. The theory stated that small-fiber afferent stimuli, particularly pain, entering the substantia gelatinosa can be modulated by large-fiber afferent stimuli and descending spinal pathways so that their transmission to ascending spinal pathways is blocked or gated.

It soon became apparent that the gate control theory could not explain many of the clinical observations associated with the use of TENS—among them, the frequently seen phenomenon of anesthesia persisting hours after stimulation and the delayed onset of analgesia experienced by some patients in pain. The neurophysiologic basis of these clinical observations remains the source of much debate—with alternative explanations such as endorphin or enkephalin release currently the most popular despite the fact that TENS analgesia is not reversed by naloxone. This lack of a scientific rationale has not deterred TENS enthusiasts, nor has it been lost on TENS critics, mainly insurance companies trying to avoid paying for this popular pain-relieving technique.

Indications for TENS

Practically every known pain syndrome has been treated with TENS because of its ease of use and lack of side effects. The true efficacy of TENS for the painful

TABLE 338–1 Clinical Indications for TENS

- Acute post-traumatic pain
- Acute postoperative pain
- Musculoskeletal pain
- Peripheral vascular insufficiency
- Functional abdominal pain
- Neuropathic pain

conditions discussed next is difficult to ascertain because true double-blind placebo-controlled trials are difficult to conduct owing to the patient's ability to perceive whether the TENS unit is delivering stimulation. Despite this fact, the following indications fall within the broad category of conditions in which TENS is, at least, worth considering. Table 338-1 summarizes the current clinical applications for TENS.

ACUTE PAIN

TENS has been shown to reduce pain and, in some cases, reduce the need for narcotic analgesics and improve pulmonary function after upper abdominal, thoracic, or orthopedic surgery as well as total hip or knee arthroplasty. TENS may also be useful following traumatic rib fracture and other acute trauma. Sterile electrodes allow placement of electrodes adjacent to lacerations or surgical incisions theoretically enhancing efficacy.

MUSCULOSKELETAL PAIN

TENS has been successfully used to reduce pain associated with osteoporosis-induced vertebral compression fractures, arthritis pain, and strains and sprains. Anecdotal reports regarding the efficacy of TENS in the management of carpal tunnel syndrome suggest a positive response in some patients who have failed conservative and surgical management of this entrapment neuropathy. The benign nature and flexibility of the modality lend themselves to these more chronic pain complaints.

PERIPHERAL VASCULAR INSUFFICIENCY

Early reports suggested that TENS had the ability to not only reduce pain associated with peripheral vascular insufficiency but also improve blood flow. Further studies have cast doubt on these claims, although there are many anecdotal reports of improvement in ulcer size and healing with the use of TENS. Given the lack of treatment options for this difficult group of patients, TENS represents a reasonable treatment option if nothing else is working.

ABDOMINAL AND VISCERAL PAIN

Most clinicians believe that TENS is not particularly useful in the treatment of chronic abdominal and visceral pain. Some investigators believe that, despite less-than-optimal pain relief, TENS may exert a salutary effect on bowel function and may also improve the obstipation associated with opioid analgesics.

NEUROPATHIC PAIN

In general, TENS has been shown to be ineffective in the treatment of most neuropathic pain states. Whether this is because of lack of sensory afferent nerve function to carry the TENS impulses to the spinal cord or because of other changes in the nervous system is unclear. There continue to be anecdotal reports of efficacy in a variety of neuropathic pain states including postherpetic neuralgia and diabetic polyneuropathy.

BEHAVIORAL PAIN

Beyond the placebo effect, there is very little to recommend TENS in the treatment of pain without an organic basis. Initial patient enthusiasm may be quickly replaced with confounding behavior surrounding the use of TENS in this clinical setting. The use of TENS without a clear clinical indication is in most cases a fruitless endeavor.

TENS Apparatus

The TENS unit consists of a battery-powered pulse generator that is capable of delivering a variety of different pulse characteristics and stimulation frequencies, leads, and a set of electrodes to deliver the stimulus to the affected area. Most investigators prefer a monophasic square wave that is delivered by a pulse generator capable of automatically sensing and compensating for the variation in impedance caused by normal and diseased skin and less than optimal electrode contact. Stimulation frequencies between 30 and 100 Hz are most comfortable for patients. Lower frequencies, which are designed to produce what is thought to be an effect more analogous to acupuncture, are recommended by some clinicians, although many patients find this stimulation frequency too uncomfortable. This discomfort may be decreased by using a pulse generator capable of producing a series of 8 to 10 rapid pulses of a lower-frequency stimulus. Reusable electrodes that require the use of conductive gel and tape have been replaced with disposable pre-gelled self-sticking electrodes.

How to Use TENS

If efficacy is to be achieved, the patient must be thoroughly familiar with the basic operation of the TENS unit and clear on how electrodes are to be placed. Although the placement of electrodes is certainly more of an art than a science, it has been my experience that giving the patient specific parameters for electrode placement works better than telling the patient to experiment with electrode placement. The clinician should generally place the electrodes in the painful area and in most instances place the electrodes within the same dermatome whenever possible. Dual-channel units are currently the norm and allow large painful areas to be treated. A form with an anatomic outline showing where the electrodes should be placed is helpful when instructing the patient on the use of the TENS unit.

Because electricity is involved, it may be useful for the clinician to first demonstrate the TENS unit by having the patient apply the electrodes to the clinician's forearm and then turning on the unit before placing electrodes on the patient. This increases patient confidence and lowers the anxiety regarding getting "shocked."

After proper electrode placement, the patient should be instructed to turn all settings on the pulse generator to zero before turning on the unit. This helps avoid any sudden shock sensation and allows the patient to slowly determine the sensation threshold necessary to feel the first sign of stimulation. In general, a level of 2.5 to 3 times the sensation threshold will be most efficacious for a variety of painful conditions. A stimulus frequency of 90 to 100 Hz is generally a good starting place and the frequency can be adjusted by the patient to comfort and efficacy, thereby giving the patient some control over one portion of his or her treatment. The clinician should demonstrate to the patient what TENS-induced muscle contractions look like and how adjusting the unit can make them stop.

Contraindications to TENS

TENS is a remarkably safe treatment modality. Without the risk of thermal injury associated with heat and cold and without the side effects associated with pharmacologic, nerve block, and surgical interventions, it is not surprising that there is a perception among many clinicians and third-party payers that TENS is being overused. There remains a small group of patients in whom TENS may produce risk (Table 338-2). These include (1) patients with pacemakers, (2) patients with significant sensory impairment (e.g., quadriplegics, due to risk of skin breakdown, patients with implantable drug delivery systems), (3) patients with spinal cord stimulators, and

TABLE 338–2 Contraindications to TENS

- Patients with pacemakers
- Patients with implantable drug delivery systems
- Patients with spinal cord stimulators
- Patients with significant impairment of sensation
- Patients who are pregnant

(4) pregnant patients, due to risk of inducement of labor. Some clinicians caution against placing TENS electrodes near the carotid sinuses or laryngeal nerves, because of the risk of vasovagal syncope and laryngospasm, although this admonition may be more theoretical than real.

Conclusion

TENS as a pain-relieving modality has appeared to stand the test of time. Despite the apparent disconnect between the enthusiastic anecdotal clinical reports and lack of demonstrable long-term efficacy of controlled studies, TENS represents a viable alternative for a variety of painful conditions. Given the favorable risk-benefit ratio and cost-benefit ratio of TENS compared with other pain-relieving options, TENS remains a part of our armamentarium in the treatment of pain.

SUGGESTED READING

Waldman SD: Transcutaneous nerve stimulation. In Waldman SD (ed): Pain Management. Philadelphia, Saunders, 2007.

CHAPTER 339

Acupuncture

Acupuncture is the best known branch of what is known as Traditional Chinese Medicine. It is estimated that approximately 40% of health care provided in China may be classified as Traditional Chinese Medicine, which, in addition to acupuncture, includes special massage techniques, moxibustion, cupping, herbal remedies, and a number of mind-body exercises. The earliest surviving texts on acupuncture date back to the second century BC. It is believed that acupuncture was brought to the Europeans by Jesuit missionaries, who coined the word "acupuncture" by combining the Latin words *acus* for "needle" and *punctum* for "puncture." Sir William Osler included the use of acupuncture in the management of sciatica in his classic text *The Principles and Practice of Medicine.*

The conceptual basis of acupuncture finds its origin in the ancient Chinese Taoist religion, which puts forth that all of nature, including humans, is simply an expression of a universal force. This universal force is believed to exist as a bipolar or dual nature, each of which represents its counterpart's opposite or extreme. Known as yin and yang, this duality is interdependent in that there can be no yin without yang. Furthermore, yin is always relational to its counterpart yang. This interdependent relationality can be best understood by thinking about the relative relationship of Chicago and the rest of the world. Chicago is west of New York City but east of Seattle, that is, Chicago cannot be only east or west, but according to Tao beliefs, must be both east and west simultaneously.

Flowing between the yin and yang of all things in nature is a life force called *oi* or *chi*. In the human, the omnipresent and dynamic life force flows through a series of pathways known as meridians. Traditional Chinese Medicine states that when there is an imbalance between the flow of *oi*, then disease may occur. It is believed that by inserting acupuncture needles into one or more of over 300 special acupuncture points along these meridians, the flow of *oi* can be adjusted to return the yin and yang to a state of equilibrium consistent with health.

In an effort to reconcile the fundamental beliefs of Traditional Chinese Medicine with modern Western medicine, several alternative explanations as to how acupuncture works have been put forth. Although skeptics initially explained away acupuncture's ability to relieve pain as simply one more example of the placebo effect, research has shown that the effects of acupuncture analgesia can be blocked with naloxone, supporting the notion that acupuncture exerts a physiologic effect on the human. This physiologic effect is thought to be mediated via the release of endorphins and enkephalins in both the spinal cord and brain, especially in the periaqueductal gray area of the midbrain. Research has also indicated that the insertion of acupuncture needles into acupuncture points can cause a release of adrenocorticotrophic hormone (ACTH) from the pituitary gland, which results in a release of cortisol from the adrenal gland.

Although among the safest analgesic techniques used in medicine today, acupuncture has been associated with rare side effects and complications. Although most patients note only minor discomfort during the insertion of acupuncture needles, an occasional patient complains of pain and refuses further treatment. Infection from improperly sterilized needles has been reported, as has bleeding in patients who are receiving platelet-inhibiting drugs or other anticoagulants. Rare occasions of damage to deep structures from acupuncture needles have also been reported.

SUGGESTED READING

Garcia MK, Chiang JS: Acupuncture. In Waldman SD (ed): Pain Management. Philadelphia, Saunders, 2007.

CHAPTER 340

Biofeedback

Biofeedback is a well-established adjunct in the treatment of a variety of painful conditions that has in the past been the province of clinical psychologists and occupational therapists. It has more recently been adopted by the growing group of practitioners who practice alternative and complementary medicine. Originally studied at Yale University in the early 1960s, biofeedback in its most basic form is a process that is designed to train the patient in techniques that are useful in gaining control of basic autonomic functions including heart rate, blood pressure, skin temperature, muscle tension, and the galvanic response. This is most often accomplished by the use of devices that provide the patient with real-time visual and/or auditory feedback as to the status of the physiologic activity being measured. Theoretically, by providing the patient with clear feedback regarding these physiologic processes of which under ambient conditions the patient is not usually aware, it is believed that the patient can learn to modify these autonomic responses to his or her benefit.

Types of devices commonly used to assist in biofeedback training include thermistor skin temperature monitors, electromyographic monitors, galvanic skin response monitors, and heart rate monitors (Table 340-1). These devices range from expensive, computer-driven models used for research to simple hand-held models designed for home use.

Thermistor skin temperature monitors are one of the most commonly used biofeedback devices and are particularly amenable for home use. Skin temperature biofeedback is useful in helping train the patient to increase the blood flow to the body part being monitored. This increase in blood flow causes a concomitant increase in skin temperature that can be detected by the skin temperature biofeedback device. Because the increased catecholamine release associated with stress causes a decrease in peripheral blood flow, by training the patient to increase peripheral blood flow, stress reduction can be theoretically accomplished. This technique has been extended to other diseases that worsen with stress, such as hypertension, ulcers, asthma, and headaches.

Electromyographic biofeedback device is also commonly used to treat pain and associated muscle spasm, as well as other diseases that tend to worsen with stress, such as asthma, headaches, and ulcers. It is also used to help reeducate muscles after stroke. The electromyographic biofeedback utilizes electrodes to measure muscle tension, and the device provides auditory and/or visual feedback to help train the patient to relax the muscles being monitored. This biofeedback approach is frequently combined with other relaxation techniques.

Galvanic skin response biofeedback utilizes electrodes to measure the amount of activity of the sweat glands,

TABLE 340–1 Commonly Used Biofeedback Devices

- Thermistor temperature-monitoring devices
- Electromyographic monitoring devices
- Galvanic skin response devices
- Heart rate monitors

which increase their activity when the patient is under stress. The electrogalvanic response that is monitored with the galvanic skin response biofeedback device can be useful in training the patient to relax. This technique has been shown to be useful in the management of stress-related diseases.

Heart rate monitors are used to monitor the patient's heart rate, which is often elevated in response to stress. Auditory and/or visual feedback from the heart rate monitor can assist in training the patient to lower his or her heart rate in response to stress.

Although there are essentially no complications associated with the use of biofeedback, a failure to address the patient's underlying causes of stress will result in less-than-optimal results. In general, biofeedback is most useful when used as part of a multidisciplinary treatment plan supervised by a health care professional who is well versed in the relationship between stress and the symptoms being treated.

SUGGESTED READING

Rinne C, Andrasik F: Relaxation techniques and guided imagery. In Waldman SD (ed): Pain Management. Philadelphia, Saunders, 2007.

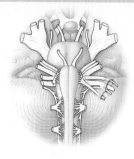

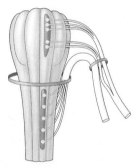

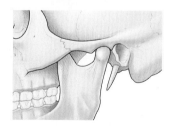

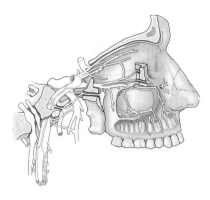

Pharmacology

CHAPTER 341

Local Anesthetics

Since the introduction of the use of cocaine to provide surgical anesthesia for eye surgery by Karl Koller in 1884, local anesthetics have become an integral part of modern medicine. Local anesthetics produce anesthesia by reversibly binding to sodium channels and rendering them inactive. This inactivation of the sodium channel causes depolarization of the nerve and produces a reversible inability of the nerve to propagate a nerve impulse. Recent research has shown that the open state of the sodium channel is the primary site of action of local anesthetics and application of local anesthetics to these open sodium channels produces what is known as a state-dependent block.

All local anesthetics have in common a similar chemical structure, which includes a lipophilic aromatic end, an intermediate connecting chain, and a hydrophilic amine end (Fig. 341-1). It is the variations in the aromatic and amine ends that determine the clinically observed properties of a specific local anesthetic under physiologic conditions. Variations in the intermediate chain portion of the basic local anesthetic molecule have resulted in the development of two basic classes of local anesthetics, the esters and the amides (see Fig. 341-1). Amino amides have an amide link between the intermediate chain and the aromatic end, whereas amino esters have an ester link between the intermediate chain and the aromatic end. These variations in the intermediate chain structure result in significant differences in the two basic classes of local anesthetics. The ester-type local anesthetics are less stable in solution, are rapidly metabolized by plasma pseudocholinesterase, and appear to be associated with rare true allergic reactions. The amide-type local anesthetics are very stable in solution, are metabolized in the liver by cytochrome P450 enzymes, and are almost never associated with true allergic reactions. Commonly used ester and amide local anesthetics are listed in Table 341-1.

Variables that affect the clinical activity of a given local anesthetic are listed in Table 341-2. These include the percent of ionization at physiologic pH, the pH of the tissues being blocked, lipid solubility, affinity for protein binding, the drug's ability to produce vasodilatation, and diffusibility. It is these properties that give each local anesthetic their unique clinical profile and, to a certain extent, their toxicity profile.

The portion of local anesthetic that exists in an ionized and nonionized form when the drug is in equilibrium is unique for each local anesthetic, as is the pH at which this equilibrium occurs. The equilibrium pH for the commonly used local anesthetics ranges from 7.6 to 8.89. Local anesthetics that have a greater unionized portion at physiologic pH will have a faster onset of action, as it is the nonionized portion of the drug that is able to diffuse across nerve membranes and block sodium channels It should be noted that this balance is also affected by the pH of the tissues in which the drug is being injected, which explains why infected tissues that have a more acidic pH are harder to block with local anesthetics.

Lipid solubility is an extremely important property affecting the clinical profile of local anesthetics, because

TABLE 341–1 Some Common Local Anesthetics

Generic Name	Trade Name
Bupivacaine	Sensorcaine, Marcaine
2-Chloroprocaine	Nesacaine
Etidocaine	Duranest
Levobupivacaine	Chirocaine
Lidocaine	Xylocaine
Mepivacaine	Carbocaine, Polocaine
Prilocaine	Citanest
Procaine	Novacaine
Ropivacaine	Naropin
Tetracaine	Pontocaine

TABLE 341–2 Properties Affecting the Clinical Properties of Local Anesthetics

- Percentage of ionization at physiologic pH
- Lipid solubility
- Affinity for protein binding
- pH of the tissues being blocked
- Drug's ability to produce vasodilatation
- Drug's diffusibility

more than 90% of the nerve cell membrane is composed of lipid and lipid-like substances. As a general rule, lipid solubility is directly proportional to the potency of a given local anesthetic, with increased lipid solubility yielding more rapid diffusion through the nerve cell membrane to allow the blocking of sodium channels. The ease with which a given local anesthetic diffuses through the tissues surrounding a nerve will also affect the time from onset to peak.

The more protein bound a local anesthetic, the longer is its duration of action as it attaches itself to protein-rich sodium channels. Conversely, with the exception of cocaine, all local anesthetics produce vasodilatation, which speeds absorption of the local anesthetic. The greater the vasodilating properties of a given local anesthetic, the shorter is its duration of action all other things being equal. The addition of vasoconstrictors such as epinephrine or Neo-Synephrine to the local anesthetic can help counteract the vasodilating properties of the drug and prolong its duration of action.

Ultimately, the toxicity of a given local anesthetic is directly related to the amount of peak circulating levels of the drug. This peak circulating blood level is affected by a number of variables including the chemical structure of the drug, how the drug is distributed, how the drug is metabolized, the speed of administration, the vascularity of the tissue being injected, the presence or absence of vasoconstrictors, and the technique of administration.

The distribution of a local anesthetic following its absorption into the blood stream follows a three-phase model. The first phase is the almost immediate distribution of the drug to highly vascular tissues including the lungs, kidneys, and liver. The second phase is the distribution of the local anesthetic to less vascular skeletal muscle and adipose tissue. The third phase is metabolism with the ester-type local anesthetics being metabolized by available plasma psuedocholinesterase and amide-type local anesthetics being metabolized by the liver.

When local anesthetic toxicity occurs, the culprit is either the inadvertent intravascular administration of the drug or simply the administration of too much drug. Most often, when either of these situations occur, the central nervous system and heart are the systems most often affected and the most problematic to treat, especially in the setting of massive intravascular injection of large amounts of local anesthetic. In such dosage ranges, both the myocardium and the cardiac conduction system are affected with resulting cardiac arrhythmias and decreased cardiac contractility. In such dosage ranges, the patient may complain of a series of neurologic complaints before losing consciousness and seizing. One of the earliest of these complains is numbness of the lips and tongue and lightheadedness. A failure to rapidly diagnose and aggressively treat local anesthetic toxicity may result in dire consequences including anoxic encephalopathy and death.

SUGGESTED READING

Heavner JE: Topical and systemic local anesthetics. In Waldman SD (ed): Pain Management. Philadelphia, Saunders, 2007.

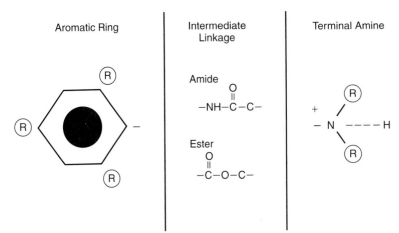

FIGURE 341–1 The basic structure of local anesthetics.

CHAPTER 342

Chemical Neurolytic Agents

Although radiofrequency destruction of nerves has largely supplanted the use of chemical neurolytic agents in many clinical situations, chemical neurolytic agents still have a place in contemporary pain management. The most commonly used chemical neurolytic agents are ethyl alcohol, phenol, glycerol, ammonium salt compounds, and hypertonic and/or hypotonic solutions (Table 342-1).

Absolute alcohol is generally administered in concentrations ranging from 50% to 95%. Higher concentration ranges are required to produce complete motor block, whereas lower concentrations may spare motor fibers while still producing varying degrees of anesthesia. Today, ethyl alcohol is most commonly used for subarachnoid, lumbar sympathetic, splanchnic, and celiac plexus block. This chemical neurolytic agent is generally avoided when destruction of the trigeminal nerves is being considered due to an unacceptable incidence of postblock neuritis known as *anesthesia dolorosa*. Postblock deafferentation pain has also been reported following intercostal block with ethyl alcohol.

Ethyl alcohol destroys nerves by denaturing lipids commonly found within neural tissue including phospholipids, cerebrosides, and cholesterol as well as causing precipitation of lipoproteins and mucoproteins. These changes result in Wallerian degeneration. When ethyl alcohol is injected into the subarachnoid space, it is hypobaric relative to the cerebrospinal fluid. Small amounts of ethyl alcohol injected into the subarachnoid space primarily affect the nerve roots and, to a lesser extent, the posterior columns and Lissauer's tract. Larger amounts of ethyl alcohol can result in significant degeneration of the spinal cord itself. Injection of ethyl alcohol in proximity of the sympathetic ganglion results in destruction of the ganglionic cell bodies and affects a postganglionic block.

When administered in lower concentrations, phenol acts as a local anesthetic. At higher concentrations, it acts as a neurolytic agent. Because of its inherent local anesthetic activity, phenol tends to be much less painful when injected compared with ethyl alcohol. Generally administered in concentrations between 6% and 8% when used for neurodestructive procedures, phenol can be mixed with glycerol to make it more hyperbaric. When administered onto neural tissue, phenol causes a concentration-dependent denaturing of the neural proteins as well as thrombosis of blood vessels. Clinical experience suggests that phenol produces a less intense destruction of neural tissue, and its effects are generally of a shorter duration than those of ethyl alcohol. Uses of phenol as a chemical neurolytic agent include subarachnoid, lumbar sympathetic, splanchnic, and celiac plexus block as well as peripheral nerve block.

Glycerol has been used primarily as a neurolytic agent for the destruction of the Gasserian ganglion. It has been used to treat both trigeminal neuralgia and pain of malignant origin that is mediated via the Gasserian ganglion. Clinical experience suggests that glycerol is more forgiving than alcohol when used for this purpose and has a much lower incidence of anesthesia dolorosa. Histologic studies of nerves exposed to glycerol reveal destructive changes similar to those seen with ethyl alcohol.

Ammonium compounds including a distillate from the pitcher plant have been used with varying degrees of success in neurodestructive procedures. Clinical experience has shown that a 6% concentration of ammonium chloride or ammonium hydroxide provides prolonged neural blockade that is generally of less intensity and shorter duration than that seen with the use of ethyl alcohol or phenol. Ammonium compounds have been used to treat intercostal neuralgia and meralgia paresthetica.

There has been a recent increased interest in use of hypertonic saline as a neurolytic agent as the Racz procedure (lysis of epidural adhesions) has gained widespread clinical acceptance. Hypertonic saline has also been administered into the subarachnoid space in an attempt to obtain prolonged neural blockade for a variety of painful conditions. This same approach has been used

TABLE 342–1 Commonly Used Chemical Neurolytic Agents

- Ethyl alcohol
- Phenol
- Glycerol
- Ammonium compounds
- Hypertonic solutions
- Hypotonic solutions

with a hypotonic solution of distilled water. Histologic examination of nerves and spinal cord segments exposed to hypertonic saline and hypotonic distilled water has not conclusively demonstrated actual neural destruction but rather osmotic swelling of the nerve bundles.

SUGGESTED READING

Jain S, Gupta R: Neurolytic agents in clinical practice. In Waldman SD (ed): Atlas of Interventional Pain Management, ed 2. Philadelphia, Saunders, 2004.

CHAPTER 343

Nonsteroidal Anti-inflammatory Drugs and the COX-2 Inhibitors

The nonsteroidal anti-inflammatory drugs (NSAIDs) are among the most widely used drugs in America today. This heterogeneous group of drugs includes aspirin, the non-acetylated salicylates, and an ever-increasing number of chemically diverse nonsalicylate compounds commonly referred to as NSAIDs and a subclass of drugs within this group that are known collectively as the cyclooxygenase (COX)-2 inhibitors. These drugs have become an integral part of the routine treatment of a variety of painful conditions.

Although it was initially assumed that the pain-relieving properties of the NSAIDs could be attributed solely to their inhibition of prostaglandins, recent research suggests that at least some of the NSAIDs may exert an antinociceptive effect separate and apart from their anti-inflammatory properties. The purpose of this chapter is to review the pharmacology, probable mechanisms of action, and adverse effects of the NSAIDs. The chapter will also provide the clinician with a practical framework for the safe and optimal use of this class of drugs.

Prostaglandin Synthesis and the Analgesic Effects of the Nonsteroidal Anti-inflammatory Drugs

It was initially believed that the pain-relieving properties of the NSAIDs were primarily the result of these drugs' ability to inhibit the peripheral formation of prostaglandins. Further understanding of how the NSAIDs produce both their beneficial and harmful effects has led to the understanding that this class of drugs most likely work by inhibition of the enzyme COX. Currently, it is known that at least two forms of the enzyme exist. These have been named COX-1 and COX-2. COX-1 activation leads to, among other things, the production of prostacyclin, which exhibits antithrombogenic and gastric cytoprotective properties. COX-2 is induced by inflammatory stimuli and cytokines and exhibits an anti-inflammatory response. The anti-inflammatory actions of the NSAIDs appear to be due to inhibition of COX-2, whereas many of the unwanted side effects of the NSAIDs (e.g., gastrointestinal bleeding) are due to inhibition of COX-1. Therefore, in theory, drugs that have the highest COX-2 activity and a more favorable COX-2:COX-1 activity ratio should have a potent anti-inflammatory activity with fewer side effects than drugs with a less favorable COX-2:COX-1 activity ratio. Although this conclusion is the logical result of years of basic science research and has led to the development of a number of new NSAIDs with this seemingly desirable profile, the recent withdrawal of rofecoxib (Vioxx) and other COX-2 inhibitors from the market due to unwanted cardiovascular side effects has called this logic into question or at least has pointed to our yet incomplete understanding of how the NSAIDs affect the various organ systems with which they interact.

Although the earlier discussion provides an explanation for how the NSAIDs can relieve pain mediated via the inflammatory response, it does not fully explain the antinociceptive properties of this group of drugs in the treatment of acute pain from a single noxious stimuli on otherwise healthy tissue. This apparent disparity between the relative anti-inflammatory and antinociceptive effects is termed "dissociation." The proposed reasons for dissociation include (1) that NSAIDs produce pain relief in the absence of the physicochemical changes induced by inflammation, (2) that the NSAIDs appear to exert some central modulation of pain via attenuation of the phenomena of "central sensitization" independent of peripheral events including prostaglandin synthesis, and (3) that there is little correlation between the efficacy of a given NSAID to relieve pain and its ability to inhibit prostaglandin synthesis. The clinical importance of these findings is currently the subject of much clinical research.

The Body's Response to Inflammation

Inflammation is the body's response to tissue injury. Many of the major events in the inflammatory process have been identified, but the reasons for these events and the roles of the different chemical mediators in this process remain unclear. Factors such as the severity of tissue injury and the patient's ability to mount an inflammatory response determine the intensity of inflammation in each individual case. Histamine mediates the initial inflammatory response by producing a transient period of vasoconstriction. Subsequently, vasodilation and increased permeability of blood vessels are a process that is sustained by prostaglandins. In addition to these vascular events, cellular events contribute to the production of inflammation. At the site of inflammation, complement activation causes the release of chemotactic peptides called "leukotrienes." These peptides diffuse into the adjoining capillaries, causing passing phagocytes to adhere to the endothelium. This process is called "pavementing." The phagocytes insert pseudopods between the endothelial cells and dissolve the basement membrane (diapedesis). The neutrophils then pass out of the blood vessel and move up the concentration gradient of the chemotactic peptides toward the site of inflammation. The end result of this phagocytic process is the eventual destruction of the neutrophil. When this occurs, intracellular free radicals and lysosomal enzymes are released from the cell into the extracellular space. These substances cause further tissue damage.

As the process continues, other chemical mediators, including complement fragments and interleukin 1, stimulate increased release of leukocytes from the bone marrow. As leukocytes, leukocyte fragments, damaged tissue, and plasma accumulate in the area of injury, an exudate (pus) forms. These events characterize acute inflammation. When the precipitating stimulus is removed or destroyed, inflammation resolves. If, however, the precipitating stimulus cannot be eliminated by these body defenses, inflammation will progress from an acute to a chronic state.

The Anti-inflammatory Drugs

SALICYLATES

Aspirin (acetylsalicylic acid) is the prototype of nonopioid anti-inflammatory drugs (Fig. 343-1). Aspirin and aspirin-like drugs are most often administered as analgesics, antipyretics, and inhibitors of platelet aggregation. To achieve anti-inflammatory activity, doses of aspirin greater than 3.6 g/day are necessary. The serum half-life of salicylates ranges from 2 hours for analgesic doses to more than 20 hours for anti-inflammatory doses.

Orally administered salicylates are rapidly absorbed from the small intestine and, to a lesser extent, from the stomach. There is no conclusive evidence that sodium bicarbonate given with aspirin (buffered aspirin) results in a faster onset of action, greater peak intensity, or longer analgesic effect. Aspirin available in buffered effervescent preparations, however, undergoes a more rapid systemic absorption and achieves higher plasma concentrations than the corresponding tablet formulations. These effervescent preparations also cause less gastrointestinal irritation. Food delays the absorption of salicylates.

Aspirin, by acetylating COX, decreases the formation of both thromboxane (a potent vasoconstrictor and stimulant of platelet aggregation) and prostacyclin (a potent vasodilator and inhibitor of platelet aggregation). Low doses of aspirin, 60 to 100 mg daily, selectively suppress the synthesis of platelet thromboxane without inhibiting the production of endothelial prostacyclin. This selective suppression may explain the favorable effect of low doses of aspirin in preventing coronary artery thrombosis. Aspirin-induced platelet dysfunction seen with higher doses of aspirin lasts for the normal life span of platelets, which is 8 to 11 days.

The decreased platelet aggregation observed with aspirin is not seen with the nonacetylated salicylate products such as choline magnesium trisalicylate (Trilisate) and salsalate (Disalcid). These nonacetylated salicylates are a much safer alternative in patients with a bleeding disorder or in those patients scheduled to undergo a surgical procedure. Aspirin should be avoided in patients with severe hepatic dysfunction, vitamin K deficiency, hypoprothrombinemia, or hemophilia because platelet inhibition in such patients can result in hemorrhage. Aspirin should also be avoided in children with chickenpox and flulike illnesses, because the drug has been implicated as a possible causative or contributory factor in the evolution of Reye's syndrome. Patients with asthma and nasal polyposis should also avoid aspirin and aspirin-like drugs, because acute allergic reactions may result.

Salicylates may cause gastric irritation and ulceration by a reduction in prostaglandins, which normally inhibits gastric acid secretion and their ability to inhibit COX-1. Alcohol ingestion may exacerbate the problem. To minimize these effects, the salicylates should be taken with food or milk or administered with cytoprotection agents. Being highly bound to albumin (80% to 90%), aspirin and aspirin-like drugs may displace other drugs such as warfarin, oral hypoglycemic, and methotrexate from protein-binding sites.

DIFLUNISAL (DOLOBID)

Diflunisal (Dolobid) is a difluorophenyl derivative of salicylic acid. This drug has a pharmacodynamic and pharmacokinetics profile similar to the other salicylates. It has been used primarily for musculoskeletal pain. It is less likely to cause the tinnitus associated with higher doses of aspirin. The initial loading dose for diflunisal is 1000 mg followed by 250 to 500 mg every 8 to 12 hours.

NONACETYLATED SALICYLATES

Choline magnesium trisalicylate (Trilisate) and salsalate (Disalcid) are two nonacetylated salicylate derivatives that appear to lack many of the side effects of the other members of the salicylate family. These drugs exert significantly fewer effects on platelets and cause fewer gastrointestinal side effects. These unique qualities are especially useful in the oncology patient who may have chemotherapy-induced clotting abnormalities. Both drugs appear to exert analgesic and anti-inflammatory effects similar to the acetylated salicylates. Choline magnesium trisalicylate is available in a liquid form, making it useful for those patients who are unable to swallow pills.

The Nonsteroidal Anti-inflammatories

Although technically the salicylates and *para*-aminophenol derivatives (acetaminophen) are included in this class of drugs, the term "nonsteroidal anti-inflammatory drug" has gained common acceptance as describing the chemically heterogeneous group of drugs that exhibit aspirin-like analgesic and anti-inflammatory properties. NSAIDs provide analgesic effects at lower doses and anti-inflammatory effects at higher doses. Many NSAIDs from a variety of chemical classes are available. More products are in various phases of clinical testing in Europe and the United States. Although the drugs referred to in common parlance as the COX-2 are also technically NSAIDs, they are considered separately next.

In general, the NSAIDs are indicated after simple analgesics have failed to relieve pain, toxic effects have developed, or inflammation is present. All NSAIDs appear to be as effective as aspirin in terms of analgesia or anti-inflammatory properties and may cause fewer gastrointestinal complaints than aspirin, although this relationship may be dose dependent. These characteristics have encouraged many physicians to select NSAIDs before aspirin despite the increased cost to the patient.

The pharmacokinetics of all individual NSAIDs are similar. All are well absorbed after oral administration, are highly protein bound (greater than 90%), and have a low volume of distribution (less than 0.2 l/kg).

The NSAIDs readily penetrate synovial fluid in concentrations approximately one-half those found in blood. Elimination is dependent on hepatic biotransformation to inactive metabolites (except sulindac, which is metabolized to an active form), with renal excretion of less than 5% of the unchanged drug.

SELECTION

Many NSAIDs are available. Busy clinicians need not be familiar with each drug, but they should have a working knowledge of one or two agents in each class of drugs. For each drug, physicians should be aware of the need for a loading dose, the time from onset of activity to peak effect, routes of administration, cost, and the side effect profile. Also, efficacy may be enhanced by choosing a drug that can be given by a nonoral route, such as rectal administration of indomethacin and intramuscular administration of ketorolac tromethamine. By capitalizing on the unique properties of each drug, physicians can tailor a treatment plan to meet each individual patient's needs. Practical suggestions for choosing an NSAID are offered in Table 343-1.

Because of the great variation in dosage ranges and dosing frequency of NSAIDs, physicians should carefully review the properties of the agent chosen. In general, dosing should be started at the low end of the recommended range and titrated upward as therapeutic response and side effects dictate. A loading dose should be used if indicated, especially when treating acute pain syndromes. Extreme caution should be exercised whenever the recommended ceiling dose is exceeded.

Patient response to NSAIDs is typically variable and highly individual. Therefore, it is reasonable to try other NSAIDs in a selected manner after an adequate trial (2 to 3 weeks) at an adequate dose (either anti-inflammatory or analgesic). Patients should always be instructed that a trial with more than one product may be necessary and compliance with the scheduled regimen is important in evaluating effectiveness. Combination of NSAIDs with other NSAIDs or aspirin increases toxic effects while providing

TABLE 343–1 Guidelines for Choosing a Nonsteroidal Anti-Inflammatory Drug

- Assess patient's renal status and prior history of peptic ulcer disease prior to starting drug.
- Determine best route of administration.
- Identify drugs that are appropriate for route of administration desired.
- Select familiar agent among these drugs whose time between onset of activity and peak effect is appropriate for pain syndrome being treated.

no added benefit. If additional analgesic effects are needed, a narcotic analgesic may be used during the acute phase of the pain problem.

SIDE EFFECTS

Considering their diversity in chemical structure, NSAIDs are extremely well tolerated and, compared with all of the other nonopioid drugs currently used to treat acute pain, have some of the most favorable risk-benefit ratios. However, as with all medications, NSAIDs can cause side effects ranging from minor annoyances (e.g., dyspepsia, diarrhea, constipation) to life-threatening conditions (e.g., gastrointestinal hemorrhage, hepatic dysfunction, renal insufficiency). Consequently, physicians need to anticipate the potential for side effects and use this important group of drugs appropriately.

NSAIDs have also been shown to cause a variety of renal complications, including peripheral edemas, transient acute renal insufficiency, tubulointerstitial nephropathy, hyperkalemia, and renal papillary necrosis. Piroxicam, tolmetin, and especially sulindac are considered less likely to have renal side effects. A higher incidence of adverse effects on kidney function has been seen with indomethacin, ibuprofen, fenoprofen, mefenamic acid, naproxen, and diclofenac. Prostaglandin-mediated renal effects are usually reversible upon discontinuation of therapy if identified early. Identifying a patient with borderline renal function purely on clinical grounds is often impossible. For this reason, a baseline measurement of the serum creatinine level should be obtained before NSAID therapy is begun. This both alerts the physician to preexisting renal problems that may be exacerbated by NSAID use and enables the physician to attribute any changes in renal function that occur during NSAID therapy in patients who had normal function prior to beginning therapy.

In general, NSAIDs should be taken with food to minimize gastrointestinal side effects. A past history of dyspepsia and gastrointestinal upset may indicate the need for the concurrent use of gastric cytoprotective agents. A past history of gastric ulceration or hemorrhage requires that NSAIDs be used only after medications that are free of gastrointestinal side effects have failed to adequately control the pain. In this event, histamine-blocking and cytoprotective agents should be given concurrently with NSAIDs and patients carefully monitored for occult gastrointestinal blood loss. NSAID therapy should be discontinued at the first sign of gastrointestinal difficulties. The concurrent use of two or more NSAIDs increases the risk of side effects (as may the concurrent use of an NSAID and a simple analgesic, such as acetaminophen). Thus, patients with acute pain must be carefully questioned about their use of over-the-counter agents.

The Cyclooxygenase-2 Inhibitors

As mentioned, as our understanding of the role the enzyme COX plays in the efficacy and side effects of the NSAIDs increased, a body of conventional wisdom developed that the majority of the side effects associated with an otherwise class of clinically useful drugs was the result of their inhibition of the COX-1 form of the COX enzyme. It was believed that if drugs could be developed that had an increased COX-2 activity, more beneficial effects and fewer side effects would result. In part, this logic was correct and a new subclass of the NSAIDs with less gastrointestinal side effects called the COX-2 inhibitors was developed. The first of these drugs, celecoxib (Celebrex), became a huge commercial success and encouraged the development and release of similar drugs. Unfortunately, with widespread clinical use, it was determined that although these new COX-2 inhibitors did produce fewer gastrointestinal side effects, they appeared to increase the risk of cardiovascular side effects, including an increased risk of myocardial infarction. Several COX-2 inhibitors were subsequently withdrawn from the market in the United States. The actual risk profile of this class of drugs has yet to be elucidated and whether these drugs should remain available for patients suffering from inflammatory arthritis and connective tissue diseases remains to be answered.

CELECOXIB (CELEBREX)

One of the first COX-2 inhibitors available for clinical use, celecoxib found widespread acceptance as an analgesic and anti-inflammatory drug. The initial promise of decreased gastrointestinal side effects, although not absolute, represented a positive development for patients and prescribing physicians alike. Supplied as 100-mg, 200-mg, and 400-mg tablets, celecoxib should be started at 100 mg BID orally or as a single 200-mg oral dose. It may be increased carefully while observing for hepatic, renal, gastrointestinal, or cardiovascular side effects to a maximum daily dose of 400 mg. Higher doses have been used for the treatment of familial polyposis but are not generally recommended for pain management indications.

Clinical experience with the drug has been positive, but the increased incidence of stroke and cardiac abnormalities led the U.S. Food and Drug Administration to mandate that the U.S. prescribing information be modified to include black-box warnings about cardiovascular and gastrointestinal risks. Whether the risk of these side effects warrants the discontinuation of this drug in patients who have tolerated it is unclear, as is whether this subclass of drugs should be used as a first-line analgesic or anti-inflammatory therapy at all.

Summary

The NSAIDs are a heterogeneous group of compounds that have been shown to be effective in the management of a variety of acute and chronic painful conditions. The clinician must understand the basic pharmacokinetics data of each NSAID that he or she prescribes in order to optimize pain relief and avoid side effects.

SUGGESTED READING

Waldman SD: Nonsteroidal anti-inflammatory drugs and COX-2 inhibitors. In Waldman SD (ed): Pain Management. Philadelphia, Saunders, 2007.

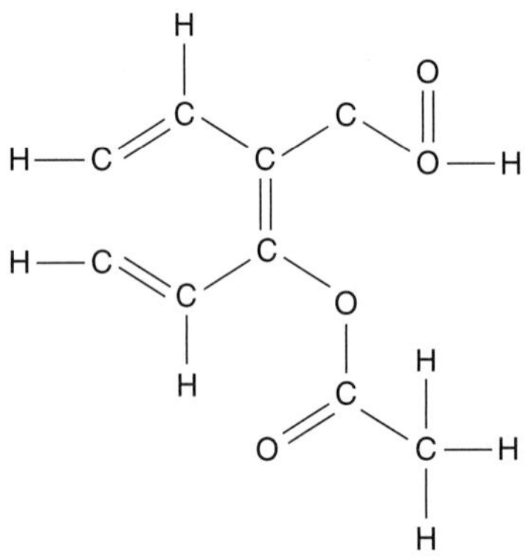

FIGURE 343–1 The chemical structure of aspirin.

Opioid Analgesics

Opioid selection is based on a variety of pharmacologic factors and patient variables. Important considerations include the division of opioids into "weak" and "strong," opioid class, differential toxicities, pharmacokinetic distinctions, and duration of effect (Table 344-1).

The so-called "weak" opioids are those typically administered orally to patients with mild to moderate pain; they include preparations containing codeine, propoxyphene, oxycodone, hydrocodone, or dihydrocodeine. Meperidine and pentazocine are sometimes used but are not recommended for the reasons discussed later.

It is important to recognize that, with the exception of pentazocine, none of these drugs has a ceiling dose, the property that would be the pharmacologic basis for their designation as "weak." Rather, their customary use at relatively low doses, which are adequate only to treat moderate pain in nontolerant patients, is based on other considerations, such as toxicity at high doses (e.g., seizures from meperidine or propoxyphene, psychotomimetic effects from pentazocine, and possible gastrointestinal intolerance from codeine), availability limited to mixtures containing acetaminophen or aspirin (e.g., hydrocodone), or historic acceptance (oxycodone). Recognition that these drugs are not inherently weak provides added therapeutic flexibility; if pain is not controlled at the usual doses and the drug is well tolerated, consideration can be given to increasing the dose, rather than switching to another drug.

In the United States, the reasonable "weak" opioid for the second rung of the analgesic ladder is typically a combination product containing an NSAID and opioid, such as 30 to 60 mg of codeine or 5 mg of oxycodone combined with 325 mg of aspirin or acetaminophen. The dose of this drug can be increased until the risks associated with the NSAID become prohibitive. With an acetaminophen- or aspirin-containing product, three tablets every 4 hours is a prudent maximum dose.

The opioids can be divided into the pure agonist class (e.g., morphine, hydromorphone, methadone, levorphanol, meperidine, and oxycodone) and the agonist-antagonist class (e.g., pentazocine, nalbuphine, dezocine, butorphanol, and buprenorphine). The latter class is characterized by a balance between agonism and competitive antagonism at one or more of the opioid receptors. Based on receptor interactions, opioids can be additionally categorized into partial agonists, of which only buprenorphine is included, and the mixed agonist-antagonists, which include pentazocine, nalbuphine, dezocine, and butorphanol.

Agonist-antagonist drugs are characterized by a lesser propensity to produce physical dependence and by a ceiling effect for respiratory depression and, probably, for analgesia. These drugs have the potential to reverse effects in patients receiving agonist opioids. Administration to patients physically dependent on an agonist drug may cause an abstinence syndrome. The mixed agonist-antagonist subclass, particularly pentazocine, also has prominent psychotomimetic effects. These characteristics, combined with the lack of oral formulations, justify the conclusion that agonist-antagonist drugs are not preferred for cancer pain management. The only exception to this generalization may be sublingual buprenorphine, which has achieved some acceptance due to the potential value of the route of administration and its relatively long duration of action.

Thus, the management of pain in the tolerant patient generally relies on the pure agonist drugs morphine, hydromorphone, methadone, and levorphanol. Oxycodone as a single entity is sometimes used as well. Meperidine is not preferred because it is metabolized to normeperidine, a compound with significant central nervous system toxicity, including myoclonus, tremulousness, and seizures.

In most countries, morphine is the first-line drug for cancer pain. Morphine is metabolized to an active compound, morphine-6-glucuronide, which is cleared by the kidney. The metabolite may contribute to the clinical effects of the parent compound, particularly in patients with relatively high concentrations due to renal insufficiency. Patients with renal failure have been reported who developed respiratory compromise during morphine treatment and were found to have high levels of the metabolite in the plasma, with almost no measurable morphine. Given the available data, it is reasonable to administer morphine cautiously to patients with stable renal insufficiency and to consider an alternative opioid in those with unstable renal function, in whom the amount of morphine-6-glucuronide may change and unpredictably influence drug effects.

The most important pharmacokinetic parameter in drug selection is its half-life. Regardless of the drug, dose, or route of administration, four to five half-lives

TABLE 344–1 Agonist Opioid Analgesics

Opioid Drug	Dose*	Peak Effect (hr)	Duration (hr)	Toxicity and Side Effects	Comments
Morphine	10 mg IM 20-60 mg PO	0.5-1 1.5-2	3-6 4-7	Constipation, nausea, sedation Constipation most common; respiratory depression most serious; itch and urinary retention uncommon	Standard comparison for opioids; multiple routes available. A switch from immediate- to controlled-release morphine should be done at the same milligram dose
Controlled-release morphine	20-60 mg PO	3-4	8-12	Same as morphine	Standard comparison for opioids; multiple routes available. A switch from immediate- to controlled-release morphine should be done at the same milligram dose
Hydromorphone hydrochloride	1.5 mg IM 7.5 mg PO	0.5-1 1-2	3-4 3-4	Same as morphine	Used for multiple routes
Oxycodone hydrochloride	30 mg PO	1	3-6	Same as morphine	
Heroin		0.5-1	4-5	Same as morphine	Analgesic action due to metabolites, predominantly morphine; not available in the United States
Levorphanol tartrate	2 mg IM 4 mg PO	0.5-1.5	4-6	Same as morphine	With long half-life, accumulation can occur after beginning or increasing dose
Methadone hydrochloride	10 mg IM 20 mg PO	0.5-1.5	4-6	Same as morphine	Risk of delayed toxicity due to accumulation is a significant problem; dosing should start on parenteral basis, with close monitoring
Codeine	130 mg IM 200 mg PO	1.5-2	3-6	Same as morphine	Usually combined with NSAID
Propoxyphene hydrochloride	65 mg PO	1.5-2	3-6	Same as morphine, plus seizures with overdose	Toxic metabolite, norpropoxyphene, accumulates with repetitive dosing but not significant at doses used clinically; often combined with NSAID
Propoxyphene napsylate	Propoxyphene napsylate 100 mg/acetaminophen 650 mg PO	1.5-2	3-6	Same as propoxyphene hydrochloride	Same as propoxyphene hydrochloride

Dose in mg that is equianalgesic to morphine sulfate 10 mg.

Continued

TABLE 344–1 Agonist Opioid Analgesics—cont'd

Opioid Drug	Dose*	Peak Effect (hr)	Duration (hr)	Toxicity and Side Effects	Comments
Hydrocodone bitartrate	Hydrocodone bitartrate 10 mg/ acetaminophen 650 mg PO	0.5-1	3-4	Same as morphine	Available only combined with acetaminophen
Oxymorphone	1 mg IM 10 mg rectally	0.5-1 1.5-3	3-6 4-6	Same as morphine	No oral formulation
Meperidine hydrochloride	75 mg IM 300 mg PO	0.5-1 1-2	3-4 3-6	Same as morphine, plus CNS excitation. Contraindicated in those taking monoamine oxidase inhibitors	Not preferred for cancer pain because of potential toxicity

are required to approach steady-state plasma levels. This becomes a clinical issue only in the case of methadone, whose half-life may be so long that drug accumulation can continue for a week or longer when dosing is instituted or the dose increased; failure to recognize this potential for accumulation has resulted in serious delayed toxicity. Levorphanol also has a relatively long half-life, but clinical experience has not suggested that delayed effects are a common problem. Nonetheless, both methadone and levorphanol should be used as second-line agents in patients with the potential for significantly prolonged drug metabolism and those who are at particular risk of adverse drug effects. Such patients include the elderly, those with organ failure (lungs, kidneys, liver, or brain), and those whose compliance or communication with the physician is in question.

Another important consideration in opioid selection is duration of analgesic effect. The short–half-life opioids, such as morphine and hydromorphone, must be administered at least every 4 hours, whereas the opioid with the longest half-life—methadone—can often be administered every 6 hours and sometimes even less frequently. Controlled-release formulations of morphine can be given every 8 to 12 hours.

In summary, morphine or hydromorphone and perhaps oxycodone are the preferred first-line drugs for severe pain in the elderly and those with major organ dysfunction. However, morphine should be used cautiously, if at all, in the patient with changing renal function. In the younger, compliant patient without organ failure, therapy can begin with morphine, or any other drug on the third rung of the "analgesic ladder." A favorable previous experience with one of these drugs may be considered in this decision. Patients who may benefit from less frequent dosing should be considered for a trial of controlled-release morphine, usually after titration with an immediate-release morphine formulation.

The physician should start with the lowest dose that produces analgesia. Relatively nontolerant patients with severe pain, including those who have failed to respond to a trial with a "weak" opioid, are generally administered an opioid at a dose equivalent to 5 to 10 mg of intramuscular morphine. Patients who are switched from a higher dose of an opioid to an alternative drug should begin at a dose that is one half to two thirds the equianalgesic dose of their current medication. This reduction is recommended in the expectation that a new drug will have relatively greater effects, due to the occurrence of incomplete cross-tolerance between opioids. To avoid side effects, elderly patients and those with compromised hepatic or renal function should receive even lower starting doses. Clinical experience also suggests that a switch to methadone should be accompanied by a greater decrement, perhaps to one third the equianalgesic dose. In all cases, the calculation of equianalgesic doses is based on well-accepted relative potencies among opioids.

Dose titration is the most important principle in opioid therapy. The dose should be gradually increased until favorable effects occur or intolerable and unmanageable side effects supervene. If pain remains severe after the initial dose, the subsequent dose can be doubled. If partial analgesia occurs, dose titration can usually follow on a daily basis. A useful approach involves concurrently administering a fixed, around-the-clock dose together with a "rescue dose," which is usually equal to 5% to 10% of the total daily dose and is offered "as needed" every one to two hours for "breakthrough" pain. This approach provides the patient with some personal control over analgesic dosing and can be used to estimate the increment in the fixed dose. For example, a patient receiving 100 mg of morphine every 4 hours, who required six "rescue" doses of 60 mg during the previous 24 hours, has demonstrated the need for at least an additional 360 mg/day; hence, it is reasonable to increase the fixed dose to 160 mg every 4 hours and simultaneously to increase the "rescue" dose to 90 mg, thereby maintaining it at 10% of the total daily dose.

For all agonist drugs except methadone, the "rescue" dose medication should be the same as the drug administered on a fixed basis. When methadone is administered on an around-the-clock basis, concurrently administering a short-half-life opioid, such as morphine or hydromorphone, will avoid unanticipated toxicity from drug accumulation.

Scheduled "around-the-clock" dosing should be used in all patients with relatively constant pain. It is important to recognize, however, that "as needed" dosing may be valuable in selected circumstances. The use of the "rescue dose" was described previously. In addition, "as needed" dosing without a concurrent fixed dosing regimen may have advantages in some settings, including (1) defining the analgesic requirement in a nontolerant patient who is beginning opioid therapy, (2) titrating methadone at less risk of drug accumulation, and (3) facilitating dose changes during rapidly changing nociception (such as that occurring with radiotherapy to a painful bony lesion).

The physician should always choose an appropriate route of administration. If the patient can swallow and absorb the drug, the oral route is always preferable. Many other routes of opioid administration are available, however, and clinicians who manage patients with pain should have knowledge of those used most frequently (Table 344-2).

The clinician must also be aware of equianalgesic doses. As noted, awareness of equianalgesic doses is necessary to safely change drugs or routes of administration. These ratios, which were developed from controlled single-dose studies of relative potency, are available for parenteral and oral dosing; the relative potency of drug administration by other routes (e.g., epidural or sublingual) is not known and complicates the management of patients treated with these approaches.

It is important to recognize that published equianalgesic doses should be viewed as broad guidelines. The dose of a new drug must be reduced in all patients due to anticipated incomplete cross-tolerance, and this reduction

TABLE 344–2 Routes of Administration

Route	Comment
Oral	Preferred in cancer pain management
Buccal	May be useful in carefully selected patients who cannot tolerate PO
Sublingual	Buprenorphine is effective when administered sublingually, while efficacy of sublingual morphine is controversial
Rectal	Available for morphine, oxymorphone, and hydromorphone. Although few studies are available, it is customarily used as if dose is equianalgesic to oral dose.
Transdermal	Transdermal fentanyl effective in selected patients
Intranasal	May be efficacious with some drugs. It is currently investigational.
Subcutaneous Repetitive bolus Continuous infusion Continuous infusion with patient-controlled analgesia (PCA)	Recent advent of ambulatory infusion pumps permits outpatient continuous infusion. Can be accomplished with any drug with a parenteral formulation.
Intravenous Repetitive bolus Continuous infusion PCA (with or without infusion)	This route indicated if other routes unavailable or not tolerated. Infusion most useful in obviating bolus effect (i.e., peak concentration toxicity or pain breakthrough at the trough).
Epidural	Clearest indication is pain in lower body with poor relief and side effects from systemic opioids. Epidural catheter can be percutaneous (from lumbar region or tunneled to abdomen) or connected to subcutaneous portal, depending on life expectancy. Intrathecal usually administered via subcutaneous pump.
Intracerebroventricular	Rarely indicated but effective in patients with no other option.

should be greater in patients predisposed to adverse effects because of advanced age or organ failure. Dose titration is almost always required after a switch to a new drug or route of administration.

Opioid side effects vary greatly among patients. Furthermore, the pattern and severity of side effects vary from drug to drug in the same patient. This observation suggests that a trial with an alternative opioid should be undertaken if intolerable side effects occur during dose titration. Early and appropriate management of side effects may enhance the patient comfort and permit dose escalation to proceed.

Common side effects include constipation, sedation, and nausea. Opioid-induced constipation is so common that many practitioners believe that laxatives should always be administered concurrently with the opioid. This probably is the best course in the elderly and others with predisposing factors for constipation (e.g., use of other drugs with constipating effects or intra-abdominal neoplasm); younger patients without these factors can be observed for the development of constipation and treated only if needed. Constipation can usually be managed by an increase in fiber consumption and the use of one of the following therapies: (1) an osmotic laxative, such as magnesium citrate, milk of magnesia, or sodium citrate, administered every 2 or 3 days; (2) chronic administration of a stool softener and a contact laxative (senna, bisacodyl, or phenolphthalein); or (3) chronic administration of lactulose, beginning at a dose of 15 to 30 mL twice daily, and titrated upward as needed. The choice of therapy should be based on the specific needs and desires of the patient. Sedation, if not transitory, can usually be reversed with a small dose of a psychostimulant, either dextroamphetamine or methylphenidate. The starting dose is 2.5 to 5 mg once or twice daily and is gradually increased if needed. Some patients also benefit from a change in the dosing interval or opioid administered.

Nausea usually can be managed by an antiemetic, such as metoclopramide, prochlorperazine, haloperidol, or hydroxyzine. Because tolerance to this effect often develops within a week or two, it is often useful to administer one of these drugs on a fixed schedule for a brief time after nausea begins, then discontinuing it to determine whether treatment is still needed. If movement-induced nausea or vertigo is prominent, an antivertiginous medication, such as meclizine, cyclizine, or scopolamine, may be helpful. Finally, if epigastric fullness or early satiety is a significant complaint, a trial of metoclopramide, a drug that enhances gastric emptying, is appropriate.

Opioid drugs can cause psychotomimetic effects (ranging from nightmares to frank psychosis), dry mouth, itch, or urinary retention (usually in men with prostatism or patients with pelvic cancer). Management includes discontinuation of other nonessential drugs with additive side effects, a change to an alternative opioid, and symptomatic treatment, if available (e.g., antihistamines for those with uncomfortable itch).

Tolerance

The physician should be aware of *tolerance*, a poorly understood phenomenon defined as a need for increasing doses to maintain opioid effects. The need for escalating doses may not reflect the primary effect of tolerance, however, and most patients who require rapidly increasing doses have progression of painful lesions or an increase in the level of psychological distress. Indeed, if progressive disease is not clinically overt, the need for increasing opioid doses should be considered a possible indication for reevaluation of the neoplasm.

When pharmacologic tolerance does occur, it typically manifests as a reduction in the duration of analgesia after a dose. This can usually be managed by dose escalation or an increase in dosing frequency. There is no limit to tolerance and, in an effort to maintain analgesia, doses can become extremely high; for example, a dose higher than that equivalent to 35,000 mg of morphine has been reported.

Tolerance usually develops rapidly to respiratory depression, and drug-induced respiratory compromise is rare in patients receiving chronic opioid therapy. Should respiratory symptoms occur, there is almost always another cause, such as pneumonia or pulmonary embolism. Patients who are receiving high opioid doses may show great sensitivity to the antagonist drugs; therefore, naloxone should be used cautiously, and only to treat symptomatic respiratory depression. In this situation, diluted naloxone (0.4 mg in 10 mL of saline) should be given slowly until the respiratory rate improves. A return to consciousness, which is often accompanied by a severe abstinence syndrome and the return of pain, should not be viewed as the goal of this intervention. Repeated doses of naloxone usually are required.

Physical dependence is a pharmacologic property of opioid drugs defined by an abstinence syndrome that occurs after abrupt discontinuation of the drug or administration of an antagonist. Presumably, all patients administered high enough doses for a long enough period of time will become physically dependent. This presents no difficulties in management if the opioid dose is tapered before discontinuation and antagonist drugs, including the agonist-antagonist analgesics, are avoided.

In contrast, addiction is a psychological and behavioral syndrome characterized by psychological dependence (drug craving and overwhelming concern with drug acquisition) and aberrant drug-related behaviors, including drug selling or hoarding, acquisition of drugs from nonmedical sources, and unsanctioned dose escalation. Unlike physical dependence, there is little evidence to support the conclusion that otherwise normal patients with painful medical diseases are at substantial risk of developing addiction from the administration of opioids in a medical context. Concern about addiction should never inhibit the aggressive management of this symptom.

SUGGESTED READING

Koyyalagunta D: The anticonvulsant compounds in clinical practice. In Waldman SD (ed): Pain Management. Philadelphia, Saunders, 2007.

CHAPTER 345

Antidepressants

Although the antidepressant compounds have been used in patients suffering from a variety of painful conditions since first released almost 50 years ago, their use in this clinical setting was predicated on the logical notion that most patients with unremitting pain were depressed. It was not until the early 1970s that Mirsky and others put forth the notion that this group of drugs might have analgesic properties separate and apart from their primary mood-altering purpose. This notion has stood the test of time, and the results of numerous controlled studies have indeed confirmed it. Given the widespread use of the antidepressant compounds as a first-line treatment for pain, one must wonder if the pharmaceutical companies that first introduced these drugs as antidepressants could turn back the hands of time, they would have introduced them as analgesics. This chapter reviews the clinical relevant pharmacology of the various antidepressant compounds that are thought to be useful in the management of pain with an eye to providing the clinician with a practical roadmap on how to implement, manage, and discontinue therapy with this heterogeneous group of drugs.

Classification of Antidepressant Compounds

For the purposes of this chapter, the antidepressant compounds can be divided into six groups: (1) the tricyclic antidepressants (TCAs), (2) the selective serotonin reuptake inhibitors (SSRIs), (3) the serotonin and noradrenergic reuptake inhibitors (SNRIs), (4) the noradrenergic and specific serotonergic antidepressants (NSSAs), (5) the noradrenergic reuptake inhibitors (NRIs), and (6) the monoamine oxidase inhibitors (MAOIs) (Table 345-1). Although many of the characteristics of the various types of antidepressant compounds are similar to the

TCAs, the unique properties of each class of drugs are discussed individually.

TRICYLIC (HETEROCYCLIC) ANTIDEPRESSANTS

The TCAs are the prototypical antidepressant compounds in clinical use for the treatment of pain and are by far the most studied. Their name is derived from their molecular structure, which is composed of three rings (Fig. 345-1). It is the modification of the middle ring and the alteration of the amine group on the terminal side chain that have resulted in a variety of clinically useful drugs. More recently, the addition of a fourth ring to the TCAs in drugs such as trazodone and amoxapine has complicated the nomenclature of this class of drugs (Fig. 345-2). As a result this class of drugs is now referred to as the heterocyclic antidepressants for sake of correctness, but the more familiar term TCAs is still used as a term of art by most clinicians to indicate the amitriptyline-like drugs regardless of their actual chemical structure and to segregate them from the SSRIs and other classes of antidepressant drugs especially the MAOIs.

Mechanism of Action

The TCAs' mechanism of action is thought to be via their ability to alter monoamine transmitter activity at the

TABLE 345–1 Classification of Antidepressant Compounds

- Tricyclic antidepressants
- Selective serotonin reuptake inhibitors
- Serotonin and noradrenergic reuptake inhibitors
- Noradrenergic and specific serotonergic antidepressants
- Noradrenergic reuptake inhibitors
- Monoamine oxidase inhibitors

synapse by blocking the reuptake of serotonin and norepinephrine. Although this pharmacologic effect begins with the first dose of the drug, most clinicians believe that clinically demonstrable improvement in the patient's pain complaints requires 2 to 3 weeks of treatment. This lag in onset of clinically demonstrable improvement suggests that there may be more at play than the simple alteration of monoamine transmitter activity. Some investigators have postulated that it is the normalization of a disturbed sleep pattern that is ultimately responsible for the analgesic properties of these drugs rather than their direct action on monoamine transmitter activity per se.

Absorption and Metabolism

The TCAs are well absorbed orally and are bound to serum proteins. This class of drugs undergoes rapid first-pass hepatic metabolism but they have relatively long elimination half-lives of 1 to 4 days due to their lipophilic nature. Diseases that affect serum proteins or decrease liver function can alter the serum levels of these drugs. These drugs are excreted in the urine and feces.

Side Effects

In addition to blocking the synaptic reuptake of serotonin and norepinephrine, the TCAs also interact with a number of other receptors, which account for the wide and varied side effect profile (Table 345-2). Many of the early TCAs, as typified by amitriptyline, exert significant anticholinergic side effects via the muscarinic receptors. Such side effects include xerostomia, xerophthalmia, constipation, urinary retention, tachycardia, decreased gastric emptying, and difficulties in visual accommodation.

TABLE 345–2 Common Side Effects of the Tricyclic Antidepressants

- Xerostomia
- Xerophthalmia
- Urinary retention
- Blurred vision
- Constipation
- Sedation
- Cardiac arrhythmias
- Sleep disruption
- Weight gain
- Headache
- Nausea
- Gastrointestinal disturbance/diarrhea
- Abdominal pain
- Inability to achieve an erection
- Inability to achieve an orgasm (men and women)
- Loss of libido
- Agitation
- Anxiety

In addition to the anticholinergic side effects of the TCAs, many of these drugs cause significant blockade of the alpha-adrenergic receptors with resulting orthostatic hypotension. The orthostatic hypotension is most likely the result of venous blood pooling in the lower extremity and viscera. This potentially dangerous side effect can range from a mild annoying sensation of transient light headedness when arising to near-syncopal episodes with falling and head injury distinct possibilities.

Other side effects include the blocking of the H_2 receptors with resultant decrease in gastric acid production as well as a variety of psychomimetic side effects that can be most upsetting to the patient. These psychomimetic side effects include vivid "Technicolor" dreams, prolonged intense dreaming, restlessness, and occasionally psychic activation. Some drugs in this class seem to produce increased appetite and weight gain, whereas others seem to suppress appetite. Increased and decreased libido as well as sexual dysfunction can occur and should be discussed with patients when assessing the efficacy of therapy with the TCA compounds. The unique side effect of priapism, which occurs in approximately 1:10,000 men when taking trazodone, should also be discussed when implementing treatment with this drug.

These side effects can usually be managed by proper dosing techniques when implementing therapy with the TCAs as discussed later but may necessitate switching to a drug with a different side effect profile to achieve patient compliance.

Abuse Potential and Side Effects on Withdrawal of the Drug

The TCAs do not appear to interact significantly with the opioid, benzodiazepine, gamma-aminobutyric acid, or beta-adrenergic receptors. There is no clinical evidence of addiction in the true sense of the word that occurs when these drugs are discontinued, but some drugs in this class have a propensity to cause a variety of symptoms including insomnia, restlessness, lack of energy, and increased cholinergic activity as manifested by excessive salivation and occasional gastrointestinal distress. These side effects can be avoided by slowly tapering the TCA over 10 to 14 days.

Overdosage

Overdosage of significant amounts of the TCAs is a serious event that, if not aggressively managed, can result in death. Although, in general, the dosages that are required to treat pain are lower than those required to treat severe depression, the advent of mail order pharmacies with their 90-day prescription requirements has made overdose a real issue as doses of amitriptyline of greater that 2000 mg can be fatal, well within the amounts prescribed in a 90-day prescription. Sedation progressing to coma combined with cardiac abnormalities, including delays in cardiac conduction as manifested by a prolonged QT interval and bizarre cardiac arrhythmia, can make the management of TCA overdose most challenging. Further complicating this clinical picture is the potential for grand mal seizures and a hypercholinergic state consisting of mydriasis, urinary retention, dry mouth and eyes, and delirium. Because of the potential for disastrous results with TCA overdosage, all such events should be taken seriously and all patients suspected of overdosage should be immediately evaluated and treated in an emergency department equipped to manage the attendant life-threatening symptoms.

Some Common Tricyclic and Tetracyclic Antidepressants

AMITRIPTYLINE (ELAVIL)

Amitriptyline is the prototype of all antidepressants. Its efficacy as an analgesic has been studied extensively, and there is significant clinical experience in this setting. Blocking both norepinephrine and serotonin, amitriptyline is an efficacious analgesic, but with significant side effects including sedation, orthostasis, and most of the troublesome anticholinergic side effects. It should be used cautiously in patients with cardiac conduction defects owing to its propensity to cause tachycardia and should not be used in patients with narrow angle glaucoma and significant prostatism. Despite its side effect profile, amitriptyline remains a reasonable starting point for implementation of TCA therapy owing to its proven efficacy, low cost, availability of liquid and parenteral formulations, ability to treat sleep disturbance, dosing flexibility, and universal availability even for those patients on Medicaid or in managed care plans with restrictive formularies. Due to its sedative properties, amitriptyline should be given as a bedtime dose starting at 10 to 25 mg at bedtime. The drug can be titrated upward as side effects allow in 10- to 25-mg doses, with care being taken to identify the increases in side effects as the dose is raised. In particular, orthostatic hypotension can be insidious in onset as the dosage of the drug is raised and may lead to falls at night when the patient gets up to use the bathroom. If analgesia is not achieved by the time the dose is raised to 150 mg, the patient should be switched to a different antidepressant compound, preferably from another class of drugs, and/or another adjuvant analgesic could be added such as gabapentin if appropriate. If the patient has partial relief of pain, this drug can be carefully titrated upward to a single bedtime dose of 300 mg.

DESIPRAMINE (NORPRAMIN) AND NORTRIPTYLINE (PAMELOR)

Both desipramine and nortriptyline are good choices for initial TCA therapy if sedation is not desired or the sedative side effects of amitriptyline are too great. Given as a morning dose, these drugs are good first choices in those patients suffering from pain who have complained of a lack of energy or who are at risk for the orthostatic side effects of amitriptyline (e.g., patients receiving warfarin sodium [Coumadin]). Dosed at 10 to 25 mg every morning and titrated upward to a maximum dose of 150 mg, pain relief will usually be seen at doses of 50 to 75 mg after 2 to 3 weeks of therapy, although improvement in sleep may occur much sooner. These drugs should be used cautiously in patients with cardiac arrhythmia and those prone to psychic activation or agitation. Such psychic activation or agitation may be exacerbated by the concomitant administration of steroids, such as epidural steroid injections.

TRAZODONE (DESYREL)

Although the unique side of effect of priapism may limit the use of this drug in men, trazodone has the sedating characteristic of amitriptyline, which is desirable in those patients suffering from sleep disturbance as part of their pain symptomatology without the cardiac, anticholinergic, and orthostatic side effects The drug should be started at a bedtime dose of 75 mg and titrated upward to 300 mg as side effects allow. Pain relief will usually occur at a dosage range of 150 to 200 mg.

SELECTIVE SEROTONIN REUPTAKE INHIBITORS

Although generally less efficacious than the tricyclic (heterocyclic) antidepressants in the treatment of pain, the SSRIs have a proven efficacy in this clinical setting. Their lack of side effects relative to the TCAs makes the SSRIs a good choice for those pain patients who cannot or will not tolerate the side effects of the TCAs, albeit at greater monetary cost.

Mechanism of Action

The SSRIs selectively block the reuptake of serotonin by blocking the sodium/potassium adenosine triphosphate (Na^+,P^+-ATP) pump resulting in increased levels of serotonin at the synaptic cleft. They also affect other serotonin receptors, most notably in the gut, which probably accounts for their propensity to cause gastrointestinal side effects, especially during initiation of therapy.

Absorption and Metabolism

The SSRIs are well absorbed orally. This class of drugs undergoes rapid first-pass hepatic metabolism by hepatic enzymes and may compete with other drugs for these enzymes resulting in increased blood levels of Coumadin and the benzodiazepines among others. These drugs have relatively long serum elimination half-lives, and given the fact that many of the SSRIs have active metabolites, side effects may persist for a long time after this class of drugs is discontinued. The SSRIs are excreted in the urine and feces.

Side Effects

As mentioned, the SSRI interaction with the serotonin receptors of the gut may result in the side effects of cramping, nausea, and diarrhea, especially during the initial implementation of therapy. These symptoms are usually self-limited and will actually decrease as the gut accommodates to the increased serotonergic milieu. In addition to the gastrointestinal side effects associated with the SSRIs, side effects associated with central nervous system activation, including tremors, insomnia, and physic activation, can limit the use of these drugs, as can the increased incidence of sexual side effects relative to the TCAs. These side effects include alterations in libido, erectile and orgasmic difficulties, ejaculatory delay, and impotence. The allegation that the SSRI fluoxetine may cause increased suicidal ideations has not appeared to be a problem with the use of this drug as an analgesic, although its relative lack of efficacy for this purpose compared with the TCAs has been a problem. It should be noted that the SSRIs can interact with the MAOIs to produce a potentially life-threatening constellation of symptoms known as the central serotonergic syndrome. The central serotonergic syndrome is characterized by hypertension, fever, myoclonus, and seizures. Tachycardia and, in extreme instances, cardiovascular collapse and death may occur. For this reason, these classes of drugs should never be used together and a long drug-free period of at least 10 half-lives should be implemented when stopping the SSRIs and starting the MAOIs. This class of drugs also appears to interact with St. John's wort, and hypertensive crises have been reported when the drugs were taken together.

Abuse Potential and Side Effects on Withdrawal of the Drug

Like the TCAs, the SSRIs do not appear to interact significantly with the opioid, benzodiazepine, gamma-aminobutyric acid, or beta-adrenergic receptors. There is no clinical evidence that addiction in the true sense of the word occurs when these drugs are discontinued, but some drugs in this class have a propensity to cause a variety of symptoms, including lack of energy, and decreased serotonergic activity as manifested by constipation and other side effects. These side effects can be avoided by slowly tapering the SSRI over 10 to 14 days.

Overdosage

In general, overdosage with the SSRIs is much less serious than overdosage with the TCAs. There have been remarkably few fatal overdoses reported in the literature or to the U.S. Food and Drug Administration involving ingestion only of an SSRI. Moderate overdoses of up to 30 times the daily dose are associated with minor or no symptoms, whereas ingestions of greater amounts typically result in drowsiness, tremor, nausea, gastrointestinal disturbances, and vomiting. At very high doses of greater than 75 times the common daily dose, the more serious adverse events, including seizures, electrocardiographic (ECG) changes, and decreased consciousness, may occur. SSRI overdoses in combination with alcohol or other drugs are associated with increased toxicity, and almost all fatalities involving SSRIs have involved ingestion of other substances.

Some Common Selective Serotonin Reuptake Inhibitors

FLUOXETINE (PROZAC, SARAFEM)

Fluoxetine is available in capsule, tablet, and liquid forms, which are usually taken once a day in the morning or twice a day, in the morning and at noon, as well as a fluoxetine delayed-release capsule that is usually taken once a week (Fig. 345-3). As the side effect profile is minimal, it is usually possible to start this drug at the lower range of the dosages thought to provide analgesia, 20 mg, and titrate upward to 60 mg as side effects allow and efficacy demands. The onset of analgesic action of fluoxetine usually occurs within 2 to 3 weeks.

PAROXETINE (PAXIL)

Well tolerated by most patients, paroxetine is another reasonable choice for patients who do not tolerate the TCAs. It comes in both an immediate-release and a controlled-release form. It is taken as a once-a-day dose or twice a day at morning and noon to minimize the side effects of tremors or irritability. There are anecdotal reports that paroxetine may have a lower incidence of ejaculatory side effects compared with fluoxetine. Paroxetine should be started at a dose of 20 mg and titrated upward to 40 mg as side effects allow and efficacy dictates.

SERTRALINE (ZOLOFT)

Sertraline is available as an immediate-release tablet or capsule as well as an oral liquid concentrate. Generally well tolerated, sertraline is taken once a day as a morning dose, starting at 50 mg and titrated upward to 200 mg as side effects and efficacy allow. This drug may also have efficacy for those patients suffering from pain who also exhibit obsessive-compulsive tendencies.

SEROTONIN AND NORADRENERGIC REUPTAKE INHIBITORS

Venlafaxine (Effexor)

Venlafaxine has been shown to be useful as an analgesic in controlled clinical trials. It has a structure that is different than that of any of the other clinically useful antidepressant compounds (Fig. 345-4). With a better side effect profile than the SSRIs, this drug is a good starting point for those patients who seem to have side effects with most adjuvant analgesics. Like amitriptyline, venlafaxine affects both serotonin and norepinephrine, which theoretically should make it more efficacious for pain than the SSRIs. It remains to be seen whether widespread clinical use will bear this out. A reasonable starting dose for pain is 25 mg of venlafaxine every 12 hours with the dose increased by 25 mg every week as side effects allow and efficacy dictate.

NORADRENERGIC REUPTAKE INHIBITORS

Reboxetine (Edronax)

The newest class of antidepressants, the noradrenergic reuptake inhibitors (NRIs), are among the least studied of the antidepressant compounds in the role as analgesics. Given the fact that reboxetine acts primarily on the noradrenergic system, theoretically it is most useful for those patients with pain who are also suffering from significant anergia and depression and cannot tolerate desipramine or nortriptyline. Not currently available in the United States but available in more than 50 other countries, reboxetine is given as a 4-mg twice-daily dose titrating upward by 1 mg each week to 10 mg as side effects allow and efficacy dictates. There are anecdotal reports that painful ejaculation can occur at higher dosages of this drug.

MONOAMINE OXIDASE INHIBITORS

Isoniazid and its derivative iproniazid were introduced in 1951 as pharmacologic treatments for tuberculosis. It was found that iproniazid inhibited the enzyme MAO and that patients with tuberculosis who were treated with this drug experienced an elevation of mood. This discovery along with the introduction of the phenothiazines ushered in the modern era of the pharmacologic treatment of psychiatric disorders. Widespread experience with this class of drugs led to an understanding that these drugs were also useful in patients suffering from chronic pain, most notably intractable headache, as well as the realization that their side effect profile limited their clinical utility. The introduction of the TCAs in the early 1960s led to the almost complete abandonment of the MAOIs except in the most severely disturbed psychiatric patients and a few recidivist headache patients. Through the almost single-handed efforts of Diamond and his colleagues at the Diamond Headache Clinic in Chicago, the efficacy and safety of the MAOIs in combination with the TCAs in the treatment of intractable headache have been firmly established.

The MAOIs are a heterogeneous group of drugs that work by blocking the oxidative deamination of the biogenic amines at the nerve synapse. This leads to the release of a larger-than-normal amount of these amines by the synapse when there is an action potential. The MAOIs are well absorbed by mouth and are metabolized in the liver primarily by acetylation. Some potential for liver damage from this class of drugs exists, and appropriate monitoring of liver function tests should be part of the patient's

TABLE 345–3 Dietary Restrictions When Taking MAO Inhibitors

- Aged foods or meats
- Overripe fruit
- Fermented foods
- Chicken livers
- Soy sauce
- Smoked or pickled meat, poultry, or fish
- Cold cuts including bologna, pepperoni, salami, summer sausage
- Alcoholic beverages (especially Chianti, sherry, liqueurs, and beer)
- Alcohol-free or reduced-alcohol beer or wine
- Anchovies
- Caviar
- Cheeses (especially strong or aged varieties)
- Figs
- Raisins, bananas
- Meat prepared with tenderizers
- Meat extracts

overall treatment plan to avoid permanent liver damage. Despite their efficacy in the treatment of intractable pain, the unpredictable and sometimes severe side effects of this class of drugs limit their use in pain management to patients for whom other, less problematic treatments have failed and are willing and able to strictly adhere to the dietary and medication restrictions required with these drugs. These restrictions are extremely important because many drugs and foods can potentiate the adrenergic and serotonergic effects of MAOIs (Tables 345-3 and 345-4).

Commonly used MAOIs include phenelzine, isocarboxazid, and tranylcypromine, which are nonselective inhibitors of MAO, with phenelzine being the one most commonly used in pain management (Fig. 345-5). Phenelzine is started at an initial morning dose of 15 mg. The dose may be increased by 15 mg per week with the second dose being given at noon as side effects allow and efficacy dictates to a total dose of 60 mg. If there is no relief of pain at this point, amitriptyline at a dose of 10 mg should be added with careful monitoring for side effects. Phenelzine should not be abruptly discontinued, and the patient should be cautioned of such, but tapered over a 2- to 3-week period.

How to Use the Antidepressant Compounds as Analgesics—Practical Considerations

There are as many ways to use antidepressants to treat pain as there are antidepressant drugs. The following is an

TABLE 345–4 Drug Interactions and MAO Inhibitors

- Allergy medicines (including nose drops or sprays)
- Appetite suppressants
- Antihistamines (Actifed DM, Benadryl, Benylin, Chlor-Trimeton, Compoz, etc.)
- Antipsychotics
- Antivert
- Asthma drugs
- Atrovent
- Blood pressure medicine
- Bucladin
- BuSpar
- Cocaine
- Cold medicines
- Demerol (deaths have occurred when combining MAOIs and a single dose of meperidine)
- Dextromethorphan, Ditropan
- Dopar, Larodopa
- Flexeril
- Insulin (MAOIs may change amount of insulin needed)
- Ludiomil
- Marezine
- Other monoamine oxidase inhibitors
- Norflex
- Norpace
- Phenergan
- Pronestyl
- Prozac and all other selective serotonin reuptake inhibitors
- Quinidex
- Ritalin
- Sinus medicine
- Symmetrel
- Tegretol
- Temaril
- Tricyclic antidepressants
- Tryptophan
- Urispas
- Wellbutrin

approach that has proved beneficial in the management of patients with a variety of painful conditions in a variety of clinical settings.

The first step in the practical implementation of antidepressant treatment for pain is to explain to the patient that you are treating pain as the primary symptom, not depression. Patients have an unfortunate tendency to attribute motive to the act of prescribing antidepressants and that motive is that the doctor thinks they are crazy enough to need medications or, in some patients, that the pain is not real and it is "all in their head." Referring to the drugs as tricyclic analgesics and providing patient information sheets that reflect this nomenclature will also help. Beware that the recent efforts by pharmacies to provide written patient information materials with each prescription may undermine the best of intentions. With patients for whom the motive for prescribing is an issue, a call to the pharmacist to enlist his or her help in patient education is beneficial.

The second step in the practical implementation of antidepressant treatment for pain is to explain to the patient that the medication will not work immediately but will take a period of weeks for the patient to experience meaningful pain relief. Explain that you are starting at a low dose and for them not to be surprised when you tell them to increase the amount of medication they are taking. This helps alleviate concerns that they are taking "too much medicine." Again, the pharmacist can be of great help in this setting.

The third step is to educate the patient in the role of normal sleep in health and its importance in pain relief.

Reinforce the salutary effects of normalization of the patient's sleep cycle as a benefit of most of the drugs discussed earlier. Let the patient know that this drug is not a "sleeping pill" but will actually help treat the sleep disturbance and, most important, the pain.

The fourth step is to discuss side effects without setting the stage for medication noncompliance. For the most part, this class of drugs is well tolerated, as the chosen drug is started at the lower range of the dosage spectrum and increases in dosage are made slowly. Preempting common early side effects of the TCAs such as xerostomia by having the patient suck on cough drops to stimulate saliva production and treating xerophthalmia with lubricating eye drops before bedtime will improve patient compliance. Telling the patient that they may feel a little "hung over" for the first few days of treatment but that this bothersome side effect will go away will also help.

The final step is to remain positive regarding the potential for the patient to obtain pain relief. Let the patient know that there will in all likelihood be some adjustment of drug dosage and in some cases that switching to another drug will be required to obtain pain relief. Most important, the message should be one of hope, not negativity.

SUGGESTED READING

Waldman SD: The antidepressant compounds. In: Pain Management. Philadelphia, Saunders, 2007.

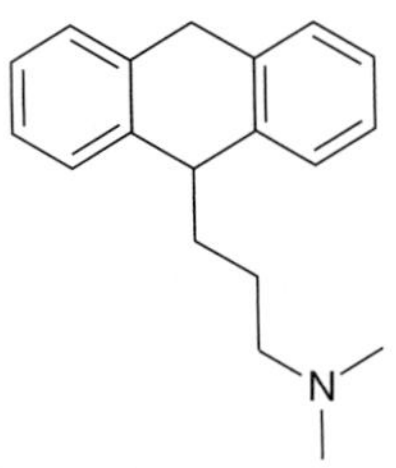

FIGURE 345–1 The chemical structure of amitriptyline.

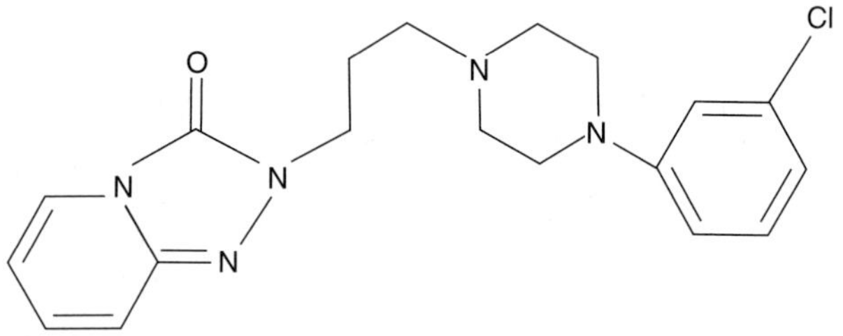

FIGURE 345–2 The chemical structure of trazodone.

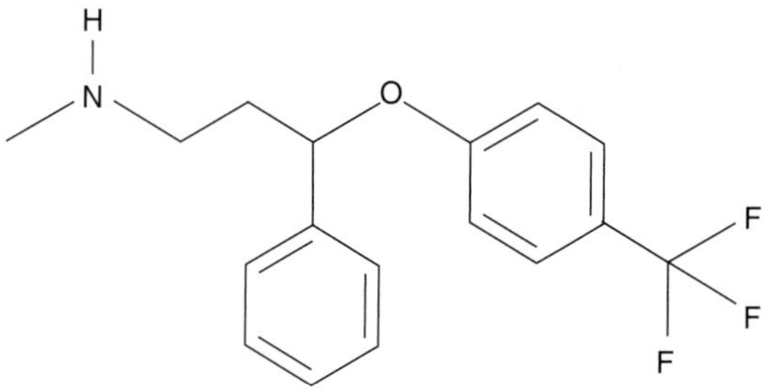

FIGURE 345–3 The chemical structure of fluoxetine.

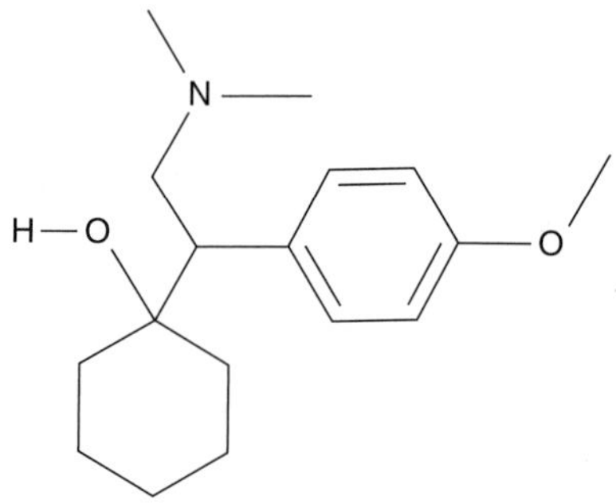

FIGURE 345–4 The chemical structure of venlafaxine.

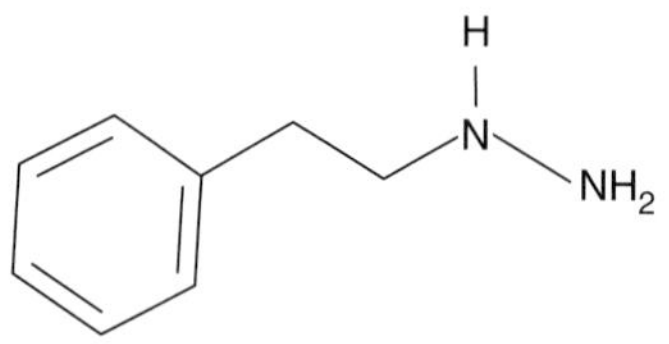

FIGURE 345–5 The chemical structure of phenelzine.

CHAPTER 346

Anticonvulsants

What is striking about the anticonvulsants that are used to treat pain is their heterogeneity. Unlike the antidepressants, which can readily be grouped into classes based on their chemical structure, such as the tricyclic antidepressants, or their mechanism of action, such as the selective serotonin reuptake inhibitors, the anticonvulsants defy simple classification. However, some generalizations can be made. The anticonvulsants that are useful in the treatment of pain can be placed into two broad categories (Table 346-1). Category 1 includes those drugs whose primary mechanism of action is to modulate the function of the voltage-dependent sodium channels, with category

2 drugs having mechanisms other than modulation of the sodium channel. Each group is discussed individually.

Category 1 Anticonvulsants—Drugs That Modulate the Voltage-Dependent Sodium Channel

While the exact mechanism of neuropathic pain has not been fully explained, some generalizations can be made that may help explain how the anticonvulsants exert their analgesic effect in this clinical setting. If one begins

TABLE 346-1 Classification of Anticonvulsants Used in the Treatment of Pain Based on Their Mechanism of Action

Category 1 Anticonvulsants—Drugs That Modulate the Voltage-Dependent Sodium Channel
• Phenytoin
• Carbamazepine
• Lamotrigine
• Topiramate
Category 2 Anticonvulsants—Drugs Whose Primary Mechanism of Action Is Unrelated to Modulation of the Voltage-Dependent Sodium Channel
• Gabapentin
• Tiagabine
• Valproic acid

TABLE 346-2 Side Effects Associated With Phenytoin

• Nystagmus
• Behavioral changes
• Peripheral neuropathy
• Gingival hyperplasia
• Gastrointestinal disturbance
• Osteomalacia
• Rash
• Stevens-Johnson syndrome
• Liver dysfunction
• Blood dyscrasias
• Pseudo-lymphoma

with an assumption that neuropathic pain is the result of abnormal nerve firing, it is reasonable to assume that anything that modulates this abnormal nerve firing downward should decrease the pain regardless of the drug's exact mechanism of action.

Conceptually, category 1 anticonvulsant drugs exert their pain-relieving effect by raising the firing threshold required to open the sodium channel and allow the nerve to reach its action potential and fire (Fig. 346-1). Although overly simplistic and ignoring the role of pain modulation at the spinal cord and central levels, the ideas that it requires more subthreshold stimuli to elicit an action potential in the presence of category 1 anticonvulsants and that there is a dose-response curve that is roughly linear fit with our overall clinical observations in this setting given the diverse nature of pain syndromes we seek to treat with the anticonvulsant drugs. Again, it must be remembered that to attribute a solely peripheral mechanism of action to the anticonvulsants is probably incorrect given the fact that all of the drugs discussed have the ability to cross the blood-brain barrier and that many of the drugs exert other pharmacologic actions at both the peripheral and higher levels, such as the ability of phenytoin to modulate the calcium and potassium channel.

SPECIFIC ANTICONVULSANT DRUGS USED TO TREAT NEUROPATHIC PAIN

Phenytoin (Dilantin)

The first modern anticonvulsant drug to be used to treat neuropathic pain, phenytoin has seen extensive use as an adjuvant analgesic over the past 60 years with mixed results (Fig. 346-2). Reasonably well absorbed after oral administration, phenytoin is extensively protein bound with only approximately 10% existing in its free state. The drug is metabolized by the liver with only a small

amount excreted in the urine. Phenytoin is available in a large array of formulations including immediate-release and sustained-release oral products in a variety of dosages as well as liquid solutions and an injectable preparation. In clinical dosage ranges, it is relatively nonsedating and reasonably well tolerated. Side effects of phenytoin are summarized in Table 346-2 and include nystagmus, behavioral changes, peripheral neuropathy, gingival hyperplasia, gastrointestinal disturbance, osteomalacia, rash, Stevens-Johnson syndrome, liver dysfunction, blood dyscrasias, and a unique side effect of pseudo-lymphoma, which is very difficult to distinguish clinically from Hodgkin's disease. Because phenytoin is so highly protein bound, any drugs that compete with the binding sites on serum albumin have the potential to increase the free fraction of the drug and can result in toxicity.

To treat neuropathic pain with phenytoin, a dose of 100 mg at bedtime is a reasonable starting place. After 1 week, an additional 100 mg morning dose may be added. If the patient is not experiencing limiting side effects, an additional 100 mg noon dose may be added. At this point, laboratory work consisting of a complete blood count and liver function tests should be performed. If the patient is tolerating the 300-mg dosing regimen and has experienced partial pain relief, the drug may be titrated upward by 30 mg per week to a maximum dose of 400 mg as side effects allow and efficacy dictates. If at the 300-mg dose the patient is experiencing no diminution of pain, it may be reasonable to switch to another anticonvulsant. Like other anticonvulsants, this drug should be discontinued slowly to avoid any rebound effect.

Carbamazepine (Tegretol)

Particularly useful in the treatment of lancinating and neuritic pain syndromes such as trigeminal neuralgia, carbamazepine has proven efficacy in the treatment of a variety of neuropathic pain syndromes including diabetic polyneuropathy, trigeminal neuralgia, glossopharyngeal neuralgia, postherpetic neuralgia, and central pain states (Fig. 346-3). There are many anecdotal reports supporting the efficacy of carbamazepine in a number of other painful conditions including HIV and chemotherapy-related neuropathic pain. Chemically related to the tricyclic antidepressants, carbamazepine is highly protein bound and is metabolized in the liver. After glucuronidation, it is excreted in the urine. Like phenytoin, interaction with other drugs that are protein-bound, such as isoniazid and warfarin sodium (Coumadin) can affect free fraction concentrations and lead to toxicity. In addition to raising the firing threshold of the voltage-dependent sodium channel, carbamazepine suppresses noradrenalin reuptake and in all likelihood exerts some of its actions centrally given its tendency to cause sedation at the higher end of the therapeutic dosage range. In addition to sedation, carbamazepine can cause a variety of central nervous system side effects including vertigo, ataxia, diplopia, dizziness, and blurred vision. Gastrointestinal side effects and rash may occur, but the most worrisome side effect of carbamazepine is its potential to cause aplastic anemia. This side effect can generally be avoided if careful and systematic monitoring of hematologic parameters is followed in all patients being considered for treatment with this drug. Table 346-3 provides a recommended monitoring protocol for patients who are to receive carbamazepine. Failure to scrupulously monitor the patient on carbamazepine can have fatal consequences. It should be noted that this drug should be used with extreme caution in those patients suffering from neuropathic pain who have previously undergone chemotherapy or radiation therapy for malignancy even if their hematologic parameters have returned to normal. These patients are extremely sensitive to hematologic side effects from carbamazepine.

Given the reasonably high incidence of central nervous system side effects associated with carbamazepine therapy, this drug should be started at a low nighttime dose of 100 mg. The drug may then be increased in 100-mg increments giving the drug on a QID dosing schedule to a maximum dose of 1200 mg as side effects allow and efficacy dictates. For patients with pain emergencies such as intractable trigeminal neuralgia that is limiting the patient's ability to maintain adequate nutrition and hydration, hospitalization is recommended so a more rapid upward titration may be safely accomplished. Regardless of the speed at which the drug is titrated upward, the monitoring protocol outlined in Table 346-3 must be followed to avoid disaster. Like all other anticonvulsants, this drug should be discontinued slowly to avoid any rebound effect.

Lamotrigine (Lamictal)

Lamotrigine is another anticonvulsant whose mechanism of action involves modulation of the voltage-dependent sodium channel. Useful in the treatment of a variety of neuropathic pain states including HIV-induced polyneuropathy, trigeminal neuralgia, and poststroke pain, lamotrigine is worth a try in those patients who have lancinating or sharp neuropathic pain that has not responded to carbamazepine or in those patients where carbamazepine is contraindicated. Lamotrigine is rapidly and completely absorbed following oral administration, reaching peak plasma concentrations 1.4 to 4.8 hours (T_{max}) post dosing. When administered with food, the rate of absorption is slightly reduced, but the effect remains unchanged. Lamotrigine is approximately 55% bound to human plasma proteins. Unlike many of the other anticonvulsants, protein binding is unaffected by therapeutic concentrations of phenytoin, phenobarbital, or valproic acid, although valproic acid significantly increases the plasma half-life of lamotrigine, and therefore the dose should be decreased with concurrent use of these drugs. Lamotrigine is metabolized predominantly in the liver by glucuronic acid conjugation. The major metabolite is an inactive 2-H-glucuronide conjugate that can be hydrolyzed by beta-glucuronidase. Approximately 70% of an oral lamotrigine dose is recovered in urine as this metabolizes. Side effects of lamotrigine include central nervous system side effects similar, although less severe, than those of carbamazepine as well as occasional gastrointestinal upset and liver function test abnormalities. Although free of the hematologic side effects associated with carbamazepine, lamotrigine has a 10% rate of significant dermatologic side effects ranging from rash to fatal Stevens-Johnson syndrome. Severe dermatologic side effects associated with lamotrigine occur with sufficient frequency that they must be carefully looked for and the drug discontinued immediately at the first sign of even the slightest rash or skin irritation. Most dermatologic side effects of lamotrigine occur within the first weeks of therapy. No monitoring of hematologic parameters is required with this drug.

TABLE 346–3 Monitoring Protocol for Carbamazepine Use

1. Obtain baseline complete blood count (CBC), chemistry profile including creatinine and liver function tests, and urinalysis *before* first dose of carbamazepine.
2. Repeat CBC and chemistry profile after week 1 of therapy.
3. Repeat CBC and chemistry profile after week 2 of therapy.
4. Repeat CBC and chemistry profile after week 4 of therapy.
5. Repeat CBC and chemistry profile after week 6 of therapy.
6. Repeat CBC after week 8 of therapy and every 2 months thereafter.

Stop carbamazepine immediately at the first sign of hematologic or liver function abnormalities.

Lamotrigine is supplied in both a chewable and oral tablet formulation in a variety of dosage strengths, making titration of the drug reasonably easy. When treating patients suffering from neuropathic pain with lamotrigine, a reasonable starting dose is 25 mg at bedtime titrating upward in 25-mg increments using a twice-daily dosing schedule to a maximum dose of 400 mg as side effects allow and efficacy dictates. Like other anticonvulsants, this drug should be discontinued slowly to avoid any rebound effect.

Topiramate (Topamax)

With demonstrated efficacy in the treatment of the pain associated with diabetic polyneuropathy, topiramate is a reasonable next choice for those patients with neuropathic pain who have not responded to the tricyclic antidepressants either alone or in combination with other anticonvulsants. Topiramate's mechanism of action is thought to be related to its ability to modulate the voltage-dependent sodium channel and in part to its ability to inhibit carbonic anhydrase. Topiramate is well absorbed orally with its absorption unaffected by food. Topiramate is not extensively metabolized, and approximately 70% is primarily eliminated unchanged in the urine. Available in a table and sprinkle formulation, topiramate is dispensed in a variety of dosages, making titration easy. A reasonable starting dose of topiramate is 25 mg at bedtime. The dosage is then increased in weekly intervals by 25 mg with a twice-daily dosing schedule to a maximum dose of 400 mg as side effects allow and efficacy dictates. Central nervous system side effects similar to those of carbamazepine occur in approximately 15% of patients taking topiramate. Like other anticonvulsants, this drug should be discontinued slowly to avoid any rebound effect.

Category 2 Anticonvulsants—Drugs Whose Primary Mechanism of Action is Unrelated to Modulation of the Voltage-Dependent Sodium Channel

GABAPENTIN (NEURONTIN)

One of the most extensively used anticonvulsants in the management of neuropathic pain, gabapentin has proven efficacy in the management of diabetic polyneuropathy, postherpetic neuralgia, phantom limb pain, and pain following spinal cord injury (Fig. 346-4). An analogue of gamma-aminobutyric acid (GABA), gabapentin is thought to exert its analgesic effect by modulating high-voltage calcium channels as well as interacting at the NMDA receptors. Generally well tolerated, gabapentin's oral absorption is not dose dependent in that as the dose administered orally increases, the proportion that is absorbed decreases. Less than 3% of orally administered gabapentin is protein bound with negligible drug metabolism. The drug is excreted unchanged in the urine. Treatment with gabapentin is begun with a 100 mg bedtime dose and then increased on a weekly basis by 100-mg increments using a qid dosing schedule. Gabapentin can be increased to a maximum dose of 3600 mg as side effects allow and efficacy dictates. Central nervous system side effects are similar to those of the other anticonvulsants but generally milder. Occasional gastrointestinal side effects including nausea and gastrointestinal upset can occur. Like other anticonvulsants, this drug should be discontinued slowly to avoid any rebound effect.

TIAGABINE (GABATRIL)

A number of anecdotal reports have suggested that tiagabine may be efficacious in the treatment of neuropathic pain. Tiagabine blocks GABA uptake into presynaptic neurons, permitting more GABA to be available for receptor binding on the surfaces of postsynaptic cells. Some investigators have suggested that tiagabine is especially effective in preventing the wind-up phenomenon often seen in many neuropathic pain states. Well absorbed orally, fatty food may decrease absorption and should be avoided when taking the drug. Like phenytoin, tiagabine is highly protein bound and the possibility for drug-drug interactions with other highly protein bound drugs exists. Tiagabine is partially metabolized in the liver and is excreted in the feces and urine. Therapy with tiagabine should begin with a 4 mg daily dose with the dose being increased in weekly intervals by 4 mg to a maximum dose of 56 mg as side effects allow and efficacy dictates. Side effects of tiagabine include dizziness, sedation, difficulty thinking, and gastrointestinal intolerance. Reports of painful urination and hematuria have also been associated with the use of tiagabine. Like other anticonvulsants, this drug should be discontinued slowly to avoid any rebound effect.

DIVALPROEX SODIUM (DEPAKOTE)

Divalproex sodium, which is metabolized to valproic acid in the gastrointestinal tract, has been used to treat a variety of neuropathic pain syndromes. Although its mechanism of action has not yet been established, it has been suggested that divalproex sodium's activity is related to its ability to increase levels of GABA. Valproic acid is well absorbed orally and rapidly distributed throughout the body, and over 90% of the drug is strongly bound to human plasma proteins, giving the potential for drug-drug interactions with other drugs that are highly protein bound. Divalproex sodium is metabolized in the liver and excreted in the urine. Central nervous system side effects are similar to those observed with tiagabine. Fatal hepatic side effects have been reported with this drug, and patients started on divalproex sodium require careful monitoring of liver function studies throughout therapy. Like other anticonvulsants, this drug should be discontinued slowly to avoid any rebound effect.

Conclusion

The anticonvulsant compounds have demonstrable efficacy in the treatment of a variety of neuropathic pain syndromes. Much like the antidepressants, the art of using these drugs correctly is paramount if high levels of patient compliance and satisfaction and the avoidance of potentially serious side effects are to be achieved.

The admonition of "start low and go slow" is quite apt when contemplating starting a patient on an anticonvulsant drug to treat neuropathic pain. Clear and frequent communication with the patient emphasizing the "trial and error" nature of the use of this class of drugs is mandatory to avoid noncompliance. Maintaining a positive and hopeful attitude toward the probability of success will often enhance the therapeutic outcome for the patient in this challenging clinical setting.

SUGGESTED READING

Waldman SD: The anticonvulsant compounds in clinical practice. In: Pain Management. Philadelphia, Saunders, 2007.

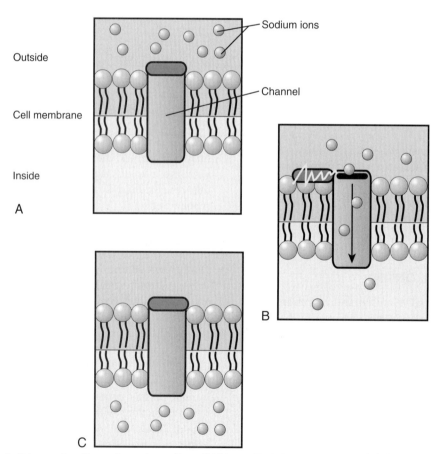

FIGURE 346–1 Category 1 anticonvulsant drugs. (From Waldman SD: Pain Management. Philadelphia, Saunders, 2007.)

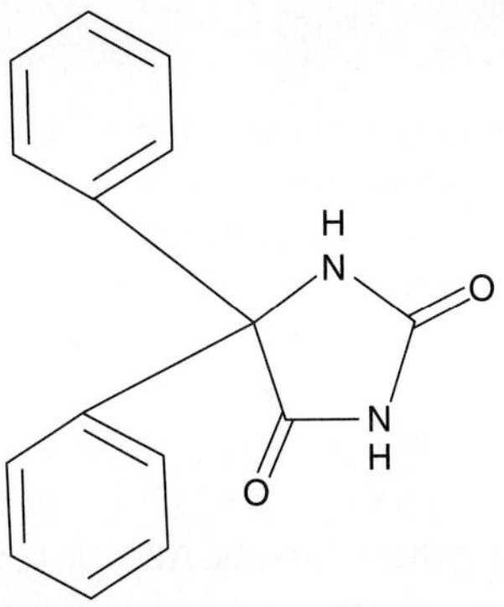

FIGURE 346–2 Chemical structure of phenytoin.

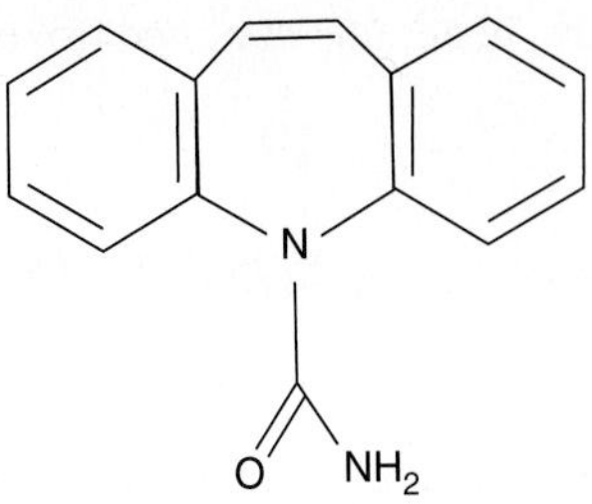

FIGURE 346–3 Chemical structure of carbamazepine.

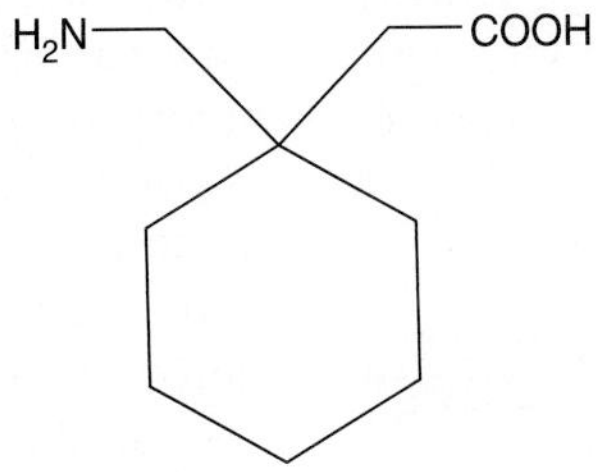

FIGURE 346–4 Chemical structure of gabapentin.

CHAPTER 347

Skeletal Muscle Relaxants

Numerous painful conditions have associated muscle spasm. These are most frequently musculoskeletal disorders (e.g., muscle strain) and central nervous system disorders associated with spasticity. Various therapeutic interventions, including pharmacologic agents, have been utilized in an attempt to reduce or obliterate muscle spasm in the belief that this will secondarily alleviate pain and improve function. Although associated with some controversy, centrally acting skeletal muscle relaxants (SMRs) are the most frequently prescribed drugs for this purpose (Table 347-1). Studies have suggested that these drugs are effective, have tolerable side effects, and can be an adjunct in the treatment of painful musculoskeletal conditions with associated muscle spasm. Their use is limited by somnolence and the potential for abuse and dependency. The SMRs should not be confused with peripherally acting skeletal muscle relaxants (e.g., curare and pancuronium), which block neuromuscular junction

TABLE 347–1 Commonly Used Skeletal Muscle Relaxants

Generic drug name	Brand drug name
Carisoprodol	Soma
Chlorphenesin carbamate	Maolate
Chlorzoxazone	Paraflex/Parafon
	Forte DSC
Cyclobenzaprine HCl	Flexeril
Metaxalone	Skelaxin
Methocarbamol	Robaxin
Orphenadrine	Norflex
Tizanidine	Zanaflex

function and are generally confined to use in surgical anesthesia.

Mechanism of Action

The exact mode of action of the SMRs is not known. The SMRs appear to preferentially depress polysynaptic reflexes. At higher dosages, the SMRs may influence monosynaptic reflexes. In animal studies, these drugs appear to produce their muscle-relaxation effects by inhibiting interneuronal activity and blocking polysynaptic neurons in the spinal cord and descending reticular formation in the brain. In humans, the SMRs do not appear to directly relax skeletal muscle. Rather, they may produce their effects through sedation, with resultant depression of neuronal activity at therapeutic doses.

Muscle Relaxants as Adjuvant Analgesics

The SMRs are generally well absorbed after oral ingestion. They have a rapid onset of action, generally within 1 hour. Some SMRs may be administered parenterally, and this route yields a more rapid onset of action. The drugs undergo biotransformation in the liver and are excreted primarily in the urine as metabolites. There is significant variability between individual drugs, plasma half-life, and duration of action.

Clinical Efficacy

There have been numerous clinical trials of SMRs. Unfortunately, study design deficiencies have made interpretation of results and comparisons between studies difficult. These deficiencies include ill-defined patient selection criteria, noncomparable musculoskeletal disorders studied, variability of disease severity and duration, and subjective assessment of the patient's response to therapy. Despite these difficulties, certain conclusions are possible. In almost all studies, SMRs were more effective than placebo in the treatment of acute painful musculoskeletal disorders and muscle spasm. Efficacy was less consistent in the treatment of chronic disorders. When used alone, SMRs were not consistently superior to simple analgesics (e.g., aspirin, acetaminophen, and nonsteroidal anti-inflammatory medications) in pain relief. However, when SMRs were used in combination with an analgesic, pain relief was superior to either drug used alone. Comparative studies of SMR efficacy have failed to document superiority of one drug over another.

Side Effects

The most commonly reported side effect of the SMRs is drowsiness. Manufacturers of these agents warn against activities that require mental alertness (e.g., driving, operation of machinery) while taking these medications. Other central nervous system (CNS) side effects include dizziness, blurred vision, confusion, hallucinations, agitation, and headaches. Gastrointestinal (GI) side effects have also been frequently reported, including anorexia, nausea, vomiting, and epigastric distress. Allergic reactions, including skin rash, pruritus, edema, and anaphylaxis, have also been observed. SMRs are generally not recommended for use in children or in pregnant or lactating women. Because SMRs undergo hepatic metabolism and renal excretion, they must be used cautiously in patients with compromised hepatic or renal function. SMRs should be used cautiously in combination with alcohol and other CNS depressants because their effects may be cumulative. Excessive doses of SMRs may result in significant toxicity with CNS depression consisting of stupor, coma, respiratory depression, and even death. On abrupt cessation of some SMRs, there may be associated withdrawal symptoms similar to barbiturate or alcohol withdrawal.

Potential for Abuse

It has been recently recognized that SMRs have the potential for abuse and dependence. Although abuse potential of the SMRs is less than that for tranquilizers or opioids, numerous incidences have been reported in the medical literature.

The SMRs may be the primary drug of abuse, presumably to obtain their sedative or mood-altering effects. More frequently, SMRs are used in combination with other CNS depressants, such as opioids or alcohol. These combinations may be taken to prolong the effect of the opioid or tranquilizer or achieve the same effect with a lesser amount of the primary drug of abuse. Prescriptions for the SMRs are more readily obtainable than prescriptions for opioids or tranquilizers and elicit less suspicion when they are frequently refilled. Because of their potential for abuse, it has been recommended that SMRs be prescribed only for acute conditions and for short periods of time. The SMRs should be used cautiously in known or suspected drug abusers, especially if they are already using other CNS depressants.

Individual Skeletal Muscle Relaxants

CARISOPRODOL (SOMA)

Carisoprodol is a precursor of meprobamate (Miltown and Equanil), and meprobamate is one of the three primary metabolites produced by hepatic biotransformation. Meprobamate dependency secondary to carisoprodol use has been reported with associated drug-seeking behavior and withdrawal symptoms. Withdrawal symptoms are similar to those seen in withdrawal from barbiturates and include restlessness, anxiety, insomnia, anorexia, and vomiting. Severe withdrawal symptoms have included agitation, hallucinations, seizures, and, rarely, death. Because of this potential for physical dependency, carisoprodol should be tapered rather than abruptly discontinued following long-term use. Idiosyncratic adverse effects include weakness, speech disturbances, temporary visual loss, ataxia, and transient paralysis.

The onset of action of carisoprodol is 30 minutes. The plasma half-life is 8 hours, and the duration of action is 4 to 6 hours. The drug is supplied as 350-mg tablets, and the recommended dose is one tablet taken 4 times daily. Carisoprodol is also available in combination with aspirin (Soma Compound) or aspirin and codeine (Soma Compound with Codeine).

CHLORZOXAZONE (PARAFON FORTE DSC)

Chlorzoxazone is similar to other SMRs, with the exception of a limited number of reported cases of significant hepatotoxicity in individuals taking this drug. Chlorzoxazone has an onset of action within 1 hour and a plasma half-life of 1 to 2 hours. The duration of action is 3 to 4 hours. The drug is available in 250- and 500-mg caplets, and the recommended adult dose is 250 to 750 mg taken 3 or 4 times daily. A pediatric dose of 20 mg/kg divided into 3 or 4 doses is suggested by the manufacturer.

CYCLOBENZAPRINE HYDROCHLORIDE (FLEXERIL)

Cyclobenzaprine is related structurally and pharmacologically to the tricyclic antidepressants (TCAs). Like other SMRs, cyclobenzaprine produces its effects within the CNS, primarily at the brainstem level. Like the TCAs, cyclobenzaprine has anticholinergic properties and may cause dry mouth, blurred vision, increased intraocular pressure, urinary retention, and constipation. The drug should, therefore, be used with caution in individuals with angle-closure glaucoma or prostatic hypertrophy. As with other TCAs, cyclobenzaprine should not be used in patients with cardiac arrhythmias, conduction disturbances, or congestive heart failure or during the acute phase of recovery from myocardial infarction. Cyclobenzaprine may interact with monoamine oxidase inhibitors and should not be used concurrently or within 14 days of discontinuation of these drugs. Withdrawal symptoms consisting of nausea, headache, and malaise have been reported following abrupt cessation of cyclobenzaprine after prolonged use.

Cyclobenzaprine has an onset of action within 1 hour. The plasma half-life is 1 to 3 days, and the duration of action is 12 to 24 hours. Cyclobenzaprine is supplied as 10-mg tablets and has a recommended dose of 10 mg 3 times per day. Up to 40 mg daily in divided doses may be prescribed. A new, controlled-release formulation of the drug is now available and appears to have a more favorable side-effect profile when compared with the immediate-release formulation.

METAXALONE (SKELAXIN)

Metaxalone is comparable in effect to the other SMRs. Adverse effects are also similar, with the exception of drug-associated hemolytic anemia and impaired liver function. Hepatotoxicity associated with metaxalone has not been as severe as that reported with chlorzoxazone. Monitoring of liver function is recommended with long-term use. Metaxalone has an onset of action of 1 hour, a plasma half-life of 2 to 3 hours, and a duration of action of 4 to 6 hours. This drug is supplied as 400-mg tablets and has a recommended dose of 800 mg 3 or 4 times daily.

METHOCARBAMOL (ROBAXIN)

Methocarbamol is available in oral and parenteral form for intravenous (IV) or intramuscular (IM) injection. Subcutaneous injection is not recommended. Taken orally, this drug is similar to the other SMRs. Parenteral use of methocarbamol has been associated with pain, sloughing of skin, and thrombophlebitis at the injection site. Additionally, overly rapid IV injection has been associated with syncope, hypotension, bradycardia, and convulsions. Because of the risk of convulsion, parenteral use of the drug is not recommended for use in patients with epilepsy.

Onset of action is 30 minutes following oral ingestion and almost immediate following parenteral administration. The plasma half-life of the drug is 1 to 2 hours. The duration of action has not been reported. Methocarbamol is produced in 500- and 750-mg tablets and has a recommended dosage range of 4000 to 4500 mg daily in 3 or 4 divided doses. For severe conditions, dosage as high as 6 to 8 g may be given for the first 48 to 72 hours. This drug is available for IV or IM injection in 10-mL single-dose vials containing 10 mg/mL. Methocarbamol tablets are also available in combination with aspirin (Robaxisal).

ORPHENADRINE CITRATE (NORFLEX)

Orphenadrine is an analogue of the antihistamine diphenhydramine (Benadryl). Orphenadrine shares some of diphenhydramine's antihistaminic and anticholinergic effects. Unlike the other SMRs, orphenadrine produces some independent analgesic effects that may contribute to its efficacy in relieving painful skeletal muscle spasm. In addition to adverse effects commonly associated with other SMRs, dry mouth, blurred vision, and urinary retention may occur as a result of the drug's anticholinergic activity. Rare instances of aplastic anemia have been reported. Like methocarbamol, orphenadrine is available for IV or IM injection. Anaphylactoid reactions have been reported following parenteral administration.

Orphenadrine has an onset of action of 1 hour following oral administration. Onset of action is approximately 5 minutes after IM injection and almost immediate with IV administration. The drug's plasma half-life is 14 hours with a duration of action of 4 to 6 hours. Orphenadrine is available in 100-mg tablets with a recommended dose of 1 tablet twice daily. Orphenadrine is available for parenteral use in 2-mL ampules containing 60 mg of the drug and is also administered once every 12 hours. Orphenadrine tablets are also produced in combination with aspirin and caffeine (Norgesic and Norgesic Forte, respectively).

TIZANIDINE HYDROCHLORIDE (ZANAFLEX)

Tizanidine hydrochloride is a centrally acting alpha$_2$-adrenergic agonist. Tizanidine is thought to exert its antispasticity properties by increased presynaptic inhibition of motor neurons, which reduces facilitation of spinal motor neuron firing. There does not appear to be any direct effect on the neuromuscular junction or any direct effect on skeletal muscle fibers by tizanidine. The drug is well absorbed after oral administration with a half-life of approximately 2.5 hours. Tizanidine is metabolized by the liver and 95% is excreted in the urine and feces. The drug is available in 2-mg and 4-mg tablets for oral administration.

Because of the drug's short half-life, it must be administered on an every 6- to 8-hours dosing schedule. Because of the common side effects of weakness and sedation, it is best to start the patient on a 2-mg bedtime dose and then titrate upward in 2-mg doses given every 6 to 8 hours every 4 to 6 days. Faster upward titration is best accomplished in an inpatient setting. The maximum daily divided dose should not exceed a total of 36 mg.

Associated Drugs Used in the Treatment of Muscle Spasm and Spasticity

Two additional drugs with muscle relaxant effects may be useful in the treatment of the pain patient, specifically the benzodiazepine diazepam and the antispasmodic agent baclofen. A third drug, dantrolene sodium, a peripherally acting spasmolytic agent, is limited to controlling chronic spasticity associated with upper motor neuron (UMN)

disorders. Finally, the cinchona alkaloid, quinine sulfate, may help to reduce nocturnal leg cramps. A discussion of each drug follows.

DIAZEPAM (VALIUM)

Diazepam is the most frequently prescribed benzodiazepine used in the treatment of muscle spasm and pain. Other available benzodiazepines have not been proved superior to diazepam for this use. Diazepam has anxiolytic, hypnotic, and antiepileptic properties in addition to its antispasmodic actions.

The muscle relaxant effects of this drug are thought to result from enhancement of gamma-aminobutyric acid (GABA)–mediated presynaptic inhibition at spinal and supraspinal sites. Numerous studies have been performed comparing diazepam to placebo and to other SMRs in the treatment of painful musculoskeletal disorders. Results have been inconsistent; in general, however, diazepam has been found to be superior to placebo but not consistently superior to other SMRs in the relief of muscle spasm and pain. Diazepam did appear to offer greater relief of associated anxiety than the other SMRs tested. Diazepam is superior, however, to other SMRs in the treatment of spasticity associated with CNS disorders such as spinal cord injury and cerebral palsy. Efficacy is similar to baclofen and dantrolene sodium for the latter use. Diazepam's long-term use in these disorders is limited primarily by sedation, abuse potential, and dependence.

Diazepam is well absorbed from the GI tract, although it may also be administered via IV or IM injection. The drug undergoes biotransformation in the liver and is excreted in the urine. Diazepam is highly lipid soluble and rapidly crosses the blood-brain barrier. Onset of action is rapid following oral and parenteral administration. Diazepam's plasma half-life is 20 to 50 hours, and active metabolites of the drug have plasma half-lives ranging from 3 to 200 hours. Duration of action is variable, depending on rate and extent of drug distribution and elimination.

Abuse and dependence have been reported with the use of diazepam and the other benzodiazepines. The incidence of these problems is somewhat controversial. The potential for abuse varies among individuals and also varies with dosages and length of therapy. Withdrawal symptoms may occur with abrupt cessation of the drug and are similar to symptoms of barbiturate or alcohol withdrawal, including anxiety, dysphoria, insomnia, diaphoresis, vomiting, diarrhea, tremor, and seizures. Diazepam may have an additive effect when taken with other CNS depressants. Diazepam may have reduced plasma clearance and an increased half-life when taken in combination with disulfiram (Antabuse) or cimetidine (Tagamet).

Diazepam's most common adverse effects are related to its CNS-depressant activity: sedation, impairment of psychomotor performance, cognitive dysfunction, confusion, dizziness, and behavioral changes. Paradoxical CNS stimulation has also been reported. Other reported adverse effects include GI complaints, skin rash, blood dyscrasias, and elevation of liver enzymes. Parenteral administration has been associated with pain and thrombophlebitis at the injection site. IV and IM administration have produced more serious side effects, especially in seriously ill or geriatric patients; these include cardiopulmonary depression, apnea, hypotension, bradycardia, and cardiac arrest.

Diazepam is available in 2-mg, 5-mg, and 10-mg tablets. The recommended dose for relief of painful musculoskeletal conditions is 2 to 10 mg 3 or 4 times daily. An extended-release 15-mg capsule (Valrelease) is produced and has a daily single dose of 1 to 2 capsules. Diazepam is available for parenteral administration in 2-mL ampules or 10-mL vials with 5 mg/mL. The recommended IM or IV dose is 5 to 10 mg every 3 to 4 hours as necessary.

BACLOFEN (LIORESAL)

Baclofen is a chemical analogue of GABA, which is an inhibitory neurotransmitter. The drug produces its effects primarily by inhibiting monosynaptic and polysynaptic transmission in the spinal cord, although some supraspinal activity may also occur. Baclofen is used chiefly in the management of spasticity associated with CNS disorders such as spinal cord lesions and multiple sclerosis. The drug is reported to be equal or superior in efficacy compared to diazepam and dantrolene sodium. It is less sedating than diazepam and has fewer serious side effects than dantrolene sodium. Baclofen may be administered intrathecally to manage severe spasticity in patients who are intolerant to, or do not respond to, oral therapy.

Baclofen has been found useful in the treatment of trigeminal neuralgia. Because of a more favorable side effect profile, some researchers consider baclofen to be the drug of first choice in the treatment of this condition. The coadministration of baclofen and carbamazepine may be more effective than either drug used singly due to a synergistic effect; however, adverse effects may be cumulative. L-Baclofen has been reported to be more effective and have fewer side effects than racemic baclofen.

Baclofen is well absorbed from the GI tract and undergoes limited hepatic biotransformation. Most of the drug is excreted unchanged in the urine. Onset of action is highly variable, ranging from hours to weeks. The drug has a plasma half-life of 2½ to 4 hours. Onset of action following intrathecal injection is 0.5 to 1 hour.

The most frequent side effects associated with the use of baclofen are drowsiness, dizziness, weakness, confusion, nausea, and hypotension. Side effects may be minimized by starting the drug at a low dose and gradually increasing it to the desired level. Abrupt discontinuation

of the drug has been associated with hallucinations, psychiatric disturbances, and seizures; therefore, the drug should be withdrawn gradually. Baclofen is produced in 10- and 20-mg tablets. The recommended starting dose is 5 mg 3 times daily for 3 days with an incremental increase of 5 mg per dose every 3 days. The therapeutic range is 40 to 80 mg daily.

DANTROLENE SODIUM (DANTRIUM)

Dantrolene sodium is a peripherally acting skeletal muscle relaxant that produces its effect on skeletal muscle by interfering with the release of calcium ions from the sarcoplasmic reticulum. The primary indication for this drug is reduction of spasticity associated with upper motor neuron disorders, including spinal cord injury, stroke, multiple sclerosis, and cerebral palsy. It is also used in the treatment of malignant hyperthermia by reducing the hypermetabolic processes associated with this disorder. Dantrolene sodium is not indicated in the treatment of other painful musculoskeletal disorders.

Dantrolene sodium is incompletely absorbed from the GI tract. It is metabolized by the liver and is excreted in the urine primarily as metabolites. Onset of action may require a week or more in the treatment of CNS-associated spasticity. The drug's plasma half-life is 8.7 hours. The most frequent side effects associated with its use are muscle weakness, drowsiness, dizziness, malaise, and diarrhea, which may be severe. Serious idiosyncratic and hypersensitive hepatocellular injury may occur that may be fulminant and fatal. This has occurred most frequently in women older than the age of 35 years. The drug is supplied in 25-mg, 50-mg, and 100-mg tablets. For treatment of spasticity, the recommended starting dose is 25 mg, which is gradually increased to a maximum daily dose of 400 mg.

QUININE SULFATE (QUINAMM)

Quinine sulfate is a cinchona alkaloid best known for its use as an antimalarial. Although controversial, many clinicians believe that the drug is useful in the treatment of nocturnal leg cramps. The drug reportedly produces its effect on skeletal muscle via an increased refractory period, reduced excitability of the motor end plate to acetylcholine, and redistribution of calcium within the muscle fiber. After oral ingestion, the drug is well absorbed, metabolized by the liver, and excreted in the urine. Quinine sulfate has a plasma half-life of 4 to 5 hours.

Some individuals are hypersensitive to quinine sulfate and develop thrombocytopenia purpura, which may be life-threatening. Visual disturbances, nausea, vomiting, and skin rash have also been reported. The drug may increase plasma levels of digoxin and may potentiate the effects of neuromuscular blocking agents due to its curariform-like effects. Cinchonism does not usually occur at doses used to treat leg cramps. The drug is supplied as 260-mg tablets, and the recommended dose is 1 or 2 tablets nightly.

Summary

The centrally acting SMRs have proved to be efficacious in the treatment of painful musculoskeletal disorders. They are generally more effective in combination with analgesics and may potentiate the effects of other CNS depressants. Their use may be limited by sedation and other undesirable side effects, as well as by their potential for abuse and dependence.

Diazepam may also be useful as a muscle relaxant and an anxiolytic, but it also causes sedation and has potential for abuse. Baclofen is used primarily to treat spasticity due to CNS lesions. It is also useful in the treatment of trigeminal neuralgia and may be the drug of first choice for this condition.

Dantrolene sodium is a peripherally acting agent used to treat spasticity. It is not useful in the treatment of other painful musculoskeletal disorders. Quinine sulfate is an antimalarial that may be useful in the treatment of nocturnal leg cramps.

Numerous evaluations have failed to demonstrate clear superiority of one skeletal muscle relaxant over another. Practitioners should base their choice of an agent on careful consideration of individual variables in a given clinical situation.

SUGGESTED READING

Waldman HJ, Waldman KA, Waldman SD: Skeletal muscle relaxants. In Waldman SD (ed): Pain Management. Philadelphia, Saunders, 2007.

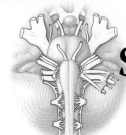

Special Patient Populations

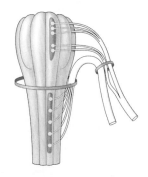

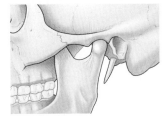

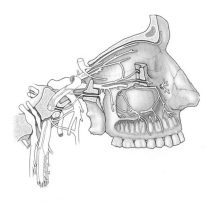

CHAPTER 348

The Parturient and Nursing Mother

Pain is a common occurrence during pregnancy due to both anatomic and physiologic changes. In general, the first tenet of the management of pain during pregnancy is to minimize the use of all drugs and to attempt to palliate the patient with reassurance and nonpharmacologic modalities. This is most crucial during the first 10 weeks of pregnancy as counted from the last menses, during the crucial period of fetal organ development.

If drug therapy is required, the pain management specialist must consider the risk to both the mother and the fetus. To aid the physician in choosing the drug with the most favorable risk to benefit ratio, the U.S. Food and Drug Administration has designed a Pregnancy Risk Classification for all approved drugs in the hope that drugs with a higher risk of teratogenic or embryotoxic effects can be avoided. Table 348-1 provides a partial list of drugs commonly used in the pain management setting.

Due to the almost universal use of nonsteroidal anti-inflammatory agents and their ready availability, it is not uncommon for a women who is unaware she is pregnant to consume a small amount of ibuprofen or naproxen. Fortunately, there is little evidence that such limited exposure poses a risk for the mother or the fetus. However, more prolonged use later in pregnancy may result in a variety of complications, including oligohydramnios and narrowing of the ductus arteriosus.

Aspirin poses problems for both the mother and the fetus owing to its inhibiting effect on platelets. The potential for epidural hematoma or peripartum hemorrhage is increased by the ingestion of regular doses of aspirin, as is the increased risk of fetal intracranial hemorrhage. Minidose aspirin for cardiac prophylaxis does not appear to carry the same risks as do higher doses of aspirin.

Although opioids when administered for a short period are a reasonably safe choice for moderate to severe acute pain in the parturient who has failed to respond to nonpharmacologic modalities, prolonged use of opioids is very problematic. Acute withdrawal of maternal opioids, especially late in pregnancy, can result in intrautero fetal withdrawal syndrome that may culminate in fetal demise. For this reason, it is recommended that opioid-dependent parturients avoid acute narcotic withdrawal until after delivery. In this setting, the newborn will almost always also be dependent on opioids and will manifest acute narcotic abstinence syndrome, and a slow tapering schedule of opioids may be required. It should be remembered that the administration of opioids in the opioid-naïve parturient will result in the potential for both maternal and fetal respiratory depression.

Although the local anesthetics lidocaine and bupivacaine are generally considered safe for the mother and

TABLE 348–1 Pregnancy Risk Classification for Some Common Pain Management Medications Based on the Food and Drug Administration Classification

FDA Classification	FDA Definition	Representative Drugs
Category A	Controlled studies indicate no risk to fetus	Multivitamins
Category B	Well-controlled human studies have shown no risk, but animal studies may have indicated teratogenic risk	Acetaminophen, fentanyl, hydrocodone, methadone, meperidine, oxycodone, morphine, ibuprofen (may decrease amniotic fluid production and narrow the ductus arteriosus)
Category C	Noncontrolled studies have indicated teratogenic risks in animals; no human controlled studies	Aspirin, ketorolac, codeine, gabapentin, pregabalin, lidocaine, propranolol, sumatriptan
Category D	Positive evidence of fetal risk, but, in certain cases, the benefits may outweigh the risks	Amitriptyline, imipramine, diazepam, phenytoin
Category X	Positive evidence of fetal risk and the risk clearly outweighs benefits	Ergotamine

the fetus, oral mexiletine is considered to be much riskier and should be used only if absolutely necessary. Epidural administration of steroids in combination with lidocaine or bupivacaine is thought to have a reasonably favorable risk-to-benefit ratio, especially in those patients who have failed to respond to less risky measures and are incapacitated by pain.

In general, the antidepressant compounds should be avoided as adjuvant analgesics during pregnancy. Some of the selective serotonin reuptake inhibitors have been associated with both fetal cardiovascular abnormalities and cleft lip and palate. The tricyclic antidepressants have also been associated with congenital abnormalities, and, given the usual ameliorating effects of pregnancy on migraine headache, they should be avoided altogether during pregnancy.

The use of anticonvulsants during pregnancy has been studied extensively in the context of seizure control, and these data have been extrapolated to the use of this class of drugs in the management of pain. Impaired folate absorption associated with phenytoin and, in all likelihood, carbamazepine and valproic acid is thought to be the cause of a significant increase in neural tube defects in the babies of mothers taking these drugs during early pregnancy. A syndrome known as fetal hydantoin syndrome consisting of mental retardation, microencephaly, and dysmorphic features has been associated with the ingestion of these drugs by parturients. In general, the use of this category of drugs as adjuvant analgesics should be avoided during pregnancy.

Medications for the treatment of headache also present special risks for the mother and her fetus. The ergot alkaloids, which are used to abort acute migraine headache, are absolutely contraindicated in pregnancy owing to both a propensity to induce uterine contractions and spontaneous abortion and the teratogenic effect on the fetus. Sumatriptan, a selective serotonin agonist drug used to abort acute migraine headache, is also associated with an increased incidence of fetal abnormalities and should not be used during pregnancy. The beta-blocker propranolol, which has gained wide acceptance as a prophylactic agent in the treatment of migraine headache, is probably safer than the other headache drugs mentioned here but should also be avoided, although it is probably safe in the lactating mother.

Drugs with high lipid solubility, lower molecular weight, low protein binding, and an active moiety that exists in an unionized state are not only transferred transplacentally but also excreted in breast milk. Although only a small percentage of the maternal dose is excreted in breast milk, the effects of these drugs on the newborn must still be kept in mind. As with pregnancy, an avoidance of any and all drugs whenever possible when the mother is breastfeeding seems a prudent course of action. If drugs need to be given to the breastfeeding mother, they should be administered so as to allow the longest time possible between the administration of the drug and the baby's next feeding. In general, drugs with longer half-lives and drugs formulated as sustained-release products should be avoided in this setting.

SUGGESTED READING

Niebyl JR: Nonanesthetic drugs during pregnancy and lactation. In Chestnut DH (ed): Obstetrical Anesthesia: Principles and Practice, ed 3. St. Louis, Mosby, 2004.

CHAPTER 349

The Pediatric Patient with Headaches

Headaches are a common complaint in the pediatric population. They tend to increase in frequency and intensity as children reach adolescence. Before puberty, headaches are more frequent in boys, but after the onset of puberty, they are more frequent in girls. As with adults, pediatric headaches are most often of benign etiology, but on occasion can be the harbinger of life-threatening disease. Despite the relative frequency of these common complaints, most physicians approach the pediatric patient suffering from headache and facial pain with great trepidation. This high degree of concern stems from two problems:

1. The vast majority of pediatric patients suffering from headache and/or facial pain have a normal physical examination and normal laboratory and radiographic findings. This lack of objective parameters from which physicians may make a diagnosis and initiate

treatment runs against the "scientific" approach that they take when evaluating and treating other disease states.

2. Physicians recognize that headache and/or facial pain may represent the harbinger of life-threatening illness; to ignore such symptoms may risk the life of the patient.

By gaining an understanding of the common types of headache and facial pain that affect children and adolescents, physicians can do much to ease their anxiety when evaluating and treating this group of patients.

Evaluation of the pediatric patient with headache begins with the taking of a targeted headache history. Special attention should be given to positive responses to factors that cause concern. Obtaining a targeted history is the most important portion of the evaluation of the patient suffering from headache and facial pain. From the history, physicians should be able to recognize the emergence of a specific constellation of symptoms that point to a working diagnosis in most patients with headache and/or facial pain. Failure to obtain a targeted history can lead not only to the implementation of an ineffective treatment plan but also, in some situations, to the failure to recognize life-threatening disease.

In most simplistic terms, the targeted history allows physicians to determine "sick" from "well." If it is determined that in all probability the patient is well (i.e., that no life-threatening illness exists), the workup and treatment plan may proceed at a more conservative pace. Obviously, if the targeted history points to a life-threatening disease process, an aggressive course of action is indicated.

The following areas of historical information should be explored not only to distinguish sick patients from well ones but also to try to ascertain the specific diagnosis:

Chronicity

The length of illness sets the direction of the initial history and carries much weight in the "sick" from "well" determination. For this reason, it serves as the starting point of the targeted history. In general, headaches that have been present for 5 to 6 years are in and of themselves not associated with progressive and life-threatening neurologic disease. This finding leads one to strongly consider a self-limited pain syndrome; hence, the "well" determination. Conversely, the sudden onset of severe headache or the sudden change in the character of a headache or facial pain syndrome that has been stable for many years must be considered to fall in the category of "sick" until proved otherwise. This type of pain manifestation has often been called the "first or worst" syndrome. Patients who fall within this category deserve a high level of concern, and their pain should be viewed as a medical emergency.

TABLE 349–1 Commonly Occurring Aurae

Ocular Symptoms
• Fortification spectra (teichopsia)
• Flashing lights (photopsia)
• Scotomata
• Hemianopia
• Visual hallucinations
Auditory Symptoms
• Auditory hallucinations
Olfactory Symptoms
• Olfactory hallucinations
Motor and Sensory Symptoms
• Weakness
• Paresthesia

Pitfalls in evaluation of chronicity include failure to (1) identify ominous changes in a longstanding stable headache or facial pain syndrome; (2) attribute the sudden onset of symptoms to a benign etiology without adequate evaluation (e.g., attributing a sudden, severe headache in a patient with generalized staphylococcal sepsis simply to fever without ruling out cerebral abscess); and (3) recognize new symptoms superimposed on chronic headache symptomatology (e.g., attributing increased headache when coughing to a patient's asthma while ignoring the fact that the patient also has a known Wilms' tumor, which could silently metastasize to the brain, causing increased intracranial pressure).

Age at Onset

Headaches that begin in childhood through the second decade of life are most often vascular in nature. Headaches and facial pain that begin later in life are statistically most commonly psychogenic or musculoskeletal ills, such as tension-type headache, nonneuralgic atypical facial pain, and fibromyalgia. Two notable exceptions to this rule are trigeminal neuralgia, which is rarely seen before the third decade unless in association with multiple sclerosis, and temporal arteritis, the incidence of which increases markedly during the fifth and sixth decades.

Pitfalls in the age-at-onset portion of the targeted history center around two facts:

1. As one gets older, the chances of systemic illness such as hypertension, glaucoma, stroke, and cancer increase.

2. Children, adolescents, and young adults can all suffer from these systemic illnesses, albeit rarely. Unfortunately, from the point of view of chronologic age, these systemic diseases are rarely suspected in this age group.

Duration and Frequency of Pain

This may provide the best clue to the classification and diagnosis. Although most headache and facial pain syndromes may occur in a seemingly sporadic and random nature, careful questioning may reveal an identifiable pattern to aid in the diagnosis. A headache diary kept for a period of 2 to 3 months may be useful to elucidate this pattern in difficult or confusing cases.

In general, vascular headaches and migraine variants such as cyclical vomiting and paroxysmal benign vertigo tend to occur in an episodic fashion, with the duration of pain and associated symptoms ranging from minutes in the case of cluster headache and trigeminal neuralgia to hours in the case of migraine and migraine equivalents. Cluster headache, although extremely rare in the pediatric and adolescent patient population, may be seasonal, with cluster headache having peak occurrences in the spring and fall. Headaches and facial pain of organic origin (e.g., sinus disease, brain tumor) tend to be continuous, with acute exacerbation caused by exercise, change in position, and Valsalva maneuver, for example. These pain syndromes will worsen over time if the underlying organic disease is not correctly diagnosed and treated or if the disease does not resolve spontaneously. Pain that is present on a daily basis and persists for months to years most likely falls under the category of tension-type headache or non-neuralgic atypical facial pain.

Onset-to-Peak Time

When coupled with the information obtained in the duration and frequency portion of the targeted history, the onset-to-peak time may help further narrow the diagnostic possibilities. A rapid onset-to-peak time (seconds to minutes) should increase suspicion of organic disease. Of particular concern are headaches that worsen with such activities as exercise, Valsalva maneuver, and bending forward. Notable exceptions to this rule are cluster headache and trigeminal neuralgia.

Migraine tends to evolve over several hours, with neurologic symptoms occurring early after onset in the migraine with aura sufferer. As mentioned earlier, cluster headache has a much more rapid onset to peak. Tension-type headache and nonneuralgic atypical facial pain evolve over a period of hours to days and then tend to remain constant.

Pitfalls when drawing conclusions regarding the onset-to-peak time of a headache or facial pain syndrome include the special situation in which a syndrome with slow onset-to-peak time (e.g., tension-type headache) may trigger a syndrome with a more rapid onset-to-peak time (e.g., migraine or migraine equivalent), producing the "coexistent" or "mixed headache" syndrome.

Location

The location of headache or facial pain may provide additional information about the classification and diagnosis of the patient's pain syndrome. Pain localized to an anatomical structure should be evaluated in the context of common disease entities for that structure (e.g., otitis media, dental pain).

Vascular headache is usually unilateral, although the side may change from attack to attack. Cluster headache is usually localized to the ocular and retro-ocular region, whereas migraine tends to involve the entire hemicranium. Temporal arteritis, which is usually associated with a generalized collagen vascular disease such as polyarteritis nodosum or dermatomyositis in the pediatric and adolescent population, is localized to the temple, but jaw claudication while chewing and generalized aching may confuse the presentation.

Tension-type headache is usually bilateral but can be unilateral, often involving the frontal, temporal, and occipital regions. Associated neck symtomatology often coexists. It may manifest as band or caplike tightness in the aforementioned anatomic areas.

Trigeminal neuralgia generally involves only one division of the trigeminal nerve (>98%). If the localization of pain overlaps anatomic distribution, non-neuralgic atypical facial pain, referred pain, or local pathology is a more likely explanation.

Pitfalls in assessing location include referred pain and sudden changes of anatomic localization during an attack. Special attention should be given to any atypical manifestation or poorly localized pain, because pain referred from tumors of the hypopharynx and posterior fossa can easily be misdiagnosed. Pain that is occipital or unilateral but becomes holocranial during Valsalva maneuver is suggestive of intracranial pathology and probable increased intracranial pressure or may be the result of benign intracranial hypertension.

Character and Severity of Pain

Although there is considerable overlap of these symptoms, some generalizations can be made when taking a targeted history. Vascular headaches tend to be throbbing and pulsatile in nature, with the pain intensity often described as intense. Cluster headache may have a deeper boring and burning quality. This pain is reputed to be among the worst pains known to humankind. Trigeminal neuralgia is typically described as paroxysmal jablike or shocklike pain in contradistinction to non-neuralgic atypical facial pain, which is more often a dull ache, nagging in character. Tension-type headache is a persistent dull aching, with a constant baseline level of pain and occasional severe exacerbations. Headache associated with lumbar puncture will worsen when the patient assumes the recumbent position.

Pitfalls in judging the character of pain include the fact that the patient may be suffering from more than one type of headache and that the most recent or most severe headache may be the one that the patient best remembers even though it is not the most common type for that patient. This is frequently the case in patients with coexistent or mixed headaches with a predominant tension-type component.

Premonitory Symptoms and Aurae

These are usually associated with vascular headaches, specifically migraine. Premonitory symptoms usually precede the migraine attack by 2 to 48 hours. Among the common premonitory symptoms experienced with migraine are fatigue, elation, depression, changes in libido, craving for certain foods, and abnormal hunger. These premonitory symptoms occur before an attack of migraine without aura (previously called common migraine) or prior to the onset of aura associated with an attack of migraine with aura (previously called classic migraine).

Aurae are manifested by focal cerebral dysfunction. Most aurae are ocular symptoms originating in the visual cortex of the occipital lobe. They are presumably due to localized ischemia of this anatomic region. Other examples of aurae include disturbances of smell, feeling, or motor function (see Table 349-1).

Pitfalls encountered include the fact that many chronic headache sufferers may "adopt" symptoms associated with chronic headaches other than that from which they suffer. These symptoms are gleaned from articles in the lay press and from repeated visits to health care professionals in an attempt to find relief. The acceptance of these symptoms at face value by a physician may lead to an erroneous diagnosis. Tumors of the occipital lobe may produce symptoms similar to migrainous aura. These symptoms are usually more persistent relative to those associated with migraine.

Associated Symptoms

The targeted history should include questions regarding other symptoms associated with the painful condition reported. Photophobia, sonophobia, nausea, vomiting, aversion to strong odors, and focal neurologic changes may be seen with migraine. These symptoms may also be seen with other headache and facial pain syndromes. Cluster headache is frequently accompanied by symptoms of complete or partial Horner's syndrome, including lacrimation, heavy rhinorrhea, and blanching of the face on the affected side.

Meningeal signs will occur rapidly after onset of subarachnoid hemorrhage, as will the focal neurologic changes of stroke. Tinnitus or hearing loss in patients with trigeminal neuralgia may indicate an underlying brainstem tumor. Weakness, bowel or bladder difficulties, and sudden visual loss in patients suffering from trigeminal neuralgia may suggest coexisting multiple sclerosis.

Precipitating Factors

Migraine headache may be triggered by change in diet or sleep habits, tyramine-containing foods, monosodium glutamate, nitrates, motion (e.g., driving in a car), alcohol, hormones and oral contraceptives, fatigue, stress, menstruation, underlying tension-type headache, strong odors, and bright sunlight. Many pediatric and adolescent headache sufferers will give a strong history of motion sickness. Tension-type headache is usually triggered by underlying environmental or physiological stress, depression, fatigue, and, occasionally, abnormalities of the cervical spine. Like migraine, cluster headache may be triggered by alcohol, high altitude, and, occasionally, vasodilating substances. Non-neuralgic atypical facial pain may be caused by stress, bruxism, prolonged dental work, and, occasionally, poorly fitting dental appliances.

Environmental Factors

As mentioned, contact with vasodilating substances by means of diet or absorption through the skin or respiratory tract may precipitate vascular headache. Stress and pressure in the workplace, video display terminals, industrial fumes, carbon monoxide, high altitude, and airborne contaminants carried by heating and cooling systems also have been implicated as precipitating factors for headache.

Family History

Migraine is a familial disease. If both parents suffer from migraine, there is a 70% to 75% chance that their children will have migraine. If only one parent suffers from the disease, the incidence in offspring drops to 45%.

Cluster headache, trigeminal neuralgia, and non-neuralgic atypical facial pain do not appear to be familial in nature.

A common pitfall encountered when exploring familial history as part of the targeted history is that headache and facial pain may be a learned behavior, which may explain the clustering of syndromes thought to be nonfamilial throughout several generations of a given family.

Pregnancy and Menstruation

Migraine may commonly occur with the onset of menses. Interestingly, it appears that pregnancy provides some amelioration of migraine headache after the first trimester. Menopause usually has the same effect; the migraine headache may disappear or decrease markedly in intensity and frequency. Hormones given at the time of menopause may prolong the headache syndrome.

Some migraine headaches worsen with the initiation of oral contraceptives. Concerns have been raised that the use of this group of drugs in migraine sufferers may increase the incidence of stroke, especially in patients who experience focal neurologic symptoms as part of an aura. This risk may be further increased if the patient also is a smoker.

Other forms of contraception usually provide a more favorable risk-benefit ratio in this group of patients; therefore, oral contraceptives should be avoided whenever possible.

A pitfall to be avoided is the assumption that all headaches associated with menses are vascular in nature. Many patients may suffer a monthly tension-type headache associated with their menses.

Medical/Surgical History

Headache can be a symptom of most systemic illnesses. Specific questioning regarding infection; previous malignancy; medications that may cause headaches (including topical nitroglycerin); trauma; previous cranial surgery; recent lumbar puncture or myelogram; diseases of the eye, ear, nose, throat, and cervical spine; anemia; thyroid disease; travel out of the country; changes in food, sleep, workplace, and job; and, most important, environmental stress may offer important clues.

Past Treatments

Many facial pain and headache sufferers have tried various treatment modalities in an effort to obtain pain relief. In evaluating the success or failure of each of these treatment techniques, one may draw a conclusion as to the type of treatment likely to be beneficial as well as the probable diagnosis of the pain syndrome being treated.

Pitfalls when exploring this part of the targeted history center around two points:

1. It is often impossible to assess the adequacy of a trial of a given treatment modality in terms of dosage, duration of treatment, and patient compliance.
2. The patient may be using the failure of multiple treatment regimens as a prelude to drug-seeking behavior. This may also manifest itself by the historical finding that the only drugs that have ever been effective in providing pain relief are controlled substances.

Previous Diagnostic Tests

Physicians must evaluate the adequacy, validity, age, and quality of previous testing when deciding whether or not additional testing is indicated. Factors that would indicate additional testing include a change in a previously stable headache or facial pain problem, onset of a new headache or facial pain problem, a discovery of new systemic illness that may be contributing to or causing the pain problem, or new neurologic findings.

Migraine Equivalents

Although migraine without aura and migraine with aura are frequently seen in the pediatric and adolescent population, many headache specialists believe that there are a group of nonheadache diseases that are migraine equivalents. These include cyclical vomiting syndrome, benign paroxysmal vertigo, and acute confusional states. Cyclical vomiting syndrome is a constellation of symptoms characterized by a unique temporal pattern of recurrent, isolated, and similar episodes of explosive vomiting that interrupt periods of completely normal health. Benign paroxysmal vertigo is characterized by a constellation of symptoms including true spinning vertigo, dizziness, nystagmus, nausea, and vomiting. Acute confusional states in children are characterized by the abrupt onset of confusion, disorientation, memory disturbance, dysarthria, and even unresponsiveness.

After obtaining a targeted headache history, the clinician should perform a targeted headache examination. Like the targeted headache history, the targeted physical examination is designed to aid the clinician in determining sick from well. Special attention should be paid to the presence of fever, which may indicate infection, or elevated blood pressure and bradycardia, which may serve as a harbinger of increased intracranial pressure. Assessment of the cranial nerves including a careful funduscopic examination is mandatory in all patients complaining of headache, as is an assessment for nuchal rigidity. Motor and sensory examination as well as an evaluation of the patient's level of consciousness should also be performed. Examination of the cranium for signs of trauma as well as a skin assessment to identify cutaneous signs of systemic disease (e.g., heliotrope rash of dermatomyositis or neurofibromatomata associated with von Recklinghausen's disease) should be performed.

Laboratory testing is indicated in any patient in this age group with unexplained headache. Lumbar puncture for evaluation of cerebrospinal fluid should be performed sooner rather than later in any patient with headache associated with unexplained fever to rule out central nervous system infection. It should be remembered that children and adolescents with strep throat can appear extremely ill and will often complain of headache and photophobia. Magnetic resonance imaging and/or computed tomographic scanning should be performed in all patients in whom factors that cause concern have been identified as well as those with unexplained headache that has not responded to conservative treatment (Table 349-2).

TABLE 349–2 Factors That Cause Concern

- New headache of recent onset ("the first")
- New headache of unusual severity ("the worst")
- Headache associated with neurologic dysfunction
- Headache associated with systemic illness (especially infection)
- Headache that peaks rapidly
- Headache associated with exertion
- Focal headache
- Sudden change in a previously stable headache pattern
- Headache associated with Valsalva maneuver
- Nocturnal headache

SUGGESTED READING

Lewis DW: Headaches in children and adolescents. Curr Probl Pediatr Adolesc Health Care 2007;37:207-246.

CHAPTER 350

The Pediatric Patient with Pain

Assessment of the pediatric patient with pain requires special skills to ensure that no child is the victim of undertreated pain. Infants and younger children may be unable to verbalize their pain complaints and older children may not have the context, vocabulary, or experience to adequately describe what they are feeling (Table 350-1). Cognitive, behavioral, and emotional impairment as well as fear may further exacerbate the situation. Further complicating the caregiver's assessment of the child's expression of pain is the patient's unique psychosocial perspective on pain that may be influenced by cultural and learned behavior. The use of observational assessment tools and/or more objective pain assessment tools such as the Wong-Baker Faces Scale may help the clinician further clarify the individual patient's clinical situation. For premature and term infants, the Premature Infant Pain Profile (PIPP) and the CRIES Postoperative Pain Scale have been demonstrated to correlate with clinically observed pain behavior in this special patient population. For patients from 2 months to 7 years of age who have

undergone surgery, the FLACC Scale has been shown to be a useful tool in the assessment of postoperative pain.

Untreated or undertreated pain can cause extreme emotional distress and anxiety in the pediatric population. It is imperative that the clinician employ simple

TABLE 350–1 Age-Normal Pain Expression in the Pediatric Population

• 18 Months to 3 years of age	Child can begin to use appropriate words to indicate he or she is in pain
• 3-5 Years of age	Child can use words to describe the pain, its location, its frequency, and its severity
• School-age children	Child can more clearly articulate the pain experience and, in absence of cognitive impairment, can use numerical pain scales

nonpharmacologic approaches in all children in pain or who are undergoing repeated painful procedures such as blood draws and injections. Simple reassurance, distraction techniques, and positive reinforcement techniques that can take the form of stickers or prizes combined with praise can be effective. Although chronic pain secondary to medical conditions is much less common in the pediatric population compared with adults, it must be managed aggressively. Patients suffering from cancer, collagen vascular diseases, cystic fibrosis, and sickle cell anemia require not only appropriate nonpharmacologic and pharmacologic management of their pain but also the behavioral support required to enable them to optimize their sense of well-being.

When considering pharmacologic management of the newborn in pain, it is important to recognize that although the newborn's anatomic development may seem complete, the functional development of the newborn's organ system is not. During the first 3 months of life (and longer if the newborn is preterm), the liver is not able to completely metabolize many common analgesic drugs such as morphine and local anesthetics, nor is the kidney fully functional at birth with decreased glomerular filtration rates. Decreased volumes of plasma albumin in the neonate may lead to an increased amount of unbound drug, resulting in unexpected side effects and toxicity.

Acetaminophen is a safe drug in the newborn and is available in liquid formulations for ease of administration. Interestingly, newborns appear to have some degree of protection against acetaminophen toxicity due to increased levels of glutathione peroxidase, which binds the toxic metabolite of acetaminophen, acetyl-*p*-benzoquinone-imine. Daily maximum oral dosing is recommended not to exceed 45 mg/kg for premature infants >34 weeks' gestational age, 60 mg/kg for term neonates <10 days of age, and 90 mg/kg for children.

The nonsteroidal anti-inflammatory agents are a reasonably safe alternative to acetaminophen after the newborn period. Pharmacokinetics and pharmacodynamics are similar to those of the healthy adult, and children appear to have a reduced incidence of renal and gastrointestinal side effects compared with adults. If a parenteral drug is needed, ketorolac at a dosage range of 0.25 to 0.5 mg/kg every 6 hours without a loading dose is a reasonable choice.

The use of opioids in newborns requires special attention to dosing and careful ongoing clinical assessment. Because of immature liver enzyme function, the half-life of morphine and other opioids such as fentanyl is essentially doubled. Decreased glomerular infiltration rates further delay elimination of metabolites. Further complicating the use of opioids in this special population is the fact that immaturity of the central respiratory control mechanisms renders normal physiologic feedback caused by hypoxia or hypercarbia less than optimal, resulting in respiratory complications.

For mild to moderate pain, codeine often in combination with acetaminophen is a reasonable starting point. Available in an elixir form, these two drugs work synergistically and are generally safe when given in doses of 10 to 15 mg/kg acetaminophen and 0.5 mg/kg codeine. For more severe pain, methadone elixir is a good choice and, given its longer half life, allows for less frequent dosing in more chronic situations such as cancer pain. Starting doses are 0.1 mg/kg every 4 to 8 hours in patients weighing less than 50 kg and 10 mg every 4 to 8 hours in patients weighing more than 50 kg.

If oral analgesics cannot be used, the intravenous route of administration is preferred over the more painful intramuscular route. Clinical experience is that children will deny they have pain simply to avoid receiving a "shot." Initial treatment of severe acute pain (e.g., burns, fractures) with intermittent intravenous boluses of morphine, hydromorphone, or fentanyl should be performed only by those familiar with the use of this class of drugs in this special population. Continuous infusions of narcotic analgesics, as well as the use of patient-controlled analgesia, represent a reasonable next step in the treatment of ongoing acute pain. Initial morphine infusion rates are 0.025 mg/kg/hr for toddlers and children. Much lower dosages are required for newborns and should be administered only in carefully monitored settings. The concept of patient-controlled analgesia can generally be understood by non–cognitively impaired children 6 to 7 years of age. This modality can be modified to nurse-controlled analgesia in the younger patient population.

Typical dosage ranges for drugs commonly used in patient-controlled analgesia in children are summarized in Table 350-2.

TABLE 350–2 Starting Dosages for Patient-Controlled Analgesia in the Pediatric Population

Typical Starting Dosages for PCA Using a 7-Minute Lockout Period			
Drug	Bolus dose (µg/kg)	Continuous rate (µg/kg/hour)	4-Hour limit (µg/kg)
Morphine	20	4-15	300
Hydromorphone	5	1-3	60
Fentanyl	0.25	0.15	4

The use of topical local anesthetics such as eutectic mixtures of local anesthetics (EMLA) such as lidocaine/prilocaine and lidocaine/tetracaine are effective in reducing pain from painful procedures such as venipuncture, intravenous line starts, and circumcision. EMLA must be applied in a heavy layer to the intact skin overlying the area and then covered. Optimal analgesia will occur within 90 to 120 minutes, so it may be prudent to have the parents apply the EMLA cream at home prior to the anticipated painful procedure.

Regional anesthesia techniques, such as field blocks following inguinal hernia repair and single-shot epidural and caudal injections, are useful in the management of postoperative pain. Continuous epidural infusions can also be used if the pain is anticipated to last for longer periods of time.

In summary, children of all ages deserve thoughtful and compassionate pain management. Failure to adequately manage pain in this special patient population can lead to needless suffering, anxiety, and a lifelong fear of doctors and other health care professionals.

SUGGESTED READING

Berde CB, Sethna NF: Analgesics for the treatment of pain in children. N Engl J Med 2002;347:1094-1103,1114.

CHAPTER 351

Pain in the Older Adult

As our population ages, the management of pain in older adults becomes increasingly important. The literature is replete with studies showing that pain in the elderly is inadequately treated, yet there are few articles providing the clinician with practical guidelines to manage pain in older adults. Failure to adequately diagnose and treat pain in this special patient population can result in sleep disturbance, decreased mobility, impaired socialization, depression, and, of course, needless suffering.

The first step in effectively managing pain in older adults is performing an age- and patient-appropriate pain assessment. Acute organic brain syndrome induced by medication of illness, cognitive impairment, dementia, and preexisting chronic pain may make this assessment more challenging. The clinician must also be aware of impairment of hearing and vision that may complicate the pain assessment. The clinician must remember that there is no scientific evidence to support the common misperception that patients in any one of these situations experience less pain than those patients of the same chronologic age who do not suffer cognitive impairment. In this setting, the clinician should use subjective clinical observations (e.g., whether the patient is grimacing, agitated, or restless) combined with more objective measures such as the Wong-Baker Faces Scale.

The second step when performing a pain assessment in the older adult is to identify comorbidities that may be contributing to the older patient's pain. Often undertreated, common pain comorbidities in the elderly that should be diligently searched for include musculoskeletal complaints such as osteoarthritis, bursitis, vertebral compression fractures and tendinitis, peripheral neuropathy and other neuropathic pain, collagen vascular diseases such as polymyalgia rheumatica and temporal arteritis, and fibromyalgia.

The third step in assessing pain in the older patient is to identify any coexistent depression that may be an integral part of the patient's pain complaint. Involvement of the caregiver and family may provide useful clues as to subtle changes in the patient's mental state that may point toward depression (Table 351-1). A failure to identify and

TABLE 351–1 Signs of Depression in the Elderly

- Irritable mood
- Bouts of temper
- Difficulty concentrating
- Memory loss
- Difficulty staying asleep
- Insomnia
- Unintentional weight loss
- Unexplained weight gain
- Feelings of worthlessness
- Loss of interest or pleasure in daily activities
- Fatigue
- Vague aches and pains
- Suicidal ideations

treat underlying depression will make the treatment of the primary pain complaint more difficult, if not impossible.

The fourth step in assessing pain in the older adult is the identification of factors that may influence how the patient perceives and/or reports pain that may be unique to the individual patient. Such factors include patient misconceptions (e.g., pain is a sign of weakness, pain is a normal part of aging, pain means cancer). Other factors unique to the individual patient may be an unfounded fear of addiction if pain medications are taken and unique religious and cultural beliefs regarding pain. All of these factors may be magnified given the prevalence of misconceptions about pain in the elderly that are held by many clinicians and caregivers.

A careful history, including the patient's past medical and surgical history, as well as an accurate list of current medications, is necessary to begin to formulate a treatment plan of the patient's pain. A careful assessment of the frequency, character, intensity, onset to peak, and duration of the pain is also useful, as is an assessment of previous treatments and medications. The clinician should always ask about the use of over-the-counter medications and/or herbal or alternative remedies that may confuse the clinical presentation of many common painful conditions or put the patient at risk for other comorbidities. Every pain management history should include the question "What have you been unable to do in the past day, week, month because of the pain?"

Physical examination of the older patient with pain should include a careful examination of the painful area with care being taken not to cause excessive pain. A thorough neurologic examination including an assessment of any cognitive impairment should be carried out.

Evaluation of the patient's ability to ambulate, rise from sitting to standing, and ambulate without shortness of breath or angina will also be useful when formulating a pain treatment plan.

Because of age-normal changes in physiologic functions involving the renal, liver, and cardiovascular systems, older adults are at particular risk for undermedication as well as overmedication. This means that the use of analgesic drugs and adjuvant analgesics in this special group of patients must be individualized and monitored closely.

As a general rule, the initial dose of analgesics should be reduced by 25% and then titrated slowly upward as the clinical situation and side effects dictate. If stronger opioid analgesics are needed, morphine is the drug of choice with hydromorphone being an acceptable alternative. Meperidine should be avoided in this special population due to the potential for accumulation of the normeperidine metabolite.

SUGGESTED READING

Gagliese L, Melzack R: Pain in the elderly. In: Wall and Melzack's Textbook of Pain, ed 5 [online edition]. Elsevier Churchill Livingstone, 2006.

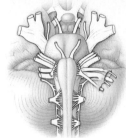

Ethical and Legal Issues in Pain Management

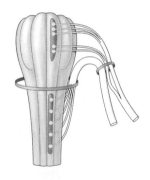

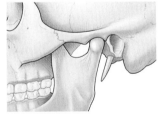

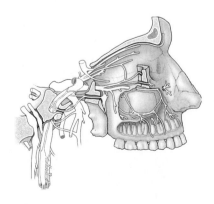

CHAPTER 352

Informed Consent and Consent to Treatment

Informed consent is the process by which a patient receives the information necessary to exercise his or her legal and ethical right to choose whether or not to undergo treatment recommended by an ethical caregiver. In order for this to occur, several elements must be included in the discussion between the caregiver and the patient. These elements include (1) the nature of the recommended treatment; (2) the benefits, side effects, risks, and uncertainties related to the recommended treatment; (3) the reasonable alternatives to the proposed treatment; (4) the benefits, side effects, risks, and uncertainties related to the alternative treatments; (5) an assessment by the caregiver of the ability of the patient to understand the information presented and to make an informed decision; and (6) the voluntary assent by the patient to undergo the proposed treatment.

Consent to treatment, although an integral element of informed consent, is also an independent part of the legal and ethical duty of the caregiver to the patient. Consent to treatment is used each time the caregiver wants to do something to the person of the patient, such as phlebotomy examination, and intravenous line start. In essence, the caregiver simply tells the patient what he or she wants to do and the patient gives or withholds a consent to treatment. The patient's consent to treatment allows the caregiver to perform what would otherwise be the intentional tort of battery. *Battery* is actionable in all 50 states and is defined as a willful harmful or offensive contact by an individual on the person of the patient.

Although most states have defined by statute or regulation what constitutes adequate informed consent, the following elements are generally assessed if there is a question if the consent provided was adequate. The first element is whether the caregiver provided the patient with information that all reasonable physicians provide to a similar patient considering a similar treatment recommendation. The second element in determining whether the information provided was adequate for the patient to provide true informed consent is whether the information included everything a typical patient similarly situated would need to know to provide informed consent.

The third element assessed is whether a reasonable caregiver would determine, with the information provided, that a similar patient would be able to understand the information presented and to make an informed decision. This third element encompasses the competence of the patient not just to understand the information presented but also to have the judgment to make a rational decision. It should be remembered that a patient's judgment may vary owing, for example, to the progression of their disease, medications administered, and psychiatric illness.

As mentioned, theoretically all treatment that requires contact with the patient requires a consent to treatment as well as an informed consent. In general, minor procedures such as a rectal or pelvic examination do not require a signed informed consent form. However, any more invasive or risky procedure (e.g., surgery, radiation therapy, and/or anesthesia) will generally involve having the patient sign a form acknowledging that he or she has received the information necessary to grant an informed consent as well as a consent to treatment.

If a patient is deemed to be incapable of providing informed consent, a surrogate decision maker must speak for him or her. Most states provide a statutory hierarchy of who may serve as a surrogate decision maker for an incompetent patient, with the patient's parents usually identified as best being able to serve in this capacity. In the absence of any appropriate surrogate decision maker, the caregiver has a duty to act in the best interests of the patient until the court can appoint a surrogate decision maker. Informed consent can only be implied or presumed in emergency situations where the patient is either unconscious or obviously incompetent and no surrogate decision maker is available.

SUGGESTED READING

Sachs GA: American Geriatrics Society Position Statement on Informed Consent. Available from the American Geriatrics Society, The Empire State Building, 350 Fifth Avenue, Suite 801, New York, NY 10118.

CHAPTER **353**

Patient Confidentiality

The doctor's duty to preserve patient confidentiality finds its basis in the fiduciary relationship between the caregiver and the patient. Although the concept of fiduciary relationship is most often thought of as arising between individuals engaged in business transactions involving money, stocks, or bonds, the fiduciary relationship exists any time a person reasonably believes and relies on the fact that a person of trust will protect that person's personal interests and/or act in that person's best interests. Perhaps nowhere else but in the doctor/patient relationship is the fiduciary duty of the person of trust more important.

Doctors are defined as being in a position of power over the patient given their knowledge, education, and social status and, perhaps, most important, society's reasonable expectation that the doctor will always honor his or her fiduciary duty to the patient. Such reliance allows patients to share with their doctor the most confidential, intimate, and often embarrassing aspects about themselves without fear that this information will be disclosed to a third party. This expectation of a trusting and confidential environment is essential if the patient is to be completely honest with the physician.

The obligation of patient confidentiality embedded in the fiduciary relationship between doctor and patient prohibits the doctor from disclosing confidential information regarding the patient to other interested parties (i.e., relatives, employers, family, the media). This obligation of confidentiality extends beyond simply not disclosing confidential information to, in fact, ensuring that the confidential information is protected so that unauthorized access to this information does not occur.

This duty has been codified into a federal law known as HIPAA, or the Healthcare Insurance Portability and Accountability Act of 1996 and its subsequent amendments. This federal law sets forth, in what has become known as The Privacy Rule, both the allowed and prohibited uses of confidential information (called *protected health information* under the act) and provides penalties for those covered under this law who do not follow it. It is important to note that protected health information includes much more than simply what a specific patient told his or her doctor in confidence. It includes any information about the patient's health care as well as all of the details surrounding the payment for said health care. The act also expands who has a duty to follow the rules regarding protected health information beyond the actual caregivers to anyone designated as a covered entity. These covered entities include hospitals, surgical centers, laboratories, imaging centers, insurers, and business associates that may have access to protected health information as defined by the act.

As important as patient confidentiality is to the provision of health care, ethicists and legal experts have set forth several limited exceptions to the doctor's absolute duty to maintain patient confidentiality. In general, these exceptions are allowed when the harm in maintaining patient confidentiality is greater than the harm that will result in the disclosing of the confidential patient information. Most states have provided laws that allow for the release of confidential patient information in this setting. Examples in which release of confidential patient information to someone other than the patient is not just allowed but required include situations in which the patient has revealed to the doctor credible plans to harm another individual or individuals or in situations in which failure to release certain confidential patient information may cause harm to the public welfare, as in the case of a patient suffering from a communicable disease such as tuberculosis or HIV.

SUGGESTED READINGS

HHS Standards for Privacy of Individually Identifiable Health Information; Final Rule: 45 CFR Parts 160 and 164.
Wilson J: Health Insurance Portability and Accountability Act privacy rule causes ongoing concerns among clinicians and researchers. Ann Intern Med 2006;145:313-316.

CHAPTER 354

Prescribing Controlled Substances

Current laws regarding the prescribing of controlled substances find their basis in the Federal Controlled Substance Act of 1970, which was the federal government's attempt to provide a unified, comprehensive set of laws to guide prescribing of controlled substances. This act, acknowledging that some controlled substances presented more risk to the public than others, introduced the concept of a schedule of clinical useful drugs.

This schedule groups drugs that have been deemed to have approved clinical uses in Schedules II through V, with Schedule I drugs being those controlled substances that have been deemed to have no current approved clinical uses (Table 354-1). The act allows the use of controlled substances for the treatment of pain but puts specific limitations on the chronic use of controlled substances to treat chemical dependence.

The act also requires those prescribing controlled substances to obtain a registration number from the Drug Enforcement Agency, commonly known as a DEA number. Many states also require a separate registration number issued by the state in addition to the federally issued DEA number. The act requires only those possessing a valid DEA number to prescribe controlled substances, and for certain schedules of controlled substances, the prescription must be written in indelible ink and dated and signed by the prescribing caregiver on the date written. In general, a practitioner may not write postdated prescriptions for controlled substances.

An emergency exception for these requirements has been promulgated by the Secretary of Health and Human Services. This exception allows for verbal orders to a pharmacist when the prescribing practitioner determines that (1) immediate administration of a controlled substance is necessary, for proper treatment of the intended ultimate user; (2) that no appropriate alternative treatment is available, including administration of a drug that is not a controlled substance under Schedule II of the act; and (3) it is not reasonably possible for the prescribing practitioner to provide a written prescription to be presented to the person dispensing the substance, prior to dispensing. This exception also requires the pharmacist to make a reasonable effort to identify the prescribing physician if not personally known to the pharmacist. Both the physician and pharmacist must clearly document the medical justification for the use of the emergency exception. Furthermore, the prescribing physician must

TABLE 354-1 Schedule of Controlled Substances

Schedule I Drugs

- High potential for abuse
- No currently accepted medical use in treatment in the United States
- Lack of accepted safety for use of the drug or other substance under medical supervision
- Examples: LSD and Peyote

Schedule II Drugs

- High potential for abuse
- Use may lead to severe physical or psychological dependence
- Prescriptions must be written in ink or typewritten and signed by the practitioner, or verbal prescriptions must be confirmed in writing within 72 hours and may be given only in a genuine emergency
- No renewals are permitted
- Examples: Fentanyl and Dilaudid

Schedule III Drugs

- Some potential for abuse
- Use may lead to low to moderate physical dependence or high psychological dependence
- Prescriptions may be oral or written
- Up to 5 renewals are permitted within 6 months
- Examples: Fiorinal and Tylenol #3

Schedule IV Drugs

- Low potential for abuse
- Use may lead to limited physical or psychological dependence
- Prescriptions may be oral or written
- Up to 5 renewals are permitted within 6 months
- Examples: Xanax and Valium

Schedule V Drugs

- Subject to state and local regulation
- Abuse potential is low
- A prescription may not be required
- Examples: Lomotil and Robitussin AC

deliver an original written prescription that complies with all of the elements required by the act for prescribing controlled substances.

SUGGESTED READINGS

Acute Pain Management Guideline Panel: Acute Pain Management: Operative or Medical Procedures and Trauma. Clinical Practice Guideline. Rockville, MD, Agency for Health Care Policy and Research, U.S. Department of Health and Human Resources, Public Health Service, February 1992. AHCPR Publication No. 92-0032.

Jacox A, Carr DB, Payne R, et al: Management of Cancer Pain. Rockville, MD, Agency for Health Care Policy and Research, U.S. Department of Health and Human Resources, Public Health Service, March 1994. Clinical Practice Guideline No. 9. AHCPR Publication No. 94-0592.

CHAPTER 355

Prevention of Drug Diversion, Abuse, and Dependence

It is the responsibility of the physician to take all steps necessary to prevent drug diversion, abuse, and dependence. Duties include maintaining control of prescription pads, not allowing office staff to write or call in prescriptions for controlled substances, the standardization of practice policies regarding the prescription of controlled substances, and careful recordkeeping.

The bulk of drug diversion involving otherwise responsible and honest physicians involves *prescription fraud*, which is defined as the illegitimate and illegal acquisition of prescription drugs for personal use or profit. The biggest factor contributing to the prevalence of prescription fraud is the increasing abuse of and addiction to prescription drugs such as opioids, stimulants, and tranquilizers. Those at risk for abuse of and addiction to prescription drugs range from younger patients who have used their family members' prescription drugs as gateway drugs to adults who become iatrogenically addicted to drugs appropriately prescribed for medical conditions and then seek to use prescription fraud to continue their supply of drugs. Healthcare workers are also at increased risk for drug addiction due to increased availability of prescription drugs and frequently turn to prescription drug fraud to maintain their supply of drugs. Statistically, women are twice as likely as men to become involved in prescription drug fraud after being prescribed a prescription drug for a legitimate medical purpose, usually anxiety or pain. Individuals who are already addicted to illegal drugs such as opioids, amphetamines, and cocaine may use prescription fraud to obtain quantities of legal prescription drugs to sell or trade for their drug of choice.

The most common form of prescription fraud involves the forging or alteration of a prescription (Table 355-1). Forging can take the form of writing what appears to be an

TABLE 355-1 Characteristics of Forged Prescriptions

1. Prescription looks "too perfect."
2. The prescriber's handwriting is too neat and legible.
3. Quantities, directions, or dosages do not conform to common medical use.
4. Prescription does not use standard format or abbreviations typical of the type of prescription being written.
5. Prescription appears to be photocopied.
6. Directions are written in full with no abbreviations.
7. Prescription written in different color inks or written in different handwriting.
8. Prescription contains cross-outs or obvious alterations.

otherwise legal prescription for a reasonable quantity of a drug with the hope that the pharmacist will fill it without questioning its validity. These forged prescriptions are often written on prescription forms stolen from a doctor's office or reproduced on high-quality home laser printers. Often the telephone number on the prescription is altered to that of the forger so the forger can confirm that the prescription is legitimate should the pharmacist call to verify that the doctor actually wrote it. Individuals impersonating a doctor or his or her office staff may attempt to obtain illegal prescriptions by calling in a prescription to an unsuspecting pharmacist. This is often done when the real doctor's office is closed, to avoid detection. Alteration of prescriptions to increase the dosage, number of pills dispensed, or the number of refills is another way that individuals obtain illegal prescriptions.

Doctor shopping is another method that individuals may use to perpetrate prescription fraud. The feigning of symptoms of painful conditions that have minimal objective findings such as migraine headache or the use of ruses such as traveling from out of town and inadvertently forgetting their prescription are but a few of the myriad tactics employed by those seeking to obtain a prescription for a legal drug by fraudulent means. Such tactics are frequently used in urgent care centers and emergency departments.

To avoid problems when prescribing drugs with the potential for diversion, abuse, or addiction, the doctor should adhere to the following approach to treating patients requesting such prescriptions. The first step in the care of a patient requesting a prescription for a drug with the potential for diversion, abuse, or addiction is taking a complete history and performing a physical examination, which must be carefully documented in the patient's medical record. Elements of this documentation should include the medical indication for the prescription, current and previous treatments for the medical condition, comorbidities that preclude the use of safer alternative drugs, and any history of substance abuse.

The second step in the care of a patient requesting a prescription for a drug with the potential for diversion, abuse, or addiction is the clear written documentation of a treatment plan stating the objectives of proposed treatment with the drug in question as well as any other concurrent treatment modalities that might be prescribed such as physical therapy or psychological counseling. Reasonable treatment objectives should be, for example, pain relief, treatment of attention deficit disorder, the improvement of sleep, and functional disability.

The third step in the care of a patient requesting a prescription for a drug with the potential for diversion, abuse, or addiction is a thorough discussion of the risks and benefits for the proposed treatment and, in some instances, a written informed consent and an agreement for treatment. The agreement for treatment should clearly and unambiguously outline the patient's responsibilities during treatment with the drug in question. Elements of

such an agreement might include that the patient will only obtain the drug from one physician, will fill the prescription at one pharmacy, that no replacements will be given for lost or damaged prescriptions, the number and frequency of prescription refills, and the reasons that the physician may terminate prescribing the drug should the patient violate the agreement.

The fourth step in the care of a patient requesting a prescription for a drug with the potential for diversion, abuse, or addiction is the careful written documentation of the prescription of the drug in question in the patient's medical record. Such documentation should include the name of the drug, the dosage, the amount prescribed, the instructions for use, any specific warnings about the use of the drug (e.g., may make drowsy), and any refills.

The fifth step in the care of a patient requesting a prescription for a drug with the potential for diversion, abuse, or addiction is for the physician to conduct a periodic review as to the appropriateness of the continued use of the drug in question. This review should include whether the previously stated treatment objectives have been met and whether new or revised treatment objectives are required. Patient compliance with the treatment plan should also be assessed. All of the information gleaned from the periodic review process should be clearly documented in writing in the patient's medical record.

It is important to note that when following these steps when prescribing a drug with the potential for diversion, abuse, or addiction, the physician must comply with all applicable federal, state, and local laws. A failure to follow such laws may subject the physician to disciplinary action by federal and state licensing agencies.

SUGGESTED READING

Spickard A, Dodd D, Swiggart W, Dixon GL, Pichert JW: Physicians who misprescribe controlled substances: A CME alternative to sanctions. Fed Bull 1998;85: 8-19.

Review Questions
and Answers

Review Questions

1. Structures of the rhinencephalon include the:
   a. olfactory receptor cells
   b. olfactory epithelium
   c. olfactory bulbs
   d. olfactory tracts and areas
   e. all of the above ✗

2. Which of the following structures is *not* a cranial nerve?
   a. trigeminal
   b. olfactory
   c. obturator ✗
   d. vagus
   e. spinal accessory

3. Which of the following statements regarding the optic nerve are *true?*
   a. It is the second cranial nerve.
   b. It contains special afferent sensory fibers.
   c. Fibers from each optic nerve cross the midline to exit the chiasm together at the opposite optic tract.
   d. Via the optic tract and optic radiations, visual information carried by the optic nerve is projected onto the occipital lobes.
   e. all of the above ✗

4. Systemic diseases that can cause visual impairment include:
   a. diabetes mellitus
   b. hypertension
   c. vitamin A deficiency
   d. vitamin B_{12} deficiency
   e. all of the above ✗

5. Diseases that may affect the oculomotor (cranial nerve III) are:
   a. brain tumors
   b. aneurysms
   c. increased intracranial pressure
   d. low cerebrospinal fluid pressure
   e. all of the above ✗

6. Clinical symptoms associated with disorders of the oculomotor nerve include:
   a. severe facial pain
   b. inactive pupil
   c. palsy of the medial rectus muscle with weak adduction
   d. b and c ✗
   e. all of the above

7. Cranial nerve IV is the:
   a. spinal accessory nerve
   b. trochlear nerve ✗
   c. trigeminal nerve
   d. glossopharyngeal nerve
   e. supraorbital nerve

8. Palsy of the trochlear nerve will present clinically as the:
   a. inability to look downward
   b. inability to look upward
   c. inability to look inward
   d. b and c
   e. a and c ✗

9. The most common disorder affecting the trigeminal nerve is:
   a. peripheral neuropathy
   b. wallerian degeneration
   c. moya moya disease
   d. trigeminal neuralgia ✗
   e. none of the above

10. Trigeminal neuralgia is:
    a. characterized by paroxysms of shocklike pain
    b. characterized by an association with multiple sclerosis in 2% to 3% of patients
    c. often caused by tortuous cranial blood vessels
    d. severe in intensity
    e. all of the above ✗

11. The most common cause of isolated abducens (cranial nerve VI) palsy is:
    a. microvascular disease associated with diabetes ○
    b. Rift Valley fever
    c. open-angle glaucoma ✗
    d. closed-angle glaucoma
    e. none of the above

12. The patient suffering from abducens (cranial nerve VI) palsy will be unable to:
    a. abduct the eye on the affected side ✗
    b. smell strong odors
    c. constrict the pupil
    d. elevate the scapula
    e. none of the above

13. The facial nerve is made up of the following types of nerve fibers:
    a. branchial motor special visceral efferent fibers
    b. visceral motor general visceral efferent fibers
    c. special sensory special afferent fibers
    d. general sensory general somatic afferent
    e. all of the above ✗

14. The most common disorder affecting the facial nerve is:
    a. trigeminal neuralgia
    b. Dercum's disease
    c. Ramsay Hunt syndrome
    d. Bell's palsy ✗
    e. none of the above

15. Abnormalities of the vestibulocochlear nerve can manifest themselves clinically as:
    a. pain in the posterior third of the tongue
    b. vertigo
    c. hearing loss
    d. b and c ✗
    e. none of the above

16. The most common disorder affecting the glossopharyngeal nerve is:
    a. trigeminal neuralgia
    b. glossopharyngeal neuralgia ✗
    c. Ramsay Hunt syndrome
    d. Bell's palsy
    e. none of the above

17. Functions related to the glossopharyngeal nerve include:
    a. the "dry mouth" associated with fear
    b. the salivation reflex associated with the smell of food
    c. taste on the posterior two-thirds of the tongue
    d. sensation of the external ear
    e. all of the above ✗

18. The vagus nerve provides innervation to:
    a. the posterior skin of the ear, the external surface of the tympanic membrane, the pharynx, and the external auditory meatus
    b. sensory information from the larynx, esophagus, trachea, and abdominal and thoracic viscera
    c. information from the stretch receptors of the aortic arch and chemoreceptors of the aortic bodies ✗
    d. innervation to the intrinsic muscles of the larynx
    e. all of the above

19. Clinical findings suggestive of compromise of the vagus nerve include:
    a. hoarseness
    b. anisocoria
    c. difficulty swallowing
    d. a and b
    e. a and c ✗

20. Disorders of the spinal accessory nerve will present clinically as:
    a. weakness of the sternocleidomastoid muscle on the affected side
    b. weakness of the intercostal muscles on the affected side
    c. weakness of the trapezius muscle on the affected side
    d. a and c ✗
    e. a and b

21. Which of the following is *not* a clinical sign of damage to the hypoglossal nerve?
    a. weakness of the intrinsic muscles of the tongue
    b. deviation of the extended tongue to the affected side.
    c. atrophy of the intrinsic muscles of the tongue on the affected side when the compromise of the hypoglossal nerve has been of long-standing
    d. weakness of elevation of the contralateral shoulder ✗
    e. all of the above

22. The greater occipital nerve:
    a. is a peripheral branch of the second and third cervical nerves
    b. supplies the medial portion of the posterior scalp as far anterior as the vertex
    c. has been implicated as one of the nerves subserving the pain of occipital neuralgia
    d. all of the above ✗
    e. none of the above

23. The sphenopalatine ganglion sends major branches to the:
    a. gasserian ganglion and trigeminal nerves
    b. carotid plexus
    c. facial nerve
    d. superior cervical ganglion
    e. all of the above ✗

24. The superficial cervical plexus:
    a. controls closure of the true vocal cords
    b. arises from fibers of the primary ventral rami of the first, second, third, and fourth cervical nerves
    c. provides only motor innervation
    d. provides innervation of the exocrine pancreas
    e. all of the above ✗

25. The deep cervical plexus:
    a. controls closure of the true vocal cords
    b. arises from fibers of the primary ventral rami of the first, second, third, and fourth cervical nerves
    c. provides only motor innervation
    d. contributes fibers to the phrenic nerve
    e. b and d ✗

26. The stellate ganglion is:
    a. located in the retrocrural space
    b. made up primarily of special efferent motor fibers
    c. formed by the fusion of the inferior cervical and the first thoracic ganglion as they meet anterior to the vertebral body of C7
    d. inferior to the celiac plexus
    e. all of the above ✗

27. The following structures are anterior to the stellate ganglion:
    a. skin
    b. subcutaneous tissue
    c. sternocleidomastoid muscle
    d. carotid sheath
    e. all of the above ✗

28. The following are *true* statements about the structure and function of the cervical vertebrae:
    a. There are seven cervical vertebrae.
    b. The first cervical vertebra is called atlas.
    c. The second cervical vertebra is called axis.
    d. The transverse foramen protects and allows passage of the vertebral artery and vein.
    e. all of the above ✗

29. Rudimentary structures found on the seventh cervical vertebra in a small number of patients are called:
    a. chorionic villi
    b. cervical ribs

c. Schmorl's nodes ✗
d. sesamoid bones
e. none of the above

30. Which of the following statements are *true* about the cervical intervertebral disc?
   a. It serves as the major shock absorbing structure of the cervical spine.
   b. It prevents impingement of the adjacent neural structures.
   c. It helps facilitate the synchronized movement of the cervical spine.
   d. It prevents impingement of the vasculature that traverse the cervical spine.
   e. all of the above ✗

31. The top and bottom of the cervical intervertebral discs are called the:
   a. syndesmotic junction
   b. nucleus pulposus
   c. end plates ✗
   d. vomer
   e. none of the above

32. The outside of the cervical intervertebral disc is made up of a woven crisscrossing matrix of fibroelastic fibers called the:
   a. annulus ✗
   b. nucleus pulposus
   c. end plates
   d. vomer
   e. none of the above

33. The center of the disc is the water-containing mucopolysaccharide gel-like substance called the:
   a. annulus
   b. nucleus pulposus ✗
   c. end plates
   d. vomer
   e. none of the above

34. The meninges are made up of three layers that include the:
   a. pia mater
   b. arachnoid mater
   c. dura mater
   d. tunica alba
   e. a, b, and c ✗

35. The cerebrospinal fluid is absorbed by the:
   a. tunica alba
   b. pineal gland
   c. arachnoid granulations
   d. lacrimal glands
   e. all of the above ✗

36. The cervical epidural space is bounded by the:
   a. fusion of the periosteal and spinal layers of dura at the foramen magnum superiorly
   b. posterior longitudinal ligament anteriorly
   c. vertebral laminae and the ligamentum flavum posteriorly
   d. vertebral pedicles and intervertebral foramina laterally
   e. all of the above ✗

37. The cervical epidural space contains:
   a. fat
   b. veins and arteries
   c. lymphatics
   d. connective tissue
   e. all of the above

38. Which of the following statements regarding the cervical facet joints is *false*?
   a. The lower cervical facet joints receive innervation from one vertebral level. ✗
   b. The atlanto-occipital and atlantoaxial joints are unique relative to the other cervical facet joints.
   c. The lower cervical facet joints receive innervation from two vertebral levels.
   d. The lower cervical facet joints are true joints as they are lined with synovium.
   e. All of the statements are false.

39. Which of the following structures aid in stabilizing the cervical spine?
   a. ligamentum nuchae
   b. interspinous ligament
   c. supraspinous ligament
   d. ligamentum flavum
   e. all of the above ✗

40. The smaller upper four thoracic vertebrae share characteristics in common with the:
   a. cervical vertebrae ✗
   b. thoracic vertebrae
   c. lumbar vertebrae
   d. sacrum
   e. none of the above

41. The larger lower four thoracic vertebrae share characteristics in common with the:
   a. cervical vertebrae
   b. thoracic vertebrae
   c. lumbar vertebrae ✗
   d. sacrum
   e. none of the above

42. A distinguishing characteristic of the first 10 thoracic vertebrae is the presence of:
   a. intervertebral foramen
   b. articular facets for the ribs ✗
   c. arachnoid granulations
   d. no end plates
   e. all of the above

43. The following structure is found at the T4 dermatome in most patients:
   a. nipple ✗
   b. jugular notch
   c. stellate ganglion
   d. umbilicus
   e. none of the above

44. The following structure is found at the T10 dermatome in most patients:
   a. nipple
   b. jugular notch

c. stellate ganglion
d. umbilicus
e. none of the above

45. The following structure is found at the T12 dermatome in most patients:
   a. nipple
   b. jugular notch
   c. iliac crest
   d. umbilicus
   e. none of the above

46. The brachial plexus is formed by the fusion of the anterior (ventral) rami of the:
   a. C5 spinal nerve
   b. C6 spinal nerve
   c. C7 spinal nerve
   d. C8 and T1 spinal nerves
   e. all of the above

47. The brachial plexus occasionally receives contributions from the anterior (ventral) rami of the:
   a. C2 spinal nerve
   b. C4 spinal nerve
   c. T2 spinal nerve
   d. b and c
   e. all of the above

48. The brachial plexus is subdivided into:
   a. roots
   b. trunks
   c. divisions and cords
   d. terminal branches
   e. all of the above

49. Injuries that are isolated to the musculocutaneous nerve present clinically as:
   a. painless weakness of elbow flexion
   b. painless weakness of elbow supination
   c. localized sensory deficit on the radial side of the forearm
   d. all of the above
   e. none of the above

50. The musculocutaneous nerve arises from the:
   a. lateral cord of the brachial plexus
   b. posterior cord of the brachial plexus
   c. medial cord of the brachial plexus
   d. all of the above
   e. none of the above

51. The ulnar nerve provides sensory innervation to the:
   a. ulnar aspect of the dorsum of the hand
   b. dorsal aspect of the little finger and the ulnar half of the ring
   c. palmar aspect of the little finger and the ulnar half of the ring finger.
   d. all of the above
   e. none of the above

52. The ulnar nerve:
   a. arises from the medial cord of the brachial plexus
   b. is made up of fibers from C6-T1 spinal roots
   c. lies anterior and inferior to the axillary artery

d. all of the above
e. none of the above

53. The median nerve provides sensory innervation to:
   a. a portion of the palmar surface of the hand
   b. the palmar surface of the thumb, index and middle fingers, and the radial portion of the ring finger
   c. distal dorsal surface of the index and middle fingers and the radial portion of the ring finger
   d. all of the above
   e. none of the above

54. The median nerve:
   a. arises from the medial and lateral cords of the brachial plexus
   b. is made up of fibers from C5-T1 spinal roots
   c. lies anterior and superior to the axillary artery
   d. all of the above
   e. none of the above

55. Entrapment of the median nerve:
   a. occurs most commonly at the wrist
   b. occurs most commonly at the elbow
   c. is known as carpal tunnel syndrome
   d. all of the above
   e. a and c

56. The radial nerve:
   a. arises from the posterior cord of the brachial plexus
   b. is made up of fibers from C5-T1 spinal roots
   c. lies posterior and inferior to the axillary artery
   d. all of the above
   e. none of the above

57. Damage to the radial nerve as it winds around the shaft of the humerus is characterized by:
   a. palsy or paralysis of all extensors of the wrist and digits
   b. palsy or paralysis of the forearm supinators
   c. numbness over the dorsoradial aspect of the hand and the dorsal aspect of the radial 3½ digits
   d. all of the above
   e. none of the above

58. Which of the following statements is *true* regarding the glenohumeral joint?
   a. The humeral head articulates with the glenoid fossa.
   b. It is a true joint.
   c. It is the most commonly dislocated joint in humans.
   d. all of the above
   e. none of the above

59. The acromioclavicular joint is formed by the:
   a. distal end of the clavicle and the anterior and medial aspect of the acromion
   b. head of the humerus and the glenoid fossa
   c. sternoclavicular space
   d. articulation of the first rib and the vertebra
   e. none of the above

60. The subdeltoid bursa lies primarily under the:
   a. acromion extending laterally between the deltoid muscle and joint capsule
   b. scapula

c. suprascapular notch
d. all of the above
e. none of the above

61. The biceps muscle:
    a. supinates the forearm
    b. flexes the elbow joint
    c. is innervated by the musculocutaneous nerve
    d. has a long and a short head
    e. all of the above

62. The muscles that comprise the rotator cuff include the:
    a. supraspinatus muscle
    b. infraspinatus muscle
    c. teres minor muscle
    d. subscapularis muscle
    e. all of the above

63. The muscles and their associated fascia and tendons of the rotator cuff:
    a. work in concert to maintain the stability of the shoulder joint throughout a wide and varied range of motion
    b. assist in deglutition
    c. are subject to tears from overuse or misuse
    d. a and c
    e. none of the above

64. The supraspinatus muscle:
    a. is the most important muscle of the rotator cuff
    b. provides shoulder joint stability
    c. along with the deltoid muscle adducts the arm at the shoulder by fixing the head of the humerus firmly against the glenoid fossa.
    d. is innervated by the suprascapular nerve
    e. all of the above

65. The infraspinatus muscle:
    a. provides shoulder joint stability
    b. along with the teres minor muscle externally rotates the arm at the shoulder
    c. is innervated by the suprascapular nerve
    d. all of the above
    e. none of the above

66. The subcoracoid bursa lies:
    a. between the joint capsule and the coracoid process
    b. just inferior to the jugular notch
    c. at the costosternal junction
    d. at the costovertebral angle
    e. none of the above

67. The intercostal nerves arise from the:
    a. stellate ganglion
    b. anterior division of the thoracic paravertebral nerves
    c. celiac plexus
    d. all of the above
    e. none of the above

68. The four branches of a typical intercostal nerve include the:
    a. unmyelinated postganglionic fibers of the gray rami communicantes
    b. posterior cutaneous branch

c. lateral cutaneous division
d. anterior cutaneous branch
e. all of the above

69. The 12th intercostal nerve is commonly known as the:
    a. subcostal nerve
    b. posterior cutaneous branch
    c. lateral cutaneous division
    d. anterior cutaneous branch
    e. all of the above

70. The first thoracic ganglion is fused with the lower cervical ganglion to help make up the:
    a. gasserian ganglion
    b. ganglion of Impar
    c. stellate ganglion
    d. all of the above
    e. none of the above

71. The major preganglionic contribution to the celiac plexus is provided by the:
    a. greater splanchnic nerves
    b. lesser splanchnic nerves
    c. least splanchnic nerves
    d. all of the above
    e. none of the above

72. The ganglia usually lie approximately at the level of:
    a. the fifth intercostal vein
    b. T6
    c. the first lumbar vertebra
    d. the third lumbar vertebra
    e. none of the above

73. The celiac plexus is:
    a. anterior to the crus of the diaphragm
    b. posterior to the crus of the diaphragm
    c. superior to the crus of the diaphragm
    d. intrathoracic
    e. none of the above

74. The superior hypogastric plexus lies in front of:
    a. L1
    b. L4
    c. T12
    d. the greater curvature of the stomach
    e. none of the above

75. The hypogastric nerves provide sympathetic innervation to the:
    a. pelvic viscera
    b. esophagus
    c. pelvic viscera
    d. a and c
    e. b and c

76. The lumbar sympathetic chain and ganglia lie:
    a. at the anterolateral margin of the lumbar vertebral bodies
    b. in the peritoneal cavity
    c. within the spinal canal
    d. within the corresponding spinal nerve roots
    e. none of the above

77. The peritoneal cavity lies lateral and anterior to the:
    a. small intestine
    b. lumbar sympathetic chain
    c. colon
    d. all of the above
    e. none of the above

78. The greater splanchnic nerve has its origin from the:
    a. T5-10 spinal roots
    b. C7-T2 spinal roots
    c. stellate ganglion
    d. all of the above
    e. none of the above

79. The lesser splanchnic nerve arises from the:
    a. T10-11 roots
    b. C7-T2 spinal roots
    c. stellate ganglion
    d. all of the above
    e. none of the above

80. The least splanchnic nerve has its origin from the:
    a. T11-12 spinal roots
    b. C7-T2 spinal roots
    c. stellate ganglion
    d. all of the above
    e. none of the above

81. The elbow joint is composed of the following bones:
    a. humerus
    b. ulna
    c. radius
    d. all of the above
    e. none of the above

82. The bursae most commonly inflamed by overuse or misuse of the elbow include the:
    a. olecranon bursa
    b. cubital bursa
    c. pes anserine bursa
    d. b and c
    e. a and b

83. The olecranon bursa lies:
    a. in the posterior aspect of the elbow joint between the olecranon process of the ulna and the overlying skin
    b. in the antecubital fossa lateral to the artery
    c. in the antecubital fossa medial to the artery
    d. under the biceps brachii muscle
    e. none of the above

84. The cubital bursa:
    a. lies in the anterior aspect of the elbow
    b. is subject to inflammation from overuse or misuse of the elbow
    c. may become infected
    d. may become calcified if the inflammation becomes chronic
    e. all of the above

85. The radial nerve at the elbow lies between the:
    a. lateral epicondyle of the humerus and the musculo-spiral groove

b. the fascia of the triceps muscle and the muscle substance
    c. fascia of the biceps muscle and the muscle substance
    d. none of the above
    e. all of the above

86. The cubital tunnel:
    a. contains the axillary artery and nerve
    b. is made up of the olecranon process and medial epicondyle of the humerus
    c. contains the radial artery and nerve
    d. a and b
    e. b and c

87. The anterior interosseous nerve:
    a. provides motor innervation to the flexor muscles of the forearm
    b. is susceptible to nerve entrapment by aberrant ligaments, muscle hypertrophy, and direct trauma
    c. is a branch of the median nerve
    d. all of the above
    e. none of the above

88. The lateral antebrachial cutaneous nerve:
    a. is a continuation of the musculocutaneous nerve
    b. is susceptible to entrapment as the nerve passes lateral to the fascia of the biceps tendon
    c. passes behind the cephalic vein, where it divides into a volar branch that continues along the radial border of the forearm
    d. provides sensory innervation to the skin over the lateral half of the volar surface of the forearm
    e. all of the above

89. The wrist allows which of the following movements?
    a. flexion/extension
    b. radial/ulnar deviation
    c. pronation/supination
    d. all of the above
    e. none of the above

90. The wrist is made up of the following joints:
    a. distal radioulnar joint
    b. radiocarpal joint and the ulnar carpal joint
    c. proximal carpal joints
    d. midcarpal joints
    e. all of the above

91. The triangular fibroelastic cartilage:
    a. is located primarily between the distal ulna and the lunate and triquetrum
    b. is made up of very strong fibroelastic fibers
    c. acts like an intervertebral disc in that it serves as the primary shock absorber of the wrist and acts like a ligament in that it serves as the primarily stabilizer for the distal radioulnar joint
    d. has a poor vascular supply and heals poorly
    e. all of the above

92. The ulnar tunnel is:
    a. the space between the pisiform and hamate bones of the wrist through which the ulnar nerve and artery pass

b. also known as the cubital tunnel
c. also known as Guyon's canal
d. a and b
e. a and c

93. The carpal tunnel:
a. is bounded on three sides by the carpal bones and is covered by the transverse carpal ligament
b. contains the radial nerve
c. contains the median nerve
d. a and b
e. a and c

94. In addition to the median nerve, the carpal tunnel also contains:
a. a number of flexor tendon sheaths
b. blood vessels
c. lymphatics
d. all of the above
e. none of the above

95. The carpometacarpal joint:
a. is a synovial, saddle-shaped joint
b. is a synovial hinge type joint
c. serves as the articulation between the trapezium and the base of the first metacarpal
d. a and b
e. a and c

96. The carpometacarpal joints of the fingers:
a. are synovial plane joints that serve as the articulation between the carpals and the metacarpals
b. also allow articulation of the bases of the metacarpal bones with one another
c. is a synovial hinge-type joint
d. a and b
e. a and c

97. The metacarpophalangeal joint:
a. is a synovial, ellipsoid-shaped joint
b. serves as the articulation between the base of the proximal phalanges and the head of its respective metacarpal
c. is a synovial hinge-type joint
d. a and b
e. a and c

98. The interphalangeal joints:
a. are synovial hinge-shaped joints
b. are synovial plane joints
c. serve as the articulation between the phalanges
d. a and b
e. a and c

99. The sciatic nerve:
a. innervates the distal lower extremity and foot with the exception of the medial aspect of the calf and foot, which are subserved by the saphenous nerve
b. is the largest nerve in the body
c. is derived from the L4, L5, and S1-3 nerve roots
d. all of the above
e. none of the above

100. Branches of the sciatic nerve include the:
a. tibial
b. common peroneal nerves
c. ganglion of Impar
d. a and b
e. a and c

101. The lumbar plexus:
a. lies within the substance of the psoas muscle
b. is made up of the ventral roots of the first four lumbar nerves and, in some patients, a contribution from the 12th thoracic nerve
c. consists of nerves that lie in front of the transverse processes of their respective vertebrae as they course inferolaterally
d. consists of nerves that divide into a number of peripheral nerves
e. all of the above

102. The femoral nerve:
a. innervates the anterior portion of the thigh and medial calf
b. is derived from the posterior branches of the L2, L3, and L4 nerve roots
c. roots fuse together in the psoas muscle and descend laterally between the psoas and iliacus muscles to enter the iliac fossa
d. gives off motor fibers to the iliac, sartorius, quadriceps femoris, and pectineus muscles
e. all of the above

103. The femoral nerve:
a. passes beneath the inguinal ligament to enter the thigh
b. is just lateral to the femoral artery as it passes beneath the inguinal ligament
c. is enclosed with the femoral artery and vein within the femoral sheath
d. provides sensory fibers to the knee joint as well as the skin overlying the anterior thigh
e. all of the above

104. The lateral femoral cutaneous nerve:
a. is formed from the posterior divisions of the L2 and L3 nerves
b. leaves the psoas muscle and courses laterally and inferiorly to pass just beneath the ilioinguinal nerve at the level of the anterior superior iliac spine and then divides into an anterior and a posterior branch
c. provides limited cutaneous sensory innervation over the anterolateral thigh through its anterior branch
d. provides cutaneous sensory innervation to the lateral thigh from just above the greater trochanter to the knee through its posterior branch
e. all of the above

105. Entrapment of the lateral femoral cutaneous nerve is known as:
a. meralgia paresthetica
b. ilioinguinal neuralgia
c. genitofemoral neuralgia

d. femoral neuralgia
e. none of the above

106. The ilioinguinal nerve:
    a. is a branch of the L1 nerve root with a contribution from T12 in some patients
    b. follows a curvilinear course that takes it from its origin of the L1 and occasionally T12 somatic nerves to inside the concavity of the ilium
    c. continues anteriorly to perforate the transverse abdominal muscle at the level of the anterior superior iliac spine.
    d. may interconnect with the iliohypogastric nerve as it continues to pass along its course medially and inferiorly, where it accompanies the spermatic cord through the inguinal ring and into the inguinal canal
    e. all of the above

107. Entrapment of the ilioinguinal nerve is known as:
    a. meralgia paresthetica
    b. ilioinguinal neuralgia
    c. genitofemoral neuralgia
    d. femoral neuralgia
    e. none of the above

108. Entrapment of the iliohypogastric nerve is known as:
    a. meralgia paresthetica
    b. iliohypogastric neuralgia
    c. genitofemoral neuralgia
    d. femoral neuralgia
    e. none of the above

109. Entrapment of the genitofemoral nerve is known as:
    a. meralgia paresthetica
    b. ilioinguinal neuralgia
    c. genitofemoral neuralgia
    d. femoral neuralgia
    e. none of the above

110. The iliohypogastric nerve:
    a. is a branch of the L1 nerve root with a contribution from T12 in some patients
    b. follows a curvilinear course that takes it from its origin of the L1 and occasionally T12 somatic nerves to inside the concavity of the ilium
    c. continues anteriorly to perforate the transverse abdominal muscle to lie between it and the external oblique muscle where it divides into an anterior and a lateral branch
    d. all of the above
    e. none of the above

111. The ilioinguinal nerve:
    a. provides cutaneous sensory innervation to the posterolateral gluteal region via its lateral branch
    b. pierces the external oblique muscle just beyond the anterior superior iliac spine to provide cutaneous sensory innervation to the abdominal skin above the pubis via its anterior branch
    c. may interconnect with the ilioinguinal nerve along its course, resulting in variation of the distribution of

the sensory innervation of the iliohypogastric and ilioinguinal nerves
    d. all of the above
    e. none of the above

112. The genitofemoral nerve:
    a. is a branch of the L1 nerve root with a contribution from T12 in some patients
    b. follows a curvilinear course that takes it from its origin of the L1 and occasionally T12 and L2 somatic nerves to inside the concavity of the ilium
    c. descends obliquely in an anterior course through the psoas major muscle to emerge on the abdominal surface opposite L3 or L4
    d. all of the above
    e. none of the above

113. The genitofemoral nerve:
    a. divides into a genital and femoral branch just above the inguinal ligament
    b. in males, the genital branch travels through the inguinal canal passing inside the deep inguinal ring to innervate the cremaster muscle and skin of the scrotum
    c. in females, the genital branch follows the course of the round ligament and provides innervation to the ipsilateral mons pubis and labia majora
    d. in males and females, the femoral branch descends lateral to the external iliac artery to pass behind the inguinal ligament to enter the femoral sheath lateral to the femoral artery to innervate the skin of the anterior superior femoral triangle
    e. all of the above

114. The obturator nerve:
    a. provides the majority of innervation to the hip joint
    b. is derived from the posterior divisions of the L2, L3, and L4 nerves
    c. leaves the medial border psoas muscle and courses inferiorly to pass the pelvis, where it joins the obturator vessels to travel via the obturator canal to enter the thigh where it then divides into an anterior and posterior branch
    d. all of the above
    e. none of the above

115. The anterior branch of the obturator nerve supplies:
    a. an articular branch to provide sensory innervation to the hip joint
    b. motor branches to the superficial hip adductors
    c. a cutaneous branch to the medial aspect of the distal thigh
    d. all of the above
    e. none of the above

116. The posterior branch of the obturator nerve provides:
    a. motor innervation to the deep hip adductors
    b. an articular branch to the posterior knee joint.
    c. motor innervation to the superficial hip abductors
    d. a and b
    e. a and c

117. The ganglion of Impar:
    a. lies in front of the coccyx just below the sacrococcygeal junction
    b. is the terminal coalescence of the sympathetic chains
    c. receives fibers from the lumbar and sacral portions of the sympathetic and parasympathetic nervous system
    d. all of the above
    e. none of the above

118. The tibial nerve:
    a. is one of the two major continuations of the sciatic nerve
    b. provides sensory innervation to the posterior portion of the calf, the heel, and the medial plantar surface
    c. splits from the sciatic nerve at the superior margin of the popliteal fossa and descends in a slightly medial course through the popliteal fossa
    d. continues its downward course, running between the two heads of the gastrocnemius muscle, passing deep to the soleus muscle
    e. all of the above

119. The tibial nerve:
    a. courses medially between the Achilles tendon and the medial malleolus, where it divides into the medial and lateral plantar nerves
    b. provides sensory innervation to the heel and medial plantar surface
    c. provides motor innervation to the extensor hallucis longus
    d. a and b
    e. a and c

120. Entrapment of the tibial nerve as it courses medially between the Achilles tendon and the medial malleolus is known as:
    a. anterior tarsal tunnel syndrome
    b. posterior tarsal tunnel syndrome
    c. hallux rigidus
    d. meralgia paresthetica
    e. none of the above

121. The common peroneal nerve:
    a. is one of the two major continuations of the sciatic nerve
    b. provides sensory innervation to the inferior portion of the knee joint and the posterior and lateral skin of the upper calf
    c. is derived from the posterior branches of the L4, the L5, and the S1 and S2 nerve roots
    d. splits from the sciatic nerve at the superior margin of the popliteal fossa and descends laterally behind the head of the fibula
    e. all of the above

122. The ischial bursa:
    a. lies between the gluteus maximus muscle and the ischial tuberosity
    b. lies between the inguinal ligament and the acetabulum

    c. lies between the tensor fascia lata and the greater trochanter
    d. all of the above
    e. none of the above

123. The hip:
    a. is a ball-and-socket type joint
    b. is composed of the femoral head and the cup-shaped acetabulum
    c. has a femoral head that is completely covered with hyaline cartilage except for a central area called the fovea, which is the point of attachment for the ligamentum teres
    d. all of the above
    e. none of the above

124. The gluteal bursae:
    a. lie between the gluteal maximus, medius, and minimus muscles as well as between these muscles and the underlying bone
    b. lie between the inguinal ligament and the acetabulum
    c. lie between the tensor fascia lata and the greater trochanter
    d. all of the above
    e. none of the above

125. The trochanteric bursa:
    a. lies between the greater trochanter and the tendon of the gluteus medius and the iliotibial tract
    b. lies between the inguinal ligament and the acetabulum
    c. lies between the tensor fascia lata and the greater trochanter
    d. all of the above
    e. none of the above

126. The SI joint:
    a. is a synovial (diarthrodial) joint
    b. is more mobile in youth than later in life
    c. becomes more fibrotic in adulthood in the upper two-thirds of the joint
    d. of the female pelvis is also more mobile to accommodate pregnancy and parturition
    e. all of the above

127. The SI joint:
    a. is densely innervated by several levels of spinal nerves (L3-S1)
    b. may produce lumbar disc–like symptoms when stimulated
    c. has muscle insertions near the joint such as the gluteus maximus and hamstrings, which may refer pain to the hip and ischial area, respectively, when stressed
    d. all of the above
    e. none of the above

128. The femoral-tibial joint:
    a. is made up of the articulation of the femur and the tibia
    b. is a synarthrodial joint

c. is not a true joint
d. all of the above
e. none of the above

129. The main extensor of the knee is:
    a. the extensor hallucis longus
    b. the quadriceps muscle that attaches to the patella via the quadriceps tendon
    c. the extensor hallucis brevis
    d. all of the above
    e. none of the above

130. The main flexors of the hip joint are the:
    a. hamstrings
    b. gastrocnemius
    c. sartorius
    d. gracilis
    e. all of the above

131. The prepatellar bursa:
    a. lies between the subcutaneous tissues and the patella
    b. lies deep to the inguinal ligament
    c. is superficial to the inguinal ligament
    d. is deep to the pes anserine bursa
    e. none of the above

132. The suprapatellar bursa:
    a. extends superiorly from beneath the patella under the quadriceps femoris muscle and its tendon.
    b. lies deep to the inguinal ligament
    c. is superficial to the inguinal ligament
    d. is deep to the pes anserine bursa
    e. none of the above

133. The deep infrapatellar bursa:
    a. lies between the ligamentum patellae and the tibia
    b. lies deep to the inguinal ligament
    c. is superficial to the inguinal ligament
    d. is deep to the infrapatellar fossa
    e. none of the above

134. The superficial infrapatellar bursa:
    a. lies between the subcutaneous tissues and the ligamentum patellae
    b. lies deep to the inguinal ligament
    c. is superficial to the inguinal ligament
    d. is deep to the infrapatellar fossa
    e. none of the above

135. The pes anserine bursa:
    a. lies between the combined tendinous insertion of the sartorius, gracilis, and semitendinosus muscles and the medial tibia
    b. lies deep to the inguinal ligament
    c. is superficial to the inguinal ligament
    d. is deep to the infrapatellar fossa
    e. none of the above

136. The iliotibial band bursa:
    a. lies between the iliotibial band and the lateral condyle of the femur
    b. lies deep to the inguinal ligament
    c. is superficial to the inguinal ligament

d. is deep to the infrapatellar fossa
e. none of the above

137. The iliotibial band:
    a. is an extension of the fascia lata that inserts at the lateral condyle of the tibia
    b. can rub backward and forward over the lateral epicondyle of the femur
    c. can irritate the iliotibial bursa beneath it
    d. all of the above
    e. none of the above

138. The distal joint between the tibia and fibula:
    a. allows very little movement with the hinge joint formed by the distal ends of the tibia and fibula and the talus providing dorsiflexion and plantar flexion needed for ambulation
    b. is stabilized by the medial and lateral malleoli, which extend along the sides of the talus to form a mortise and prevents ankle rotation
    c. is further strengthened by the deltoid ligament medially and the anterior talofibular, posterior talofibular, and calcaneofibular ligaments laterally
    d. all of the above
    e. none of the above

139. The talocalcaneal joint:
    a. lies between the talus and calcaneus
    b. allows for additional range of motion of the ankle joint and makes up for the limitations of motions placed on the joint by the mortise structure of the talus and medial and lateral malleoli
    c. permits approximately 30 degrees of foot inversion
    d. permits 15 to 20 degrees of foot eversion, which allows walking on uneven surfaces
    e. all of the above

140. The deltoid ligament:
    a. has two layers
    b. attaches above to the medial malleolus
    c. has a deep layer that attaches below to the medial body of the talus
    d. superficial fibers attach to the medial talus and the sustentaculum tali of the calcaneus and the navicular tuberosity
    e. all of the above

141. The anterior talofibular ligament:
    a. runs from the anterior border of the lateral malleolus to the lateral surface of the talus
    b. attaches above to the medial malleolus
    c. has a deep layer that attaches below to the medial body of the talus
    d. superficial fibers attach to the medial talus and the sustentaculum tali of the calcaneus and the navicular tuberosity
    e. all of the above

142. The posterior tarsal tunnel:
    a. is made up of the flexor retinaculum, the bones of the ankle, and the lacunate ligament
    b. is the site of compression of the tibial nerve

c. contains the posterior tibial artery and a number of flexor tendons
d. all of the above
e. none of the above

143. The deep branch of the peroneal nerve:
   a. continues down the leg in conjunction with the tibial artery and vein to provide sensory innervation to the web space of the first and second toes and adjacent dorsum of the foot
   b. provides motor innervation to all of the toe extensors
   c. passes beneath the dense superficial fascia of the ankle where it is subject to entrapment called anterior tarsal tunnel syndrome
   d. all of the above
   e. none of the above

144. The Achilles tendon:
   a. is the thickest and strongest tendon in the body, yet also very susceptible to rupture
   b. is the common tendon of the gastrocnemius muscle
   c. begins at mid-calf and continues downward to attach to the posterior calcaneus, where it may become inflamed
   d. narrows during its downward course, becoming most narrow approximately 5 cm above its calcaneal insertion
   e. all of the above

145. The Achilles bursa:
   a. lies between the Achilles tendon and the base of the tibia and the posterior calcaneus
   b. is rarely inflamed
   c. lies superficial to the Achilles tendon and the base of the tibia and the posterior calcaneus
   d. all of the above
   e. none of the above

146. The Achilles bursa:
   a. may become inflamed with overuse or misuse
   b. is located in the anterior tarsal tunnel
   c. may become inflamed in association with Achilles tendonitis
   d. a and b
   e. a and c

147. The shallow longitudinal indentation along the length of the dorsal surface of the spinal cord is called the:
   a. anterior median fissure
   b. posterior median sulcus
   c. central canal
   d. filum terminale
   e. none of the above

148. The deep longitudinal indentation along the ventral surface of the spinal cord is called the:
   a. anterior median fissure
   b. posterior median sulcus
   c. central canal
   d. filum terminale
   e. none of the above

149. The cervical enlargement:
   a. contains interneurons for the nerves that supply the upper extremities and pectoral girdle as well as fibers from regions inferior to the cervical region, e.g., thoracic, lumbar, and sacral
   b. contains the geniculate ganglion
   c. contains the ganglion of Gasser
   d. all of the above
   e. none of the above

150. The lumbar enlargement contains:
   a. interneurons for the nerves that supply the lower extremities and pelvis as well as fibers from the more inferior sacral region
   b. the geniculate ganglion
   c. the ganglion of Gasser
   d. all of the above
   e. none of the above

151. The end of the spinal cord tapers to a point that is called the:
   a. cervical enlargement
   b. lumbar enlargement
   c. hypogastric plexus
   d. conus medullaris

152. The conus medullaris is at the:
   a. third segment of the sacrum
   b. sacral hiatus
   c. level of the first lumbar vertebra
   d. foramen ovale
   e. none of the above

153. The distal spinal cord is tethered distally by the:
   a. filum terminale
   b. sacral hiatus
   c. first lumbar vertebra
   d. foramen ovale
   e. none of the above

154. The dorsal root ganglia:
   a. contain the nerve cell bodies of the corresponding sensory neurons
   b. contain the nerve cell bodies of the corresponding motor neurons
   c. contain the origins of the ganglion of Gasser
   d. all of the above
   e. none of the above

155. The ventral nerve root carries primarily:
   a. sensory neurons
   b. motor neurons
   c. parasympathetic ganglia
   d. all of the above
   e. none of the above

156. The spinal nerve root:
   a. is a mixed nerve that carries both motor and sensory information
   b. is formed from the coalescence of the dorsal and ventral nerve roots
   c. exits via the intervertebral foramen

d. all of the above

e. none of the above

157. In the center of the spinal cord is an H-shaped structure made up primarily of:
    a. gray matter consisting of nerve cell bodies and glial cells
    b. white matter consisting of nerve cell bodies and glial cells
    c. connective tissue
    d. veins and lymphatics
    e. all of the above

158. The concept that dorsal roots carry sensory information and the ventral roots carry motor information is known as the:
    a. Herring-Brewer law
    b. Mason-Dixon law
    c. Bell-Magendie law
    d. Marbury-Madison law
    e. none of the above

159. The first pair of spinal nerves is designated C1 and they:
    a. exit between the skull and the first cervical vertebra
    b. exit between the first and second cervical vertebrae
    c. exit via the jugular foramen
    d. exit via the foramen magnum
    e. none of the above

160. The last pair of cervical nerves exit between the seventh cervical vertebra and the first thoracic vertebra and are designated:
    a. C7
    b. C8
    c. the cervical plexus
    d. the stellate ganglion
    e. none of the above

161. The first thoracic spinal nerve T1 exits:
    a. just beneath the seventh cervical vertebra
    b. just beneath the first thoracic vertebra
    c. via the jugular foramen
    d. via the foramen magnum
    e. none of the above

162. Each spinal nerve is invested with three layers of connective tissue, which include the:
    a. outermost epineurium
    b. central perineurium
    c. innermost epineurium
    d. all of the above
    e. none of the above

163. The white ramus:
    a. carries visceral motor fibers to the nearby autonomic ganglia associated with the sympathetic chain
    b. carries special sensory fibers
    c. is made up of myelinated fibers
    d. a and c
    e. b and c

164. Reflexes:
    a. are immediate involuntary motor responses to a specific stimulus that are designed to help maintain homeostasis across a wide range of conditions
    b. can be modulated at the spinal cord level
    c. can be modulated by the brain
    d. all of the above
    e. none of the above

165. The posterior column pathway carries:
    a. fine touch information
    b. pressure information
    c. vibratory information
    d. proprioceptive information
    e. all of the above

166. First-order neurons carrying fine touch, pressure, vibratory, and proprioceptive information from the upper extremities enter the central nervous system via the dorsal roots and ascend via the:
    a. stellate ganglion
    b. fasciculus cuneatus
    c. ganglion of Gasser
    d. fasciculus gracilis
    e. none of the above

167. First-order neurons carrying fine touch, pressure, vibratory, and proprioceptive information from the lower extremities enter the central nervous system via the dorsal roots and ascend via the:
    a. stellate ganglion
    b. fasciculus cuneatus
    c. ganglion of Gasser
    d. fasciculus gracilis
    e. none of the above

168. Second-order neurons of the posterior column pathway leave the medulla oblongata and immediately cross to the opposite side of the brainstem to relay transmitted information via the:
    a. ribbon-like medial lemniscus
    b. ribbon-like lateral lemniscus
    c. stellate ganglion
    d. trigeminal nucleus
    e. none of the above

169. Fine touch information that comes from stimulus of the left great toe is projected onto the:
    a. ipsilateral primary sensory cortex
    b. contralateral primary sensory cortex
    c. ipsilateral frontal lobe
    d. contralateral frontal lobe
    e. none of the above

170. The tract cells of the spinothalamic pathway:
    a. decussate at the brainstem level to the contralateral thalamus via the anterior white tract
    b. decussate to the opposite side of the spinal cord via the anterior white commissure to the contralateral anterolateral spinal cord
    c. travel up the ipsilateral side of the spinal cord in the ventral region of the spinal cord

d. travel up the ipsilateral side of the spinal cord in the dorsal region of the spinal cord
e. none of the above

171. The anterior spinothalamic tract carries:
a. pain and temperature information
b. vibratory information
c. crude touch
d. proprioception
e. none of the above

172. The lateral spinothalamic tract carries:
a. pain and temperature information
b. vibratory information
c. crude touch
d. proprioception
e. none of the above

173. The pyramidal system is made up of the:
a. corticobulbar tracts
b. lateral corticospinal tracts
c. anterior corticospinal tracts
d. all of the above
e. none of the above

174. Approximately 85% of these primary motor axons decussate at the level of the medulla to cross to the contralateral spinal cord to enter the:
a. lateral corticospinal tracts
b. anterior corticospinal tracts
c. medial lemniscal tract
d. anterior lemniscal tract
e. none of the above

175. Approximately 15% of these primary motor axons do not decussate at the level of the medulla to remain on the ipsilateral side of the spinal cord to enter the:
a. lateral corticospinal tracts
b. anterior corticospinal tracts
c. medial lemniscal tract
d. anterior lemniscal tract
e. none of the above

176. The extrapyramidal system is the name used to describe a number of centers and their associated tracts whose primary function is to coordinate and process:
a. motor commands performed at a subconscious level
b. sudomotor responses
c. vasomotor responses
d. all of the above
e. none of the above

177. The extrapyramidal processing centers produce output to a variety of targets including:
a. the primary motor cortex to modulate the activities of the pyramidal system
b. the cranial nerve nuclei to coordinate reflex activities in response to visual, auditory, and equilibrium input
c. descending pathways into the spinal cord including the vestibulospinal tracts, the tectospinal tracts, the rubrospinal tracts, and the reticulospinal tracts

d. all of the above
e. none of the above

178. Functions of the cerebellum include the:
a. processing and integration of the functioning of the pyramidal and extrapyramidal systems
b. maintenance of motor tone for the muscles of posture
c. processing of proprioceptive information
d. all of the above
e. none of the above

179. The sympathetic chain ganglia:
a. are responsible for the sympathetic activity of the thoracic cavity, chest and abdominal wall, the head, neck, and the extremities
b. are located on each side of the vertebral columns
c. on each side average 3 cervical, 11 or 12 thoracic, 3 to 5 lumbar, and 4 or 5 sacral ganglia
d. of the coccyx from each sympathetic chain are fused to form a single terminal ganglion known as the ganglion of Impar
e. all of the above

180. The myelinated sympathetic fibers from the spinal nerve roots:
a. may synapse within the sympathetic chain ganglion at the same level at which the fibers entered the ganglion
b. may ascend or descend within the sympathetic chain and then synapse with a sympathetic ganglion at a level different from the level of fiber entry
c. may simply pass through the sympathetic chain without synapsing with any sympathetic chain ganglion to ultimately synapse with a collateral ganglion or the adrenal medulla
d. all of the above
e. none of the above

181. The sympathetic division of the autonomic nervous system is best characterized by the concept of:
a. convergence
b. divergence
c. reverberating circuitry
d. ultra-short axons
e. none of the above

182. The sympathetic collateral ganglia:
a. most often lie anterolateral to the descending aorta
b. include the celiac ganglion
c. include the superior and inferior mesenteric ganglia
d. give off postganglionic fibers that provide sympathetic innervation to the abdominopelvic viscera
e. all of the above

183. The sympathetic nerves located in the center of the adrenal medulla:
a. release epinephrine and norepinephrine into the capillary bed of the adrenal medulla
b. allow tissues not innervated by postganglionic sympathetic fibers to receive stimulation by the

sympathetic nervous system providing they have receptors sensitive to epinephrine and norepinephrine
c. are stimulated by preganglionic sympathetic nerves that do not synapse in the ganglia of the sympathetic chain
d. all of the above
e. none of the above

184. The parasympathetic division of the autonomic nervous system has:
a. preganglionic neurons and nuclei that are located in the brain, mesencephalon, pons, and medulla oblongata
b. autonomic nuclei that reside in the lateral gray horns of spinal segments S2-4
c. preganglionic fibers that travel within cranial nerves III, VII, IX, and X to synapse at the ciliary, sphenopalatine, otic, and submandibular ganglia
d. short postganglion fibers that carry parasympathetic commands to their respective target organs
e. all of the above

185. Stimulation of these parasympathetic nerves results in:
a. the release of acetylcholine by all preganglionic parasympathetic neurons, which causes stimulation of all nicotinic receptors
b. stimulation of muscarinic receptors
c. inhibition of muscarinic receptors
d. all of the above
e. none of the above

186. The autonomic nervous system is characterized by:
a. one nerve–one fiber innervation
b. discrete innervation
c. an antagonistic dual innervation system
d. an all-sort axon configuration
e. all of the above

187. Nociceptors are freely distributed in the:
a. outer layers of the skin
b. walls of blood vessels
c. periosteum of bone
d. joint capsules
e. all of the above

188. When nociceptors are initially stimulated, the first response is the firing of the receptors to produce an immediate message to the central nervous system that results in the perception known as:
a. dull pain
b. slow pain
c. fast pain
d. internuncial pain
e. none of the above

189. Fast pain information is carried by:
a. C fibers
b. A delta fibers
c. the white communicantes
d. the gray communicantes
e. all of the above

190. Slow pain information is carried by:
a. C fibers
b. A delta fibers
c. the white communicantes
d. the gray communicantes
e. all of the above

191. C fibers are:
a. heavily myelinated
b. pure sympathetic fibers
c. unmyelinated
d. only found in the pelvis
e. none of the above

192. Pain and temperature impulses are carried to the central nervous system via the:
a. lateral spinothalamic tract
b. anterior spinothalamic tract
c. Meissner corpuscles
d. all of the above
e. none of the above

193. Mechanoreceptors include:
a. tactile receptors
b. baroreceptors
c. proprioceptors
d. all of the above
e. none of the above

194. Baroreceptors are commonly found in the:
a. aorta and carotid arteries
b. urinary bladder and ureters
c. respiratory system
d. digestive system
e. all of the above

195. Encapsulated tactile receptors include:
a. Meissner's corpuscles
b. Pacinian corpuscles
c. Ruffinian corpuscles
d. all of the above
e. none of the above

196. Unencapsulated receptors include:
a. Merkel's discs
b. free nerve endings
c. root hair plexuses
d. the digestive system
e. all of the above

197. Proprioceptors are located in:
a. muscle spindles
b. the Golgi tendon apparatus
c. joint capsules
d. ligaments
e. all of the above

198. Examples of specialized proprioceptors include:
a. the muscle spindle apparatus
b. Meissner's corpuscles
c. the Golgi tendon apparatus
d. a and b
e. a and c

199. The major chemoreceptors are located in the:
    a. medulla oblongata
    b. carotid bodies
    c. aortic bodies
    d. all of the above
    e. none of the above

200. Chemoreceptors located in the medulla oblongata respond to changes in the:
    a. hydrogen ion concentrations in the cerebrospinal fluid
    b. protein concentration in the cerebrospinal fluid
    c. carbon dioxide concentrations in the cerebrospinal fluid
    d. a and b
    e. a and c

201. The phenomenon of wind-up:
    a. is modulated in large part by modulatory neurotransmitter peptides
    b. is an example of how modulatory neurotransmitter peptides can result in increased transmission of nociceptive information
    c. occurs primarily at the spinal cord level
    d. often results in increased perception of pain
    e. all of the above

202. Examples of modulatory neurotransmitter peptides include:
    a. substance P
    b. somatostatin
    c. vasoactive intestinal polypeptide
    d. calcitonin gene–related peptide
    e. all of the above

203. The two cerebral hemispheres are divided by the:
    a. medial longitudinal fissure
    b. Sylvian fissure
    c. postcentral gyrus
    d. precentral gyrus
    e. putamen

204. The primary area for afferent sensory processing of the cerebrum is:
    a. medial longitudinal fissure
    b. Sylvian fissure
    c. postcentral gyrus
    d. precentral gyrus
    e. putamen

205. The primary area for efferent motor processing of the cerebrum is:
    a. medial longitudinal fissure
    b. Sylvian fissure
    c. postcentral gyrus
    d. precentral gyrus
    e. putamen

206. The central white matter is made up of:
    a. unmyelinated fibers
    b. myelinated fibers
    c. ganglionic cell bodies

    d. small-diameter sympathetic fibers
    e. all of the above

207. Efferent motor impulses originating in the precentral gyrus of the left cerebral hemisphere control the:
    a. right side of the body
    b. left side of the body
    c. both sides of the body
    d. all of the above
    e. none of the above

208. The functions of the limbic system are complex and include:
    a. the establishment of baseline emotional states
    b. behavior drives
    c. facilitation of storage and retrieval of memories
    d. the coordination and linkage of the complex conscious functions of the cerebral cortex with the unconscious and autonomic functions
    e. all of the above

209. Afferent sensory impulses originating on the left side of the body are perceived by the:
    a. right postcentral gyrus
    b. left postcentral gyrus
    c. postcentral gyri of both cerebral hemispheres
    d. all of the above
    e. none of the above

210. Inhibition of pain impulses may also occur by stimulation of:
    a. periaqueductal gray matter that surrounds the third ventricle and cerebral aqueduct
    b. trigone of the bladder
    c. pulmonary vasculature
    d. all of the above
    e. none of the above

211. The ventral posterior portion of the ventral nuclei is the primary relay station for the transmission of:
    a. fine touch
    b. pain
    c. temperature
    d. pressure and proprioception
    e. all of the above

212. The posterior nuclei is made up of the:
    a. pulvinar
    b. lateral geniculate nuclei
    c. medial geniculate nuclei
    d. all of the above
    e. none of the above

213. The thalamic nuclei include the:
    a. lateral nuclei and medial nuclei
    b. anterior nuclei
    c. ventral nuclei
    d. posterior nuclei
    e. all of the above

214. The thalamus is located in the:
    a. rhinencephalon
    b. norencephalon

   c. mesencephalon
   d. diencephalons
   e. none of the above

215. Functions of the hypothalamus include:
   a. raising or lowering of body temperature
   b. causing the release of antidiuretic hormone to signal the kidneys to restrict water loss
   c. causing the release of oxytocin to stimulate contractions of the uterus and prostate as well as the myo-epithelial cells of the breasts
   d. coordination of circadian rhythms
   e. all of the above

216. Functions of the hypothalamus include the:
   a. coordination and modulation of autonomic functions including blood pressure, heart rate, blood pressure, and respiration
   b. coordination and modulation of involuntary somatic motor activities associated with pain, pleasure, rage, and sexual arousal
   c. coordination of the complex interactions between the neuroendocrine system and the pituitary gland
   d. coordination and modulation of voluntary and involuntary behavioral patterns including thirst and hunger
   e. all of the above

217. Structures of the mesencephalon include the:
   a. red nuclei
   b. substantia nigra
   c. superior and inferior colliculus
   d. reticular activating system
   e. all of the above

218. The pons contains the following structures:
   a. the apneustic center and the pneumotaxic centers
   b. the sensory and motor nuclei of cranial nerves V, VI, VII, and VIII
   c. the nuclei that process and relay afferent information from the cerebellum that arrives in the pons via the middle cerebral peduncles
   d. tracts of ascending, descending, and transverse fibers that carry information from the spinal cord to the brain and from the brain to the spinal cord and the information from opposite cerebral hemispheres
   e. all of the above

219. The apneustic center and the pneumotaxic centers control:
   a. voluntary respiration
   b. involuntary respiration
   c. heart rate
   d. all of the above
   e. none of the above

220. Important nuclei and centers that sort, relay, and modulate a variety of activities necessary for the maintenance of homeostasis which are located in the medulla oblongata include the:
   a. respiratory rhythmicity center
   b. cardiovascular center

   c. olivary nuclei
   d. nucleus gracilis and cuneatus
   e. all of the above

221. Clinical characteristics include:
   a. bilateral or occasionally unilateral pain involving the frontal, temporal, and occipital regions
   b. bandlike nonpulsatile ache or tightness
   c. associated neck symptomatology
   d. pain that evolves over a period of hours or days and then tends to remain constant without progressive symptomatology
   e. all of the above

222. The following statements are *true* about tension-type headache.
   a. There is no aura associated with tension-type headache.
   b. Significant sleep disturbance is usually present.
   c. It affects females more than males.
   d. all of the above
   e. none of the above

223. Effective treatments for tension-type headache include:
   a. tricyclic antidepressants
   b. cervical steroid epidural nerve blocks
   c. biofeedback
   d. all of the above
   e. none of the above

224. Effective prophylactic treatments for migraine headaches include:
   a. beta-blockers
   b. calcium channel blockers
   c. nonsteroidal anti-inflammatory agents
   d. valproic acid
   e. all of the above

225. The main risk of the use of abortive therapies in the treatment of migraine headache includes:
   a. analgesic rebound headache
   b. peripheral vascular ischemia
   c. coronary artery ischemia
   d. all of the above
   e. none of the above

226. Clinical signs and symptoms of migraine headache include:
   a. unilateral pounding headache
   b. nausea and vomiting
   c. pallor
   d. photophobia and sonophobia
   e. all of the above

227. The painless neurologic phenomenon associated with migraine with aura includes:
   a. Braxton-Hicks contractions
   b. Cullen's sign
   c. aura
   d. all of the above
   e. none of the above

228. Clinical signs and symptoms of cluster headache include:
    a. severe retro-orbital and temporal headache
    b. deep, boring quality
    c. unilateral
    d. Horner's syndrome and rhinorrhea
    e. all of the above

229. Effective treatments for cluster headaches include:
    a. prednisone
    b. sphenopalatine ganglion blocks
    c. lithium carbonate
    d. methysergide
    e. all of the above

230. In contradistinction to migraine and tension-type headache, cluster headache is unique in its:
    a. female predominance
    b. association with sickle cell disease
    c. male predominance
    d. long onset-to-peak
    e. none of the above

231. The headache with the shortest onset-to-peak is:
    a. migraine headache
    b. cluster headache
    c. tension-type headache
    d. analgesic rebound headache
    e. none of the above

232. The diagnostic criteria for pseudotumor cerebri include:
    a. signs and symptoms suggestive of increased intracranial pressure including papilledema
    b. normal magnetic resonance imaging (MRI) or computed tomography (CT) of the brain performed with and without contrast media
    c. increased cerebrospinal fluid pressure documented by lumbar puncture
    d. normal cerebrospinal fluid chemistry, cultures, and cytology
    e. all of the above

233. The typical patient suffering from papilledema is:
    a. female
    b. obese
    c. between 20 and 45 years old
    d. complaining of headache
    e. all of the above

234. Drugs implicated in the evolution of pseudotumor cerebri include:
    a. vitamin A
    b. tetracyclines
    c. nalidixic acid
    d. corticosteroids
    e. all of the above

235. Clinical disorders associated with pseudotumor cerebri include:
    a. anemias
    b. endocrinopathies
    c. blood dyscrasias

d. chronic respiratory insufficiency
    e. all of the above

236. Common causes of ocular pain include:
    a. conjunctivitis
    b. corneal abrasions
    c. glaucoma
    d. uveitis
    e. all of the above

237. The *sine qua non* of post-dural puncture headache is:
    a. postural headache
    b. fever
    c. unilateral nature
    d. all of the above
    e. none of the above

238. Causes of trigeminal neuralgia include:
    a. acoustic neuromas
    b. cholesteatomas and bony abnormalities
    c. aneurysms and angiomas
    d. compression by aberrant or tortuous blood vessels
    e. all of the above

239. Medication treatment options for trigeminal neuralgia include:
    a. carbamazepine
    b. baclofen
    c. gabapentin
    d. all of the above
    e. none of the above

240. Surgical treatment options for trigeminal neuralgia include:
    a. trigeminal nerve block
    b. retrogasserian injection of glycerol
    c. radiofrequency lesioning of the gasserian ganglion
    d. microvascular decompression of the trigeminal root
    e. all of the above

241. The following symptom is pathognomonic for temporal arteritis:
    a. tinnitus
    b. papilledema
    c. jaw claudication
    d. areflexia
    e. none of the above

242. Temporal arteritis is a:
    a. disease of the sixth decade
    b. disease associated with polymyalgia rheumatica in approximately 50% of patients
    c. disease that affects females three times more often than males
    d. disease that affects almost exclusively whites
    e. all of the above

243. Over 90% of patients with temporal arteritis have a significantly elevated:
    a. hemoglobin
    b. erythrocyte sedimentation rate
    c. uric acid

    d. all of the above
    e. none of the above

244. Common causes of otalgia include:
    a. cellulitis and/or abscess of the auricle
    b. otitis externa
    c. otitis media
    d. meningitis
    e. all of the above

245. Herpes zoster infection involving the geniculate ganglion and external auditory canal and auricle is called:
    a. Boerhaave's syndrome
    b. zoster sine herpes
    c. zoster ophthalmicus dura
    d. zoster polio juvenalis
    e. none of the above

246. The ear receives innervation from the:
    a. facial nerve
    b. glossopharyngeal nerve
    c. auriculotemporal branch of the mandibular nerve
    d. superficial petrosal nerve
    e. all of the above

247. Nose pain is commonly caused by:
    a. infections including folliculitis
    b. foreign bodies
    c. malignancies
    d. all of the above
    e. none of the above

248. Midface pain may be caused by:
    a. sinusitis
    b. osteomyelitis of the facial bones
    c. squamous cell carcinomas
    d. nasopharyngiomas
    e. all of the above

249. Referred pain to the ear, midface, and throat can be caused by:
    a. tumors of the nasopharynx
    b. deep infections of the pharynx including retropharyngeal abscess
    c. dental infections
    d. Eagle's syndrome
    e. all of the above

250. The greater occipital nerve:
    a. arises from fibers of the dorsal primary ramus of the second cervical nerve
    b. arises, to a lesser extent, from fibers from the third cervical nerve
    c. pierces the fascia just below the superior nuchal ridge along with the occipital artery
    d. supplies the medial portion of the posterior scalp as far anterior as the vertex
    e. all of the above

251. The lesser occipital nerve:
    a. arises from the ventral primary rami of the second and third cervical nerves
    b. passes superiorly along the posterior border of the sternocleidomastoid muscle, dividing into cutaneous branches that innervate the lateral portion of the posterior scalp and the cranial surface of the pinna of the ear
    c. is relatively easy to block with local anesthetic and steroid
    d. all of the above
    e. none of the above

252. Cervical radiculopathy is best treated with a multi-modality approach including:
    a. physical therapy including heat modalities and deep sedative massage
    b. nonsteroidal anti-inflammatory agents
    c. skeletal muscle relaxants
    d. cervical steroid epidural nerve blocks with local anesthetic and steroid
    e. all of the above

253. Pain syndromes that may mimic cervical radiculopathy include:
    a. cervicalgia
    b. cervical bursitis and cervical fibromyositis
    c. inflammatory arthritis
    d. disorders of the cervical spinal cord, roots, plexus, and nerves
    e. all of the above

254. The causes of cervical radiculopathy include:
    a. herniated disc
    b. foraminal stenosis and osteophyte formation
    c. tumor
    d. infection
    e. all of the above

255. The patient suffering from cervical radiculopathy may experience:
    a. pain in a dermatomal distribution
    b. numbness
    c. weakness
    d. loss of reflexes
    e. all of the above

256. Patients will commonly place the hand of the affected extremity on the top of the head in order to obtain relief when suffering from compromise of which of the following cervical nerve roots?
    a. C5
    b. C6
    c. C7
    d. C8
    e. none of the above

257. The clinical hallmark of cervical strain is:
    a. neck pain
    b. pain in a dermatomal distribution
    c. myelopathy
    d. all of the above
    e. none of the above

258. The pain of cervical strain:
    a. often begins in the occipital region
    b. radiates in a nondermatomal pattern into the shoulders and intrascapular region

c. is often exacerbated by movement of the cervical spine and shoulders

d. is often accompanied by headaches and sleep disturbance

e. all of the above

259. Physical examination results of the patient suffering from cervical strain may include:
   a. tenderness on palpation of the paraspinous musculature and trapezius
   b. spasm of the paraspinous musculature and trapezius
   c. decreased range of motion of the cervical spine
   d. normal neurologic examination of the upper extremities
   e. all of the above

260. Cervical strain is best treated with a multimodality approach including:
   a. physical therapy with heat modalities and deep sedative massage
   b. nonsteroidal anti-inflammatory agents
   c. skeletal muscle relaxants
   d. cervical facet blocks with local anesthetic and steroid
   e. all of the above

261. The patient suffering from cervicothoracic bursitis will present with:
   a. the complaint of dull, poorly localized pain in the lower cervical and upper thoracic region
   b. nonradicular pain that spreads from the midline to the adjacent paraspinous area
   c. the patient holding the cervical spine rigid with the head thrust forward to splint the affected ligament and bursae
   d. pain that is exacerbated by flexion and extension of the lower cervical spine and upper thoracic spine
   e. all of the above

262. The pathognomonic lesion of fibromyalgia pain is the:
   a. goblet cell
   b. trigger point
   c. delta cell
   d. beta cell
   e. none of the above

263. Cervicothoracic bursitis is best treated with a multimodality approach including:
   a. physical therapy with heat modalities and deep sedative massage
   b. nonsteroidal anti-inflammatory agents
   c. skeletal muscle relaxants
   d. injection of the cervicothoracic bursae with local anesthetic and steroid
   e. all of the above

264. Fibromyalgia of the cervical spine is best treated with a multimodality approach including:
   a. techniques that will help eliminate the trigger point
   b. tricyclic antidepressant compounds
   c. trigger point injections
   d. all of the above
   e. none of the above

265. Each facet joint receives fibers from the:
   a. dorsal ramus at the same level as the vertebra
   b. ventral ramus at the same level as the vertebra
   c. dorsal ramus of the vertebra above
   d. a and b
   e. a and c

266. Cervical facet syndrome is a constellation of symptoms consisting of:
   a. neck, head, shoulder, and proximal upper extremity pain that radiates in a nondermatomal pattern
   b. pain that is dull and ill defined in character
   c. pain that may be unilateral or bilateral
   d. pain that is exacerbated by flexion, extension, and lateral bending of the cervical spine
   e. all of the above

267. Cervical facet syndrome is best treated with a multimodality approach including:
   a. physical therapy with heat modalities
   b. nonsteroidal anti-inflammatory agents
   c. skeletal muscle relaxants
   d. injection of the cervical facet joints with local anesthetic and steroid
   e. all of the above

268. Common causes of thoracic radiculopathy include:
   a. herniated disc
   b. foraminal stenosis and osteophyte formation
   c. tumor and infection
   d. vertebral compression fractures
   e. all of the above

269. The patient suffering from thoracic radiculopathy may experience:
   a. pain in a dermatomal distribution
   b. numbness and paresthesias
   c. weakness
   d. loss of superficial abdominal reflexes
   e. all of the above

270. Thoracic myelopathy is most commonly due to:
   a. midline herniated thoracic disc
   b. spinal stenosis
   c. demyelinating disease
   d. tumor or, rarely, infection
   e. all of the above

271. Intercostal neuralgia is best treated with a multimodality approach including:
   a. tricyclic antidepressant compounds
   b. nonsteroidal anti-inflammatory agents
   c. gabapentin
   d. injection of the intercostal nerves with local anesthetic and steroid
   e. all of the above

272. Physical examination of the patient suffering from costosternal syndrome will reveal that:
   a. the patient will vigorously attempt to splint the joints by keeping the shoulders stiffly in neutral position

b. pain is reproduced with active protraction or retraction of the shoulder, deep inspiration, as well as full elevation of the arm

c. the costosternal joints and adjacent intercostal muscles may be tender to palpation

d. the patient may also complain of a clicking sensation with movement of the joint

e. all of the above

273. Physical examination of the patient suffering from manubriosternal joint syndrome will reveal that:
a. the patient will vigorously attempt to splint the joints by keeping the shoulders stiffly in neutral position
b. pain is reproduced with active protraction or retraction of the shoulder, deep inspiration, and full elevation of the arm
c. the manubriosternal joint may feel hot and inflamed
d. shrugging of the shoulder may also reproduce the pain
e. all of the above

274. Symptoms associated with compression fractures of the thoracic vertebra include:
a. pain that is aggravated by deep inspiration, coughing, and any movement of the dorsal spine
b. pain and spasm of the paraspinous muscles elicited by palpation of the affected vertebra
c. hematoma and ecchymosis overlying the fracture site if trauma has occurred
d. abdominal ileus and severe pain with resulting splinting of the paraspinous muscles of the dorsal spine further compromising the patient's ability to walk and their pulmonary status
e. all of the above

275. Initial treatment of pain secondary to compression fracture of the thoracic spine should include:
a. combination of simple analgesics and the nonsteroidal anti-inflammatory drugs or opioids if the pain is uncontrolled
b. the local application of heat and cold, which may also be beneficial to provide symptomatic relief of the pain of vertebral compression fracture
c. the use of an orthotic, such as the CASH brace
d. thoracic epidural block using local anesthetic and steroid
e. all of the above

276. The patient suffering from lumbar radiculopathy will complain of:
a. pain, numbness, tingling, and paresthesias in the distribution of the affected nerve root or roots
b. weakness and lack of coordination in the affected extremity
c. muscle spasms and back pain as well as pain referred into the buttocks
d. reflex changes are demonstrated on physical examination and a reflex shifting of the trunk to one side called a list
e. all of the above

277. Lumbar radiculopathy is best treated with a multimodality approach including:
a. physical therapy with heat modalities
b. nonsteroidal anti-inflammatory agents
c. skeletal muscle relaxants
d. lumbar epidural or caudal injection of the affected nerve roots with local anesthetic and steroid
e. all of the above

278. Lumbar myelopathy is most commonly due to:
a. midline herniated lumbar disc
b. spinal stenosis
c. tumor or, rarely, infection
d. all of the above
e. none of the above

279. Patients suffering from lumbar myelopathy or cauda equina syndrome will experience:
a. varying degrees of lower extremity weakness
b. bowel symptomatology
c. bladder symptomatology
d. all of the above
e. none of the above

280. The patient suffering from coccydynia will exhibit:
a. point tenderness over the coccyx with the pain being increased with movement of the coccyx
b. movement of the coccyx may cause sharp paresthesias into the rectum
c. on rectal exam, the levator ani, piriformis, and coccygeus muscles may feel indurated and palpation of these muscles may induce severe spasm
d. sitting may exacerbate the pain of coccydynia, and the patient may attempt to sit on one buttock to avoid pressure on the coccyx
e. all of the above

281. The following pathologic conditions may mimic the pain of coccydynia:
a. primary pathology of the rectum and anus
b. primary tumors or metastatic lesions of the sacrum and/or coccyx
c. proctalgia fugax
d. insufficiency fractures of the pelvis and sacrum
e. all of the above

282. Proctalgia fugax can be distinguished from coccydynia in that patients suffering from proctalgia fugax will exhibit:
a. no increase in pain with movement of the coccyx
b. an increase in pain with movement of the coccyx
c. blood in stool
d. a and c
e. none of the above

283. Reflex sympathetic dystrophy is characterized by:
a. burning facial pain
b. sudomotor changes
c. vasomotor changes
d. trophic skin changes
e. all of the above

284. The clinical symptomatology of reflex sympathetic dystrophy of the face may often be confused with:
    a. pain of dental origin
    b. pain of sinus origin
    c. atypical facial pain
    d. trigeminal neuralgia
    e. all of the above

285. Characteristic symptoms of a typical post-dural puncture headache include:
    a. rapid onset of headache when the patient moves from the horizontal to the upright position
    b. constant holocranial headache when the patient is supine
    c. headache that abates when the patient resumes a horizontal position
    d. a and b
    e. a and c

286. Untreated post-dural puncture headache may result in:
    a. glossopharyngeal neuralgia
    b. persistent cranial nerve palsies
    c. increased serum potassium
    d. increased serum sodium
    e. none of the above

287. Medication treatment options for glossopharyngeal neuralgia include:
    a. carbamazepine
    b. baclofen
    c. gabapentin
    d. all of the above
    e. none of the above

288. Surgical treatment options for glossopharyngeal neuralgia include:
    a. glossopharyngeal nerve block
    b. radiofrequency lesioning of the glossopharyngeal nerve
    c. microvascular decompression of the trigeminal root
    d. all of the above
    e. none of the above

289. Varieties of spasmodic torticollis include:
    a. tonic spasmodic torticollis
    b. clonic spasmodic torticollis
    c. tonic/clonic spasmodic torticollis
    d. all of the above
    e. none of the above

290. Patients suffering from brachial plexopathy will complain of:
    a. pain radiating to the supraclavicular region and upper extremity
    b. neuritic pain that may take on a deep, boring quality with invasion of the plexus by tumor
    c. movement of the neck and shoulder that exacerbates the pain
    d. all of the above
    e. none of the above

291. Common causes of brachial plexopathy include:
    a. compression of the plexus by cervical ribs or abnormal muscles
    b. invasion of the plexus by tumor, e.g., Pancoast's syndrome
    c. direct trauma to the plexus, e.g., stretch injuries and avulsions
    d. inflammatory causes, e.g., Parsonage-Turner syndrome and postradiation plexopathy
    e. all of the above

292. Adson's maneuver is helpful in the diagnosis of thoracic outlet syndrome and is performed by:
    a. palpating the radial pulse on the affected side with the patient's neck extended and the head turned toward the affected side
    b. occluding both the ulnar and radial arteries at the wrist
    c. forcibly flexing the cervical spine
    d. active pronation of the affected extremity
    e. none of the above

293. Signs and symptoms of thoracic outlet syndrome include:
    a. paresthesias of the upper extremity radiating into the distribution of the ulnar nerve
    b. aching and incoordination of the affected extremity
    c. edema or discoloration of the arm
    d. in rare instances venous or arterial thrombosis
    e. all of the above

294. Provocation of the symptoms of thoracic outlet syndrome may be elicited by a variety of maneuvers including the:
    a. Adson test
    b. elevated arm stress test
    c. Allen test
    d. a and b
    e. a and c

295. Invasive treatments useful in the palliation of the pain associated with Pancoast's tumor include:
    a. brachial plexus block
    b. dorsal root entry zone lesioning
    c. radiofrequency lesioning of the brachial plexus
    d. cordotomy
    e. all of the above

296. Pharmacologic treatment useful in the palliation of the pain associated with Pancoast's tumor includes:
    a. gabapentin
    b. carbamazepine
    c. baclofen
    d. opioid analgesics
    e. all of the above

297. Patients suffering from Pancoast's tumor syndrome will complain of:
    a. neuritic pain radiating to the supraclavicular region and upper extremity.
    b. initial pain in the upper thoracic and lower cervical dermatomes as the lower portion of the brachial plexus is involved as the tumor grows from below

c. exacerbation of pain with movement of the neck and shoulder
d. Horner's syndrome in some patients
e. all of the above

298. Pancoast's tumor syndrome:
a. is the result of local growth of tumor from the apex of the lung directly into the brachial plexus
b. usually involves the first and second thoracic nerves as well as the eighth cervical nerve producing a classic clinical syndrome consisting of severe arm pain and, in some patients, Horner's syndrome
c. often results in destruction of the first and second ribs
d. all of the above
e. none of the above

299. Tennis elbow is also known as:
a. medial epicondylitis
b. lateral epicondylitis
c. radial tunnel syndrome
d. pronator syndrome
e. none of the above

300. Which of the following painful conditions may be misdiagnosed as tennis elbow?
a. radial tunnel syndrome
b. pronator syndrome
c. C6-7 radiculopathy
d. a and b
e. a and c

301. Treatments effective in the management of tennis elbow include:
a. nonsteroidal anti-inflammatory agents
b. local application of heat and cold
c. physical therapy
d. injection of the lateral epicondyle with local anesthetic and steroid
e. all of the above

302. Patients suffering from tennis elbow will complain of:
a. pain that is localized to the region of the lateral epicondyle
b. pain that is constant and is made worse with active contraction of the wrist
c. the inability to hold a coffee cup or hammer with weakened grip strength
d. pain when undergoing a tennis elbow test
e. all of the above

303. Golfer's elbow is also known as:
a. medial epicondylitis
b. lateral epicondylitis
c. radial tunnel syndrome
d. pronator syndrome
e. none of the above

304. Which of the following painful conditions can be misdiagnosed as golfer's elbow?
a. radial tunnel syndrome
b. gout, arthritis, and bursitis
c. C6-7 radiculopathy

d. a and b
e. b and c

305. Treatments effective in the management of golfer's elbow include:
a. nonsteroidal anti-inflammatory agents
b. local application of heat and cold
c. physical therapy
d. injection of the medial epicondyle with local anesthetic and steroid
e. all of the above

306. Patients suffering from golfer's elbow will complain of:
a. pain that is localized to the region of the medial epicondyle
b. pain that is constant and is made worse with active contraction of the wrist
c. the inability to hold a coffee cup or hammer with weakened grip strength
d. pain when undergoing a Golfer's elbow test
e. all of the above

307. In radial tunnel syndrome, the:
a. posterior interosseous branch of the radial nerve is entrapped
b. anterior interosseous branch of the radial nerve is entrapped
c. lateral interosseous branch of the radial nerve is entrapped
d. medial interosseous branch of the radial nerve is entrapped
e. none of the above

308. Mechanisms implicated in the compression of the radial nerve in radial tunnel syndrome include:
a. aberrant fibrous bands in front of the radial head
b. anomalous blood vessels that compress the nerve
c. a sharp tendinous margin of the extensor carpi radialis brevis
d. all of the above
e. none of the above

309. Clinical features of radial tunnel syndrome include:
a. aching lateral elbow pain
b. pain that is localized to the deep extensor muscle mass
c. pain that may radiate proximally and distally into the upper arm and forearm
d. all of the above
e. none of the above

310. Which of the following painful conditions can be misdiagnosed as radial tunnel syndrome?
a. tennis elbow
b. pronator syndrome
c. C5-6 radiculopathy
d. a and b
e. a and c

311. Ulnar nerve entrapment at the elbow is also called:
a. tardy ulnar palsy
b. cubital tunnel syndrome
c. ulnar nerve neuritis.

d. all of the above

e. none of the above

312. Physical findings of ulnar nerve entrapment at the elbow may include:
    a. tenderness over the ulnar nerve at the elbow
    b. positive Tinel's sign over the ulnar nerve as it passes beneath the aponeuroses
    c. weakness of the intrinsic muscles of the forearm and hand that are innervated by the ulnar nerve
    d. loss of sensation on the ulnar side of the little finger
    e. all of the above

313. The pain and muscle weakness of anterior interosseous syndrome can be caused by:
    a. median nerve compression of the nerve just below the elbow by the tendinous origins of the pronator teres muscle and flexor digitorum superficialis muscle of the long finger
    b. aberrant blood vessels
    c. inflammatory causes
    d. all of the above
    e. none of the above

314. Clinically, anterior interosseous syndrome presents as:
    a. acute pain in the proximal forearm and deep in the wrist
    b. heavy sensation in the forearm with minimal activity
    c. inability to pinch items between the thumb and index finger due to paralysis of the flexor pollicis longis and the flexor digitorum profundus
    d. all of the above
    e. none of the above

315. The following statement(s) regarding olecranon bursitis is (are) *true*.
    a. Olecranon bursitis may develop gradually due to repetitive irritation of the olecranon bursa or acutely due to trauma or infection.
    b. The olecranon bursa lies in the posterior aspect of the elbow between the olecranon process of the ulna and the overlying skin.
    c. The olecranon bursa may exist as a single bursal sac or, in some patients, as a multisegmented series of sacs that may be loculated in nature.
    d. With overuse or misuse, these bursae may become inflamed, enlarged, and, on rare occasions, infected.
    e. all of the above

316. The following statement(s) regarding olecranon bursitis is(are) *true*.
    a. The patient suffering from olecranon bursitis will frequently complain of pain and swelling with any movement of the elbow, but especially with extension.
    b. The pain of olecranon bursitis is localized to the olecranon area with referred pain often noted above the elbow joint.
    c. Physical examination will reveal point tenderness over the olecranon and swelling of the bursa, which at times can be quite extensive.

d. Passive extension and resisted flexion shoulder will reproduce the pain, as will any pressure over the bursa.

e. all of the above

317. Carpal tunnel syndrome is the most common entrapment neuropathy encountered in clinical practice and is caused by compression of the:
    a. median nerve as it passes through the carpal canal at the wrist
    b. radial nerve as it passes through the carpal canal at the wrist
    c. ulnar nerve as it passes through the carpal canal at the wrist
    d. median nerve as it passes through the Vesuvian canal at the wrist
    e. none of the above

318. The most common causes of carpal tunnel syndrome include:
    a. flexor tenosynovitis
    b. rheumatoid arthritis
    c. pregnancy
    d. amyloidosis and other space-occupying lesions that compromise the median nerve as it passes though this closed space
    e. all of the above

319. Carpal tunnel syndrome presents as:
    a. pain, numbness, paresthesias, and associated weakness in the hand and wrist
    b. pain, numbness, paresthesias, and associated weakness that radiates to the thumb, index, middle, and radial half of the ring fingers
    c. pain, numbness, and paresthesias that radiate proximal to the entrapment into the forearm
    d. all of the above
    e. none of the above

320. Signs and symptoms of carpal tunnel syndrome include:
    a. a positive Tinel's sign over the median nerve at the wrist
    b. a positive Phalen's sign
    c. weakness of thumb opposition
    d. wasting of the thenar eminence
    e. all of the above

321. Cheiralgia paresthetica is caused by compression of the:
    a. sensory branch of the radial nerve at the wrist
    b. sensory branch of the median nerve at the wrist
    c. sensory branch of the ulnar nerve at the wrist
    d. motor branch of the radial nerve at the wrist
    e. none of the above

322. de Quervain's tenosynovitis is caused by an:
    a. inflammation and swelling of the tendons of the adductor pollicis longus and flexor pollicis longus at the level of the radial styloid process
    b. inflammation and swelling of the tendons of the abductor pollicis longus and extensor pollicis brevis at the level of the radial styloid process

c. inflammation and swelling of the tendons of the abductor pollicis brevis and extensor pollicis longus at the level of the radial styloid process

d. all of the above

e. none of the above

323. Signs and symptoms associated with Dupuytren's contracture include:

a. hard fibrotic nodules along the path of the flexor tendons

b. taut fibrous bands that may cross the metacarpophalangeal joint and ultimately the proximal interphalangeal joint

c. limitation of finger extension

d. relatively normal finger flexion

e. all of the above

324. Dupuytren's contracture:

a. is thought to have a genetic basis

b. occurs most frequently in males of northern Scandinavian descent

c. may be associated with trauma to the palm

d. may be associated with diabetes, alcoholism, and chronic barbiturate use

e. all of the above

325. The nonsurgical treatment of the pain and functional disability associated with Dupuytren's contracture should include:

a. nonsteroidal anti-inflammatory drugs

b. the use of physical modalities including local heat as well as gentle range-of-motion exercises

c. a nighttime splint to protect the fingers, which may help relieve symptoms

d. injection of Dupuytren's contracture with local anesthetic and steroid, which may also be effective in the management of the symptoms associated with Dupuytren's contracture

e. all of the above

326. Disorders that may mimic the symptoms of diabetic truncal neuropathies include:

a. Hansen's disease

b. Lyme disease

c. HIV

d. toxic neuropathies

e. all of the above

327. Disorders that may mimic the symptoms of diabetic truncal neuropathies include:

a. heavy metal poisoning

b. neuropathy secondary to chemotherapy

c. heritable neuropathies including Charcot-Marie-Tooth disease

d. vitamin deficiencies

e. all of the above

328. Disorders that may mimic the symptoms of diabetic truncal neuropathies include:

a. sarcoidosis

b. amyloidosis

c. intercostal neuralgia

d. intra-abdominal and intrathoracic pathology

e. all of the above

329. Medical treatment of diabetic truncal neuropathy should include:

a. anticonvulsants

b. antidepressants

c. antiarrhythmics

d. tight control of blood sugars

e. all of the above

330. Topical agents shown to be useful in the palliation of pain secondary to the pain of diabetic truncal neuropathy include:

a. capsaicin

b. topical lidocaine creme

c. lidocaine transdermal patch

d. all of the above

e. none of the above

331. Signs and symptoms associated with Tietze's syndrome include:

a. tenderness and swelling of the second and third costosternal joints

b. tenderness of intercostal muscles adjacent to the second and third costosternal joints

c. increased pain with retraction of the shoulders

d. a clicking sensation with movement of the affected costosternal joints

e. all of the above

332. Treatment of the pain and functional disability associated with Tietze's syndrome should include:

a. nonsteroidal anti-inflammatory drugs

b. the local application of heat and cold

c. the use of an elastic rib belt

d. injection of the costosternal joints using local anesthetic and steroid

e. all of the above

333. Causes of post-thoracotomy syndrome include:

a. direct surgical trauma to the intercostal nerves and/or cutaneous neuroma formation

b. fractured ribs due to the rib spreader

c. compressive neuropathy of the intercostal nerves due to direct compression to the intercostal nerves by retractors

d. stretch injuries to the intercostal nerves at the costovertebral junction

e. all of the above

334. Treatment of post-thoracotomy syndrome includes:

a. nonsteroidal anti-inflammatory agents and simple analgesics

b. anticonvulsants and antidepressant compounds

c. application of local heat and cold

d. injection of the structures causing the pain with local anesthetic and steroid

e. all of the above

335. Treatment of post-mastectomy syndrome includes:

a. nonsteroidal anti-inflammatory agents and simple analgesics

b. anticonvulsants and antidepressant compounds

c. application of local heat and cold

d. injection of the intercostal nerves and/or thoracic epidural nerves with local anesthetic and steroid

e. all of the above

336. The following statement(s) regarding herpes zoster is (are) *true*.

a. Herpes zoster is an infectious disease that is caused by the varicella-zoster virus.

b. The thoracic nerve roots are the most common site for the development of acute herpes zoster.

c. Primary infection with the varicella-zoster virus in the nonimmune host manifests itself clinically as chickenpox.

d. During the course of primary infection with varicella-zoster virus, the virus migrates to the dorsal root of the thoracic nerves where it remains dormant.

e. all of the above

337. Patients with the following diseases are more likely than the general population to develop acute herpes zoster:

a. patients with lymphoma

b. patients on steroids

c. patients undergoing chemotherapy or receiving immunosuppressive drugs

d. patients undergoing radiation therapy

e. all of the above

338. The initial treatment of acute herpes zoster should include:

a. sympathetic nerve blocks

b. antiviral agents

c. opioid analgesics

d. adjuvant analgesics including gabapentin and antidepressant compounds

e. all of the above

339. The initial treatment of postherpetic neuralgia should include:

a. sympathetic and somatic nerve blocks

b. gabapentin

c. opioid analgesics

d. adjuvant analgesics including antidepressants and antidepressant compounds

e. all of the above

340. The initial evaluation of epidural abscess should include:

a. stat blood and urine cultures

b. immediate CT and/or MRI

c. myelography if CT or MRI is equivocal or unavailable

d. all of the above

e. none of the above

341. Spondylolisthesis:

a. is a degenerative disease of the lumbar spine

b. occurs more commonly in women

c. is most often seen after the age of 40

d. is caused by the slippage of one vertebral body onto another due to degeneration of the facet joints and intervertebral disc

e. all of the above

342. In spondylolisthesis:

a. the upper vertebral body moves anteriorly relative to the vertebral body below it

b. the slippage of one vertebra onto another usually causes narrowing of the spinal canal

c. there is often a relative spinal stenosis and back pain

d. occasionally, the upper vertebral body slides posteriorly relative to the vertebral body below it, which compromises the neural foramina

e. all of the above

343. Ankylosing spondylitis is also known as:

a. Osgood-Schlatter disease

b. Marie-Strümpell disease

c. Osgood-Weber-Rendu disease

d. Dubin-Johnson-Sprint disease

e. none of the above

344. Ankylosing spondylitis:

a. is associated with an approximately 90% presence of histocompatibility antigen HLA-B27 compared with 7% of the general population

b. occurs three times more frequently in men

c. symptoms usually appear by the third decade of life

d. rarely has its onset beyond 40 years of age

e. all of the above

345. Ankylosing spondylitis is best treated with a multimodality approach including:

a. physical therapy including exercises to maintain function, heat modalities, and deep sedative massage

b. nonsteroidal anti-inflammatory agents and skeletal muscle relaxants

c. sulfasalazine

d. the addition of caudal or lumbar epidural blocks with a local anesthetic and steroid

e. all of the above

346. Acute pancreatitis is characterized by:

a. mild to severe abdominal pain

b. steady, boring epigastric pain that radiates to the flanks and chest

c. pain that is worse with the supine position

d. nausea, vomiting, and anorexia

e. all of the above

347. The patient with acute pancreatitis will exhibit the following signs and symptoms:

a. tachycardia and hypotension due to hypovolemia and low-grade fever

b. saponification of subcutaneous fat

c. pulmonary complications including pleural effusions and pleuritic pain that may compromise respiration

d. diffuse abdominal tenderness with peritoneal signs are invariably present

e. all of the above

348. Findings of hemorrhagic pancreatitis include:

a. periumbilical ecchymosis (Cullen's sign)

b. flank ecchymosis (Turner's sign)

c. absent startle reflex

d. a and b
e. a and c

349. The abnormal laboratory finding that is the *sine qua non* of acute pancreatitis is:
   a. elevated SGOT
   b. lowered SGOT
   c. elevated serum amylase
   d. elevated serum calcium
   e. none of the above

350. Common causes of acute pancreatitis include:
   a. alcohol
   b. gallstones
   c. viral infections
   d. medications
   e. all of the above

351. Common causes of acute pancreatitis include:
   a. metabolic causes
   b. connective tissue diseases
   c. obstruction of the ampulla of Vater by tumor
   d. heredity
   e. all of the above

352. Chronic pancreatitis is commonly caused by:
   a. alcohol
   b. cystic fibrosis
   c. pancreatic malignancies
   d. hereditary causes such as alpha$_1$-antitrypsin deficiency
   e. all of the above

353. Which of the following can mimic the signs and symptoms of ilioinguinal neuralgia?
   a. lesions of the lumbar plexus
   b. tumors involving the lumbar plexus
   c. diabetic neuropathy
   d. inflammation of the ilioinguinal nerve
   e. all of the above

354. Signs and symptoms associated with ilioinguinal neuralgia include:
   a. paresthesias, burning pain, and occasionally numbness over the lower abdomen that radiates into the scrotum or labia and occasionally into the inner upper thigh
   b. pain that does not radiate below the knee
   c. pain that is made worse by extension of the lumbar spine
   d. a bent-forward "novice skier's" position
   e. all of the above

355. Physical findings of genitofemoral neuralgia include:
   a. sensory deficit in the inner thigh, base of the scrotum, or labia majora in the distribution of the genitofemoral nerve
   b. weakness of the anterior abdominal wall musculature
   c. Tinel's sign that may be elicited by tapping over the genitofemoral nerve at the point it passes beneath the inguinal ligament
   d. a bent-forward "novice skier's" position
   d. all of the above

356. Meralgia paresthetica is caused by compression of the:
   a. lateral femoral cutaneous nerve
   b. femoral nerve
   c. sciatic nerve
   d. iliohypogastric nerve
   e. none of the above

357. Signs and symptoms associated with meralgia paresthetica include:
   a. tenderness over the lateral femoral cutaneous nerve at the origin of the inguinal ligament at the anterior superior iliac spine
   b. a positive Tinel's sign over the lateral femoral cutaneous nerve as it passes beneath the inguinal ligament
   c. a sensory deficit in the distribution of the lateral femoral cutaneous nerve
   d. all of the above
   e. none of the above

358. The pain of spinal stenosis usually presents in a characteristic manner as pain and weakness in the legs and calves when walking that is known as:
   a. pseudoclaudication
   b. neurogenic claudication
   c. vascular claudication
   d. a and b
   e. none of the above

359. The patient suffering from spinal stenosis:
   a. will complain of calf and leg pain and fatigue with walking, standing, or lying supine
   b. will note that the calf and leg pain and fatigue will disappear if the patient flexes the lumbar spine or assumes the sitting position
   c. will note that extension of the spine may also cause and increase the symptoms
   d. may experience weakness and reflex changes in the affected dermatomes
   e. all of the above

360. Occasionally, patients suffering from spinal stenosis may suffer from myelopathy or cauda equina syndrome. In this setting, the:
   a. onset of symptoms may be insidious
   b. patient may experience bladder symptomatology
   c. patient may experience bowel sympatomatology
   d. findings of myelopathy or cauda equina syndrome should be considered a neurosurgical emergency
   e. all of the above

361. Pain syndromes that may mimic spinal stenosis include:
   a. low back strain
   b. lumbar bursitis and lumbar fibromyositis
   c. inflammatory arthritis of the lumbosacral spine
   d. disorders of the lumbar spinal cord, roots, plexus, and nerves including diabetic femoral neuropathy
   e. all of the above

362. Pain syndromes that may mimic arachnoiditis include:
   a. tumors of the spinal cord
   b. infection involving the meninges or contents of the spinal canal

c. disorders of the lumbar spinal cord and nerve roots
d. disorders of the cervical or lumbar plexi
e. all of the above

363. Patients suffering from arachnoiditis will complain of:
a. pain in the distribution of the affected nerve root or roots
b. numbness, tingling, and paresthesias in the distribution of the affected nerve root or roots
c. weakness and lack of coordination in the affected extremity/extremities
d. reflex changes
e. all of the above

364. Common extrascrotal causes of chronic orchialgia include:
a. ureteral calculi
b. inguinal hernia
c. ilioinguinal and genitofemoral nerve entrapment
d. diseases of the lumbar spine and roots
e. all of the above

365. Common intrascrotal causes of chronic orchialgia include:
a. tumor
b. chronic epididymitis
c. hydrocele
d. varicocele
e. all of the above

366. Common extravulva pathologic processes that can mimic vulvadynia include:
a. malignancy involving the pelvic contents other than the vulva
b. tumors involving the lumbar plexus, cauda equina, and/or the hypogastric plexus
c. ilioinguinal and genitofemoral neuralgia
d. postradiation neuropathy
e. all of the above

367. Treatment of vulvadynia should include:
a. nonsteroidal anti-inflammatory agents
b. antidepressant compounds
c. empiric treatment of occult urinary tract and yeast infections
d. psychological evaluations
e. all of the above

368. Diseases that may mimic proctalgia fugax include:
a. proctitis
b. inflammatory bowel disease
c. prostatitis and prostadynia
d. hemorrhoids
e. all of the above

369. Proctalgia fugax is:
a. a disease of unknown etiology
b. characterized by paroxysms of rectal pain with pain-free periods between attacks
c. characterized, like cluster headache, by spontaneous remissions of the disease that may last weeks to years
d. more common in females
e. all of the above

370. The signs and symptoms of osteitis pubis include:
a. localized tenderness over the symphysis pubis
b. pain radiating into the inner thigh
c. waddling gait
d. characteristic radiographic changes consisting of erosion, sclerosis, and widening of the symphysis pubis
e. all of the above

371. Osteitis pubis:
a. occurs more commonly in females
b. is a disease of the second to fourth decade
c. most commonly follows bladder, inguinal, or prostate surgery and is thought to be due to hematogenous spread of infection to the relatively avascular symphysis pubis
d. can appear without an obvious inciting factor or infection
e. all of the above

372. Piriformis syndrome is caused by compression of the:
a. sciatic nerve by the piriformis muscle
b. piriformis nerve by the piriformis muscle
c. common peroneal nerve by the piriformis muscle
d. tibial nerve by the piriformis muscle
e. none of the above

373. Physical findings of piriformis syndrome include:
a. tenderness over the sciatic notch
b. positive Tinel's sign over the sciatic nerve as it passes beneath the piriformis muscle
c. tender and swollen, indurated piriformis muscle belly
d. weakness of affected gluteal muscles and lower extremity and ultimately muscle wasting
e. all of the above

374. Initial treatment of the pain and functional disability associated with piriformis syndrome should include:
a. a combination of nonsteroidal anti-inflammatory drugs and physical therapy
b. the local application of heat and cold, which may also be beneficial
c. avoidance of any repetitive activity that may exacerbate the patient's symptomatology
d. injection with local anesthetic and steroid in the region of the sciatic nerve at the level of the piriformis muscle
e. all of the above

375. Common causes of arthritis of the hip include:
a. osteoarthritis
b. rheumatoid arthritis
c. post-traumatic arthritis
d. all of the above
e. none of the above

376. Less common causes of arthritis of the hip include:
a. villonodular synovitis
b. collagen vascular diseases
c. Lyme disease
d. infections
e. all of the above

377. Arthritis of the hip should be treated with a multimodality approach including:
    a. nonsteroidal anti-inflammatory drugs
    b. physical therapy
    c. the local application of heat and cold
    d. intra-articular injection of local anesthetic and steroid
    e. all of the above

378. Femoral neuropathy may be due to compression of the femoral nerve by a(n):
    a. tumor
    b. retroperitoneal hemorrhage
    c. abscess
    d. all of the above
    e. none of the above

379. Other causes of femoral neuropathy include:
    a. stretch injuries to the femoral nerve as it passes under the inguinal ligament from extreme extension or flexion at the hip
    b. direct trauma to the nerve from surgery or during cardiac catheterization
    c. diabetes
    d. all of the above
    e. none of the above

380. Treatment of phantom limb pain should include:
    a. nerve blocks
    b. adjuvant analgesics including anticonvulsants
    c. adjuvant analgesics including antidepressants
    d. application of ice packs and/or transcutaneous stimulation
    e. all of the above

381. The patient suffering from trochanteric bursitis:
    a. will frequently complain of pain in the lateral hip that can radiate down the leg mimicking sciatica
    b. will complain of pain that is localized to the area over the greater trochanter
    c. will frequently complain of sleep disturbance
    d. may complain of a sharp, catching sensation with range of motion of the hip, especially on first arising
    e. all of the above

382. The treatment of trochanteric bursitis should include:
    a. nonsteroidal anti-inflammatory drugs
    b. physical therapy
    c. the local application of heat and cold
    d. injection of local anesthetic and steroid around the trochanteric bursa
    e. all of the above

383. Common causes of arthritis of the knee include:
    a. osteoarthritis
    b. rheumatoid arthritis
    c. post-traumatic arthritis
    d. all of the above
    e. none of the above

384. Less common causes of arthritis of the knee include:
    a. villonodular synovitis
    b. collagen vascular diseases
    c. Lyme disease
    d. infections
    e. all of the above

385. Arthritis of the knee should be treated with a multimodal approach including:
    a. nonsteroidal anti-inflammatory drugs
    b. physical therapy
    c. the local application of heat and cold
    d. intra-articular injection of local anesthetic and steroid
    e. all of the above

386. On physical examination, the patient suffering from Baker's cyst:
    a. will have a cystic swelling in the medial aspect of the popliteal fossa (Baker's cysts can become quite large)
    b. will experience an increase in symptoms when squatting or walking
    c. will experience pain that is constant and characterized as aching in nature
    d. may experience a spontaneous rupture and there may be rubor and color in the calf that may mimic thrombophlebitis
    e. all of the above

387. The incidence of Baker's cyst is greater in patients suffering from:
    a. thyrotoxicosis
    b. rheumatoid arthritis
    c. prepatellar bursitis
    d. all of the above
    e. none of the above

388. The bursae of the knee are vulnerable to:
    a. injury from both acute trauma and repeated microtrauma
    b. may exist as single bursal sacs or as a multisegmented series of loculated sacs
    c. acute injuries in the form of direct trauma to the bursa via falls or blows directly to the knee or from patellar, tibial plateau, and proximal fibular trauma
    d. calcification process in chronic inflammatory disease
    e. all of the above

389. The patient suffering from suprapatellar bursitis will frequently complain of:
    a. pain in the anterior knee above the patella
    b. pain that can radiate superiorly into the distal anterior thigh
    c. the inability to kneel or walk down stairs
    d. a sharp, catching sensation with range of motion of the knee, especially on first arising
    e. all of the above

390. Prepatellar bursitis is also known as:
    a. housemaid's knee
    b. Marie-Strümpell disease
    c. a joint mouse
    d. Dubin-Johnson-Sprint disease
    e. none of the above

391. Treatment of bursitis of the knee should include:
    a. nonsteroidal anti-inflammatory drugs
    b. physical therapy

c. the local application of heat and cold

d. injection of the inflamed bursa with local anesthetic and steroid

e. all of the above

392. Patients with pes anserine bursitis:
a. will present with pain over the medial knee joint
b. have increased pain on passive valgus and external rotation of the knee
c. will complain that activity, especially involving flexion and external rotation of the knee will make the pain worse
d. will note that rest and heat provide some relief
e. all of the above

393. Anterior tarsal tunnel syndrome presents with:
a. pain, numbness, and paresthesias of the dorsum of the foot
b. pain that radiates into the first dorsal web space
c. pain that may also radiate proximal to the entrapment into the anterior ankle
d. nighttime foot pain analogous to the nocturnal pain of carpal tunnel syndrome
e. all of the above

394. Anterior tarsal tunnel syndrome is caused by compression of the:
a. deep peroneal nerve as it passes beneath the superficial fascia of the ankle
b. tibial nerve as it passes beneath the superficial fascia of the ankle
c. superficial peroneal nerve as it passes beneath the superficial fascia of the ankle
d. sural nerve as it passes beneath the superficial fascia of the ankle
e. none of the above

395. Common causes of anterior tarsal tunnel syndrome include:
a. direct trauma to the deep peroneal nerve as it passes beneath the superficial fascia of the ankle
b. severe, acute plantar flexion of the ankle
c. the wearing of overly tight shoes
d. squatting and bending forward
e. all of the above

396. Posterior tarsal tunnel syndrome presents with:
a. pain, numbness, and paresthesias of the sole of the foot
b. weakness of the toe flexors and instability of the foot due to weakness of the lumbrical muscles
c. nighttime foot pain analogous to the nocturnal pain of carpal tunnel syndrome
d. all of the above
e. none of the above

397. Posterior tarsal tunnel syndrome is caused by compression of the:
a. deep peroneal nerve as it passes beneath the superficial fascia of the ankle
b. posterior tibial nerve as it passes through the posterior tarsal tunnel
c. superficial peroneal nerve as it passes beneath the superficial fascia of the ankle

d. sural nerve as it passes beneath the superficial fascia of the ankle
e. none of the above

398. Common causes of posterior tarsal tunnel syndrome include:
a. direct trauma to the posterior nerve as it passes through the posterior tarsal tunnel
b. thrombophlebitis involving the posterior tibial artery
c. rheumatoid arthritis
d. all of the above
e. none of the above

399. Treatment of Achilles tendinitis should include:
a. nonsteroidal anti-inflammatory agents
b. injection of the tendon with local anesthetic and steroid
c. use of heat and cold
d. avoidance of repetitive activities responsible for the evolution of the tendinitis
e. all of the above

400. Causes of Achilles tendinitis include:
a. overuse or misuse of the ankle
b. activities with sudden stopping and starting
c. improper stretching of the tendon
d. all of the above
e. none of the above

401. The signs and symptoms associated with Achilles tendonitis include:
a. pain in the posterior ankle
b. sleep disturbance
c. creaking or catching with movement of the tendon
d. pain with resisted plantar flexion of the foot
e. all of the above

402. The signs and symptoms of metarsalgia include:
a. pain that can be reproduced by pressure on the metatarsal heads
b. callus formation over the heads of the second and third metatarsal heads
c. an antalgic gait
d. ligamentous laxity and flattening of the transverse arch giving the foot a splayed-out appearance
e. all of the above

403. Other pathologic processes that may mimic metatarsalgia include:
a. gout
b. occult fractures of the metatarsals
c. tumors of the metatarsals
d. sesamoiditis
e. all of the above

404. The signs and symptoms of plantar fasciitis include:
a. foot pain that is most severe upon first walking after non–weight bearing
b. pain that is made worse by prolonged standing or walking
c. point tenderness over the plantar medial calcaneal tuberosity

d. pain that is increased by dorsiflexing the toes, which pulls the plantar fascia taut, and then palpating along the fascia from the heel to the forefoot

e. all of the above

405. Plantar fasciitis:
   a. is characterized by pain and tenderness over the plantar surface of the calcaneus
   b. occurs twice as commonly in women
   c. can be part of a systemic inflammatory condition such as rheumatoid arthritis, Reiter's syndrome, or gout
   d. can be associated with obesity and/or going barefoot or wearing house shoes
   e. all of the above

406. Treatment of plantar fasciitis should include:
   a. nonsteroidal anti-inflammatory drugs
   b. wearing shoes that provide good support
   c. the local application of heat and cold
   d. injection of the inflamed fascia with local anesthetic and steroid
   e. all of the above

407. Complex regional pain syndrome (CRPS):
   a. is divided into two types: CRPS I and CRPS II
   b. occurs more commonly in females
   c. has a peak occurrence in the fourth and fifth decades
   d. all of the above
   e. none of the above

408. Both CRPS type I and type II share a unique constellation of signs and symptoms including:
   a. allodynia and hyperalgesia
   b. spontaneous pain hyperalgesia
   c. autonomic dysfunction including sudomotor and vasomotor changes
   d. edema and trophic changes
   e. all of the above

409. Treatments useful in the management of CRPS include:
   a. sympathetic nerve blocks
   b. spinal cord stimulation
   c. gabapentin
   d. antidepressants
   e. all of the above

410. Abnormalities on three-phase radionuclide bone scanning include:
   a. a homogeneous unilateral hyperperfusion in the affected body part at 30 seconds post-injection during the perfusion phase
   b. a homogeneous unilateral hyperperfusion in the affected body part at 2 minutes during the blood pool phase
   c. most often unilateral periarticular isotope uptake during the mineralization phase that is scanned at 3 hours post-injection
   d. all of the above
   e. none of the above

411. Rheumatoid arthritis:
   a. is the most common of the connective tissue diseases
   b. has a cause that is unknown

c. can occur at any age, with the juvenile variant termed Still's disease
   d. affects women 2.5 times more often than men
   e. all of the above

412. The first symptoms of rheumatoid arthritis include:
   a. easy fatigability
   b. malaise
   c. myalgias
   d. anorexia and generalized weakness
   e. all of the above

413. Other early symptoms of rheumatoid arthritis include:
   a. ill-defined morning stiffness
   b. symmetrical joint pain with color
   c. tenosynovitis
   d. fusiform joint effusions
   e. all of the above

414. The most common joints affected in patients suffering from rheumatoid arthritis include the:
   a. wrists
   b. knees
   c. fingers
   d. bones of the feet
   e. all of the above

415. The classic joint deformity associated with rheumatoid arthritis is:
   a. ulnar drift
   b. radial drift
   c. gibbus formation
   d. Legg-Perthes deformity
   e. none of the above

416. Extra-articular manifestations associated with rheumatoid arthritis include:
   a. carpal tunnel syndrome
   b. Baker's cysts
   c. uveitis and iritis
   d. rheumatoid nodules
   e. all of the above

417. Treatment of rheumatoid arthritis should include:
   a. nonsteroidal anti-inflammatory agents
   b. corticosteroids
   c. nighttime splinting
   d. joint protection
   e. all of the above

418. Disease-modifying drugs that are useful in the treatment of rheumatoid arthritis include:
   a. methotrexate
   b. gold
   c. penicillamine
   d. sulfasalazine
   e. all of the above

419. Laboratory findings commonly seen in patients suffering from rheumatoid arthritis include a(n):
   a. normocytic normochromic anemia
   b. elevated erythrocyte sedimentation rate
   c. elevated RF agglutination factor

d. elevated C-reactive protein
e. all of the above

420. The signs and symptoms of systemic lupus erythematosus include:
   a. polyarthritis
   b. butterfly rash
   c. focal alopecia
   d. mouth ulcers
   e. all of the above

421. Common extra-articular manifestations of systemic lupus erythematosus include:
   a. vasculitis
   b. pleuritis and pneumonitis
   c. myocarditis, endocarditis, and pericarditis
   d. glomerulonephritis and hepatitis
   e. all of the above

422. Hematologic side effects of systemic lupus erythematosus include
   a. pancytopenia
   b. thrombocytopenia
   c. leukopenia
   d. hypercoagulable state
   e. all of the above

423. The laboratory test that is highly diagnostic for systemic lupus erythematosus is:
   a. highly elevated C-reactive protein
   b. presence of high levels of antinuclear antibody
   c. inversion of the SGOT/SGPT ratio
   d. all of the above
   e. none of the above

424. Scleroderma–systemic sclerosis is a disease of unknown etiology that is characterized by:
   a. diffuse fibrosis of the skin and connective tissue
   b. vascular damage
   c. arthritis
   d. abnormalities of the esophagus, gastrointestinal tract, kidneys, heart, and lungs
   e. all of the above

425. Facts about scleroderma–systemic sclerosis include that:
   a. the severity and course of the disease varies widely from patient to patient
   b. scleroderma is 4 times more common in women than in men
   c. its onset is rare before the age of 30 or after the age of 50
   d. exposure to contaminated cooking oils, polyvinyl chloride, and silica has also been implicated as a risk factor for the development of scleroderma
   e. all of the above

426. The initial complaints of patients suffering from scleroderma include:
   a. pain or deformity associated with swelling and loss of range of motion of the digits (sclerodactyly)
   b. associated Raynaud's phenomenon
   c. polyarthralgias and dysphagia

d. cutaneous fibrosis
e. all of the above

427. CREST syndrome, a variant of scleroderma–systemic sclerosis, is characterized by:
   a. calcinosis
   b. Raynaud's phenomenon
   c. esophageal dysfunction
   d. sclerodactyly and telangiectasia
   e. all of the above

428. Facts about polymyositis include:
   a. polymyositis is less common than rheumatoid arthritis, systemic lupus erythematosus, or scleroderma
   b. the disease is characterized by muscle inflammation that progresses to degenerative muscle disease and atrophy
   c. there are many variants of polymyositis, including dermatomyositis, which is, from a clinical viewpoint, simply polymyositis with significant cutaneous manifestations
   d. polymyositis affects women twice as frequently as men
   e. all of the above

429. Polymyositis is associated with an increased incidence of:
   a. occult malignancy
   b. childhood febrile exanthema
   c. exposure to mercury-containing vaccines in childhood
   d. all of the above
   e. none of the above

430. Signs and symptoms associated with the onset of polymyositis include:
   a. rash
   b. muscle weakness, which is generally the presenting symptom with the proximal muscle groups generally affected initially more commonly that the distal muscle groups
   c. myalgias and polyarthralgias
   d. febrile illness resembling a viral infection
   e. all of the above

431. The following sign is pathognomonic for dermatomyositis:
   a. Schacher's lines
   b. butterfly rash
   c. heliotrope periorbital blush
   d. Cullen's sign
   e. none of the above

432. Immunosuppressive drugs useful in treatment of polymyositis include:
   a. methotrexate
   b. cyclosporine
   c. azathioprine
   d. cyclophosphamide
   e. all of the above

433. Polymyalgia rheumatica is connective tissue disease of unknown etiology that:
   a. occurs primarily in patients over 60 years of age
   b. occurs in females twice as commonly as males
   c. may be associated with temporal arteritis

d. is associated with little proximal muscle weakness
e. all of the above

434. Polymyalgia rheumatica is characterized by a constellation of musculoskeletal symptoms that include:
   a. deep, aching pain of the cervical, pectoral and pelvic regions
   b. morning stiffness
   c. arthralgias
   d. stiffness after inactivity (gelling phenomenon)
   e. all of the above

435. Constitutional symptoms associated with polymyalgia rheumatica include:
   a. malaise
   b. fever
   c. anorexia
   d. weight loss and depression
   e. all of the above

436. Common causes of central pain include:
   a. thalamic infarcts and hemorrhage
   b. vascular malformations, infarcts, and hemorrhage of the brain and brainstem
   c. traumatic brain injury
   d. brain tumors
   e. all of the above

437. The portion of the thalamus that is most often associated with central pain is the:
   a. ventroposterior portion
   b. ventroanterior portion
   c. lateroposterior portion
   d. anteriocaudal portion
   e. all of the above

438. Common causes of central pain include:
   a. multiple sclerosis
   b. infections and inflammation of the spinal cord
   c. syringomyelia
   d. spinal cord tumors
   e. all of the above

439. Generally accepted pharmacologic treatments for central pain include:
   a. antidepressants and neuroleptics
   b. anticonvulsants
   c. analgesics
   d. local anesthetics and antiarrhythmics
   e. all of the above

440. Generally accepted invasive treatments for central pain include:
   a. spinal cord stimulations
   b. deep brain stimulation and surface motor area cortex stimulation
   c. cordotomy
   d. dorsal root entry lesioning
   e. all of the above

441. Signs and symptoms frequently associated with conversion disorder include:
   a. weakness
   b. involuntary motor movements
   c. sensory disturbances
   d. pseudoseizures
   e. all of the above

442. Signs and symptoms frequently associated with conversion disorder include:
   a. blindness
   b. deafness
   c. aphonia
   d. la belle indifférence
   e. all of the above

443. La belle indifference:
   a. is an inappropriate lack of concern for the impact and severity of somatic symptomatology associated with conversion disorder
   b. is associated with the complete denial of any psychological problems associated with the somatic difficulties of a conversion disorder
   c. can occur with organic based neurologic disorders
   d. all of the above
   e. none of the above

444. Conversion disorder is classified as a(n):
   a. somatiform disorder
   b. anxiety neurosis
   c. depressive neurosis
   d. all of the above
   e. none of the above

445. The somatic symptoms associated with a conversion disorder are:
   a. under the voluntary control of the patient
   b. under the involuntary control of the patient
   c. due to an organic lesion or disease
   d. all of the above
   e. none of the above

446. Patients suffering from Munchausen syndrome:
   a. are conscious of their confabulations
   b. are not conscious of their confabulations
   c. often have associated personality disorders
   d. a and b
   e. a and c

447. Patients suffering from Munchausen syndrome:
   a. receive no obvious primary gain
   b. receive no obvious secondary gain
   c. often create fictitious illness to produce real signs and symptoms
   d. know they are lying
   e. all of the above

448. Management of thermal injuries should include:
   a. an assessment of the classification of thermal injury
   b. an assessment of the amount of body surface affected by second-degree burns
   c. cleansing of the wound
   d. débridement of nonviable tissue
   e. all of the above

449. Fluid replacement is required with more serious burns and is guided by:
   a. the Parkland formula
   b. urine output

c. vital signs
d. all of the above
e. none of the above

450. Types of electrical injuries include:
    a. low-voltage injuries
    b. high-voltage injuries
    c. lightning injuries
    d. all of the above
    e. a and b

451. The pathognomonic cutaneous sign associated with lightning injuries is known as the:
    a. Lichtenberg figure
    b. Sturge-Weber sign
    c. vericolor rubor sign
    d. dermatographia sign
    e. none of the above

452. Tissues that have a high degree of electrical conductivity include:
    a. nerves
    b. arteries
    c. veins
    d. all of the above
    e. none of the above

453. Signs and symptoms associated with post-polio syndrome include:
    a. new asymmetrical muscle weakness in muscles that were not affected by the original infection
    b. new muscle atrophy
    c. myalgias
    d. arthralgias
    e. all of the above

454. Signs and symptoms associated with post-polio syndrome include:
    a. generalized fatigue
    b. difficulty breathing and swallowing
    c. centrally mediated sleep disorders
    d. decreased tolerance to cold ambient temperatures
    e. all of the above

455. Diseases that may mimic post-polio syndrome include:
    a. amyotrophic lateral sclerosis
    b. cervical myelopathy
    c. inflammatory myopathies
    d. hypothyroidism
    e. all of the above

456. Multiple sclerosis:
    a. is more common in women
    b. rarely occurs before the age of 20
    c. occurs more commonly in Caucasians
    d. all of the above
    e. none of the above

457. Multiple sclerosis occurs more commonly in:
    a. tropical climates
    b. temperate climates
    c. the Western Hemisphere
    d. a and b
    e. b and c

458. The classic pathologic lesion associated with multiple sclerosis is the:
    a. bullous pemphigoid
    b. plaque
    c. Golgi body
    d. Charcot-Leyden crystal
    e. None of the above

459. The following will exacerbate the symptoms of multiple sclerosis:
    a. a hot meal
    b. vigorous exercise
    c. a hot bath
    d. all of the above
    e. none of the above

460. The most common clinical presentations of multiple sclerosis include:
    a. optic neuritis
    b. transverse myelitis
    c. internuclear ophthalmoplegia
    d. pain and paresthesias
    e. all of the above

461. Tissues commonly affected by multiple sclerosis include the:
    a. optic nerve
    b. periventricular white matter of the cerebellum
    c. brainstem and the basal ganglia
    d. spinal cord
    e. all of the above

462. A hallmark physical finding of acute classic Guillain-Barré syndrome is:
    a. areflexia
    b. hyperreflexia
    c. increased cremasteric reflex
    d. increased light reflex
    e. none of the above

463. Diseases that may mimic acute classic Guillain-Barré syndrome include:
    a. multiple sclerosis
    b. heavy metal poisoning
    c. organophosphate poisoning
    d. inflammatory muscle disease
    e. all of the above

464. Diagnostic tests that may help confirm acute classic Guillain-Barré syndrome include:
    a. spinal fluid protein
    b. spinal fluid cell count
    c. gadolinium-enhanced MRI of the spinal nerves
    d. all of the above
    e. none of the above

465. Complications associated with acute classic Guillain-Barré syndrome include:
    a. thrombophlebitis
    b. respiratory insufficiency
    c. cardiac arrhythmias
    d. autonomic dysfunction
    e. all of the above

466. Sickle cell disease is most common in people whose ancestors hail from:
    a. sub-Saharan Africa
    b. the Mediterranean
    c. India
    d. the Middle East
    e. all of the above

467. Sickle cell disease is caused by:
    a. a hemoglobinopathy
    b. renal abnormalities
    c. a disorder of porphyrin metabolism
    d. all of the above
    e. none of the above

468. Complications associated with sickle cell disease include:
    a. vaso-occlusive crises
    b. splenic sequestration syndrome
    c. aplastic crises
    d. autosplenectomy
    e. all of the above

469. Treatment of sickle cell disease includes:
    a. palliation of mild to moderate pain with nonsteroidal anti-inflammatory agents
    b. palliation of severe pain with opioid analgesics
    c. oxygen
    d. zinc and hydroxyurea
    e. all of the above

470. Dependence:
    a. is defined as a physiologic state where continued intake of a substance is required to maintain homeostasis
    b. is frequently confused with addiction
    c. can be caused by drugs that are not traditionally associated with addiction, e.g., antihypertensives, antidepressants, beta-blockers, etc.
    d. can be divided into physiologic and psychological subsets
    e. all of the above

471. Tolerance:
    a. is a physiologic phenomenon in which the organism adapts to the effects of the drug and over time there is a diminution of one or more of the drug's actions
    b. of the drug's actions can be limited to its beneficial therapeutic effects
    c. can affect only the side effects of a drug
    d. can affect both the beneficial therapeutic effects and the side effects of a drug
    e. all of the above

472. Centers thought to involved in the phenomenon of addiction include the:
    a. mesolimbic pathway
    b. ventral trigeminal area of the midbrain
    c. prefrontal cortex
    d. nucleus accumbens
    e. all of the above

473. The neurotransmitter(s) thought to be *most* involved in the phenomenon of addiction include(s):
    a. dopamine
    b. MDMA
    c. acetylcholine
    d. all of the above
    e. none of the above

474. The placebo response is:
    a. the patient's psychological and behavioral response of analgesia following the administration of the sham treatment
    b. patient's psychological and behavioral response of pain following administration of the sham treatment
    c. present in 75% of patients given a sham treatment
    d. a and c
    e. b and c

475. The placebo response may be influenced by the:
    a. normal waxing and waning of the patient's perception of pain
    b. patient's interaction with the practitioner administering the placebo
    c. patient's expectancy of pain relief
    d. all of the above
    e. none of the above

476. The nocebo response is the term applied to the:
    a. patient's psychological and behavioral response of analgesia following the administration of the sham treatment
    b. patient's psychological and behavioral response of pain following the administration of the sham treatment
    c. patient's expectancy of pain relief
    d. all of the above
    e. none of the above

477. The x-ray cassette is made up of:
    a. a light tight structure
    b. a radiolucent panel that admits x-ray photons
    c. two image-intensifying panels that lie against each side of the film
    d. a Mylar sheet coated on each side with a silver halide emulsion
    e. all of the above

478. The major form of energy conversion in the typical x-ray vacuum tube is:
    a. x-ray photons
    b. heat
    c. gamma rays
    d. visible light on the blue end of the spectrum
    e. none of the above

479. The tissue with the highest density to x-ray photons is:
    a. bone
    b. muscle
    c. fat
    d. arteries
    e. none of the above

480. Commonly used intravenous radionuclides include:
    a. gallium-67
    b. iodine-123
    c. indium-111
    d. iodine-131
    e. all of the above

481. The substance that carries a radionuclide to a specific tissue is called a:
    a. SPECT scan
    b. gamma particle
    c. tracer
    d. beta particle
    e. none of the above

482. Routes of administration of radiopharmaceuticals commonly used in clinical medicine include:
    a. intravenous
    b. inhalation
    c. oral
    d. all of the above
    e. none of the above

483. The radiodensities of body tissues are assigned a number representing their relative x-ray photon attenuation value known as:
    a. pixels
    b. Hounsfield units
    c. voxels
    d. gray scale atomic number
    e. none of the above

484. Processing of the data acquired during a CT scan is accomplished in part by dividing each area of a given CT slice into small volumetric areas known as:
    a. pixels
    b. Hounsfield units
    c. voxels
    d. gray scale atomic number
    e. none of the above

485. Tissues that are more radiodense such as bone are by convention represented on a digital CT image as:
    a. white
    b. black
    c. gray
    d. all of the above
    e. none of the above

486. The paramagnetic contrast agent gadolinium should be used with caution in patients with:
    a. brain tumors
    b. seizures
    c. renal failure
    d. malignancies of the hemopoietic system
    e. none of the above

487. MRI relies on _____ to produce clinically useful images.
    a. x-ray photons
    b. the release of energy from hydrogen protons
    c. gamma rays
    d. ionizing radiation
    e. none of the above

488. Complications of discography include:
    a. discitis
    b. epidural abscess
    c. trauma to neural structures
    d. pneumothorax
    e. all of the above

489. Indications for discography include:
    a. the diagnosis of discogenic pain
    b. the identification of the disc responsible for a patient's pain in the setting of normal or equivocal imaging studies
    c. an aid to help determine which spinal levels need to be fused
    d. all of the above
    e. none of the above

490. Symptoms associated with myopathy include:
    a. symmetrical proximal muscle weakness
    b. fever
    c. muscle aches
    d. a normal sensory examination
    e. all of the above

491. Diseases associated with myopathy include:
    a. polymyositis
    b. acute alcohol intoxication
    c. hypothyroidism
    d. Cushing disease
    e. all of the above

492. Diseases associated with peripheral neuropathy include:
    a. diabetes
    b. renal disease
    c. autoimmune diseases
    d. HIV/AIDS
    e. all of the above

493. The classic finding on nerve conduction studies in patients suffering from moderately severe peripheral neuropathy is:
    a. slowing of the nerve conduction velocity
    b. enhancement of the nerve conduction velocity
    c. a Kondrake phenomenon with repetitive stimulation
    d. all of the above
    e. none of the above

494. Causes of plexopathy include:
    a. idiopathic inflammatory plexitis
    b. tumor
    c. hematoma and abscess
    d. trauma
    e. all of the above

495. Visual evoked potentials are useful in the diagnosis of:
    a. multiple sclerosis
    b. abnormalities of the optic nerve
    c. inflammatory conditions of the eye and ocular pathways
    d. tumors involving the eye and ocular pathways
    e. all of the above

496. Brainstem auditory evoked potentials are useful in the diagnosis of:
    a. multiple sclerosis
    b. acoustic neuromas
    c. cerebellopontine angle tumors
    d. strokes involving the auditory pathways
    e. all of the above

497. Somatosensory evoked potentials are useful in the diagnosis of:
    a. syringomyelia
    b. spinal cord tumors
    c. multiple sclerosis
    d. Huntington's chorea
    e. all of the above

498. Evoked potential testing:
    a. is a neurophysiologic test similar to electro-myography
    b. uses a recording electrode placed on the scalp in a manner analogous to electroencephalography
    c. uses a computer to average "time-locked" signals and cancel out noise
    d. all of the above
    e. none of the above

499. The peak of greatest interest in visual evoked potential testing is called the:
    a. P100 peak
    b. P200 peak
    c. P300 peak
    d. peak of inverse latency
    e. a and d

500. Examples of unidimensional pain assessment tools that are useful in the evaluation of adult patients in pain include the:
    a. visual analog scale
    b. numerical pain intensity scale
    c. verbal descriptor scale
    d. all of the above
    e. none of the above

501. Examples of multidimensional pain assessment tools that are useful in the evaluation of adult patients in pain include the:
    a. McGill Pain Questionnaire
    b. Brief Pain Inventory
    c. Memorial Pain Assessment Card
    d. Multidimensional Affect and Pain Survey
    e. all of the above

502. Examples of pain assessment tools that are useful in the evaluation of pain in children include:
    a. CRIES
    b. COMFORT
    c. Wong-Baker Faces Scale
    d. Oucher Scale
    e. all of the above

503. The atlanto-occipital joint:
    a. is not a true joint
    b. allows the head to nod forward and backward with an isolated range of motion of approximately 35 degrees

c. is located anterior to the posterolateral columns of the spinal cord
    d. all of the above
    e. none of the above

504. Complications associated with atlanto-occipital block include:
    a. needle-induced trauma to the brainstem
    b. ataxia due to vascular absorption
    c. seizures secondary to intravascular injection
    d. all of the above
    e. none of the above

505. The atlantoaxial joint:
    a. is not a true joint
    b. allows the head to flex and extend approximately 10 degrees, but it allows more than 60 degrees of rotation in the horizontal plane
    c. relies almost entirely on ligaments for its integrity
    d. all of the above
    e. none of the above

506. Complications associated with atlantoaxial block include:
    a. needle-induced trauma to the brainstem
    b. ataxia due to vascular absorption
    c. seizures secondary to intravascular injection
    d. all of the above
    e. none of the above

507. Complications associated with sphenopalatine ganglion block include:
    a. epistaxis
    b. orthostatic hypotension
    c. intravascular injection
    d. inadvertent blockade of the maxillary nerve when performing the lateral approach
    e. all of the above

508. Other names for the sphenopalatine ganglion include:
    a. Meckel's ganglion
    b. gasserian ganglion
    c. pterygopalatine ganglion
    d. a and c
    e. all of the above

509. Complications associated with greater and lesser occipital nerve block include:
    a. trauma to the occipital artery
    b. needle placement into the foramen magnum
    c. intravascular injection
    d. all of the above
    e. none of the above

510. Useful landmarks for the performance of greater and lesser occipital nerve block include the:
    a. nuchal ridge
    b. supraorbital foramen
    c. occipital artery
    d. a and c
    e. all of the above

511. The sensory branches of the gasserian ganglion include the:
    a. ophthalmic branch
    b. maxillary branch

c. mandibular branch
d. all of the above
e. none of the above

512. Access to the gasserian ganglion is via the:
   a. foramen ovale
   b. foramen rotundum
   c. maxillary foramen
   d. pterygopalatine foramen
   e. none of the above

513. Complications and side effects of gasserian ganglion block include:
   a. corneal anesthesia
   b. subscleral hematoma formation
   c. subarachnoid injection
   d. damage to arteries
   e. all of the above

514. A dreaded complication of destruction of the gasserian ganglion is:
   a. anesthesia phlegmosa
   b. prolonged anesthesia
   c. anesthesia dolorosa
   d. all of the above
   e. none of the above

515. Methods that can be used to destroy the gasserian ganglion include:
   a. neurolytic injections with phenol
   b. neurolytic injections with glycerol
   c. balloon compression of the ganglion
   d. radiofrequency lesioning
   e. all of the above

516. Complications and side effects of trigeminal nerve block via the coronoid include:
   a. intravascular uptake of local anesthetic
   b. hematoma formation
   c. weakness of the masseter muscles
   d. facial asymmetry due to loss of proprioception
   e. all of the above

517. The following branches of the trigeminal nerve have motor and sensory function:
   a. ophthalmic nerve
   b. maxillary nerve
   c. mandibular nerve
   d. b and c
   e. none of the above

518. The supraorbital nerve:
   a. arises from fibers of the frontal nerve
   b. is a terminal branch of the ophthalmic division of the trigeminal nerve
   c. sends fibers all the way to the vertex of the scalp and provides sensory innervation to the forehead, upper eyelid, and anterior scalp
   d. all of the above
   e. none of the above

519. The supraorbital nerve:
   a. arises from fibers of the frontal nerve
   b. is a terminal branch of the ophthalmic division of the trigeminal nerve

c. provides sensory innervation to the inferomedial section of the forehead, the bridge of the nose, and the medial portion of the upper eyelid
   d. all of the above
   e. none of the above

520. Complications of infraorbital nerve block include:
   a. compression or trauma of the infraorbital nerve if the needle enters the infraorbital foramen
   b. hematoma
   c. intravascular injection
   d. all of the above
   e. none of the above

521. The mental nerve:
   a. arises from fibers of the mandibular nerve
   b. exits the mandible via the mental foramen at the level of the second premolar, where it makes a sharp turn superiorly
   c. provides cutaneous branches that innervate the lower lip, chin, and corresponding oral mucosa
   d. all of the above
   e. none of the above

522. The muscles involved in temporomandibular joint dysfunction often include the:
   a. temporalis
   b. masseter
   c. external pterygoid
   d. internal pterygoid
   e. all of the above

523. When injecting the temporomandibular joint, if the needle is placed through the joint, the following nerve may be blocked:
   a. trigeminal nerve
   b. facial nerve
   c. spinal accessory nerve
   d. hypoglossal nerve
   e. none of the above

524. The key landmark for extraoral glossopharyngeal nerve block is the:
   a. coronoid notch
   b. vomer
   c. styloid process of the temporal bone
   d. temporomandibular joint
   e. none of the above

525. Complications of glossopharyngeal nerve block include:
   a. intravascular injection
   b. trauma to the internal jugular vein
   c. trauma to the carotid artery
   d. inadvertent vagal nerve block
   e. all of the above

526. The vagus nerve:
   a. contains both motor and sensory fibers
   b. contains motor fibers that innervate the pharyngeal muscle and provide fibers for the superior and recurrent laryngeal nerves
   c. contains sensory fibers that innervate the dura mater of the posterior fossa, the posterior aspect of the

external auditory meatus, the inferior aspect of the tympanic membrane, and the mucosa of the larynx below the vocal cords
d. provides fibers to the intrathoracic contents, including the heart, lungs, and major vasculature
e. all of the above

527. The major complication associated with vagus nerve block:
a. is related to trauma to the internal jugular vein and carotid artery including hematoma formation
b. includes intravascular injection of local anesthetic
c. includes blockade of the motor portion of the vagus nerve that can result in dysphonia and difficulty coughing due to blockade of the superior and recurrent laryngeal nerves
d. includes a reflex tachycardia secondary to vagal nerve block
e. all of the above

528. The spinal accessory nerve:
a. arises from the nucleus ambiguus
b. has two roots, which leave the cranium together along with the vagus nerve via the jugular foramen
c. has fibers of the spinal root pass inferiorly and posteriorly to provide motor innervation to the superior portion of the sternocleidomastoid muscle
d. provides, in combination with the cervical plexus, innervation to the trapezius muscle
e. all of the above

529. Complications of spinal accessory nerve block include:
a. inadvertent subdural, epidural, or surbarachnoid block
b. inadvertent block of the recurrent laryngeal nerve
c. inadvertent block of the glossopharyngeal nerve
d. hematoma and ecchymosis
e. all of the above

530. The phrenic nerve:
a. arises from fibers of the primary ventral ramus of the fourth cervical nerve, with contributions from the third and fifth cervical nerves
b. exits the root of the neck between the subclavian artery and vein to enter the mediastinum
c. on the right follows the course of the vena cava to provide motor innervation to the right hemidiaphragm
d. on the left descends to provide motor innervation to the left hemidiaphragm in a course parallel to that of the vagus nerve
e. all of the above

531. Complications of phrenic nerve block include:
a. inadvertent subdural, epidural, or surbarachnoid block
b. inadvertent block of the recurrent laryngeal nerve
c. respiratory embarrassment in the presence of respiratory disease
d. hematoma and ecchymosis
e. all of the above

532. The facial nerve:
a. provides both motor and sensory fibers to the head
b. arises from the brainstem at the inferior margin of the pons with the sensory portion of the facial nerve
c. exits the base of the skull via the stylomastoid foramen
d. passes downward and then turns forward to pass through the parotid gland, where it divides into fibers that provide innervation to the muscles of facial expression
e. all of the above

533. As it leaves the pons, the nervus intermedius is susceptible to compression producing a "trigeminal neuralgia–like" syndrome called:
a. geniculate neuralgia
b. vidian neuralgia
c. Sluder's neuralgia
d. Morton's neuralgia
e. none of the above

534. The superficial cervical plexus:
a. arises from fibers of the primary ventral rami of the first, second, third, and fourth cervical nerves with each nerve dividing into an ascending and a descending branch providing fibers to the nerves above and below, respectively
b. provides both sensory and motor innervation
c. has as its most important motor branch the phrenic nerve, with the plexus also providing motor fibers to the spinal accessory nerve and to the paravertebral and deep muscles of the neck
d. provides, with the exception of the first cervical nerve, significant cutaneous sensory innervation to the skin of the lower mandible, neck, and supraclavicular fossa
e. all of the above

535. Complications of superficial cervical plexus block include:
a. inadvertent subdural, epidural, or subarachnoid block
b. inadvertent block of the recurrent laryngeal nerve
c. respiratory embarrassment in the presence of respiratory disease
d. hematoma and ecchymosis
e. all of the above

536. The deep cervical plexus:
a. arises from fibers of the primary ventral rami of the first, second, third, and fourth cervical nerves with each nerve dividing into an ascending and a descending branch providing fibers to the nerves above and below, respectively
b. provides both sensory and motor innervation, with its most important motor branch being the phrenic nerve
c. also provides motor fibers to the spinal accessory nerve and to the paravertebral and deep muscles of the neck
d. provides significant cutaneous sensory innervation with the terminal sensory fibers of the deep cervical

plexus contributing fibers to the greater auricular and lesser occipital nerves
e. all of the above

537. Complications of superficial cervical plexus block include:
a. inadvertent subdural, epidural, or subarachnoid block
b. inadvertent block of the recurrent laryngeal nerve
c. respiratory embarrassment in the presence of respiratory disease
d. hematoma and ecchymosis
e. all of the above

538. The right and left recurrent laryngeal nerves:
a. arise from the vagus nerve and follow different paths to reach the larynx and trachea
b. on the right loops underneath the innominate artery and then ascends in the lateral groove between the trachea and esophagus to enter the inferior portion of the larynx
c. on the left loops below the arch of the aorta and then ascends in the lateral groove between the trachea and esophagus to enter the inferior portion of the larynx
d. provide the innervation to all the intrinsic muscles of the larynx except the cricothyroid muscle as well as providing the sensory innervation for the mucosa below the vocal cords
e. all of the above

539. Bilateral blockade of the recurrent laryngeal nerves will result in:
a. numbness of the posterior two-thirds of the tongue
b. bilateral vocal cord paralysis
c. numbness of the larynx above the vocal cords
d. all of the above
e. none of the above

540. Complications and side effects of stellate ganglion block include:
a. the development of Horner's syndrome
b. difficulty swallowing and a feeling like there is a lump in one's throat
c. pneumothorax
d. intravascular injection
e. all of the above

541. Inadvertent block of the recurrent laryngeal nerve when performing stellate ganglion block may cause:
a. hoarseness
b. difficulty swallowing
c. difficulty coughing
d. all of the above
e. none of the above

542. Inadvertent blockade of the superior cervical sympathetic ganglion when performing stellate ganglion block may result in:
a. contralateral vocal cord paralysis
b. ipsilateral vocal cord paralysis
c. Horner's syndrome
d. all of the above
e. none of the above

543. The stellate ganglion:
a. is located on the anterior surface of the longus colli muscle
b. lies just anterior to the transverse processes of the seventh cervical and first thoracic vertebrae
c. is made up of the fused portion of the seventh cervical and first thoracic sympathetic ganglia
d. all of the above
e. none of the above

544. The stellate ganglion:
a. lies anteromedial to the vertebral artery
b. is medial to the common carotid artery and jugular vein
c. is lateral to the trachea and esophagus
d. all of the above
e. none of the above

545. Improper needle placement during stellate ganglion block can result in:
a. inadvertent epidural injection
b. inadvertent subdural injection
c. inadvertent subarachnoid injection
d. intravascular injection
e. all of the above

546. Complications of radiofrequency lesioning of the stellate ganglion include:
a. permanent damage to neuroaxial structures
b. permanent recurrent laryngeal nerve paralysis
c. pneumothorax
d. damage to the carotid artery or internal jugular vein
e. all of the above

547. Each facet joint:
a. receives innervation from two spinal levels
b. receives fibers from the dorsal ramus at the same level as the vertebra as well as fibers from the dorsal ramus of the vertebra above
c. has a dorsal ramus that provides a medial branch that wraps around the convexity of the articular pillar of its respective vertebra
d. has a medial branch whose location is constant for the C4-7 nerves
e. all of the above

548. Complications of facet joint block include:
a. damage to the spinal cord
b. damage to the vertebral artery
c. intravascular injection
d. inadvertent subdural, epidural, or subarachnoid block
e. all of the above

549. Ligamentous structures that an epidural needle will traverse prior to entering the cervical epidural space include the:
a. ligamentum nuchae
b. interspinous ligament
c. ligamentum flavum
d. all of the above
e. none of the above

550. Complications of cervical epidural nerve block include:
    a. damage to the spinal cord
    b. infection
    c. intravascular injection
    d. inadvertent subdural or subarachnoid block
    e. all of the above

551. Cervical selective nerve root block is:
    a. performed by placing the needle just outside the neural foramina of the nerve root being blocked
    b. performed in a manner analogous to the transforaminal approach to the cervical epidural space
    c. often associated with a paresthesia if the needle impinges on the cervical nerve root being blocked
    d. all of the above
    e. none of the above

552. The brachial plexus:
    a. is formed by the fusion of the anterior rami of the C5, C6, C7, C8, and T1 spinal nerves
    b. may also have a contribution of fibers from C4 and T2 spinal nerves
    c. is formed by nerves that exit the lateral aspect of the cervical spine and pass downward and laterally in conjunction with the subclavian artery
    d. nerves and the subclavian artery run between the anterior scalene and middle scalene muscles, passing inferiorly behind the middle of the clavicle and above the top of the first rib to reach the axilla
    e. all of the above

553. Nerves from the brachial plexus that surround the axillary artery that can be blocked when performing brachial plexus block using the axillary approach include the:
    a. median nerve
    b. radial nerve
    c. ulnar nerve
    d. musculocutaneous nerve
    e. all of the above

554. The suprascapular nerve:
    a. is formed from fibers originating from the C5 and C6 nerve roots of the brachial plexus with some contribution of fibers from the C4 root in most patients
    b. passes inferiorly and posteriorly from the brachial plexus to pass underneath the coracoclavicular ligament through the suprascapular notch
    c. is accompanied by the suprascapular artery and vein through the suprascapular notch
    d. provides much of the sensory innervation to the shoulder joint and provides innervation to two of the muscles of the rotator cuff, the supraspinatus and infraspinatus muscles
    e. all of the above

555. Complications of suprascapular nerve block include:
    a. trauma to the suprascapular nerve
    b. intravascular injection
    c. pneumothorax
    d. all of the above
    e. none of the above

556. The radial nerve:
    a. is made up of fibers from C5-T1 spinal roots
    b. exits the axilla and passes between the medial and long heads of the triceps muscle supplying a motor branch to the triceps and gives off a number of sensory branches to the upper arm
    c. at a point between the lateral epicondyle of the humerus and the musculospiral groove divides into its two terminal branches with the superficial branch continuing down the arm along with the radial artery and provides sensory innervation to the dorsum of the wrist and the dorsal aspects of a portion of the thumb and index and middle fingers
    d. has a deep branch that provides the majority of the motor innervation to the extensors of the forearm
    e. all of the above

557. The median nerve:
    a. is made up of fibers from C5-T1 spinal roots
    b. exits the axilla and descends into the upper arm along with the brachial artery
    c. is, at the level of the elbow, just medial to the biceps muscle and brachial artery
    d. proceeds downward into the forearm giving off numerous branches that provide motor innervation to the flexor muscles of the forearm
    e. all of the above

558. The terminal branches of the median nerve provide sensory innervation to:
    a. a portion of the palmar surface of the hand
    b. the palmar surface of the thumb, index and middle fingers, and the radial portion of the ring finger
    c. the distal dorsal surface of the index and middle fingers and the radial portion of the ring finger.
    d. all of the above
    e. none of the above

559. The ulnar nerve:
    a. is made up of fibers from C6-T1 spinal roots
    b. exits the axilla and descends into the upper arm along with the brachial artery.
    c. courses medially at mid-arm to pass between the olecranon process and medial epicondyle of the humerus
    d. passes between the heads of the flexor carpi ulnaris muscle continuing downward, moving radially along with the ulnar artery
    e. all of the above

560. The ulnar nerve:
    a. at a point approximately 1 inch proximal to the crease of the wrist divides into the dorsal and palmar branches
    b. dorsal branch provides sensation to the ulnar aspect of the dorsum of the hand and the dorsal aspect of the little finger and the ulnar half of the ring finger
    c. palmar branch provides sensory innervation to the ulnar aspect of the palm of the hand and the palmar aspect of the little finger and the ulnar half of the ring finger

d. all of the above
e. none of the above

561. Ulnar nerve block at the elbow must be performed with caution:
    a. to avoid persistent paresthesia
    b. because the nerve is enclosed by a dense fibrous band as it passes through the ulnar nerve sulcus
    c. because the nerve passes through a closed space and is susceptible to compression
    d. all of the above
    e. none of the above

562. When performing radial nerve block at the wrist:
    a. the needle is inserted in a perpendicular trajectory just lateral to the flexor carpi radialis tendon
    b. the needle is inserted in a perpendicular trajectory just medial to the radial artery at the level of the distal radial prominence
    c. the needle is advanced slowly to avoid trauma to the radial nerve
    d. careful aspiration is mandatory to avoid inadvertent intravascular injection
    e. all of the above

563. When performing median nerve block at the wrist:
    a. the needle is inserted in a perpendicular trajectory just medial to the palmaris longus tendon
    b. the needle is inserted in a perpendicular trajectory at the crease of the wrist
    c. the needle is advanced slowly to avoid trauma to the median nerve
    d. careful aspiration is mandatory to avoid inadvertent intravascular injection
    e. all of the above

564. When performing ulnar nerve block at the wrist:
    a. the needle is inserted in a slightly caudad trajectory on the radial side of the flexor carpi ulnaris tendon
    b. the needle is inserted at the level of the styloid process
    c. the needle is advanced slowly to avoid trauma to the ulnar nerve
    d. careful aspiration is mandatory to avoid inadvertent intravascular injection
    e. all of the above

565. The common digital nerves:
    a. arise from fibers of the median and ulnar nerves with the thumb also having a contribution from superficial branches of the radial nerve
    b. pass along the metacarpal bones and divide into the palmar and dorsal as they reach the distal palm
    c. divide as they pass along the metacarpal bones with the palmar digital nerves supplying the majority of sensory innervation to the fingers and running along the ventrolateral aspect of the finger beside the digital vein and artery
    d. divide as they pass along the metacarpal bones, with the smaller dorsal digital nerves containing fibers from the ulnar and radial nerves and supplying the dorsum of the fingers as far as the proximal joints
    e. all of the above

566. Diseases that may mimic multiple sclerosis include:
    a. amyotrophic lateral sclerosis
    b. Guillain-Barré syndrome
    c. small vessel cerebrovascular disease
    d. central nervous system infections
    e. all of the above

567. Side effects of intravenous regional anesthesia include:
    a. phlebitis at the injection site especially with ester-type local anesthetics
    b. petechial hemorrhages distal to the tourniquet in patients taking aspirin
    c. inadvertent release of large volumes of local anesthetics due to tourniquet failure
    d. all of the above
    e. none of the above

568. Limiting factors when performing intravenous regional anesthesia include the:
    a. total amount of local anesthetic that can be safely administered
    b. size of the tourniquet utilized
    c. length of time that the circulation of the extremity can be occluded by the tourniquet
    d. a and c
    e. b and c

569. The major ligaments of the shoulder joint are the:
    a. glenohumeral ligaments in front of the capsule
    b. transverse humeral ligament between the humeral tuberosities
    c. coracohumeral ligament which stretches from the coracoid process to the greater tuberosity of the humerus
    d. all of the above
    e. none of the above

570. The cubital fossa:
    a. lies in the anterior aspect of the elbow joint
    b. is bounded laterally by the brachioradialis muscle
    c. is bounded medially by the pronator teres
    d. contains the median nerve
    e. all of the above

571. Complications of injection of the cubital bursa include:
    a. damage to the median nerve
    b. infection
    c. inadvertent intravascular injection
    d. all of the above
    e. none of the above

572. The wrist joint allows:
    a. flexion
    b. extension
    c. abduction and adduction
    d. circumduction
    e. all of the above

573. Complications of injection of the wrist joint include:
    a. damage to the ulnar nerve
    b. infection
    c. inadvertent intravascular injection

  d. all of the above
  e. none of the above

574. The inferior radioulnar joint
  a. is a synovial, pivot-type joint
  b. serves as the articulation between the rounded head of the ulna and the ulnar notch of the radius
  c. allows pronation and supination of the forearm
  d. is innervated primarily by the anterior and posterior interosseous nerves
  e. all of the above

575. The carpometacarpal joints of the fingers:
  a. are synovial plane joints that serve as the articulation between the carpals and the metacarpals
  b. allow articulation of the bases of the metacarpal bones with one another
  c. have movement limited to a slight gliding motion, with the carpometacarpal joint of the little finger possessing the greatest range of motion
  d. function primarily to optimize the grip function of the hand
  e. all of the above

576. The metacarpophalangeal joint:
  a. is a synovial, ellipsoid-shaped joint that serves as the articulation between the base of the proximal phalanges and the head of its respective metacarpal
  b. has as its primary role to optimize the gripping function of the hand
  c. allows flexion, extension, abduction, and adduction
  d. is covered by a capsule that surrounds the entire joint and is susceptible to trauma if the joint is subluxed
  e. all of the above

577. The median nerve:
  a. passes beneath the flexor retinaculum
  b. passes through the carpal tunnel
  c. has its terminal branches providing sensory innervation to a portion of the palmar surface of the hand as well as the palmar surface of the thumb, index, middle, and the radial portion of the ring finger
  d. provides sensory innervation to the distal dorsal surface of the index and middle finger and the radial portion of the ring finger
  e. all of the above

578. The carpal tunnel is:
  a. bounded on three sides by the carpal bones
  b. covered by the transverse carpal ligament
  c. the most common site of entrapment neuropathy
  d. all of the above
  e. none of the above

579. The carpal tunnel contains:
  a. the median nerve
  b. a number of flexor tendon sheaths
  c. blood vessels
  d. lymphatics
  e. all of the above

580. Complications of injection of the carpal tunnel include:
  a. infection
  b. a transient increase in pain
  c. trauma to the median nerve
  d. inadvertent intravascular injection
  e. all of the above

581. The ulnar tunnel is:
  a. a closed space
  b. bounded on one side by the pisiform and the other side by the hook of the hamate
  c. a site that is associated with entrapment neuropathy of the ulnar nerve
  d. all of the above
  e. none of the above

582. The ulnar tunnel contains:
  a. the ulnar nerve
  b. the ulnar artery
  c. flexor tendon sheaths
  d. a and b
  e. all of the above

583. Complications of thoracic epidural nerve block include:
  a. damage to the spinal cord
  b. infection
  c. intravascular injection
  d. inadvertent subdural or surbarachnoid block
  e. all of the above

584. The following approach is best suited for performing thoracic epidural block in the middle thoracic interspaces:
  a. midline approach
  b. paramedian approach
  c. the no-man's land approach
  d. the anterior approach
  e. none of the above

585. Absolute contraindications to thoracic epidural block include:
  a. local infection
  b. sepsis
  c. anticoagulation
  d. all of the above
  e. none of the above

586. The thoracic paravertebral nerves:
  a. exit their respective intervertebral foramina just beneath the transverse process of the vertebra
  b. exit the intervertebral foramen, the thoracic paravertebral nerve gives off a recurrent branch that loops back through the foramen to provide innervation to the spinal ligaments, meninges, and its respective vertebra
  c. interface with the thoracic sympathetic chain via the myelinated preganglionic fibers of the white rami communicantes as well as the unmyelinated postganglionic fibers of the gray rami communicantes
  d. divide into a posterior and an anterior primary division.
  e. all of the above

587. The thoracic paravertebral nerve:
    a. gives off a posterior division, courses posteriorly and, along with its branches, provides innervation to the facet joints and the muscles and skin of the back
    b. gives off a larger, anterior division, courses laterally to pass into the subcostal groove beneath the rib to become the respective intercostal nerves
    c. runs beneath the 12th thoracic nerve and is called the subcostal nerve
    d. all of the above
    e. none of the above

588. When performing thoracic paravertebral block, the following structures will be blocked:
    a. the anterior division of the paravertebral nerve
    b. the posterior division of the paravertebral nerve
    c. the recurrent branch that loops back through the foramen to provide innervation to the spinal ligaments, meninges, and its respective vertebra
    d. the sympathetic components of each respective thoracic paravertebral nerve
    e. all of the above

589. Complications of thoracic paravertebral nerve block include:
    a. pneumothorax
    b. infection
    c. trauma to spinal nerve roots
    d. trauma to the spinal cord
    e. all of the above

590. The thoracic facet joints are:
    a. formed by the articulations of the superior and inferior articular facets of adjacent vertebrae
    b. true joints in that they are lined with synovium and possess a true joint capsule
    c. richly innervated and support the notion of the facet joint as a pain generator
    d. susceptible to arthritic changes and trauma secondary to acceleration-deceleration injuries
    e. all of the above

591. Each thoracic facet joint receives:
    a. innervation from two spinal levels
    b. fibers from the dorsal ramus at the same level as the vertebra
    c. fibers from the dorsal ramus of the vertebra above
    d. all of the above
    e. none of the above

592. Complications of thoracic paravertebral nerve block include:
    a. pneumothorax
    b. infection
    c. trauma to spinal nerve roots and spinal cord
    d. inadvertent epidural, subdural, or subarachnoid block
    e. all of the above

593. The preganglionic fibers of the thoracic sympathetics:
    a. exit the intervertebral foramen along with the respective thoracic paravertebral nerves
    b. give off a recurrent branch that loops back through the foramen to provide innervation to the spinal ligaments, meninges, and its respective vertebra
    c. interface with the thoracic sympathetic chain via the myelinated preganglionic fibers of the white rami communicantes
    d. interface with the thoracic sympathetic chain via the gray rami communicantes
    e. all of the above

594. The preganglionic fibers of the thoracic sympathetics provide sympathetic innervation to the:
    a. vasculature
    b. sweat glands
    c. pilomotor muscles of the skin
    d. to the cardiac plexus
    e. all of the above

595. A typical intercostal nerve has four major branches that include the:
    a. first branch, which is the unmyelinated postganglionic fibers of the gray rami communicantes, which interface with the sympathetic chain
    b. second branch, which is the posterior cutaneous branch, which innervates the muscles and skin of the paraspinal area
    c. third branch, which is the lateral cutaneous division, which arises in the anterior axillary line which provides the majority of the cutaneous innervation of the chest and abdominal wall
    d. fourth branch, which is the anterior cutaneous branch supplying innervation to the midline of the chest and abdominal wall
    e. all of the above

596. Complications of intercostal nerve block include:
    a. intravascular injection
    b. infection
    c. pneumothorax
    d. all of the above
    e. none of the above

597. Complications of interpleural nerve block include:
    a. intravascular injection
    b. infection
    c. pneumothorax
    d. all of the above
    e. none of the above

598. Complications of injection of the sternoclavicular joint include:
    a. intravascular injection
    b. infection
    c. pneumothorax
    d. trauma to the great vessels
    e. all of the above

599. The sternoclavicular joint:
    a. is a double gliding joint with an actual synovial cavity
    b. provides articulation occurs between the sternal end of the clavicle, the sternal manubrium, and the cartilage of the first rib

c. is reinforced in front and back by the sternoclavicular ligaments and by the costoclavicular ligament
d. is dually innervated by both the supraclavicular nerve and the nerve supplying the subclavius muscle
e. all of the above

600. Posterior to the sternoclavicular joint are a number of large arteries and veins including the:
a. left common carotid
b. brachiocephalic vein
c. right brachiocephalic artery
d. all of the above
e. none of the above

601. Movement at the sternoclavicular joint is provided by the:
a. serratus anterior muscle, which produces forward movement of the clavicle
b. rhomboid and trapezius muscles, which produce backward movement
c. sternocleidomastoid, rhomboid, and levator scapulae, which produce elevation of the clavicle
d. pectoralis minor and subclavius muscles, which produce depression of the clavicle
e. all of the above

602. The suprascapular nerve:
a. is formed from fibers originating from the C5 and C6 nerve roots of the brachial plexus, with some contribution of fibers from the C4 root in most patients
b. passes inferiorly and posteriorly from the brachial plexus to pass underneath the coricoclavicular ligament through the suprascapular notch
c. is accompanied through the notch by the suprascapular artery
d. provides much of the sensory innervation to the shoulder joint and provides innervation to two of the muscles of the rotator cuff, the supraspinatus and infraspinatus
e. all of the above

603. Complications of injection of the sternoclavicular joint include:
a. intravascular injection
b. infection
c. pneumothorax
d. local anesthetic toxicity
e. all of the above

604. Complications associated with injection of the costosternal joints include trauma to the:
a. lung
b. esophagus
c. trachea
d. heart
e. all of the above

605. The anterior cutaneous branch of the intercostal nerve:
a. pierces the fascia of the abdominal wall at the lateral border of the rectus abdominis muscle
b. turns sharply in an anterior direction to provide innervation to the anterior wall

c. passes through a firm fibrous ring as it pierces the fascia, and it is at this point that the nerve is subject to entrapment
d. is accompanied through the fascia by an epigastric artery and vein
e. all of the above

606. Complications of injection of the costosternal joint include:
a. intravascular injection
b. infection
c. pneumothorax
d. damage to the abdominal viscera
e. all of the above

607. Complications of splanchnic nerve block include:
a. trauma to the thoracic duct
b. trauma to the great vessels
c. pneumothorax
d. trauma to abdominal viscera
e. all of the above

608. Complications of splanchnic nerve block include *inadvertent:*
a. epidural injection
b. subdural injection
c. subarachnoid injection
d. intravascular injection
e. all of the above

609. Complications of splanchnic nerve block include:
a. trauma to abdominal viscera
b. inadvertent injection into intravertebral disc
c. discitis
d. damage to the kidney and ureter
e. all of the above

610. If the needle is placed too anterior when performing splanchnic nerve block:
a. the tip may rest in the precrural space
b. the splanchnic nerves may not be blocked
c. trauma to the abdominal viscera may occur
d. all of the above
e. none of the above

611. Contraindications to celiac plexus block include:
a. coagulopathy
b. patients on anticoagulants
c. local infection
d. all of the above
e. none of the above

612. Side effects of celiac plexus block include:
a. hypotension
b. increased bowel motility
c. diarrhea
d. all of the above
e. none of the above

613. The major preganglionic innervation of the celiac plexus arises from the:
a. lesser splanchnic nerve
b. least splanchnic nerve

c. greater splanchnic nerve
d. all of the above
e. none of the above

614. The celiac ganglia:
    a. vary from one to five and range in diameter from 0.5 to 4.5 cm
    b. lie anterior and anterolateral to the aorta.
    c. located on the left are uniformly more inferior than their right-sided counterparts by as much as a vertebral level
    d. on both the left and right lie below the level of the celiac artery at the level of the first lumbar vertebra
    e. all of the above

615. The celiac plexus provides innervation to the:
    a. distal esophagus
    b. stomach and duodenum
    c. small intestine
    d. ascending and proximal transverse colon
    e. all of the above

616. The celiac plexus provides innervation to the:
    a. adrenal glands
    b. pancreas
    c. spleen and liver
    d. biliary system
    e. all of the above

617. When performing celiac plexus block, if the needle is placed in the retrocrural space:
    a. it is more likely that the splanchnic nerves will be blocked
    b. the needle tip will be preaortic
    c. it is more likely that the upper lumbar spinal nerves will be blocked
    d. a and b
    e. a and c

618. Complications of ilioinguinal nerve block include:
    a. perforation of the abdominal viscera
    b. ecchymosis
    c. hematoma formation
    d. infection
    e. all of the above

619. Landmarks utilized in performing ilioinguinal nerve block include:
    a. the anterior superior iliac spine
    b. a point 2 inches medial from the anterior superior iliac spine
    c. a point 2 inches below a point 2 inches medial to the anterior superior iliac spine
    d. all of the above
    e. none of the above

620. The ilioinguinal nerve provides sensory innervation to the:
    a. upper portion of the skin of the inner thigh
    b. root of the penis
    c. upper scrotum in men
    d. mons pubis and lateral labia in women
    e. all of the above

621. The iliohyogastric nerve provides sensory innervation to the:
    a. posterolateral gluteal region
    b. the skin above the pubis
    c. lower scrotum in men
    d. a and b
    e. b and c

622. The genitofemoral nerve provides innervation to the:
    a. cremaster muscle
    b. skin of the anterior superior femoral triangle
    c. ipsilateral labia majora
    d. ipsilateral mons pubis
    e. all of the above

623. Complications associated with lumbar sympathetic ganglion block include:
    a. infection
    b. discitis
    c. trauma to the abdominal viscera
    d. intravascular injection
    e. all of the above

624. Placement of the needle medially when performing lumbar sympathetic ganglion block may result in *inadvertent:*
    a. subarachnoid injection
    b. subdural injection
    c. epidural injection
    d. all of the above
    e. none of the above

625. The lumbar paravertebral nerves:
    a. exit their respective intervertebral foramina just beneath the transverse process of the vertebra
    b. give off a recurrent branch that loops back through the foramen to provide innervation to the spinal ligaments, meninges, and its respective vertebra
    c. divide into posterior and anterior primary divisions with the posterior division coursing posteriorly and, along with its branches, provide innervation to the facet joints and the muscles and skin of the back
    d. divide into a posterior and larger anterior division, which courses laterally and inferiorly to enter the body of the psoas muscle
    e. all of the above

626. The lumbar plexus receives contributions from the:
    a. first four lumbar paravertebral nerves
    b. third through fifth sacral nerves
    c. twelfth thoracic paravertebral nerve
    d. a and b
    e. a and c

627. The lumbar plexus provides innervation to the:
    a. lower abdominal wall
    b. groin
    c. portions of the external genitalia
    d. portions of the lower extremity
    e. all of the above

628. Complications associated with lumbar facet medial branch block include:
    a. infection
    b. inadvertent subdural injection
    c. inadvertent subarachnoid injection
    d. inadvertent epidural injection
    e. all of the above

629. The lumbar facet joints are:
    a. formed by the articulations of the superior and inferior articular facets of adjacent vertebrae
    b. true joints in that they are lined with synovium and possess a true joint capsule
    c. susceptible to arthritic changes and trauma secondary to acceleration-deceleration injuries
    d. all of the above
    e. none of the above

630. Each lumbar facet joint:
    a. receives innervation from two spinal levels
    b. receives fibers from the dorsal ramus at the same level as the vertebra as well as fibers from the dorsal ramus of the vertebra above
    c. may be blocked by either the medial branch or intra-articular technique
    d. all of the above
    e. none of the above

631. Complications associated with the transforaminal approach to the lumbar epidural space include:
    a. trauma to the spinal cord
    b. trauma to the exiting nerve root
    c. inadvertent injection into a segmental artery
    d. all of the above
    e. none of the above

632. Complications associated with lumbar epidural block include:
    a. inadvertent intravascular injection
    b. infection
    c. trauma to the spinal cord
    d. inadvertent dural puncture
    e. all of the above

633. Complications associated with lumbar epidural block include *inadvertent*:
    a. subdural injection
    b. epidural injection
    c. subarachnoid injection
    d. all of the above
    e. none of the above

634. The spinal cord:
    a. ends at L2 in adults
    b. ends at L4 in infants
    c. is surrounded by cerebrospinal fluid
    d. all of the above
    e. none of the above

635. Common reasons for the failure to place a needle into the subarachnoid space include:
    a. failure to identify the midline
    b. underestimating the added depth of needle insertion necessary to reach the subarachnoid space

c. allowing the needle to cross the midline by using too lateral a trajectory
    d. all of the above
    e. none of the above

636. Complications associated with subarachnoid block include:
    a. infection
    b. trauma to the spinal cord
    c. trauma to the nerve roots
    d. hypotension
    e. all of the above

637. Contraindications to performing a subarachnoid block include:
    a. local infection
    b. sepsis
    c. anticoagulated state
    d. coagulopathy
    e. all of the above

638. The sacral canal contains:
    a. blood vessels and fat
    b. the filum terminale
    c. the sacral nerve roots
    d. the coccygeal nerves
    e. all of the above

639. Caudal epidural nerve block is performed by placing the needle through the:
    a. foramen rotundum
    b. sacral hiatus
    c. foramen ovale
    d. hiatus of Munro
    e. none of the above

640. Complications associated with caudal epidural block include:
    a. inadvertent subarachnoid injection
    b. infection
    c. inadvertent vascular injection
    d. trauma to structures surrounding the sacrum and coccyx
    e. all of the above

641. Incorrect needle placement during caudal epidural block can include placement of the needle:
    a. outside the sacrum into the subcutaneous tissues
    b. under the periostium of the sacrum
    c. into the substance of the sacrococcygeal ligament
    d. through the sacrum into the pelvis
    e. all of the above

642. Indications for lysis of adhesions include:
    a. perineural fibrosis
    b. epidural scarring after infection
    c. herniated disc
    d. vertebral body compression fracture
    e. all of the above

643. Complications associated with epidural lysis of adhesions include:
    a. persistent sensory deficits
    b. bowel and bladder difficulties

c. sexual dysfunction
d. infection
e. all of the above

644. The sacral nerve roots provide:
   a. motor innervation to the external anal sphincter and levator ani muscles
   b. sensory innervation to the anorectal region
   c. visceral innervation to the bladder and urethra
   d. sensory innervation to the external genitalia
   e. all of the above

645. Side effects and complications associated with blockade of the sacral nerve roots include:
   a. inadvertent intravascular injection
   b. trauma to the vasculature
   c. infection
   d. bladder and bowel dysfunction
   e. all of the above

646. Complications associated with hypogastric plexus block include:
   a. trauma to the iliac vessels
   b. trauma to the pelvic viscera
   c. trauma to the cauda equina
   d. infection
   e. all of the above

647. Complications associated with hypogastric plexus block include inadvertent:
   a. subdural injection
   b. epidural injection
   c. subarachnoid injection
   d. all of the above
   e. none of the above

648. Complications of blockade of the ganglion of Walther (Impar) include:
   a. rectal fistula formation
   b. infection
   c. trauma to the cauda equina
   d. all of the above
   e. none of the above

649. Complications of blockade of the pudendal nerve include:
   a. rectal fistula formation
   b. infection
   c. trauma to the pudendal nerve and artery
   d. intravascular injection into the pudendal nerve and artery
   e. all of the above

650. The pudendal nerve:
   a. is made up of fibers from the S2, S3, and S4 nerves
   b. passes inferiorly between the piriformis and coccygeal muscles
   c. leaves the pelvis via the greater sciatic foramen along with the pudendal artery and nerve
   d. passes around the medial portion of the ischial spine to reenter the pelvis through the lesser sciatic foramen
   e. all of the above

651. The pudendal nerve branches into the:
   a. inferior rectal nerve, which provides innervation to the anal sphincter and perianal region
   b. perineal nerve, which supplies the posterior two thirds of the scrotum or labia majora and muscles of the urogenital triangle
   c. dorsal nerve of the penis or clitoris, which supplies sensory innervation to the dorsum of the penis or clitoris
   d. all of the above
   e. none of the above

652. The sacroiliac joint:
   a. is formed by the articular surfaces of the sacrum and iliac bones
   b. bears the weight of the trunk and are thus subject to the development of strain and arthritis
   c. receives its innervation from L3 to S3 nerve roots, with L4 and L5 providing the greatest contribution to the innervation of the joint
   d. has a very limited range of motion and that motion is induced by changes in the forces placed on the joint by shifts in posture and joint loading
   e. all of the above

653. Complications and side effects of injection of the sacroiliac joint include:
   a. infection
   b. trauma to the sciatic nerve
   c. increased pain following injection
   d. all of the above
   e. none of the above

654. The hip joint is innervated by the:
   a. femoral nerve
   b. obturator nerve
   c. sciatic nerves
   d. all of the above
   e. none of the above

655. The major ligaments of the hip joint include the:
   a. iliofemoral ligament
   b. pubofemoral ligament
   c. ischiofemoral ligament
   d. transverse acetabular ligament
   e. all of the above

656. Complications and side effects of injection of the ischial bursa include:
   a. infection
   b. trauma to the sciatic nerve
   c. increased pain following injection
   d. all of the above
   e. none of the above

657. Causes of ischial bursitis include:
   a. direct trauma to the bursa
   b. overuse syndromes
   c. prolonged sitting
   d. running on sand or uneven surfaces
   e. all of the above

658. The gluteal bursae lie between the:
   a. gluteus maximus muscle
   b. gluteus medius muscle

    c. gluteus minimus muscle
    d. all of the above
    e. none of the above

659. Complications associated with injection of the psoas bursa include:
    a. trauma to the femoral nerve
    b. trauma to the femoral vein
    c. trauma to femoral artery
    d. infection
    e. all of the above

660. Physical examination of patients suffering from psoas bursitis will reveal:
    a. point tenderness in the upper thigh just below the crease of the groin
    b. reproduction of the pain with passive flexion of the affected lower extremity at the hip
    c. reproduction of the pain with passive adduction of the affected lower extremity at the hip
    d. reproduction of the pain with passive abduction of the affected lower extremity at the hip
    e. all of the above

661. The iliopectinate bursa lies between the:
    a. psoas muscle
    b. iliacus muscle
    c. iliopectinate eminence
    d. all of the above
    e. none of the above

662. When performing injection of the iliopectinate bursa, a paresthesia is occasionally elicited when the needle impinges on the:
    a. femoral nerve
    b. sciatic nerve
    c. iliac nerve
    d. the common peroneal nerve
    e. none of the above

663. Patients suffering from trochanteric bursitis will frequently complain of:
    a. pain in the hip region radiating down the affected extremity
    b. a catching sensation when walking
    c. an inability to sleep on the affected side
    d. difficulty walking up stairs
    e. all of the above

664. When performing injection of the trochanteric bursa, a paresthesia is occasionally elicited when the needle impinges on the:
    a. femoral nerve
    b. sciatic nerve
    c. iliac nerve
    d. the common peroneal nerve
    e. none of the above

665. Physical examination of the patient suffering from trochanteric bursitis will reveal:
    a. point tenderness in the lateral thigh
    b. no sensory deficit
    c. pain on active resisted abduction of the affected extremity

    d. all of the above
    e. none of the above

666. Meralgia paresthetica is caused by entrapment of the:
    a. femoral nerve
    b. sciatic nerve
    c. lateral femoral cutaneous nerve
    d. common peroneal nerve
    e. none of the above

667. Physical findings of meralgia paresthetica include:
    a. tenderness over the lateral femoral cutaneous nerve at the origin of the inguinal ligament at the anterior superior iliac spine
    b. a positive Tinel's sign may be present over the lateral femoral cutaneous nerve as it passes beneath the inguinal ligament
    c. a sensory deficit in the distribution of the lateral femoral cutaneous nerve
    d. no motor deficit should be present
    e. all of the above

668. The following have been implicated in the evolution of meralgia paresthetica:
    a. wearing of wide belts
    b. sitting for long periods
    c. squatting for long periods
    d. tight waistbands
    e. all of the above

669. Piriformis syndrome presents as:
    a. pain in the distribution of the sciatic nerve
    b. numbness in the distribution of the sciatic nerve
    c. weakness in the distribution of the sciatic nerve
    d. paresthesias in the distribution of the sciatic nerve
    e. none of the above

670. Piriformis syndrome is caused by compression of the _____ nerve by the piriformis muscle:
    a. femoral
    b. sciatic
    c. lateral femoral cutaneous
    d. common peroneal
    e. none of the above

671. Complications and side effects of blockade of the lumbar plexus using the Winnie 3-in-1 technique include:
    a. trauma to the femoral nerve
    b. trauma to the femoral vein
    c. trauma to femoral artery
    d. infection
    e. all of the above

672. Complications and side effects of blockade of the lumbar plexus using the psoas technique include inadvertent:
    a. subdural injection
    b. epidural injection
    c. subarachnoid injection
    d. all of the above
    e. none of the above

673. Complications and side effects of blockade of the femoral nerve include:
    a. trauma to the femoral nerve
    b. trauma to the femoral vein
    c. trauma to the femoral artery
    d. infection
    e. all of the above

674. The femoral nerve provides motor innervation to the:
    a. sartorius muscle
    b. quadriceps femoris muscle
    c. pectineus muscle
    d. all of the above
    e. none of the above

675. The femoral nerve provides sensory innervation to the:
    a. knee joint
    b. skin overlying the anterior thigh
    c. skin of the medial thigh
    d. all of the above
    e. none of the above

676. Indications for obturator nerve block include:
    a. obturator nerve entrapment
    b. hip pain
    c. relief of adductor spasm to facilitate perineal care
    d. an aid to physical therapy following hip surgery
    e. all of the above

677. Complications and side effects of blockade of the obturator nerve include:
    a. trauma to the obturator nerve
    b. trauma to the obturator vein
    c. trauma to the obturator artery
    d. infection
    e. all of the above

678. The sciatic nerve:
    a. is the largest nerve in the body
    b. roots fuse together in front of the anterior surface of the lateral sacrum on the anterior surface of the piriform muscle
    c. travels inferiorly and leaves the pelvis just below the piriform muscle via the sciatic notch
    d. courses downward past the lesser trochanter to lie posterior and medial to the femur
    e. all of the above

679. The femoral nerve divides into the:
    a. tibial nerve
    b. common peroneal nerve
    c. quadriceps minor nerve
    d. a and b
    e. b and c

680. The tibial nerve provides sensory innervation to the:
    a. posterior portion of the calf
    b. heel
    c. medial plantar surface
    d. all of the above
    e. none of the above

681. The tibial nerve:
    a. splits from the sciatic nerve at the superior margin of the popliteal fossa
    b. descends in a slightly medial course through the popliteal fossa
    c. at the knee lies just beneath the popliteal fascia and is readily accessible for neural blockade
    d. runs between the two heads of the gastrocnemius muscle, passing deep to the soleus muscle
    e. all of the above

682. The saphenous nerve:
    a. is the largest sensory branch of the femoral nerve
    b. is derived primarily from the fibers of the L3 and L4 nerve roots
    c. travels along with the femoral artery through Hunter's canal
    d. passes over the medial condyle of the femur, splitting into terminal sensory branches
    e. all of the above

683. The saphenous nerve provides sensory innervation to the:
    a. medial malleolus
    b. medial calf
    c. medial arch of the foot
    d. all of the above
    e. none of the above

684. The common peroneal nerve:
    a. is a continuation of the sciatic nerve
    b. is derived from the posterior branches of the L4, the L5, and the S1 and S2 nerve roots
    c. splits from the sciatic nerve at the superior margin of the popliteal fossa
    d. descends laterally behind the head of the fibula
    e. all of the above

685. The common peroneal nerve is:
    a. subject to entrapment as it descends laterally behind the head of the fibula
    b. on occasion compressed by casts
    c. on occasion compressed by tourniquets
    d. all of the above
    e. none of the above

686. When performing deep peroneal nerve block at the ankle, a paresthesia is often elicited:
    a. in the skin between the great and second toe
    b. over the lateral malleolus
    c. over the medial malleolus
    d. over the distal little toe
    e. none of the above

687. The superficial branch of the superficial peroneal nerve:
    a. continues down the leg in conjunction with the extensor digitorum longus muscle
    b. divides into terminal branches at a point just above the ankle
    c. has fibers of the terminal branches that provide sensory innervation to most of the dorsum of the foot except for the area adjacent to the web space of the

first and second toes, which is supplied by the deep peroneal nerve

d. provides sensory innervation to the toes except for the area between the first and second toe, which is supplied by the deep peroneal nerve

e. all of the above

688. The sural nerve:
a. is a branch of the posterior tibial nerve
b. passes from the posterior calf around the lateral malleolus to provide sensor innervation of the posterior lateral aspect of the calf and the lateral surface of the foot and fifth toe and the plantar surface of the heel
c. is subject to compression at the ankle and is known as boot syndrome
d. all of the above
e. none of the above

689. Complications associated with metatarsal and digital nerve block include:
a. infection
b. vascular compromise caused by injection of large volumes of local anesthetic into a closed space
c. vascular compromise caused by the use of epinephrine containing local anesthetics
d. all of the above
e. none of the above

690. The knee joint is susceptible to the development of:
a. arthritis
b. bursitis
c. disruption of the ligaments
d. disruption of the cartilage
e. all of the above

691. The suprapatellar tendon is subject to inflammation from:
a. misuse
b. overuse
c. direct trauma
d. all of the above
e. none of the above

692. Findings of suprapatellar bursitis include:
a. swelling in the suprapatellar region
b. tenderness to palpation of the suprapatellar region
c. increased pain on passive flexion of the knee
d. pain on active resisted extension of the knee
e. all of the above

693. Patients suffering from suprapatellar bursitis will frequently complain of:
a. anterior knee pain
b. pain that radiates into the anterior distal thigh
c. an inability to walk stairs
d. an inability to kneel
e. all of the above

694. Symptoms of infection of the prepatellar bursitis include:
a. fever
b. malaise
c. rubor

d. color
e. all of the above

695. The prepatellar bursa:
a. is subject to the development of bursitis from misuse, overuse, or direct trauma
b. lies beneath the subcutaneous tissues
c. lies above the patella
d. is held in place by the ligamentum patellae
e. all of the above

696. Physical examination of patients suffering from superficial infrapatellar bursitis will reveal:
a. pain to palpation of the infrapatellar region
b. swelling and fluid accumulation around the bursa
c. pain on passive flexion
d. pain of active resisted extension
e. all of the above

697. Symptoms of infection of the superficial infrapatellar bursitis include:
a. fever
b. malaise
c. rubor
d. color
e. all of the above

698. The ligamentum patellae is made of a continuation of fibers of the:
a. femoral tuberosity
b. quadriceps tendon
c. prepatellar bursa
d. all of the above
e. none of the above

699. The major ligaments of the ankle joint include the:
a. deltoid ligament
b. anterior talofibular ligament
c. calcaneofibular ligament
d. posterior talofibular ligament
e. all of the above

700. Neurologic complications associated with subarachnoid neurolytic block include:
a. needle-induced trauma to the spinal cord
b. needle-induced trauma to the nerve roots
c. chemical irritation of the meninges
d. chemical irritation of the spinal cord and nerve roots
e. all of the above

701. Complications associated with subarachnoid neurolytic block include:
a. unexpected motor deficits
b. unexpected sensory deficits
c. infection
d. bowel and bladder dysfunction
e. all of the above

702. Side effects and complications associated with subarachnoid neurolytic block include:
a. hypotension
b. inadvertent epidural injection
c. inadvertent subdural injection

d. all of the above
e. none of the above

703. When performing hyperbaric subarachnoid neurolytic block, the patient is positioned:
    a. with the affected side up
    b. with the affected side down
    c. in the jackknife position
    d. a and b
    e. b and c

704. When performing hyperbaric subarachnoid neurolytic block, the patient is positioned:
    a. with the affected side up
    b. with the affected side down
    c. in the supine position
    d. a and b
    e. b and c

705. Contraindications to discography include:
    a. presence of anticoagulation
    b. coagulopathy
    c. sepsis
    d. local infection at the injection site
    e. all of the above

706. Complications of lumbar discography include:
    a. discitis
    b. epidural abscess
    c. trauma to the spinal cord
    d. trauma to the nerve roots
    e. all of the above

707. Complications of lumbar discography include:
    a. infection
    b. pneumothorax
    c. trauma to the kidney
    d. trauma to the great vessels
    e. all of the above

708. Indications for vertebroplasty include:
    a. osteoporosis-induced vertebral compression fractures
    b. tumors of the vertebral body
    c. hemangiomas of the vertebral body
    d. traumatic vertebral compression fractures
    e. all of the above

709. The best results from vertebroplasty can be expected when:
    a. there is limited compression of the vertebral body
    b. the fracture is less than 12 months old
    c. if the lesion is greater than 12 months old, the radionuclide bone scan is still "hot," indicating continued active disease
    d. all of the above
    e. none of the above

710. Complications associated with vertebroplasty include:
    a. intravascular injection of cement
    b. spread of cement into the spinal canal
    c. spread of cement into the neural foramina
    d. fracture of the pedicle during the procedure
    e. all of the above

711. Indications supporting a trial of spinal cord stimulation include:
    a. reflex sympathetic dystrophy and causalgia
    b. ischemic pain secondary to peripheral vascular insufficiency
    c. radiculopathies
    d. failed back syndrome
    e. all of the above

712. Indications supporting a trial of spinal cord stimulation include:
    a. arachnoiditis
    b. postherpetic neuralgia
    c. phantom limb pain
    d. intractable angina
    e. all of the above

713. Contraindications to a trial of spinal cord stimulation include:
    a. sepsis
    b. local infection at needle entry site
    c. presence of anticoagulation
    d. coagulopathy
    e. all of the above

714. Complications associated with spinal cord stimulation include:
    a. infection
    b. trauma to the spinal cord
    c. trauma to the nerve roots
    d. epidural hematoma formation
    e. all of the above

715. Indications for implantation of a totally implantable infusion pump include:
    a. the administration of epidural drugs for the palliation of pain in cancer patients with a life expectancy of months to years
    b. carefully selected patients who suffer from chronic benign pain who have experienced palliation of their pain with trial doses of spinal opioids and who have failed to respond to other more conservative treatments
    c. those patients suffering from spasticity who have experienced decreased spasms after trial doses of subarachnoid administration of baclofen
    d. all of the above
    e. none of the above

716. Indications for therapeutic ultrasound include:
    a. tendinitis
    b. bursitis
    c. nonacutely inflamed arthritis
    d. frozen joints
    e. all of the above

717. Indications for therapeutic ultrasound include:
    a. contractures
    b. degenerative arthritis
    c. fractures
    d. plantar fasciitis
    e. all of the above

718. Contraindications to subarachnoid neurolytic block include:
   a. presence of anticoagulation
   b. coagulopathy
   c. sepsis
   d. local infection at the injection site
   e. all of the above

719. Indications for therapeutic heat include:
   a. pain
   b. muscle spasm
   c. bursitis
   d. tenosynovitis
   e. all of the above

720. Indications for therapeutic heat include:
   a. collagen vascular diseases
   b. contracture
   c. fibromyalgia
   d. induction of hyperemia
   e. all of the above

721. Indications for therapeutic heat include:
   a. hematoma resolution
   b. superficial thrombophlebitis
   c. reflex sympathetic dystrophy
   d. all of the above
   e. none of the above

722. Heat modalities that rely on conduction include:
   a. hydrocollator packs
   b. circulating water heating pads
   c. chemical heating pads
   d. paraffin baths
   e. all of the above

723. Heat modalities that rely on conversion include:
   a. ultrasound
   b. short wave diathermy
   c. microwave diathermy
   d. all of the above
   e. none of the above

724. Relative contraindications to therapeutic heat include:
   a. scar tissue
   b. lack of or reduced sensation
   c. demyelinating diseases
   d. acute inflammation
   e. all of the above

725. Relative contraindications to therapeutic heat include:
   a. bleeding disorders
   b. hemorrhage
   c. malignancy
   d. inability to communicate or respond to pain
   e. all of the above

726. Physiologic effects of therapeutic heat include:
   a. increased blood flow
   b. decreased muscle spasm
   c. increased extensibility of connective tissues
   d. all of the above
   e. none of the above

727. Physiologic effects of therapeutic heat include:
   a. decreased joint stiffness
   b. reduction of edema
   c. analgesia
   d. all of the above
   e. none of the above

728. Precautions and contraindications to the use of therapeutic cold include:
   a. ischemia
   b. lack of or reduced sensation
   c. cold intolerance
   d. Raynaud's disease
   e. all of the above

729. Indications for therapeutic cold include:
   a. pain
   b. muscle spasm
   c. bursitis
   d. tendinitis
   e. all of the above

730. Contraindications to the use of transcutaneous electrical nerve stimulators include:
   a. pacemakers
   b. spinal cord stimulators
   c. insensate patients
   d. pregnancy
   e. all of the above

731. Indications for the use of transcutaneous nerve stimulators include:
   a. acute post-traumatic pain
   b. acute postoperative pain
   c. peripheral vascular insufficiency
   d. all of the above
   e. none of the above

732. Indications for the use of transcutaneous nerve stimulators include:
   a. functional abdominal pain
   b. musculoskeletal pain
   c. neuropathic pain
   d. all of the above
   e. none of the above

733. Types of biofeedback devices include:
   a. heart rate monitors
   b. electromyographic monitors
   c. galvanic skin response monitors
   d. thermostat temperature monitors
   e. all of the above

734. Factors affecting the clinical properties of local anesthetics include:
   a. percentage of ionization at physiologic pH
   b. lipid solubility
   c. affinity for protein binding
   d. all of the above
   e. none of the above

735. Factors affecting the clinical properties of local anesthetics include the:
    a. pH of the tissue being blocked
    b. drug's ability to produce vasodilatation
    c. drug's diffusibility
    d. all of the above
    e. none of the above

736. Common to the structure of all local anesthetics is a(n):
    a. terminal amine
    b. intermediate chain
    c. aromatic end
    d. all of the above
    e. none of the above

737. Neurolytic agents commonly used in clinical practice include:
    a. ethyl alcohol
    b. phenol
    c. ammonium compounds
    d. hypertonic and hypotonic solutions
    e. all of the above

738. A dreaded complication of alcohol block of the trigeminal nerve is:
    a. anesthesia dolorosa
    b. anesthesia phlegmosa
    c. anesthesia albicans
    d. all of the above
    e. none of the above

739. When alcohol is administered onto a nerve, which of the following occurs?
    a. denaturation of cerebrosides
    b. denaturation of phospholipids
    c. denaturation of lipoproteins
    d. denaturation of mucoproteins
    e. all of the above

740. When administered into the subarachnoid space, relative to cerebrospinal fluid, ethyl alcohol is:
    a. isobaric
    b. hyperbaric
    c. hypobaric
    d. radiopaque
    e. none of the above

741. The nonsteroidal anti-inflammatory drug's primary mechanism of action is the inhibition of:
    a. cyclooxygenase enzymes
    b. centrally mediated cytokines
    c. C-reactive protein type 1
    d. C-reactive protein type 2
    e. all of the above

742. Actions of aspirin include:
    a. inhibition of platelet aggregation
    b. antipyretic activity
    c. analgesic activity
    d. anti-inflammatory activity
    e. all of the above

743. The following class of analgesics has recently been associated with a higher incidence of cardiovascular side effects compared with other classes of analgesics:
    a. opioids
    b. aspirin
    c. COX-2 inhibitors
    d. nonsalicylated aspirin-like drugs
    e. none of the above

744. Commonly used skeletal muscle relaxants include:
    a. methocarbamol
    b. cyclobenzaprine
    c. orphenadrine
    d. tizanidine
    e. all of the above

745. Meprobamate dependence has been associated with the prolonged use of which of the following muscle relaxants?
    a. methocarbamol
    b. cyclobenzaprine
    c. carisoprodol
    d. tizanidine
    e. all of the above

746. Drugs that must be avoided when taking monoamine oxidase inhibitors include:
    a. meperidine
    b. antihistamines
    c. cocaine
    d. many antipsychotic medications
    e. all of the above

747. Foods that should be avoided when taking monoamine oxidase inhibitors include:
    a. aged cheeses
    b. Chianti wine
    c. figs
    d. overripe fruit
    e. all of the above

748. Foods that should be avoided when taking monoamine oxidase inhibitors include:
    a. smoked meats
    b. chicken liver
    c. soy sauce
    d. aged meats
    e. all of the above

749. Foods that should be avoided when taking monoamine oxidase inhibitors include:
    a. caviar
    b. meat extracts
    c. bananas
    d. raisins
    e. all of the above

750. Side effects of the tricyclic antidepressants include:
    a. sedation
    b. cardiac arrhythmias
    c. xerostomia
    d. xeroophthalmia
    e. all of the above

751. Side effects of the tricyclic antidepressants include:
    a. constipation
    b. urinary retention
    c. anorgasmia
    d. impotence
    e. all of the above

752. Category 1 anticonvulsants, drugs that modulate the voltage-dependent sodium channel, include:
    a. phenytoin
    b. carbamazepine
    c. lamotrigine
    d. topiramate
    e. all of the above

753. Category 2 anticonvulsants, drugs whose primary mechanism of action is unrelated to modulation of the voltage-dependent sodium channel, include:
    a. gabapentin
    b. tiagabine
    c. valproic acid
    d. all of the above
    e. none of the above

754. Side effects associated with phenytoin include:
    a. nystagmus
    b. liver dysfunction
    c. rash
    d. Stevens-Johnson syndrome
    e. all of the above

755. Side effects associated with phenytoin include:
    a. liver dysfunction
    b. gum hyperplasia
    c. peripheral neuropathy
    d. osteomalacia
    e. all of the above

756. The anticonvulsant compound that has been associated with a pseudolymphoma indistinguishable from Hodgkin's lymphoma is:
    a. carbamazepine
    b. phenytoin
    c. gabapentin
    d. phenobarbital
    e. all of the above

757. Alternative routes of administration of opioid analgesics include:
    a. rectal
    b. buccal
    c. sublingual
    d. transdermal
    e. all of the above

758. Side effects of opioid analgesics include:
    a. nausea
    b. constipation
    c. psychotomimetic effects
    d. itching
    e. all of the above

759. Factors that facilitate transplacental transfer of drugs include:
    a. high lipid solubility
    b. lower molecular weight
    c. low protein binding
    d. an active moiety that exists in an unionized state
    e. all of the above

760. Factors that facilitate transfer of drugs into breast milk include:
    a. high lipid solubility
    b. lower molecular weight
    c. low protein binding
    d. an active moiety that exists in an unionized state
    e. all of the above

761. Phenytoin has been associated with fetal abnormalities:
    a. that may be associated with impaired folate absorption
    b. that are known as the hydantoin syndrome
    c. including microcephaly, micrognathia, and dysmorphism
    d. all of the above
    e. none of the above

762. Common signs of depression in the elderly include:
    a. insomnia
    b. anger and irritability
    c. unexplained weight loss
    d. unexplained weight gain
    e. all of the above

763. Common signs of depression in the elderly include:
    a. fatigue
    b. frequent awakening
    c. difficulty concentrating
    d. loss of pleasure in daily activities
    e. all of the above

764. Unique physiologic abnormalities in the newborn that may affect how narcotic analgesics are used include:
    a. immature liver enzyme system
    b. decreased glomerular filtration rates
    c. immature central respiratory receptor system
    d. all of the above
    e. none of the above

765. The following analgesics are generally considered safe in the pediatric population:
    a. acetaminophen
    b. morphine
    c. codeine
    d. ketorolac
    e. all of the above

766. The following clinical syndromes are considered migraine equivalents:
    a. cyclical vomiting syndrome
    b. benign paroxysmal vertigo
    c. acute confusional state disorder
    d. all of the above
    e. none of the above

767. The following are considered factors that cause concern when evaluating a patient with headache:
    a. first or worst headache
    b. headache made worse with the Valsalva maneuver
    c. headache associated with fever
    d. headache associated with neurologic dysfunction
    e. all of the above

Answers

1. E	54. D	107. B	160. B
2. C	55. E	108. B	161. B
3. E	56. D	109. C	162. D
4. E	57. D	110. D	163. D
5. E	58. D	111. D	164. D
6. D	59. A	112. D	165. E
7. B	60. A	113. E	166. B
8. E	61. E	114. D	167. D
9. D	62. E	115. D	168. A
10. E	63. D	116. D	169. B
11. A	64. E	117. E	170. B
12. A	65. D	118. E	171. C
13. E	66. A	119. D	172. A
14. D	67. B	120. B	173. D
15. D	68. E	121. E	174. A
16. B	69. A	122. A	175. B
17. E	70. C	123. E	176. A
18. E	71. D	124. A	177. D
19. E	72. C	125. A	178. D
20. D	73. A	126. E	179. E
21. D	74. B	127. D	180. D
22. D	75. C	128. A	181. B
23. E	76. A	129. B	182. E
24. B	77. B	130. E	183. D
25. E	78. A	131. A	184. E
26. C	79. A	132. A	185. D
27. E	80. A	133. A	186. C
28. E	81. D	134. A	187. E
29. B	82. E	135. A	188. C
30. E	83. A	136. A	189. B
31. C	84. E	137. D	190. A
32. A	85. A	138. D	191. C
33. B	86. B	139. E	192. A
34. E	87. D	140. E	193. D
35. C	88. E	141. A	194. E
36. E	89. D	142. D	195. D
37. E	90. E	143. D	196. E
38. A	91. E	144. E	197. E
39. E	92. E	145. A	198. E
40. A	93. E	146. E	199. D
41. C	94. D	147. B	200. E
42. B	95. E	148. A	201. E
43. A	96. D	149. A	202. E
44. D	97. D	150. A	203. A
45. C	98. E	151. D	204. C
46. E	99. D	152. C	205. D
47. D	100. D	153. A	206. B
48. E	101. E	154. A	207. A
49. D	102. E	155. B	208. E
50. A	103. E	156. D	209. A
51. D	104. E	157. A	210. A
52. D	105. A	158. C	211. E
53. D	106. E	159. A	212. D

213. E	272. E	331. E	390. A
214. D	273. E	332. E	391. E
215. E	274. E	333. E	392. E
216. E	275. E	334. E	393. E
217. E	276. E	335. E	394. A
218. E	277. E	336. E	395. E
219. B	278. D	337. E	396. D
220. E	279. D	338. E	397. B
221. E	280. E	339. E	398. D
222. D	281. E	340. D	399. E
223. D	282. A	341. E	400. D
224. E	283. E	342. E	401. E
225. D	284. E	343. B	402. E
226. E	285. E	344. E	403. E
227. C	286. B	345. E	404. E
228. E	287. D	346. E	405. E
229. E	288. D	347. E	406. E
230. C	289. D	348. D	407. D
231. B	290. E	349. C	408. E
232. E	291. E	350. E	409. E
233. E	292. A	351. E	410. D
234. E	293. E	352. E	411. E
235. E	294. D	353. E	412. E
236. E	295. E	354. E	413. E
237. A	296. E	355. E	414. E
238. E	297. E	356. A	415. A
239. D	298. D	357. D	416. E
240. E	299. B	358. D	417. E
241. C	300. E	359. E	418. E
242. E	301. E	360. E	419. E
243. B	302. E	361. E	420. E
244. E	303. A	362. E	421. E
245. E	304. E	363. E	422. E
246. E	305. E	364. E	423. B
247. D	306. E	365. E	424. E
248. E	307. A	366. E	425. E
249. E	308. D	367. E	426. E
250. E	309. D	368. E	427. E
251. D	310. A	369. E	428. E
252. E	311. D	370. E	429. A
253. E	312. E	371. E	430. E
254. E	313. D	372. A	431. C
255. E	314. D	373. E	432. E
256. C	315. E	374. E	433. E
257. A	316. E	375. D	434. E
258. E	317. A	376. E	435. E
259. E	318. E	377. E	436. E
260. E	319. D	378. D	437. A
261. E	320. E	379. D	438. E
262. B	321. A	380. E	439. E
263. E	322. B	381. E	440. E
264. D	323. E	382. E	441. E
265. E	324. E	383. D	442. E
266. E	325. E	384. E	443. D
267. E	326. E	385. E	444. A
268. E	327. E	386. E	445. B
269. E	328. E	387. B	446. E
270. E	329. E	388. E	447. E
271. E	330. D	389. E	448. E

449. D	508. D	567. D	626. E
450. D	509. D	568. D	627. E
451. A	510. D	569. D	628. E
452. D	511. D	570. E	629. D
453. E	512. A	571. D	630. D
454. E	513. E	572. E	631. D
455. E	514. C	573. D	632. E
456. D	515. E	574. E	633. D
457. E	516. E	575. E	634. D
458. B	517. C	576. E	635. D
459. D	518. D	577. E	636. E
460. E	519. E	578. D	637. E
461. E	520. D	579. E	638. E
462. A	521. D	580. E	639. B
463. E	522. E	581. D	640. E
464. D	523. B	582. D	641. E
465. E	524. C	583. E	642. E
466. E	525. E	584. B	643. E
467. A	526. E	585. D	644. E
468. E	527. E	586. E	645. E
469. E	528. E	587. D	646. E
470. E	529. E	588. E	647. D
471. E	530. E	589. E	648. D
472. E	531. E	590. E	649. E
473. A	532. E	591. D	650. E
474. A	533. A	592. E	651. D
475. D	534. E	593. E	652. E
476. B	535. E	594. E	653. D
477. E	536. E	595. E	654. D
478. B	537. E	596. D	655. E
479. A	538. E	597. D	656. D
480. E	539. B	598. E	657. E
481. C	540. E	599. E	658. D
482. D	541. D	600. D	659. E
483. B	542. C	601. E	660. E
484. C	543. D	602. E	661. D
485. A	544. D	603. E	662. A
486. E	545. E	604. E	663. E
487. B	546. E	605. E	664. B
488. E	547. E	606. E	665. D
489. D	548. E	607. E	666. C
490. E	549. D	608. E	667. E
491. E	550. E	609. E	668. E
492. E	551. D	610. D	669. E
493. A	552. E	611. D	670. B
494. E	553. E	612. D	671. E
495. E	554. E	613. D	672. D
496. E	555. D	614. E	673. E
497. E	556. E	615. E	674. D
498. D	557. E	616. E	675. D
499. A	558. D	617. E	676. E
500. D	559. E	618. E	677. E
501. E	560. D	619. D	678. E
502. E	561. D	620. E	679. D
503. D	562. E	621. D	680. D
504. D	563. E	622. E	681. E
505. D	564. E	623. E	682. E
506. D	565. E	624. D	683. D
507. E	566. E	625. E	684. E

685. D
686. A
687. E
688. D
689. D
690. E
691. D
692. E
693. E
694. E
695. E
696. E
697. E
698. B
699. E
700. E
701. E
702. D
703. B
704. A
705. E

706. E
707. E
708. E
709. D
710. E
711. E
712. E
713. E
714. E
715. D
716. E
717. E
718. E
719. E
720. E
721. D
722. E
723. D
724. E
725. E
726. D

727. D
728. E
729. E
730. E
731. D
732. D
733. E
734. D
735. D
736. D
737. E
738. A
739. E
740. C
741. A
742. E
743. C
744. E
745. C
746. E
747. E

748. E
749. E
750. E
751. E
752. E
753. D
754. E
755. E
756. B
757. E
758. E
759. E
760. E
761. D
762. E
763. E
764. D
765. E
766. D
767. E

Index

Note: Page numbers followed by *f* and *t* indicate figures and tables, respectively.

A

Abdominal pain
  in acute pancreatitis, 295–296
  in chronic pancreatitis, 297
  lower
    in genitofemoral neuralgia, 299–300
    in ilioinguinal neuralgia, 298–299
Abducens nerve (CN 6), 4*f*, 10, 17–18, 25*f*, 35*f*
  course of, 13, 14*f*, 17, 18*f*
  disorders of, 17
  and lateral rectus muscle, 17, 18*f*
Abducens nucleus, 17
Abductor pollicis longus muscle, 100
A-beta fibers, 197
Abscess
  auricular, 228
  epidural, 291–292
    after discography, 368–369
  parapharyngeal, 231
  retropharyngeal, 231
Accommodation, visual, 11
Acetabular fossa, synovial membrane of, 136*f*
Acetabulum, 135, 136*f*, 143*f*
Acetaminophen
  for diabetic truncal neuropathy, 281
  safety of, for neonates, 666
Acetazolamide, for pseudotumor cerebri, 218
Acetylcholine, 185
Achilles bursa, 162, 162*f*
Achilles bursitis, 162
Achilles tendinitis, 161, 161*f*, 162, 325
Achilles tendon, 161, 161*f*, 162, 162*f*
  injection therapy for, 325
Acoustic nerve. *See* Vestibulocochlear nerve (CN 8)
Acoustic neuroma, 227
Acromioclavicular joint, 80, 81*f*, 82, 82*f*, 83
  volume of, 82
Acromioclavicular ligament(s), 82, 83
Acupuncture, 622–623
Acute intermittent porphyria, and peripheral neuropathy, 280
Acyclovir, for acute herpes zoster of thoracic dermatomes, 288
Addiction
  definition of, 357
  neurobiology of, 357–358
  to opioids, 639–640
  risk factors for, 357, 358*t*
Adductor brevis muscle, 135

Adductor longus muscle, 135
Adductor magnus tendon, 147*f*
Adductor pollicis muscle, 102*f*
A-delta fibers, 187, 190, 197, 198*f*
Adenosine triphosphate, 196
Adie's pupil, 11
Adjuvant analgesics
  for cancer pain, 349
  skeletal muscle relaxants as, 652
Adrenal medulla, 181, 182, 183*f*
  anatomy of, 184*f*
Adson's test, 260, 262
Akathisia, 180
Akinesia, 180
Alar ligament(s), of cervical spine, 59, 60*f*
Albuterol, for proctalgia fugax, 308
Alcohol
  and acute pancreatitis, 295, 295*t*
  and chronic pancreatitis, 297
Allodynia
  in central pain states, 341
  in complex regional pain syndrome, 328
  with reflex sympathetic dystrophy of face, 253
Alpha-1-antitrypsin deficiency, and chronic pancreatitis, 297
Aluminum sulfate, topical, for acute herpes zoster of thoracic dermatomes, 288
American College of Rheumatology (ACR), clinical classification criteria for rheumatoid arthritis, 330, 330*t*
Amitriptyline
  adverse effects and side effects of, 308
  chemical structure of, 646*f*
  for diabetic truncal neuropathy, 280
  for headache prophylaxis, 212
  for intercostal neuralgia, 244–245
  pharmacology of, 642
  for postmastectomy syndrome, 285–286
  for post-thoracotomy pain syndrome, 284
  for proctalgia fugax, 308
Ammonium compounds, as chemical neurolytic agents, 629–630, 629*t*
Amputation, and phantom limb pain, 313–314
Amygdala, 201*f*
Amygdaloid body, 5*f*, 199
Amyloidosis
  and peripheral neuropathy, 280
  and rheumatoid arthritis, differentiation of, 332

Analgesic ladder, 349, 637
Analgesic rebound headache, 213, 215, 219–220
  differential diagnosis of, 219
  drugs implicated in, 219, 219*t*
    discontinuation of, 219–220
  signs and symptoms of, 219
  testing for, 219
  treatment of, 219–220
Analgesics
  for bursitis syndromes of knee, 319, 320, 321
  for carpal tunnel syndrome, 274
  for coccydynia, 253
  for diabetic truncal neuropathy, 281
  for femoral neuropathy, 312
  for genitofemoral neuralgia, 300
  in Guillain-Barré syndrome, 355
  for ilioinguinal neuralgia, 299
  for intercostal neuralgia, 244
  for meralgia paresthetica, 301
  for olecranon bursitis, 273
  for postmastectomy syndrome, 285
  for post-polio syndrome, 353
  for post-thoracotomy syndrome, 284
  precautions with, in diabetes, 281
  for proctalgia fugax, 308
  for sickle cell disease, 356
  for tarsal tunnel syndrome, 323, 324
  for tension-type headache, 212
  for thoracic compression fracture, 249
  for trochanteric bursitis, 315
  for ulnar nerve entrapment at elbow, 270
Anconeus muscle, 93*f*, 94*f*
Angiotensin-converting enzyme inhibitors, for scleroderma, 338
Angle of Louis, 247
Anisocoria, 11
Ankle joint, 156*f*, 157, 158
  arthritis of, 323, 324
  functional anatomy of, 155–156, 156*f*
  functional units of, 155
  innervation of, 157, 158
  intra-articular injection of, technique for, 590, 591*f*
  ligaments of, 157, 158
  motion of, 155
  stress fractures of, 325
Ankle splint, for tarsal tunnel syndrome, 323, 324
Ankylosing spondylitis, 294–295
  clinical features of, 294